VENOUS DISORDERS

Edited by

JOHN J. BERGAN, M.D.

Scripps Memorial Hospital
La Jolla, California

JAMES S.T. YAO, M.D., Ph.D.

Chief of the Division of Vascular Surgery
Northwestern University Medical School
Chicago, Illinois

1991

W.B. SAUNDERS COMPANY
Harcourt Brace Jovanovich, Inc.

Philadelphia, London, Toronto, Montreal, Sydney, Tokyo

W. B. SAUNDERS COMPANY
Harcourt Brace Jovanovich, Inc.

The Curtis Center
Independence Square West
Philadelphia, PA 19106

Library of Congress Cataloging-in-Publication Data

Venous disorders / edited by John J. Bergan, James. S. T. Yao.
    p. cm.
   ISBN 0-7216-3747-7
   1. Veins—Surgery. 2. Veins—Diseases—Treatment. 3. Veins—
Wounds and injuries—Treatment. I. Bergan, John J.
II. Yao, James S. T.
   [DNLM: 1. Vascular Diseases—diagnosis. 2. Vascular Diseases—
therapy. 3. Veins—physiopathology. 4. Veins—surgery. WG 600
V4645]
RD598.7.V46 1991
617.4'14—dc20
DNLM/DLC
for Library of Congress   90-9094
                                             CIP

Editor: Edward H. Wickland, Jr.

VENOUS DISORDERS   ISBN   0-7216-3747-7

Printed in the United States of America.

Last digit is the print number: 9   8   7   6   5   4   3   2   1

CONTRIBUTORS

AMINE BAHNINI, M.D.

Assistant Professor, Department of Vascular Surgery, Groupe Hospitalier Pitie-Salpetriere, Paris, France

Nonthrombotic Disease of the Inferior Vena Cava: Surgical Management of 24 Patients

B. TIMOTHY BAXTER, M.D.

Assistant Professor of Surgery, University of Nebraska Medical Center, Omaha, Nebraska

Venous Angiodysplasia and Venous Malformations

JOHN J. BERGAN, M.D., F.A.C.S.

Professor of Surgery, Emeritus, Northwestern University Medical School, Chicago, Illinois; Clinical Professor of Surgery, University of California, San Diego, California

Historical Highlights in Teaching Venous Insufficiency; Surgical Procedures for Varicose Veins; Changing Concepts and Present-Day Etiology of Upper Extremity Venous Thrombosis

GARY BREITBART, M.D.

Assistant Clinical Professor of Surgery, Section of Vascular Surgery, UMDNJ-New Jersey Medical School, Newark, New Jersey

Current Status of Duplex Ultrasonography in the Diagnosis of Acute Deep Venous Thrombosis

DIMITRIS C. CHRISTOPOULOS, M.D., Ph.D.

Senior Lecturer in General and Vascular Surgery, University of Thessaloniki Medical School, Thessaloniki, Greece

Methods of Quantitation of Chronic Venous Insufficiency

JAMES A. COFFEY, M.D.

Assistant Professor of Surgery, Uniformed Services University of the Health Sciences, Bethesda, Maryland; Staff, Vascular Surgery Service, Walter Reed Army Medical Center, Washington, DC

Involvement of the Lymphatic System in Chronic Venous Insufficiency

P. D. COLERIDGE SMITH, M.S., B.M.B.Ch., F.R.C.S.

Senior Lecturer, Department of Surgery, University College and Middlesex Hospital School of Medicine, The Middlesex Hospital, London, England

Current Views on the Pathogenesis of Venous Ulceration

JOHN J. CRANLEY, M.D.

Director Emeritus, Department of Surgery and Director, Vascular Laboratory, Good Samaritan Hospital, Cincinnati, Ohio

Diagnosis of Upper Extremity Venous Thrombosis by Duplex Scanning

ROBERT D. CRANLEY, M.D.

Attending Staff, Good Samaritan Hospital, Cincinnati, Ohio

Diagnosis of Upper Extremity Venous Thrombosis by Duplex Scanning

PAT O. DAILY, M.D.

Clinical Professor of Surgery, University of California, San Diego, California; Director of Cardiovascular Surgery, Sharp Memorial Hospital, San Diego, California

Embolectomy for Acute Pulmonary Embolism; Surgical Management of Chronic Pulmonary Embolism

SIMON G. DARKE, M.S., F.R.C.S.

Honorary Lecturer, Southampton Medical School; Consultant Vascular Surgeon, Bournemouth General Hospital, Dorset, England

Recurrent Varicose Veins and Short Saphenous Insufficiency: Evaluation and Treatment

RALPH G. DePALMA, M.D., F.A.C.S.

Professor and Chairman, Department of Surgery, George Washington University School of Medicine; VA Medical Center, Washington, DC

Surgical Treatment of Chronic Venous Ulceration

JAMES A. DeWEESE, M.D.

Professor of Cardiothoracic Surgery, University of Rochester Medical School; Chairman, Division of Cardiothoracic Surgery, Strong Memorial Hospital, Rochester, New York

Results of Surgical Treatment of Axillary-Subclavian Venous Thrombosis

MARTIN I. ELLENBY, M.D.

Resident Physician, Division of General Surgery, Department of Surgery, University of Illinois and Cook County Hospitals, Chicago, Illinois

Repair or Ligation in Extremity Venous Injuries

DAVID V. FELICIANO, M.D.

Director and Vice-Chairman, Department of Surgery, University of Rochester; Attending Surgeon and S.I.C.U. Director, Strong Memorial Hospital, Rochester, New York

Management of Intraabdominal Venous Injuries

PETER GLOVICZKI, M.D.

Consultant, Section of Vascular Surgery, Mayo Clinic and Foundation; Assistant Professor of Surgery, Mayo Medical School, Rochester, Minnesota

Microsurgical Treatment for Chronic Lymphedema: An Unfulfilled Promise?

MITCHEL P. GOLDMAN, M.D.

Assistant Clinical Professor of Medicine/Dermatology, University of California, San Diego; Consulting Medical Staff, Scripps Memorial Hospital, La Jolla and Encinitas, California

Compression Sclerotherapy and its Complications

EDWARD R. GOMEZ, M.D.

Assistant Professor of Surgery, Uniformed Services University of the Health Sciences, Bethesda, Maryland; Chief, Vascular Surgery Service, Walter Reed Army Medical Center, Washington, DC

Involvement of the Lymphatic System in Chronic Venous Insufficiency; Long-Term Follow-Up of Venous Reconstruction Following Trauma

ROBERT A. GRAOR, M.D.

Staff, Department of Vascular Medicine, Division of Medicine, Cleveland Clinic, Cleveland, Ohio

Thrombolytic Therapy for Deep Vein Thrombosis and Pulmonary Emboli

LAZAR J. GREENFIELD, M.D.

F. A. Coller Professor of Surgery, Chairman of the Department of Surgery, Ann Arbor, Michigan

Vena Cava Interruption: Devices and Results

JOERG D. GRUSS, M.D.

Professor of Surgery, Professor of the University of Kassel, Head of the Department for Vascular Surgery, Kurhessisches Diakonissenhaus Kassel, Federal Republic of Germany

Venous Bypass for Chronic Venous Insufficiency

SHARON L. HAMMOND, M.D.

Instructor in Surgery, Uniformed Services University of the Health Sciences, Bethesda, Maryland; Staff, Vascular Surgery Service, Fitsimmons Army Medical Center, Aurora, Colorado

Involvement of the Lymphatic System in Chronic Venous Insufficiency; Long-Term Follow-Up of Venous Reconstruction Following Trauma

JACK HIRSH, M.D., F.R.C.P.(C), F.A.C.P.

Professor of Medicine, McMaster University; Director, Hamilton Civic Hospitals Research Centre, Hamilton, Ontario, Canada

Prophylaxis of Deep Vein Thrombosis: Current Techniques

JOHN T. HOBBS, M.D.

St. Mary's Hospital, London, England

The Treatment of Vulval and Pelvic Varices

ROBERT W. HOBSON II, M.D.

Professor of Surgery, Chief, Section of Vascular Surgery, UMDNJ-New Jersey Medical School, Newark, New Jersey

Current Status of Duplex Ultrasonography in the Diagnosis of Acute Deep Venous Thrombosis

JOHN R. HOCH, M.D.

General Vascular Resident, Department of Surgery, University of Missouri-Columbia Health Sciences Center, Columbia, Missouri

Hematologic Factors, Anticoagulation, and Anticoagulant Complications in Venous Thromboembolism

KIM J. HODGSON, M.D.

Assistant Professor of Surgery, Director of Noninvasive Vascular Laboratories, Southern Illinois University School of Medicine, Springfield, Illinois

Study of Deep Venous Thrombosis in High-Risk Patients Using Color Flow Doppler

LARRY H. HOLLIER, M.D.

Clinical Professor of Surgery, Louisiana State University Medical Center and Tulane University Medical Center; Chairman, Department of Surgery, Ochsner Clinic and Alton Ochsner Medical Foundation, New Orleans, Louisiana

Reconstruction of the Superior Vena Cava and Central Veins

ZAFAR JAMIL, M.D.

Associate Clinical Professor of Surgery, Section of Vascular Surgery, UMDNJ-New Jersey Medical School, Newark, New Jersey

Current Status of Duplex Ultrasonography in the Diagnosis of Acute Deep Venous Thrombosis

GEORGE JOHNSON, Jr., M.D.

Attending Surgeon, University of North Carolina Hospitals; Roscoe B. G. Cowper Distinguished Professor of Surgery, The University of North Carolina at Chapel Hill, Chapel Hill, North Carolina

Role of Elastic Support in Treatment of the Chronically Swollen Limb

THOMAS M. KERR, M.D.

Consulting Vascular Surgeon, St. Elizabeth Medical Center; Attending Vascular Surgeon, Teaching Staff, Good Samaritan Hospital, Cincinnati, Ohio

Diagnosis of Upper Extremity Venous Thrombosis by Duplex Scanning

EDOUARD KIEFFER, M.D.

Chief, Department of Vascular Surgery, Groupe Hospitalier Pitie-Salpetriere, Paris, France

Nonthrombotic Disease of the Inferior Vena Cava: Surgical Management of 24 Patients

ROBERT L. KISTNER, M.D.

Clinical Professor of Surgery, John A. Burns School of Medicine, University of Hawaii; Department of Surgery, Straub Clinic and Hospital, Honolulu, Hawaii

Valve Repair and Segment Transposition in Primary Valvular Insufficiency

FABIEN KOSKAS, M.D.

Assistant Professor of Vascular Surgery, Groupe Hospitalier Pitie-Saltpetriere, Paris, France

Nonthrombotic Disease of the Inferior Vena Cava: Surgical Management of 24 Patients

CARL G. LAUER, M.D.

Instructor of Surgery, Uniformed Services University of the Health Sciences, Bethesda, Maryland; Fellow, Peripheral Vascular Surgery Service, Walter Reed Army Medical Center, Washington, DC

Involvement of the Lymphatic System in Chronic Venous Insufficiency; Long-Term Follow-Up of Venous Reconstruction Following Trauma

M. LEA THOMAS, M.A., Ph.D., F.R.C.P.

Honorary Lecturer, United Medical and Dental Schools of Guy's and Thomas' Hospitals, University of London; Senior Physician in Radiology, St. Thomas Hospital, London, England

Routine and Special Phlebography in the Evaluation of Venous Problems

DARR W. LEUTZ, M.D.

Resident in Orthopaedic Surgery, Southern Illinois University School of Medicine, Springfield, Illinois

Study of Deep Venous Thrombosis in High-Risk Patients Using Color Flow Doppler

GREGG L. LONDREY, M.D.

Fellow in Vascular Surgery, Southern Illinois University School of Medicine, Springfield, Illinois

Study of Deep Venous Thrombosis in High-Risk Patients Using Color Flow Doppler

KENNETH S. LUTTER, M.D.

Senior Vascular Fellow, Good Samaritan Hospital, Cincinnati, Ohio

Diagnosis of Upper Extremity Venous Thrombosis by Duplex Scanning

HERBERT I. MACHLEDER, M.D.

Professor of Surgery, Vascular Surgery Service, UCLA Medical School, UCLA Medical Center, Los Angeles, California

Thrombolytic Therapy and Thoracic Outlet Decompression in Subclavian-Axillary Venous Thrombosis

JOHN C. MAYBERRY, M.D.

Vascular Research Fellow, Division of Vascular Surgery, Oregon Health Sciences University, Portland, Oregon

Nonoperative Treatment of Venous Stasis Ulcer

WALTER J. McCARTHY, M.D.

Assistant Professor of Surgery, Northwestern University Medical School; Attending Staff, Northwestern Memorial Hospital; Attending Surgeon, VA Lakeside Medical Center, Chicago, Illinois

Changing Concepts and Present-Day Etiology of Upper Extremity Venous Thrombosis; Reconstructive Venous Surgery; Venous Angiodysplasia and Venous Malformations

BRUCE L. MINTZ, D.O.

Chief, Vascular Medicine and Noninvasive Vascular Laboratory, St. Clares-Riverside Medical Center, Danville, New Jersey

Current Status of Duplex Ultrasonography in the Diagnosis of Acute Deep Venous Thrombosis

GREGORY L. MONETA, M.D.

Assistant Professor of Surgery, Oregon Health Sciences University Hospital, VA Hospital, Portland, Oregon

Nonoperative Treatment of Venous Stasis Ulcer

WILLIAM M. MOORE, Jr., M.D.

Fellow in Vascular Surgery, Ochsner Clinic and Alton Ochsner Medical Foundation, New Orleans, Louisiana

Reconstruction of the Superior Vena Cava and Central Veins

BERNARD HANS NACHBUR, M.D.

Chief, Department of Thoracic and Cardiovascular Surgery, University of Berne, Inselspital, Berne, Switzerland

Thrombectomy in Acute Deep Vein Thrombosis: Long-Term Follow-Up

ANDREW N. NICOLAIDES, M.D., F.R.C.S., F.R.C.S.E.

Professor of Vascular Surgery, Vascular Section, Academic Surgical Unit, St. Mary's Hospital Medical School, London, England

Methods of Quantitation of Chronic Venous Insufficiency

THOMAS F. O'DONNELL, Jr., M.D., F.A.C.S.

Professor of Surgery, Tufts University School of Medicine; Chief of Vascular Surgery, New England Medical Center, Boston, Massachusetts

Popliteal Vein Valve Transplantation for Deep Venous Valvular Reflux: Rationale, Method, and Long-Term Clinical, Hemodynamic, and Anatomic Results

WILLIAM H. PEARCE, M.D.

Associate Professor of Surgery, Northwestern University Medical School; Attending Surgeon, Northwestern Memorial Hospital and VA Lakeside Medical Center, Chicago, Illinois

Reconstructive Venous Surgery; Venous Angiodysplasia and Venous Malformations

JOHN M. PORTER, M.D.

Professor of Surgery, Oregon Health Sciences University, Portland, Oregon

Nonoperative Treatment of Venous Stasis Ulcer

SESHADRI RAJU, M.D.

Professor of Surgery, University of Mississippi Medical School; Staff Physician, VA Hospital; Attending Surgeon, University Medical Center; Director, Doppler Vascular Laboratory; Director, Mississippi Transplant Program, University Medical Center, Jackson, Mississippi

Experience with Venous Reconstruction in Patients with Chronic Venous Insufficiency

NORMAN M. RICH, M.D.

Professor and Chairman, Department of Surgery, Uniformed Services University of the Health Sciences, Bethesda, Maryland; Co-Director, Vascular Surgery Fellowship, Walter Reed Army Medical Center, Washington, DC

Involvement of the Lymphatic System in Chronic Venous Insufficiency; Long-Term Follow-Up of Venous Reconstruction Following Trauma

HANS-BEAT RIS, M.D.

Department of Thoracic and Cardiovascular Surgery, University of Berne, Berne, Switzerland

Thrombectomy in Acute Deep Vein Thrombosis: Long-Term Follow-Up

JAMES J. SCHULER, M.D.

Associate Professor of Surgery, University of Illinois College of Medicine; Attending Surgeon, Cook County Hospital; Chief of Vascular Surgery Service, West Side VA Hospital, Chicago, Illinois

Repair or Ligation in Extremity Venous Injuries

JOHN H. SCURR, B.Sc., M.B., B.S., F.R.C.S.

Senior Lecturer, University of London at the University College and Middlesex Hospitals Medical School; Consultant Surgeon, Middlesex Hospital, London, England

Current Views on the Pathogenesis of Venous Ulceration

DONALD SILVER, M.D.

Professor of Surgery and Chairman, Department of Surgery, University of Missouri-Columbia School of Medicine; Surgeon in Chief, University of Missouri Hospital and Clinics, Columbia, Missouri

Hematologic Factors, Anticoagulation, and Anticoagulant Complications in Venous Thromboembolism

DONALD P. SPADONE, M.D.

Assistant Professor of Surgery, University of Missouri, Columbia, Missouri

Study of Deep Venous Thrombosis in High-Risk Patients Using Color Flow Doppler

D. E. STRANDNESS, Jr., M.D.

Professor of Surgery; Head, Section of Vascular Surgery, University of Washington School of Medicine; Attending Staff, University Hospital and VA Hospital, Seattle, Washington

Quantitation of Venous Reflux Using Duplex Scanning

E. SHANNON STAUFFER, M.D.

Professor and Chairman, Division of Orthopaedics and Rehabilitation, Southern Illinois University School of Medicine, Springfield, Illinois

Study of Deep Venous Thrombosis in High-Risk Patients Using Color Flow Doppler

DAVID S. SUMNER, M.D.

Professor of Surgery and Chief, Section of Peripheral Vascular Surgery, Southern Illinois University School of Medicine, Springfield, Illinois

Study of Deep Venous Thrombosis in High-Risk Patients Using Color Flow Doppler

LLOYD M. TAYLOR, Jr., M.D.

Associate Professor of Surgery, Oregon Health Sciences University, Portland, Oregon

Nonoperative Treatment of Venous Stasis Ulcer

PAUL VAN BEMMELEN, M.D.

Department of Vascular Surgery, St. Antonius Ziekenhuis, Nieuwegein, Netherlands

Quantitation of Venous Reflux Using Duplex Scanning

J. LEONEL VILLAVICENCIO, M.D., F.A.C.S.

Professor of Surgery, Uniformed Services University of the Health Sciences, Bethesda, Maryland; Staff and Director of Vein Clinic, Walter Reed Army Medical Center, Washington, DC

Involvement of the Lymphatic System in Chronic Venous Insufficiency; Long-Term Follow-Up of Venous Reconstruction Following Trauma

ROBERT L. VOGELZANG, M.D.

Associate Professor of Clinical Radiology, Northwestern University Medical School; Director of Angiography and Interventional Radiology, Northwestern Memorial Hospital, Chicago, Illinois

Changing Concepts and Present-Day Etiology of Upper Extremity Venous Thrombosis; Computed Tomography and Magnetic Resonance Imaging of Venous Disorders

JAMES S. T. YAO, M.D., Ph.D.

Magerstadt Professor of Surgery and Chief, Division of Vascular Surgery, Northwestern University Medical School; Attending Vascular Surgeon and Director, Blood Flow Laboratory, Northwestern Memorial Hospital, Chicago, Illinois

Reconstructive Venous Surgery; Venous Angiodysplasia and Venous Malformations

PREFACE

At the time of compilation and organization of chapters for this volume, there were 15 announcements of forthcoming vascular meetings in the 'Events of Interest' section of a leading vascular journal. There was the usual smattering of announcements of national and international meetings. Some, concerning biomechanics, "Very Ultra Low Dosage" and impotence research seemed to have little to do with everyday vascular surgery. Others which called attention to annual meetings of various societies would have a predictable format. They would display a predictable parade of authors who would detail results of research on a variety, but predictable array, of vascular subjects. But in that announcement section, one's attention was inevitably called not to those notices but to announcements of six meetings that would deal exclusively with venous disorders. Veins have never had such exposure before. What happened?

It takes little thought to recall that several very successful meetings on venous subjects have been held within the past few months in sites as diverse as Chicago, Phoenix, and San Diego. Perhaps interest in the veins and in disorders of veins is being recycled. In North America alone, there are now three successful organizations that deal exclusively with venous subjects. Older societies of phlebology meet regularly in France, Australasia, and Germany. The Fifth European-American Congress on Venous Disorders is scheduled for late 1990 and looks to be a very informative and successful convocation.

When arterial vascular surgery flourished in the years after prosthetic grafts became available and the bypass principle was accepted, veins became less interesting to surgeons. Instead of dominating the program of the Society for Vascular Surgery as in the 1940s, vein problems were relegated to an occasional paper on an occasional program. In the hospital when vein surgery was scheduled, it drew a raised eyebrow. Vein stripping became dirty words in an era of use of the saphenous vein for arterial bypass. While surgical residents trained for practice without instruction in vein surgery, surgeons who had practiced that art abandoned it or simply retired.

This book was planned at a time when the editors perceived two important truths. The first was that well-trained physicians must take renewed interest in the very common problems of the venous system. Second was that a timely volume encompassing the field of venous problems might assist in kindling that interest. From the first, it was acknowledged that venous problems were not the exclusive domain of the surgeon. Neither the general surgeon nor the vascular surgeon could lay legitimate claim to the entire field of venous problems. In fact, it was recognized that those problems occurred in every variety of clinical practice. Thus, every physician should have at least some knowledge of proper diagnosis and care of those vein problems which might come into his practice.

Renewed interest in venous problems comes at a fortuitous time in the panorama of modern medical history. Never before has imaging of the venous system been done so well by such a variety of techniques nor has quantitation of venous physiology and pathophysiology ever been so precise. These modalities enhance diagnosis, describe epidemiology, and monitor results of therapy. Therapy itself has been revolutionized. Venous reconstruction can be done; it is even recognized in CPT coding. Venous ablation, when necessary, is done with minimal body invasion. Even the ancient art of sclerotherapy has profited by needle technology as well as by the chance discovery that a powerful local anesthetic agent is an efficient sclerosant.

This volume chronicles many of these modern changes in approaches to venous problems. If it assists in stirring interest in veins and in stimulating bright minds to be concerned with venous research, it will have achieved one important purpose. If it improves and refines venous diagnosis and, in turn, betters patient care, it will have succeeded in the editors' principal purpose.

J. J. BERGAN, M.D.
La Jolla, California

J. S. T. YAO, M.D., PH.D.
Chicago, Illinois

CONTENTS

IV

MANAGEMENT OF ACUTE DEEP VEIN THROMBOSIS

V

TREATMENT OF SUPERFICIAL VENOUS INSUFFICIENCY

VIII
MANAGEMENT OF CHRONIC VENOUS ULCERS

IX
UPPER EXTREMITY VENOUS PROBLEMS

X
SURGICAL MANAGEMENT OF VENOUS INJURIES

I

SURGERY OF THE VEINS

1

HISTORICAL HIGHLIGHTS IN TREATING VENOUS INSUFFICIENCY

John J. Bergan

In the case of an ulcer, it is not expedient to stand; more especially if the ulcer be situated in the leg.

HIPPOCRATES (460–377 BC) (1)

The study of the history of medicine is fascinating for many reasons. Names of great physicians ring down the hallways of time. Their persisting truthful observations demonstrate penetrating vision. In contrast, like interwining echoes, fabricated theories of etiology and fanciful explanations of disease processes, when looked at from a 20th-century perspective, give humor to ancient profound discourse. The fact remains that it is in the truths confirmed by history that the great lessons of the past contribute to modern knowledge.

Laufman said that "one can make a good case for the premise that anatomic research on the venous system was responsible for the entire parade of advances, from the discovery of the circulation of blood to today's marvels of cardiovascular medicine and surgery" (2). He substantiates this premise by pointing out that biohistorians agree that the landmark studies of Fabricius on venous valves led directly to William Harvey's discovery of the circulation. Also, Harvey, in the only conversation he had with Robert Boyle, said that it was a consideration of the venous valves that first induced him to think of a circulation. The background for Harvey's discoveries was laid as early as 1550 BC in the Eber's papyrus, which states that "certain serpentine windings" are not to be operated upon because that would be "head on the ground." This phrase, often quoted, has been interpreted to mean that fatal hemorrhage from incision into varicosities would cause the head to be laid on the ground in death. As shown in the record of Hippocrates' work, care of venous stasis and venous ulcer were a concern of the physician in the third and fourth century before Christ (Fig. 1–1).

An enduring record of varicose veins is seen in a votive offering in the national museum in Athens, also much reproduced (3). In this votive offering, a dedication is made to Dr. Amynous by the patient, Lysimachidis, presumably in thanks for successful treatment (Fig. 1–2).

These mentions of venous disease are historical curiosities. It is in the ob-

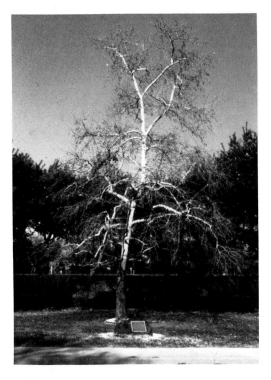

Figure 1–1. The tree of Hippocrates (*Plantus orientalis*), taken as a cutting from the parent tree under which Hippocrates is said to have held classes. Thus, Hippocrates' teachings of care of venous problems have been transmitted directly from the island of Cos to America. This tree stands on the grounds of the National Library of Medicine, where it was planted in 1961. (Photograph contributed by James Salander, M.D.)

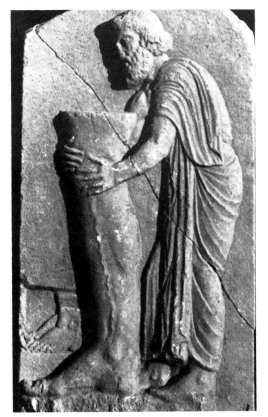

Figure 1–2. Votive offerings such as this were given to physicians by grateful patients after successful treatment. As shown here, the condition treated or organ affected was depicted in the sculpture.

servations of anatomy that Harvey's contribution was founded and studies of venous physiology begun.

CONCEPTS OF VENOUS PHYSIOLOGY

When Harvey was a student, his most influential teacher had to be Hieronymus Fabricius (1533–1620). Fabricius, in turn, had inherited the chair of surgery and anatomy held by Vesalius. Vesalius's "De Humani Corporis Fabrica," published in 1543, was the first volume to accurately illustrate anatomy. Its artistic elegance is attributable to the drawings of Jan Stefan van Kalkan, who set the anatomy in a recognizable landscape. Fabricius's publication in 1603 named the valves of the veins (4), illustrated their intervals of occurrence, and stated the theory that these were placed to delay the blood from "flooding into the feet or hands and fingers and collecting there" (Fig. 1–3). Harvey's studies with Fabricius could not have excluded such pithy observations from the master. It was a short step to the synthesis of these concepts and others that allowed Harvey to consolidate his ideas into an explanation of circulation, which he did upon returning to England in 1606. However, rapid publication was not the rule in the 17th century. Harvey's first paper on the circulation was published in 1616, and the definitive work, "Exercitatio Anatomica De Motu Cordis et Sanguinis," was not published until 1628.

The fundamental observations of Harvey are clearly illustrated in his demonstration of the blood flow and valvular arrest of venous circulation in the arm

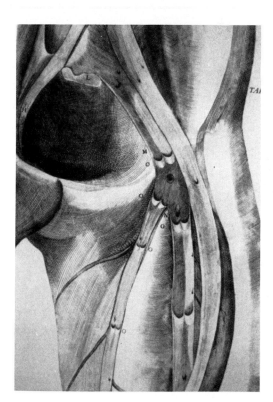

Figure 1–3. Fabricius' studies were illustrated by clear drawings that supported his theories of function of venous valves.

of man (Fig. 1–4). Indeed, it was the study of veins and their valves that uncovered the truth about blood flow and cardiac action.

It is the combination of physiology with anatomy that leads to understanding of function. While an accurate description of the physiology of the venous system is not found in Vesalius, an accurate description of the anatomy is. Earlier and often erroneous contributions had been depicted by artists, not anatomists. The best of these are seen in the work of Leonardo da Vinci (1452). Good reproductions

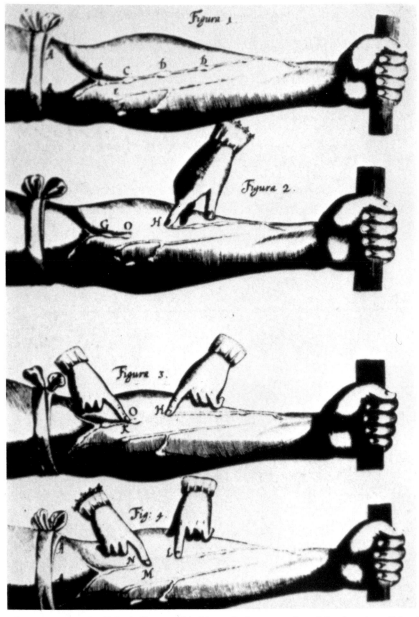

Figure 1–4.   Elegant simplicity is illustrated in Harvey's demonstration of the direction of blood flow in the arm of man. His logic was irrefutable.

of these are included in Browse et al.'s book, which duplicates drawings from the Royal Library of Windsor Castle (3). These authors pointed out that Leonardo's drawings of the superficial veins of the lower limb do not include a posterior arch vein (often called Leonardo's vein), but that his drawings of the superficial veins of the arm are similar to those found in "De Motu Cordis." The drawings of the tributaries of the long saphenous vein in the groin could serve today in a modern textbook.

Unfortunately, Galen's theory of humors dominated medical thought for some 15 centuries. During that time, varicose elongation, tortuosity, and dilation were attributed to the weight of stagnant blood on the walls of the veins (not a bad thought). Bandaging for varicose veins was known before Galen. However, it was thought that since varicosities contained black bile, so long as this was kept sidetracked outside the main venous channels, the patient would then be safe. In contrast, when bandages pressed the black bilious humors into the circulation, this might lead to "madness or other disasters" (1).

Mixed with erroneous philosophy about venous stasis were flashes of brilliant observation, including a statement by Fernel (1604), who wrote "it [the varix] comes also from a blow, from a contusion, frome excessive effort." (5). This information is useful in practice in the 20th century. On the other hand, Marianus Sanctus's theory that "standing too much before kings" was a chief cause of varicose veins is hardly useful at all in view of today's modes of governemnt (6).

Throughout recorded history, the association of varicose veins with pregnancy is accurately recorded. Sanctus related varicose veins to childbearing, and Ambroise Paré (1510–1590) observed that "women with child are commonly troubled with them" (7).

PHILOSOPHIES OF TREATMENT

Compression therapy is important to treatment of venous disorders. Compression therapy is referred to in the Old Testament (Isaiah 1:6) and receives mention in Hippocrates as well. Celsus used linen and plaster bandages much as Unna did in the 1890s. Caustic agents such as white lead and litharage were used by Virgo, who then applied circular bandages for pressure, and Roman soldiers at the time of Christ recognized that lower extremity fatigue could be ameliorated by application of tight leg strappings (10).

Compression therapy is mentioned in more recent history, including that from the Middle Ages. However, Galen's black bile theory permeated the philosophy of treatment of venous ulcer for an inordinate time. Many physicians were convinced that healing of the ulcer would be catastrophic. Avicenna before 1037, Le Dran in 1731, Heisler in 1738, Benjamin Bell in 1789, and many patinets in country districts in Ireland today believe that healing of the ulcer may cause "melancholy, madness, dropsy, palpitation . . . and other things" (8). Paré, for all of his brilliance in reintroducing the ligature, eliminating treatment of amputations by boiling with oil, and healing the leg ulcer of his captor, Lord Vaudeville, did not always believe that healing of the ulcer was beneficial. Nevertheless his advice, though 400 years old, holds true today, "[in bandaging] roule the leg beginning at the foote and finishing at the knee, not forgetting a little bolster upon the varicose veins" (7).

As early as the 14th century, not all workers in the field believed that healing of ulcers was deleterious to one's health. Henri de Mondeville, writing between 1306 and 1320, offered the opinion that a bandage embracing the whole limb was advantageous because it "drives back the evil, harmful humors infiltrated in the leg and ulcer" (9). This is perhaps the first correct statement of the theory that elimination of edema allows healing of venous ulcerations. Guy de Chauliac (1363) employed plaster bandages to treat venous ulcerations, and, as indicated above, Ambrose Paré, when taken prisoner in 1553 while acting as surgeon to Henri II, then cured the leg ulcer of his captor.

In the history of compression for venous stasis disease, one must make special mention of the work of Richard Wiseman, Sargeant Surgeon to Charles II. It was Wiseman who developed the term "varicose ulcer" and introduced what was at the time a new method of compressing the leg affected by such an ulcer (11). His laced stocking, as illustrated by Meister, was made of soft leather such as dog skin (Fig. 1–5). This was applied loose, from ankle to knee, then laced tightly to compress the leg and eliminate edema. Wiseman's methods was widely practiced in England and on the continent. Wiseman was an assistant to the surgeon at St. Thomas Hospital, where Browse had "often considered reintroducing his lace-up stocking" in his own practice (3). Theden also used a modification of lace-up leather stockings, giving credit to Fabrizio d'Aguapendente.

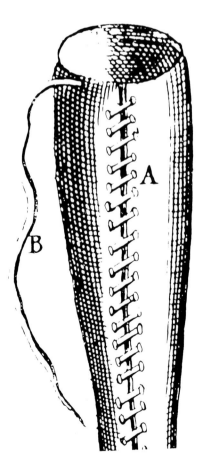

Figure 1–5. Compression therapy delivered by Wiseman's laced-up leather stocking was, and is, effective in ameliorating symptomatic venous stasis.

Further development of compression as a form of therapy necessarily awaited development of elastic fiber, subsequent covering of this fiber with silk or cotton, and then development of synthetic twisted fibers with memory in the modern era (10).

DEVELOPMENT OF VENOUS TESTING

Compression therapy was simply a logical extension of observations upon varicose veins themselves. Fabry, in describing a leg ulcer encountered in 1589, described blood in the veins receding immediately craniad when the leg was elevated and descending instantly when the leg was placed in the dependent position, as though the blood was "in a tube" (12). Brodie, in 1846, described such downward descent of blood through valveless veins in the test that bears his name, saying "the patient being in erect position, I removed the pressure from the vein, the valves being of no use, the blood rushed downward of its own weight" (13). The observations of Fabry, Brodie, and even Gay later were crystallized into the observations of Trendelenburg, who described, in 1890, the test that is still performed today (14). Trendelenburg used his powers of observation and manipulated the limb. Today, we use the powers of the continuous-wave Doppler instrument and manipulate the blood flow through it by augmentation and Valsalva maneuver.

Table 1–1 shows the gradual development of tests of venous physiology. All of these are dependent upon careful observation by an experienced physician interested in the physiologic function of the superficial and communicating venous valves and the interplay of the muscle pump. This begins with Fabry's observations and includes Home's description of congestion of granulation tissue in venous ulcers in leg dependency (15).

The modern era of venous testing perhaps began with the lectures on varicose veins and ulcers of the legs by Sir Benjamin Brodie in 1846 (13). These begin with the famous phrase, "Mary Ann Richardson, 48 years of age, was admitted on the 11th of October with ulcers of the leg." It is within this lecture that Brodie called the ulcerations varicose ulcers, ascribed varicose veins to standing occupations, and described the symptoms of venous stasis, including itching, fullness, muscle cramps, and the thrombophlebitis of superficial venous clusters. Although it is common to refer to Brodie's observations as a test, in fact he advocated using these observations in treatment. His method began with the patient standing so that the varicose clusters could be identified. He called attention to the point of

TABLE 1–1. Historical Development of Venous Testing

1589	Fabry's observations
1801	Home's observations
1846	Brodie test
1888	Schwartz's test
1891	Trendelenburg test
1895	Perthes' test
1931	McPheeter's modification of Schwartz's test
1936	Mahorne-Ochsner test
1940	Heyerdale variation of Schwartz's test
1941	Pratt's test

control and then, allowing the patient to recline with the foot raised in order to empty the varices, placed adhesive plaster across the control point to "prevent the vein from becoming distended when the patient stands erect."

In the Schwartz test, the patient is examined standing with the observing hand placed on the proximal saphenous vein and the active hand percussing the varices (16). While this test validates the communication of the clusters of varices with the proximal saphenous vein, in fact the percussion wave can pass through competent as well as incompetent valves, an observation that stimulated the development of the later modifications of this test.

Trendelenburg's contribution should probably be referred to as the Brodie-Trendelenburg test.

The first of the tests of muscle pump function was the Perthes test, performed with the superficial veins constricted proximally and with the patient utilizing the muscle pump during walking (17). Perhaps cautioned the observer to look for the disappearance of the varices; if this occured, it was the saphenous sytem that was causing the varicose veins, because the deep system valves were competent to remove the blood flow during muscle pump function.

The McPheeter modification of the Schwartz test was described in 1931 and accompanied physiologic observations of venous pressure and the effects of exercise, respiration, and position on such pressure (18). The object of the percussion test was to identify the course of the greater saphenous vein so that it could be treated by sclerotherapy. McPheeters came to the erroneous conclusion that the test had not been described before and termed his version the "percussion pulse transmittal test."

Ochsner and Mahorne's test was a modification of the Perthes test in which additional information was derived. The tourniquet was placed first on the upper part of the thigh, then across the middle part of the thigh, and then just below the knee. The objective was to determine the exact location of incompetent communicating veins between the superficial and deep system. It has been referred to as the "comparative tourniquet test" (19).

The Heyerdale modification of the Schwartz test eliminated the problem of the percussion wave passing through competent valves. The test was described by McCallig and Heyerdale, and consisted of creating percussion over the saphenous vein in the upper part of the thigh and palpating the varices in the calf at the same time (20). This, of course, would be a more reliable method of testing for valve competency, but recall that Schwartz was simply trying to identify the location of the saphenous vein for subsequent sclerotherapy.

Pratt's 1941 description of a different method of testing was most pragmatic (21). The objective was to study the patient so as to plan the operative procedure that would effectively remove the varicosities. Pratt said, "with the patient lying down, the leg to be tested is elevated and with light massage, the veins are emptied. A tourniquet is placed sufficiently high in the thigh to close off the saphenous vein. An Ace bandage is then applied from the toes to the tourniquet. The patient then stands up and the Ace bandage is slowly unwound from above down. With the tourniquet above preventing reflux of femoral blood through the saphenous vein, and with the Ace bandage below compressing the remainder of the saphenous vein, a bulge or blowout indicates an incompetent communicating branch vein . . . ." Such a perforating vein, if poorly identified, could be missed by the surgical procedure.

Today, we recognize that such observation is crucial to modern varicose vein surgery, and can be made without the elaborate method of testing described by Pratt, simply by using visual inspection and the hand-held continuous-wave Doppler instrument.

SURGICAL TREATMENT OF VARICOSE VEINS

Table 1–2 lists the steps in development of varicose vein surgery. It indicates that few options are available. These range from multiple punctures to hook avulsion, cautery, simple division with or without bandaging, and/or removal by the intraluminal or extraluminal route.

As in many other medical events, Hippocrates gets first credit for varicose vein treatment. He recommended multiple punctures and cautioned against cutting directly into the varicosity and engorged tissues. Present-day stab avulsion techniques had their origins in the methods of Galen (22), who used a hook for avulsion; 400 years later, Aegineta recommended ligation, division, and compression therapy (23). Albucasis performed a type of internal stripping in the 11th century: "introduce a needle with a strong double thread, tie it and pull it up; and insert a probe under it, and twist it all round until it comes out" (24). Paré, 500 years later, returned to ligation and division of varicosities in addition to the pressure bandaging mentioned previously.

Heister suggested bleeding through the varicosities, bandaging, and a starvation diet (25). A curious method of transcutaneous obliteration was practiced by Davat, who passed several needles through the skin and the affected vein and followed this by tying figure-of-eight ligatures around both ends of each needle (26). The inflammatory reaction produced by the inevitable infection obliterated the veins. Schede was more daring and proposed ligation and sectioning the varicosities at multiple points, passing ligatures under the vein, and tying the ligatures over a rubber tube on the surface of the skin (27). Predictably, these results proved unsatisfactory.

The origins of total greater saphenous vein stripping reside in the works of Madelung (28). He used an incision similar to the saphenectomy incision employed

TABLE 1–2. Historical Development of Varicose Vein Surgery[a]

370 BC	Hippocrates	Multiple punctures
50 AD	Celsus	Cautery and/or excision
200	Galen	Hook avulsion
650	Aegineta	Saphenous diviision, bandaging
1050	Albucasis	Venous stripping (intraluminal)
1550	Paré	Ligation, division
1700	Heister	Bleeding, starvation
1833	Davat	Transcutaneous puncture
1844	Madelung	Saphenous stripping, ligation
1877	Schede	Transcutaneous ligature
1890	Trendelenburg	Saphenous division
1904	Tavel	Saphenous division, injection
1905	Keller	Intraluminal stripping
1906	Mayo	Extraluminal stripping
1907	Babcock	Intraluminal stripping

[a] Several early dates are approximate.

today by coronary artery bypass surgeons. In the 1880s, this was a formidable procedure entailing considerable hospitalization and morbidity. Perhaps because of this, Trendelenburg suggested ligation and division of the greater saphenous vein in the middle third of the thigh (14).

Combinations of low-ligation surgery and sclerotherapy were suggested in the early 1900s by Tavel (29), who used a two-step procedure, and by Schiassi, who recommended simultaneous ligation and injection (30). Others, notably Nobili (31) and Unger (32), also used this technique and modified it, as is the wont of most surgeons. Intraluminal stripping was reintroduced by Keller (33) and extraluminal stripping in 1906 by Charles Mayo (34) (Fig. 1–6). Almost simultaneously, Babcock in New York devised the intraluminal stripper, which is remarkably reminiscent of today's disposable plastic stripping devices (35).

The most horrible example of varicose vein surgery is the procedure of Rindfleisch (36), which was also proposed by Friedel (37). In this horrendous procedure, the greater saphenous vein was excised in the thigh, then a spiral incision was made from the knee to the foot (Fig. 1–7). This incision encircled the leg four to seven times and was made through the skin and subcutaneous tissue, down to and including the deep fascia. The hideous wound that resulted was allowed to heal by granulation tissue. Fortunately, the results of this mutilating operation proved so unsatisfactory that it is forgotten today.

One wonders whether or not the operation proposed by Delbet (38) in 1895 was ever objectively reviewed after its performance. This operation was designed to transplant the greater saphenous vein to a position below a competent valve

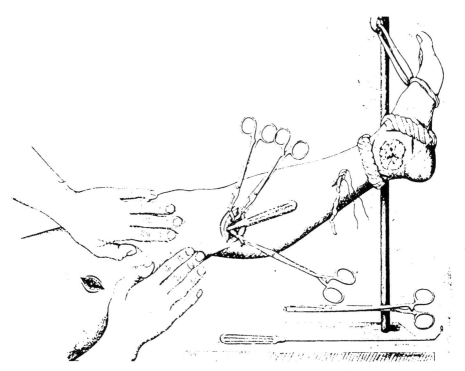

Figure 1–6.   The extraluminal Mayo stripper was a genuinely original contribution to venous ablation. As shown in this 1906 drawing, the leg is elevated to reduce venous congestion.

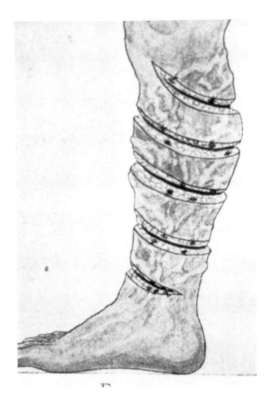

Figure 1–7. The Rindfleish operation, honored by discontinuance.

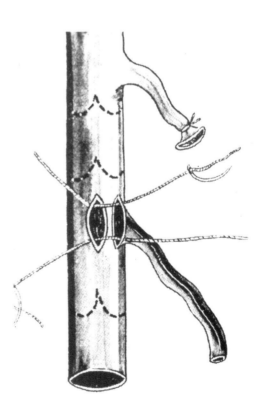

Figure 1–8. Delbet's prescient contribution is a precursor of venous transposition and was a first attempt at venous reconstruction.

(Fig. 1–8). The direct anastomosis or venovenotomy simply must have failed. If so, the procedure should have been listed as a simple ligation and division of greater saphenous vein. We know today this would be doomed to failure. The procedure was revised by Hesse and Schaack in 1921, but the results were never verified.

CONCLUSIONS

This summary of the historical highlights in the treatment of venous insufficiency includes those clinical observations made by astute physicians and the early operations that derived from that knowledge. The stage was set by these observations and treatments for physiologic studies of venous pressure, venous volume, and calf volume; noninvasive determination of venous filling recovery time, to be correlated with venous pressure recovery time; and direct imaging by duplex scan, the color flow scanning, and finally magnetic resonance imaging. Similarly, the stage was set by the early clinical work for development of venous reconstructive operations, which would go forward another step in treating venous stasis disease. These topics are detailed in the chapters that follow in this volume.

REFERENCES

1. Hippocrates: The Genuine Works of Hippocrates (Adarns EF, transl), vol 2. New York, Wm. Wood & Co, 1886; 305.
2. Laufman H: The Veins. Austin, TX, Silvergirl, Inc, 1986.
3. Browse NL, Burnand KG, Lea Thomas M: Diseases of the Veins. London, EH Arnold Publishers, 1988.
4. Fabricius: Hieronymus de Aquapendente Anatomici Patavini de Venarum Ostiolis. *In* Laufman H, ed: The Veins. Austin, TX, Silvergirl, Inc, 1986; 14.
5. Fernel J: Universa Medicina, Ambiana Pathologiae Coloniae Allobroqum, 1604.
6. Sanctus: Cited by Dodd H, Cockett FB: The Pathology and Surgery of the Veins of the Lower Limb. Edinburgh, E&S Livingstone Ltd, 1956; 8.
7. Malgaigne JF: Oeuvres Completes d'Ambroise Paré. Paris, J-B Baillière, 1840; 269.
8. Dodd H, Cockett FB: The Pathology and Surgery of the Veins of the Lower Limb. Edinburgh, E&S Livingston Ltd, 1956.
9. Mondeville H de: Chirurgie de Maître Henri de Mondeville Composée de 1306 à 1320 (Nicaise A, transl). Paris, Alcan, 1893.
10. Goldman M: Sclerotherapy. St. Louis, CV Mosby Co, 1990.
11. Wiseman R: Severall Chirurgical Treatises. London, Rogston & Took, 1676.
12. Fabry W: Observationeum et Curationum Chirurgiacarum Centuriae. Basel, Huguetam, 1606–1641.
13. Brodie BC: Lectures Illustrative of Various Subjects in Pathology and Surgery. London, Longman, Brown, Green & Longman, 1846.
14. Trendelenburg F: Über die Unterbindung der Vena saphena magna bei Unterschenkelvaricen. Beitr Klin Chir 1890; 7:195–210.
15. Home E: Practical observations on the treatment of ulcers of the legs. London, Bulmer, 1801.
16. Schwartz E: Du traitement des varices par la ligature multiple de la veine saphene interne l'extirpation. Rev Gen Clin Ther 1888; 2:65–68.
17. Perthes G: Über die Operation der Unterschenkelvaricen nach Trendelenburg. Dtsch Med Wochenschr 1895;21:253–257.
18. McPheeters HO, Merkert CE, Lundblad RA: Causes of failure of injection treatment of varicose veins. JAMA 1931;96:1114–1117.
19. Ochsner A, Mahorne H: Varicose Veins. St. Louis, CV Mosby Co, 1939.
20. McCallig JJ, Heyerdale WW: Basic understanding of varicose veins. *JAMA* 1940;115:97–100.
21. Pratt GH: Test for incompleted communicating branches in the surgical treatment of varicose veins. JAMA 1941;117:100–101.

22. Galen: Quoted by Aegineta: The Seven Books of Paulus Aegineta (Adams F, transl), London, The Sydenham Society, 1846.

23. Aegineta: The Seven Books of Paulus Aegineta (Adams F, transl), vol 2. London, The Sydenham Society, 1846;406–409.

24. Albucasis: Quoted by Ochsner A, Mahorner H: The modern treatment of varicose veins. Surgery 1937; *2*:889–894.

25. Heister L: Quoted by Ochsner A, Mahorner H: Varicose Veins. St. Louis, CV Mosby Co, 1939.

26. Davat: Quoted by Ochsner A, Mahorner H: Varicose Veins. St. Louis, CV Mosby Co, 1939.

27. Schede M: Über die operative Behandlung der Unterschenkel-varicen. Beitr Klin Wochenschr 1877;*14*:85–89.

28. Madelung H: Über die Ausschalung cirsoider Varicen an den unteren Extremitaten. Verhandl dentsch Gesellsch Chir 1884; *13*:114–117.

29. Tavel: Quoted by Ochsner A, Mahorner H: Varicose Veins. St. Louis, CV Mosby Co, 1939.

30. Schiassi B: Quoted by Ochsner A, Mahorner H: Varicose Veins, St. Louis, CV Mosby Co, 1939.

31. Nobili U: Contributo alla cura delle varici dell'arto inferiore con speciale riguardo al metedo Schiassi. Polyclinico (Sez Chir) 1921;*28*:149–159.

32. Unger E: Zur Technik der Varicenbehandlung. Zentralbl Chir 1927;*54*:3273–3274.

33. Keller WL: A new method of extirpating the internal saphenous and similar veins in varicose conditions: A preliminary report. NY Med J 1905;*82*:385–386.

34. Mayo CH: Treatment of varicose veins. Surg Gynecol Obstet 1906;*2*:385–388.

35. Babcock WW: A new operation for extirpation of varicose veins of the leg. NY Med J 1907;*86*:153–156.

36. Rindfleisch W: Quoted by Friedel G: Operative behandlung der varicen, Elephantiasis, und ulcer crurus. Arch Klin Chir 1908;*86*:143–159.

37. Friedel G: Operative behandlung der varicen, Elephantiasis, und ulcer crurus. Arch Klin Chir 1908;*86*:143–159.

38. Delbet. Quoted by Ochsner A, Mahorne H: Varicose Veins. St. Louis, CV Mosby Co, 1939.

II

BASIC
CONSIDERATIONS

2

HEMATOLOGIC FACTORS, ANTICOAGULATION, AND ANTICOAGULANT COMPLICATIONS IN VENOUS THROMBOEMBOLISM

John R. Hoch and Donald Silver

Venous thromboembolism is the product of the interaction of rheologic, structural, and hematologic factors. Virchow identified venous stasis, injury to vessel walls, and the hypercoagulability of blood as events capable of precipitating thrombosis. The etiologies of venous thrombosis have, in recent years, been expanded to include hypofibrinolysis.

Venous thromboses form in regions of low or disturbed flow and are composed primarily of red cells in a fibrin matrix. Endothelial injury and venostasis or activated coagulation proteins and venostasis reliably produce venous thromboses in experimental animals. Activation of the coagulation system in association with venostasis appears responsible for most clinical venous thromboses. The thromboses begin as small platelet aggregates that are deposited in the vein valve cusps or on regions of injured vein walls. Whether these aggregates evolve into thromboses, disaggregate, or undergo lysis depends on the rate of blood flow and the balance between the body's coagulation, anticoagulation, and fibrinolytic systems.

This chapter will first review those components and activities of the coagulation, anticoagulation, and fibrinolytic systems that predispose patients to thrombosis. The normal physiology of these systems will be reviewed and the inherited and acquired clinical disorders associated with venous thromboembolism will be discussed. The latter portion of the chapter will review the use of anticoagulant drugs in the prophylaxis and management of venous thromboembolism.

PLATELETS

Although platelets are responsible for primary hemostasis, they normally do not adhere to endothelial cells or to each other. Platelets activated, by exposure either to subendothelial collagen following vein wall trauma or to thrombin, will adhere to the vein wall. The adherence of platelets is often followed by the aggregation of more platelets to form a platelet plug. The early platelet plug is held together by fibrinogen bridges that dissociate unless thrombin-stimulated fibrin stabilization of the plug occurs. Activated platelets aid in the generation of thrombin by releasing factor V and providing phospholipid membrane binding sites for activated (a) factors Xa and Va. The prothrombinase complex formed on the platelet membrane accelerates the conversion of prothrombin to thrombin (1).

Many acquired clinical conditions predispose to venous thrombosis by activating platelets; some are associated with thrombocytosis. Myeloproliferative diseases, hyperlipidemia, diabetes mellitus, and sepsis all predispose patients to thrombosis at least partly because of their effects on platelets.

Myeloproliferative disorders, a group of related diseases of the bone marrow stem cell, include polycythemia vera, essential thrombocytosis, myeloid metaplasia, chronic myelogenous leukemia, and myelofibrosis. Although thrombocytosis may accompany these disorders, qualitative platelet abnormalities are the more important pathophysiologic factors predisposing patients to thrombosis (2). The abnormalities of the bone marrow stem cell affect the megakaryocytes, which results in the production of defective platelets (3). Qualitative platelet abnormalities include abnormal arachidonic acid metabolism; deranged ultrastructure; loss of α-adrenergic, prostaglandin, and Fc receptors; and acquired storage pool diseases (2).

Patients with myeloproliferative disorders are predisposed to venous and arterial thromboses that present in unusual anatomic sites, including the splenic, portal, hepatic, and mesenteric vessels. The myeloproliferative disorders and paroxysmal nocturnal hemoglobinuria together are the most frequently diagnosed conditions responsible for hepatic vein thrombosis (Budd-Chiari syndrome) (4). Platelets of patients with nocturnal paroxysmal hemoglobinuria are more sensitive than normal platelets to complement-mediated platelet activation (5).

Hyperlipidemia may predispose patients to thrombosis by activating platelets via one of several mechanisms. Platelets from patients with type IIa hyperlipoproteinemia demonstrate increased sensitivity to aggregating agents as a result of increased membrane cholesterol concentration (6). Cholesterol-loading of platelets in vitro has demonstrated an increased release of thromboxane that correlated with platelet hyperaggregability (7). Hyperlipidemias may also activate platelets by modulating their adenylate cyclase activity (8). Since platelet membrane cholesterol content is dependent upon plasma cholesterol content (9), reduction of plasma cholesterol may reduce a patient's risk of thrombosis.

The increased thrombotic risk of patients with diabetes mellitus is related to increased platelet hypersensitivity and subsequent activation by aggregating stimuli. Diabetes mellitus affects platelets and the vein wall by increasing the release of thromboxane A_2, von Willebrand's factor, and fibrinogen while decreasing platelet sensitivity to prostacyclin (10,11). Hyperaggregability has been directly related to hyperglycemia and therefore "tight" diabetic control may limit thrombotic sequelae (12). It is unclear whether platelet activaton in diabetes mellitus is a defect primarily of platelets or of the vessel wall. The glycosylated collagen of diabetics is a more potent activator of platelets than is collagen from normal subjects; this may partly be responsible for the platelet hyperaggregability found in the diabetic (13).

Sepsis may predispose to thrombosis by several mechanisms. Gram-positive bacteria may directly activate platelets to aggregate. Gram-negative bacterial endotoxin may stimulate platelet aggregation but also interacts with leukocytes and endothelial cells, resulting in tissue factor–like activation of the coagulation system.

Heparin-Induced Thrombocytopenia

Two types of heparin-associated thrombocytopenia have been identified, but only one is associated with thrombotic complications. The first type, occurring in up to 15 per cent of patients within 2 to 3 days of heparin exposure, is transient in nature and without clinical sequelae (14). The second type of heparin-induced thrombocytopenia (HIT) occurs in 4 per cent of patients receiving heparin (15). The onset of thrombocytopenia is delayed, occurring after 4 to 15 days (mean 8 days) of initial heparin therapy, and is independent of the amount, the route of administration, or the type of heparin used (16). This is an idiosyncratic reaction that is generally believed to be mediated by an immune mechanism. Normal platelets mixed with plasma from patients with HIT will aggregate when heparin is added to the mixture. Increased levels of immunoglobulin (Ig) G and complement (C) 3 have been demonstrated on the platelets of patients with HIT (17). A heparin-dependent antiplatelet antibody or an antibody to a heparin-platelet complex appears to stimulate platelet aggregation either by triggering the platelet release reaction or by other mechanisms (18–20). The thrombocytopenia is assumed to be due to peripheral consumption or immune destruction of platelets.

The HIT syndrome is associated with heparin-initiated arterial and venous thrombosis, thromboembolism, and, rarely, hemorrhage. A 61 per cent morbidity and 23 per cent mortality have been reported in this syndrome. However, with early recognition and treatment, the morbidity and mortality can be reduced to 22.5 and 12 per cent respectively (21). Thrombosis has been assumed to be caused by intravascular platelet aggregation leading initially to small platelet aggregates that propagate to large aggregates—the so-called white clot syndrome. Recently, it has been suggested that immune-mediated endothelial cell injury, in addition to platelet injury, may play a role in the development of these thromboses (17).

HIT should be suspected in all patients receiving herapin who have falling platelet counts (30 per cent reduction, or less than 100,000/cu mm), increasing resistance to heparin, or new thrombohemorrhagic complications. Platelet aggregometry studies establish the diagnosis, which is confirmed by the prompt increase in platelet count when all sources of heparin are eliminated. Management includes immediate cessation of all forms of heparin and the administration of platelet function–inhibiting drugs (aspirin 325 mg twice a day). If the need for anticoagulation continues, alternative anticoagulants such as warfarin, dextran, or ancrod should be used. It is recommended that all patients receiving heparin be monitored with daily platelet counts.

COAGULATION AND ANTICOAGULATION MECHANISMS

Increased activation of the blood's coagulation proteins or decreased activity of the natural anticoagulants may create hypercoagulable states. This section will review the blood coagulation and anticoagulant systems and discuss inherited and acquired disorders that predispose patients to venous thromboembolism.

Coagulation System

The series of linked proteolytic reactions leading to thrombin generation has been termed the "coagulation cascade." The cascade is activated when the inactive coagulation proteins (zymogens) are converted to their serine proteases, which then can catalyze subsequent zymogen–serine protease conversions. This is a self-amplifying system in which a small stimulus produces large quantities of thrombin. Two "pathways" have classically been described as capable of initiating the coagulation cascade. The intrinsic pathway is initiated by contact activation of factor XII, whereas the extrinsic pathway is initiated by tissue factor in association with factor VII (Fig. 2–1). Once believed to operate independently, the two pathways have complex, linked interactions.

The intrinsic pathway is initiated when factor XII is activated (XIIa) by an interaction with a negatively charged surface, such as collagen, subendothelium, or endotoxin, in the presence of high-molecular-weight kallikrein and prekallikrein. Factor XIIIa converts factor XI to its serine protease form (XIa), which proteolytically activates factor IX (IXa). Factor X is activated by factor IXa in

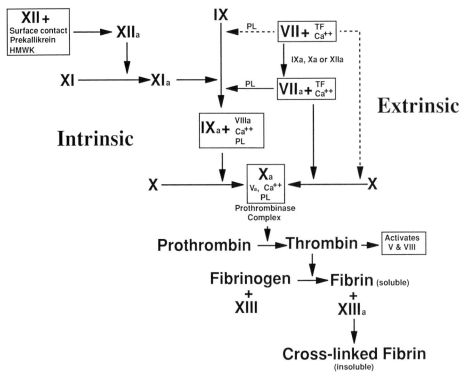

Figure 2–1. The intrinsic and extrinsic pathways of coagulation. The intrinsic pathway is initiated by surface contact whereas the extrinsic pathway is initiated by the release of tissue factor (TF) from tissues injured during surgery or trauma. The pathways are interrelated and operate in tandem to achieve hemostasis. HMWK, high-molecular-weight kallikrein; PL, phospholipid from activated platelet or endothelial membranes. (From Hoch JR, Silver D: Hemostasis and thrombosis. *In* Moore WS, ed: Vascular Surgery: A Comprehensive Review, 3rd ed. Philadelphia, WB Saunders Company, 1990.)

a reaction that takes place on platelet or endothelial cell membranes and requires factor VIIIa and calcium. The two pathways merge with the activation of factor X into a final common pathway.

The extrinsic pathway is initiated by the release of tissue factor (TF), or tissue thromboplastin, from injured tissues; the TF binds to factor VII in the presence of calcium (TF.VII). TF.VII is capable of activating factors IX and X, effectively linking the extrinsic to the intrinsic pathway. TF.VII is activated by factors IXa, Xa, and XIIa, resulting in a complex (TF.VIIa) possessing a 100-fold greater proteolytic potential than TF.VII (22).

In the common pathway, factor Xa assembles with factor Va and calcium on a platelet or endothelial cell phospholipid membrane into a prothrombinase complex that greatly accelerates the conversion of prothrombin to thrombin. Thrombin proteolytically cleaves fibrinopeptides A and B from fibrinogen to form fibrin, which then polymerizes to form a gel. Factor XIII, activated by thrombin, covalently cross-links adjacent fibrin monomers to form a stable clot.

Prethrombotic Conditions

Many clinical conditions predispose patients to venous thrombosis by overwhelming natural anticoagulant mechanisms, by increasing the plasma levels of one or more coagulation proteins, or by the excessive activation of the coagulation system. Trauma, thermal injuries, and operative dissection all release tissue thromboplastin and thus activate the extrinsic coagulation pathway. Gram-negative bacterial endotoxin may also cause TF-like activation of the coagulation system by interaction with leukocytes and endothelial cells. Intravascular hemolysis may lead to activation of the intrinsic pathway by increasing plasma concentrations of phospholipids.

A strong association between malignancy and venous thrombosis has been recognized since Trousseau described, in 1865, the syndrome of recurrent migratory thrombophlebitis in cancer patients (23). Between 5 and 15 per cent of cancer patients will develop venous thrombosis; however, the incidence may be as high as 50 per cent in patients with pancreatic carcinoma (24). Malignancies may predispose to thrombosis by synthesis of TF-like substances by monocytes and macrophages, which are stimulated by tumor antigens; tumor cell synthesis of proteases, which may directly activate the coagulation system; and platelet activation by tumor cells (24). TF-like activity has been noted in patients with multiple myeloma, promyelocytic leukemia, and mucin-secreting adenocarcinomas. Colonic, vaginal, and breast carcinomas can release proteases that directly activate factor X (25). Abnormal laboratory findings in cancer patients include elevated concentrations of factors V, VIII, IX, and X and fibronigen; decreased concentrations of antithrombin III (AT III); increased turnover of fibrinogen and platelets; and accelerated fibrinolysis (26). These findings may be interpreted as reflecting the activation of both the coagulation and fibrinolytic systems coupled with decreased anticoagulant activity in cancer patients (i.e., a state of chronic intravascular coagulation). The balance between coagulation and fibrinolysis determines whether thrombotic or hemorrhagic complications ensue.

During the puerperium and when taking exogenous estrogens, women are at increased risk for thromboembolism. During the third trimester, pregnant women demonstrate increased concentrations of factors VII, VIII, IX, and X and fibrinogen, whereas AT III levels gradually drop. This prethrombotic state is enhanced by decreased activity of the plasminogen activator system (27). Women who develop venous thrombosis during pregnancy should be treated with heparin because, unlike warfarin, it does not cross the placenta. Warfarin places the fetus at risk for hemorrhage and may be teratogenic. Exogenous estrogens, especially in oral contraceptives, have been shown to decrease AT III levels and increase the concentration of factors VII and X and are clearly associated with an increased incidence of venous thrombosis, pulmonary embolism, and postoperative thrombosis (2).

Natural Anticoagulants

Three natural anticoagulant proteins balance the activities of the coagulation cascade: AT III, protein C, and heparin cofactor II. AT III is a serine protease inhibitor that binds to and then neutralizes the activity of thrombin and the other serine proteases of the coagulation system. Circulating heparin or heparin-like substances bound on the surface of endothelial cells complex with AT III and dramatically accelerate the rate of AT III–serine protease complex formation and the rate of serine protease neutralization. Once the enzyme is neutralized, heparin is released to complex with other AT III molecules (28).

Protein C is a vitamin K–dependent proenzyme that, when converted to its active serine protease form (protein Ca), becomes a potent anticoagulant. Only thrombin can activate protein C; however, it does so slowly. Conversion of protein C to protein Ca can be increaed 20,000-fold if the thrombin first complexes with an endothelial cell membrane receptor known as thrombomodulin. Protein Ca cleaves factors Va and VIIIa, destroying the cofactors of the two rate-limiting steps of coagulation and preventing the assembly of the prothrombinase complex. This reaction takes place on platelet phospholipid membranes in the presence of calcium and another vitamin K–dependent protein, protein S, which acts as a cofactor for protein C (29). In addition, activated protein C enhances fibrinolytic activity by stimulating the release of tissue plasminogen activator.

Heparin cofactor II is a glycoprotein that acts to form a stable 1:1 complex with thrombin that effectively inhibits thrombin's activity. Unlike AT III, heparin cofactor II cannot neutralize other clotting factors. The role of heparin cofactor II in thrombosis prevention has not been well defined (30).

Deficiencies of Natural Anticoagulants

Deficiencies of anticoagulant proteins predispose patients to thrombosis by decreasing the body's natural restraints on the coagulation system. Deficiencies may be caused by inherited or acquired disorders. Congenital deficiencies are inherited as autosomal dominant traits; the homozygous condition is usually incompatible with life.

Congenital deficiency of AT III has an incidence in the general population between 1:2000 and 1:5000. The AT III level in heterozygotes varies between 25 and 60 per cent of normal. A second subgroup of patients has been identified with normal plasma AT III concentrations but reduced functional activity, suggesting that manufacturing of defective AT III molecules. Patients with AT III deficiency are predisposed to venous thrombosis, pulmonary embolism, and rarely, arterial thrombosis. Thromboembolism usually develops during or after the second decade and is usually associated with a precipitating event, such as surgery, trauma, pregnancy, or the use of oral contraceptives. Over 60 per cent of patients will develop thromboembolic disease by age 40 and over half will die as a result of pulmonary embolism or mesenteric venous thrombosis (31).

Acquired forms of AT III deficiency also predispose to thrombosis. Hepatic insufficiency, disseminated intravascular coagulation, sepsis, nephrotic syndrome, pregnancy, and the use of exogenous estrogens all lower AT III levels and place patients at increased risk for venous thrombosis.

The optimum plasma concentration of AT III to prevent thrombosis is unknown, but it is thought that functional activity 80 per cent of normal is protective and should be achieved prior to surgical procedures (32). AT III deficiency may be corrected by transfusion of fresh-frozen plasma or cryoprecipitate. The treatment of patients with AT III deficiencies who develop venous thrombosis consists of administering intravenous heparin with fresh-frozen plasma (28). Two units of fresh-frozen plasma every 8 hr is recommended during the acute episode. Lifelong warfarin therapy is recommended for patients with AT III deficiencies who have experienced thrombotic events.

The incidence of congenital protein C deficiency may be as high as 1:200 of the population (33). Thrombosis develops in more than half of affected patients before the age of 30 years, often without any precipitating event (34). The clinical spectrum of recurrent thrombotic episodes includes deep venous thrombosis, pulmonary embolism, superficial thrombophlebitis, and, rarely, arterial thrombosis. Acquired deficiencies of protein C may develop secondary to hepatic insuffciency, chronic renal failure, operative trauma, vitamin K deficiency, and warfarin therapy. Functional and immunologic assays are available to establish the diagnosis.

Initial treatment of acute thromboembolic disease in patients with protein C deficiency is intravenous heparin followed by lifelong warfarin therapy.

Protein S deficiency may be more prevalent than deficiencies of AT III or protein C (35). Approximately 70 per cent of protein S–deficient individuals will have a venous thrombosis by 35 years of age (36). The pattern of thrombotic episodes is similar to that seen in patients with protein C deficiency. Functional and immunologic assays are required to establish the diagnosis. Management of patients with protein S deficiency is the same as that described for protein C deficiency.

Congenital deficiencies of heparin cofactor II have been reported in several families and appear to also predispose affected individuals to thrombosis (37,38). The incidence of this deficiency is unknown, but patients are heterozygous and have only 50 per cent of the normal plasma concentration of heparin cofactor II. Acute thrombotic events have been successfully treated with intravenous heparin, presumably because these patients had normal plasma concentrations of AT III. Lifelong warfarin therapy is recommended for patients with heparin cofactor II deficiency who have had a thrombotic event.

Fibrinolytic System and Inhibitors

The fibrinolytic system functions to remove and/or limit fibrin deposition. Its actions are balanced by inhibitors of fibrinolytic activity. Quantitative or qualitative defects in the components of the fibrinolytic system or increased concentrations of fibrinolytic inhibitors predispose affected individuals to thrombosis.

Activation of the fibrinolytic system leads to fibrin degradation by the proteolytic enzyme plasmin. Plasmin is generated by proteolytic activation of its inactive zymogen plasminogen. Thrombin, in addition to cleaving fibrinogen to form fibrin, stimulates the release of tissue plasminogen activator (tPA) from endothelial cells. Plasminogen circulates bound to fibrinogen and remains bound to fibrin in the thrombus. tPA and other circulating plasminogen activators convert plasminogen to plasmin at the fibrin surface. Plasmin then acts to cleave fibrin into small polypeptides known as fibrin degradation products (FDPs). FDPs have an inhibitory effect on fibrin polymerization and platelet activation.

Plasmin formed in plasma is rapidly inhibited by α_2-plasmin inhibitor (39). Plasmin within the fibrin clot functions longer because the concentration of α_2-plasmin inhibitor is lower. Circulating α_2-macroglobulin is a second inhibitor of plasmin, but acts more slowly than α_2-plasmin inhibitor.

Plasminogen activator inhibitors have been identified in various tissues. Plasminogen activator inhibitor-1 (PAI-1) is produced by endothelial cells and inactivates tPA (40). PAI-1 probably functions in vivo to balance the actions of tPA, because both are synthesized and stored in endothelial cells.

Prethrombotic Conditions and the Fibrinolytic System

Congenital disorders exist that reduce fibrinolytic activity or increase inhibition of fibrinolysis. Patients have been reported with histories of recurrent episodes of venous thrombosis who were found to have a hereditary molecular defect in their plasminogen molecules. These patients have normal concentrations of plasminogen but only 50 per cent of the normal activity (41). Isolated cases of hypoplasminogenemia predisposing patients to thromboembolism have also been reported (42).

Patients with recurrent thromboembolism have been identified who have decreased synthesis of tPA or defective release of activators from endothelial cells (43). Defective fibrinolysis creating a hypercoagulable state has also been attributed to increased concentrations of plasminogen activator inhibitors (43).

The congenital dysfibrinogenemias are a group of autosomal-dominant disorders characterized by the synthesis of functionally abnormal fibrinogen. The majority of patients manifest bleeding disorders. However, some molecular forms cause hypercoagulable states. The abnormal fibrinogen molecule in these patients forms fibrin polymers that are rigid and extremely resistant to the actions of plasmin (44).

Because all patients with defective fibrinolytic systems are prone to recurrent episodes of thrombosis, lifelong warfarin therapy is recommended. Heparin is the initial therapy for acute thrombosis and for the first 3 to 4 days of warfarin therapy (28).

Coagulation and Fibrinolysis

Diseases exist that alter the function of both the coagulation and fibrinolytic mechanisms, causing hypercoagulable states in affected individuals. Perhaps the most classic example of the interaction between the coagulation and fibrinolytic systems is the acquired disorder disseminated intravascular coagulation (DIC).

DIC is characterized by intravascular coagulation with the consumption of coagulation factors and platelets and secondary activation of the fibrinolytic system. DIC is associated with a large number of disorders, including septicemia, trauma, transfusion reactions, hepatic insufficiency, malignancy, and obstetric complications. The DIC is more severe if complicated by hypotension, acidosis, and hypoxemia. Endothelial cells, monocytes, and macrophages express TF on their surfaces after exposure to stimuli associated with the disorders. TF expression leads to coagulation activation by the extrinsic pathway (45). The activation of the fibrinolytic system is a protective mechanism that maintains patency of the microcirculation and reduces organ ischemia. The activity of the fibrinolytic system can be up- or down-regulated by the disease-causing agents or mediators. Down-regulation of fibrinolysis results in progression of microvascular thrombosis, leading to endothelial and organ damage. Up-regulation of fibrinolysis coupled with the consumption of coagulation factors and platelets predisposes patients to hemorrhagic complications.

Chronic DIC, often seen in patients with malignancies, arteriovenous fistulas, and large hemangiomas, represents an equilibrium between the consumption and replacement of coagulation factors and the activation of the fibrinolytic system.

The initial management of DIC is the elimination of the causative process, which allows return of normal hemostasis. Fresh-frozen plasma and platelet transfusions are indicated if hemorrhage continues or to restore the coagulation system prior to surgery. Heparin administration may halt the consumptive process of DIC. Heparin has been used in patients, even with persistent bleeding, to restore the coagulation proteins toward normal (46).

Lupus Anticoagulant

The lupus anticoagulant is an IgG or IgM antiphospholipid antibody that attacks the phospholipid moieties of platelet and endothelial cell membranes. Spontaneous thrombotic complications occur in 23 to 69 per cent of patients with these antibodies (28). Patients with systemic lupus erythematosus or other autoimmune disorders, with some malignancies, or receiving certain drugs (e.g., hydralazine and procainamide) may have this immunoglobulin, which prolongs their activated partial thromboplastin time but poses no hemorrhagic risk. The mechanism of thrombosis is unclear, but it is probably multifactorial, involving elements of the coagulation and fibrinolytic systems. Theories include inhibition of AT III, inhibition of plasminogen conversion to plasmin, platelet damage causing increased adhesiveness, inhibition of prostacycline production by endothelial cells, and inhibition of thrombomodulin leading to decreased protein C anticoagulant activity. Because of these diverse possible mechanisms, the optimal therapy for patients with lupus anticoagulant is not well defined. Recommendations for management have included some combination of steroids, anticoagulants, and platelet-inhibitory drugs. Most often the patients are managed with long-term warfarin therapy.

ANTICOAGULANT AND COMPLICATIONS OF ANTICOAGULANT THERAPY

The remainder of this chapter will review the use of anticoagulant drugs for the prophylaxis and management of venous thromboembolism. The pharmacol-

ogy, route of administration, duration, and known complications of the anticoagulants will be discussed.

Heparin

Heparin is a negatively charged, sulfated polysaccharide that clinically is a
heterogeneous mixture of polymerized polysaccharide units with molecular
weights ranging from 4000 to 40,000. Heparin is extracted from beef lung or pork
gut mucosa. It is available as a sodium or calcium salt.

Heparin's immediate anticoagulant effect is dependent on the presence of
AT III. Heparin catalyzes the inhibition of thrombin and factors IXa, Xa, XIa,
and XIIa (the active serine proteases) by AT III. Factor Xa is the factor most
sensitive to inhibition by the heparin–AT III complex. Inhibition of one unit of
factor Xa prevents the generation of 50 units of thrombin. The effectiveness of
low-dose subcutaneous heparin has been attributed to factor Xa's sensitivity to
inhibition by heparin–AT III.

AT III levels will decrease by as much as 33 per cent with prolonged heparin
use while the AT III remains complexed with the serine proteases being inhibited
(47). Heparin has limited anticoagulant activity in patients with AT III deficiencies; transfusion of these patients with fresh-frozen plasma will restore AT III
levels and improve anticoagulation with heparin.

Heparin also catalyzes the inhibition of thrombin by heparin cofactor II.
There is evidence that heparin–AT III activity declines at plasma heparin concentration greater than 0.50 units/ml, whereas the activity of heparin cofactor II
is maintained (48). Thus heparin's action with heparin cofactor II may be clinically
relevant in situations in which high concentrations of heparin are administered.

Heparin may be administered either subcutaneously or intravenously. The
anticoagulant effect of intravenous heparin is immediate, whereas subcutaneous
absorption achieves peak effects after 4 to 6 hr with anticoagulation lasting 8 to
12 hr depending on the heparin dose. The plasma half-life of intravenous heparin
is 90 min. Clearance follows nonlinear, dose-dependent pharmacokinetics and
appears to be dependent on the reticuloendothelial system. Renal failure and
hepatic insufficiency have little effect on heparin clearance.

The efficacy of low-dose subcutaneous heparin prophylaxis in reducing the
incidence of proximal venous thrombosis and fatal pulmonary embolism in general
surgical patients has been confirmed by a large number of controlled studies.
Pooled data from randomized clinical trials evaluating venous thrombosis prophylaxis were recently analyzed by metaanalysis (49). The incidence of thrombosis diagnosed by fibrinogen scan or phlebogram was reduced from 19.1 per cent
(288/1507) in controls to 6 per cent (50/831) in patients receiving low-dose subcutaneous heparin. Pooled data from 24 randomized clinical trials were similarly
analyzed to document a 0.2 per cent incidence of fatal pulmonary embolism in
patients receiving low-dose heparin versus a 0.7 per cent incidence in controls
($p < .001$) (49).

The low-dose heparin regimen consists of administering 5000 units subcutaneously 2 hr preoperatively, followed by 5000 units every 8 to 12 hr postoperatively. Laboratory monitoring of the activated partial thromboplastin time
(aPPT) is not necessary.

The combination of 5000 units heparin with 0.5 mg dihydroergotamine has
been compared to low-dose heparin prophylaxis alone in several randomized

trials. Dihydroergotamine increases venous flow in capacitance vessels and may stimulate plasminogen activator activity. When data from over 1600 patients were analyzed by metaanalysis, the incidence of venous thrombosis by fibrinogen scan was significantly lower in the dihydroergotamine/heparin group (9 per cent) than in the group treated with heparin alone (14.5 per cent) (49). No difference in the incidence of fatal pulmonary embolism was found between groups. The dihydroergotamine/heparin-treated patients had fewer major bleeding complications (0.26 versus 1.6 per cent), than the heparin-alone group. Dihydroergotamine, however, has been associated with a 0.2 per cent risk of clinical ergotism and severe arterial vasoconstriction. These vasoconstrictive events have dampened the enthusiasm for dihydroergotamine/heparin in the managment of venous thromboembolism.

Heparin remains the drug of choice in the initial management of venous thromboembolism. Prospective trials suggest that a continuous intravenous infusion of heparin is associated with the fewest hemorrhagic complications and requires smaller amounts of heparin than do bolus injections (50). An initial intravenous bolus of 150 to 250 units of heparin/kg should be followed by a continuous infusion of 1000 to 2000 units/hr. Response to heparin anticoagulation should be monitored by either the aPTT or the activated clotting time (ACT) and the dose of heparin adjusted accordingly. The aPTT should be maintained in a range between 1.5 and 2.0 times the control value. Patients whose aPTTs are less than 1.5 times the control value during the first 24 hr of therapy have a 15-fold greater frequency of recurrent thromboembolism compared to patients whose aPTTs are maintained at 1.5 or more times the control (51). Patients with aPTTs greater than 2.5 times control are at increased risk of developing hemorrhagic complications (47). The ACT has the advantage of a linear response to increasing heparin dose; it should be maintained in the range of 150 to 200 sec to assure anticoagulation. The aPTT or ACT should be obtained every 4 hr until the heparin dose is stable and then daily thereafter. Patients should have daily platelet counts to monitor the possible development of heparin-associated antiplatelet antibodies while receiving any form of heparin.

Traditionally, intravenous heparin administration has been recommended for 7 to 14 days before the patient is changed to oral anticoagulant therapy because animal studies had shown that venous thromboses take about 10 days to organize and that heparin was more effective than warfarin in preventing thrombus propagation (52). A recent prospective study of 226 patients with submassive thromboembolism randomized subjects to begin receiving warfarin on either day 1 or day 7 of heparin infusion (53). The mean durations of heparin therapy were 4.1 and 9.5 days, respectively, with no difference in recurrence of thromboembolism being found in 3 to 6 months of follow-up. While this study suggests that a shorter duration of heparin therapy is safe, we continue to administer 7 to 10 days of intravenous heparin therapy to patients suffering a massive thromboembolic episode before converting to oral anticoagulant therapy. Many times we use minidose heparin (5000 units subcutaneously, two or three times a day) instead of warfarin after the 7 to 10 days of intensive heparin therapy.

Contraindications to heparin therapy include serious active bleeding, a recent neurosurgical procedure, malignant hypertension, or cerebral or subarachnoid hemorrhage. Relative contraindications include recent surgery, gastrointestinal bleeding, hemorrhagic diathesis, or a recent stroke.

Hemorrhage, the most common complication of heparin therapy, occurs in

5 to 20 per cent of patients receiving continuous intravenous therapy (47,49,50). The incidence of hemorrhage, however, may approach 50 per cent in patients with renal failure, underlying hemostatic defects, or thrombocytopenia. Hemorrhage may vary from mucosal oozing to severe intracranial, gastrointestinal, or urinary bleeding. The risk of fatal hemorrhage secondary to low-dose subcutaneous heparin is negligible. Discontinuing heparin is the best management for non–life threatening hemorrhage, and the administration of protamine sulfate should be considered for life-threatening hemorrhage. The amount of protamine necessary to reverse heparin may be calculated by the protamine titration test or ACT, or, alternatively, 1.0 to 1.5 mg of protamine may be given to reverse each 100 units of heparin in the circulation. Diluted portions of the calculated dose, 30 to 50 per cent, are given slowly to reduce the known risks of hypotension, bradycardia, and vasodilatation (47).

The second life-threatening complication of heparin therapy is the development of heparin-induced thrombocytopenia and thrombosis. As discussed earlier in this chapter, this syndrome occurs in 4 to 5 per cent of patients receiving heparin. Therapy consists of the immediate cessation of all forms of heparin and administration of drugs that inhibit platelet function.

Osteoporosis is a rare complication that occurs in patients receiving long-term heparin. The majority of cases have occurred in patients receiving greater than 15,000 units of heparin daily for longer than 3 months. Osteoporosis and pathologic fractures may involve the vertebrae, ribs, or long bones.

Sensitivity reactions to heparin may occur in 2 to 5 per cent of patients. Urticaria or other skin rashes, lacrimation, bronchial constriction, and rarely anaphylaxis may occur. Alopecia is another uncommon complication of heparin use. Hair growth usually resumes after heparin has been discontinued.

Warfarin

Warfarin is the most commonly used oral anticoagulant. Following gastrointestinal absorption, 97 per cent of warfarin is bound to albumin while the remaining 3 per cent is responsible for its anticoagulant activity. Warfarin's plasma half-life is 36 to 40 hr, and peak plasma levels are obtained 2 to 12 hr after oral administration.

Warfarin intereferes with the vitamin K–dependent synthesis of factors II, VII, IX, and X by the liver. Its anticoagulation effect is achieved as the concentrations of normally functioning clotting factors are decreased by natural "turnover." Factor VII's half-life is only 6 hr, whereas that of prothrombin is 36 hr. Steady state levels for factor VII are obtained after 2 days, whereas it may take 7 to 10 days for prothrobmin to reach a steady, low level. Because of the rapid decrease in factor VII, "therapeutic" prothrombin times may be obtained after a few days while the patient remains at risk of thrombosis because of continued elevation of intrinsic pathway clotting factors. Thus, it is recommended that heparin therapy continue for the first 3 to 5 days of warfarin use.

Concentrations of proteins C and S are also reduced by warfarin. Protein C's half-life is only 4 to 6 hr; thus levels are reduced early in warfarin therapy, creating the potential for a transient procoagulation state, especially in patients with preexisting protein C deficiencies. Therapeutic anticoagulation with heparin should therefore be obtained prior to warfarin administration and should be continued for 3 to 5 days until low steady state levels of the coagulation factors are achieved.

Warfarin has been demonstrated to be effective in the prophylaxis of post-operative venous thromboembolism and in the prevention of recurrent thromboembolism. For prophylaxis, warfarin should be started 2 to 4 days prior to surgery to achieve a prothrombin time 1.5 times the control on the day of surgery. Because the risk of hemorrhage with warfarin is higher than that of low-dose heparin, warfarin should only be used in clinical situations in which low-dose heparin prophylaxis has proven ineffective (54). Examples might be patients with recent hip or femur fractures, patients with malignancies, or patients undergoing hip replacement.

Long-term anticoagulation with warfarin is usually begun after 5 to 7 days of intravenous heparin therapy after a massive thromboembolic event. However, recent data suggest earlier administration of warfarin is safe following submassive thromboembolism (53). The initial warfarin dose is 7.5 to 10 mg daily; subsequent daily doses are adjusted to maintain the prothrombin time at 1.5 to 2.0 times the control value (rabbit brain thromboplastin). Recent prospective data suggest that maintaining the prothrombin time ratio as low as 1.25, compared to 1.5 to 2.0 times the control value, provides similar protection against recurrent thromboembolism (2 per cent incidence in both groups) while being associated with a lower incidence of hemorrhagic complications (4 versus 22 per cent) (55). Patients who are elderly, have hepatic insufficiency, or have vitamin K deficiencies should receive reduced initial doses of warfarin. Anticoagulation is continued for 3 months, after which time the risk of hemorrhage usually exceeds the incidence of recurrent thrombosis (47). We recommend 6 months of warfarin following major pulmonary embolism or recurrent venous thrombosis.

Hemorrhage is the commonest complication of warfarin therapy. Spontaneous bleeding may be severe and life threatening and often involves gastrointestinal, urinary, nasal, and intracerebral sites. The bleeding is most often associated with excessive warfarin dosing. Spontaneous bleeding may be prevented by maintaining the prothrombin time around 1.3 to 1.5 times the control. Bleeding may occur in patients with surgery, trauma, peptic ulceration, or neoplasm while they are receiving properly controlled doses of warfarin. We do not hesitate to perform extracavitary surgical procedures (e.g., carotid endarterectomy and femorolpopliteal bypass), on patients with prothrombin times 1.3 to 1.5 times the control. A variety of drugs that may potentiate warfarin's actions and precipitate the bleeding include phenytoin, clofibrate, phenylbutazone, indomethacin, tolbutamide, and cholysteramine. The effects of warfarin may be reversed within 24 hr by the intravenous administration of 20 mg of vitamin K; alternatively, the transfusion of fresh-frozen plasma will reverse the effect promptly in cases of life-threatening hemorrhage.

Dermal gangrene is a rare and potentially devastating complication of warfarin therapy. Its etiology has been attributed to dermal microvascular thrombosis, which occurs early after warfarin administration when protein C levels are decreased while the intrinsic coagulation pathway remains intact; patients with congenital or acquired protein C deficiency are at greater risk for these thromboses. Simultaneous heparin administration at the beginning of warfarin therapy prevents this complication. The skin of the thigh, breast, and buttocks is most often involved with the gangrene.

Other adverse effects of warfarin are rare and include alopecia, urticaria, dermatitis, fever, nausea, diarrhea, and hypersensitivity reactions. Warfarin should not be used during the first trimester of pregnancy because of its teratogenicity.

Dextran

Dextran is a polysaccharide that has been effectively used in the prophylaxis and management of venous thromboembolism. Both low-molecular-weight (dextran 40) and high-molecular-weight (dextran 70) dextran have proven effective. They appear to act through a poorly defined dual mechanism, exerting both rheologic and antithrombotic properties. Dextran's action as a plasma volume expander increases blood flow and reduces venostasis. Dextran appears to decrease platelet adhesiveness and alter the release reaction, resulting in decreased platelet aggregation. Dextran also reduces plamsa factor VIII:von Willebrand factor levels. Finally, dextran appears to interefere with fibrin polymerization, thus increasing fibrin's susceptibility to lysis by plasmin (56).

Dextran is indicated in the management of thromboembolism in patients who cannot receive heparin because of risk of heparin-induced thrombocytopenia or who have increased risks for hemorrhage. A slow infusion of dextran 40, 25 to 40 ml/hr, is recommended for prophylaxis and management of thromboembolism. Total infusion volume should not exceed 10 per cent of a patient's blood volume during a 24-hr period in order to avoid volume overload and increased hemorrhagic risk.

Major complications are more frequently associated with dextran 70 than with dextran 40, although their antithrombotic properties appear equal (57). Pulmonary edema secondary to plasma volume expansion is a major complication of dextran therapy. Allergic reactions are not infrequent and range from skin rashes to anaphylactoid reactions.

Ancrod

Ancrod, the venom of the Malayan pit viper (*Agkistrodon rhodostoma*), achieves its anticoagulant effect by cleaving the A fibrinopeptides (A, AY, and AP) from the fibrinogen molecule to form a product incapable of clot formation (58). Ancrod appears to deplete circulating fibrinogen selectively and has little effect on formed thromboses. Platelet counts and coagulation proteins are unaffected by ancrod. Blood viscosity is lowered because of the hypofibrinogenemia, thus improving blood flow and reducing venous stasis.

Acrod is ideally suited for use with patients who develop heparin-induced thrombocytopenia and who require continued systemic anticoagulation. Alternatively, patients with a history of HIT who subsequently require anticoagulation for recurrent thromboembolism or coronary artery bypass surgery can be safely anticoagulated with ancrod (58,59). Patients with AT III deficiencies who require anticoagulation for thromboembolism may be effectively managed with ancrod.

Although ancrod can be administered subcutaneously, the intravenous route is preferred for easier titration of the induced hypofibrinogenemia. Infusion of 70 units (one ampule) over 2 to 4 hr results in fibrinogen levels less than 40 mg/100 ml within 6 to 12 hr. Slower infusion of 70 units over 18 to 36 hr should produce similar defibrinogenation. A continuous infusion of 70 units over 24 to 36 hr is recommended to maintain anticoagulation. Ancrod's circulating half-life is 3 to 5 hr and is excreted unchanged in the urine. Serum fibrinogen levels should be obtained frequently (every 12 hr) at the start of therapy and the rate of infusion adjusted to keep levels between 20 and 40 mg/100 ml.

Complications including fever and minor allergic reactions have been reported following subcutaneous administration. Hemorrhagic complications have been reported, but patients have safely undergone surgery while receiving ancrod. Ancrod's effects can be rapidly reversed by administering cryoprecipitate to restore hemostatic levels of fibrinogen (>50 mg/100 ml).

REFERENCES

1. Walsh PN: The role of platelts in the contact phase of blood coagulation. Br J Haematol 1972;22:237–254.
2. Shafer AI: The hypercoagulable states. Ann Intern Med 1985;102:814–828.
3. Schafer AI: Bleeding and thrombosis in the myeloproliferative disorders. Blood 1984;64:1–12.
4. Mitchell MC, Boitnott JK, Kaufman S, et al: Budd-Chiari syndrome: Etiology, diagnosis and management. Medicine 1982;61:199–218.
5. Dixon RH, Rosse WF: Mechanisms of complement mediated activation of human blood platelets in-vitro: Comparison of normal and paroxysmal nocturnal hemoglobinuria platelets. J Clin Invest 1977;59:360–368.
6. Tremoli E, Maderna P, Sirtori M, et al: Platelet aggregation and malondialdehyde formation in type II-A hypercholesterolanemic patients. Haemostasis 1979;8:47–53.
7. Stuart MJ, Gerrard JM, White JG: Effect of cholesterol on production of TXB2 by platelets in-vitro. N Engl J Med 1980;302:6–10.
8. Sinha AK, Shattil SJ, Colman RW: Cyclic AMP metabolism in cholesterol-rich platelets. J Biol Chem 1977;252:3310–3314.
9. Shatttil SJ, Anaya-Galindo R, Bennett J, et al: Platelet hypersensitivity induced by cholesterol incorporation. J Clin Invest 1975;55:636–643.
10. Betteridge DJ, El Tahir KEH, Reckless JPD, et al: Platelets from diabetic subjects show diminished sensitivity to prostacycline. Eur J Clin Invest 1982;12:395–398.
11. Cowell JA, Winocour PD, Lopes-Virella M, et al: New concepts about the pathogenesis of atherosclerosis in diabetes mellitus. Am J Med 1983;75:67–80.
12. Petterson CM, Jones RL, Koenig RJ, et al: Reversible hematologic sequelae of diabetes mellitus. Ann Intern Med 1977;86:425–429.
13. Lelape A, Gutman N, Guitton JD, et al: Nonenzymatic glycosylation increases platelet aggregation potency of collagen from placenta of diabetic human beings. Biochem Biophys Res Commun 1983;111:602–610.
14. Green D, Martin GJ, Shoichet SH, et al: Thrombocytopenia in a prospective, randomized, double-blind trial of bovine and porcine heparin. Am J Med Sci 1984;288:60–64.
15. Kelton JG, Levine MN: Heparin-induced thrombocytopenia. Semin Thromb Hemost 1986;12:59–62.
16. Silver D: Heparin induced thrombocytopenia and thrombosis. Semin Vasc Surg 1988;1:228–232.
17. Cines DB, Kaywin P, Bina M, et al: Heparin induced thrombocytopenia. N Engl J Med 1980;303:788–795.
18. Rhodes GR, Dixon RH, Silver D: Heparin induced thrombocytopenia: Eight cases with thrombotic-hemorrhagic complications. Ann Surg 1977;186:752–758.
19. Green D, Harris K, Reynolds N, et al: Heparin immune thrombocytopenia: Evidence for a heparin platelet complex as the antigenic determinant. J Lab Clin Med 1978;91:167–175.
20. Chong BH, Grace CS, Rozenberg MC: Heparin-induced thrombocytopenia: Effect of heparin platelet antibody on platelets. Br J Haematol 1981;49:531–540.
21. Laster J, Cikrit D, Walker N, et al: The heparin-induced thrombocytopenia syndrome: An update. Surgery 1987;102:763–770.
22. Zur M, Radcliffe RD, Oberdick J, et al: The dual role of factor VII in blood coagulation. Initiation and inhibition of a proteolytic system by a zymogen. J Biol Chem 1982;257:5623–5631.
23. Trousseau A: Phlegmasia alba dolens. Clinical Medicine, Hotel de Paris 1865;3:94.
24. Rickles FR, Edwards RL: Activation of blood coagulation in cancer: Trousseau's syndrome revisited. Blood 1963;62:14–31.
25. Pineo GF, Brain MC, Gallus AS, et al: Tumors, mucus production and hypercoagulability. Ann NY Acad Sci 1974;230:262–270.
26. Kies MS, Posch JJ, Giolma JP, et al: Hemostatic function in cancer patients. Cancer 1980;46:831–837.

27. Tooke JE, McNichol GP: Thrombotic disorders associated with pregnancy and the pill. Clin Haematol 1981;*10*:613–630.

28. Ahn SS: The hypercoagulable states: A comprehensive review for the vascular surgeon. Semin Vasc Surg 1990;*3*:6–20.

29. Esmon CT, Owen WG: Identification of an endothelial cell cofactor for the thrombin-catalyzed activation of protein C. Proc Natl Acad Sci USA 1981;*78*:2249–2252.

30. Tollefsen DM, Blank MK: Detection of a new heparin-dependent inhibitor of thrombin in plasma. J Clin Invest 1982;*68*:589–596.

31. Cosgriff TM, Bishop DT, Hershgold EJ, et al: Familial antithrombin III deficiency: Its natural history, genetics, diagnosis and treatment. Medicine 1983;*62*:209–220.

32. Sager S, Nairn D, Stamatakis JD, et al: Efficacy of low-dose heparin in prevention of extensive deep-vein thrombosis in patients undergoing hip replacement. Lancet 1976;*1*:1151–1154.

33. Miletich J, Sherman L, Broze G: Absence of thrombosis in subjects with heterozygous protein C deficiency. N Engl J Med 1987;*317*:991–996.

34. Broekmans AW, Veltcamp JJ, Bertina RM: Congenital protein C deficiency and venous thromboembolism: A study of three Dutch families. N Engl J Med 1983;*309*:340–344.

35. Gladson CL, Scharrer I, Hach V, et al: The frequency of type I heterozygous protein S and protein C deficiency in 141 unrelated young patients with venous thrombosis. Thromb Haemost 1988;*59*:18–22.

36. Engesser KL, Broekmans AW, Briet E, et al: Protein S deficiency: Clinical manifestations. Ann Intern Med 1987;*106*:677–682.

37. Tran TH, Marbet GA, Duckert F: Association of hereditary heparin co-factor II deficiency with thrombosis. Lancet 1985;*2*:413–414.

38. Sie P, Pichon J, Dupoui D, et al: Constitutional heparin co-factor II deficiency associated with recurrent thrombosis. Lancet 1985;*2*:414–416.

39. Collen D: On the regulation and control of fibrinolysis. Thromb Haemost 1980;*43*:77–89.

40. Kun-yu Wu K, Frasier-Scott K, Hatzakis H: Endothelial cell function in hemostasis and thrombosis. Adv Exp Med Biol 1987;*242*:127–133.

41. Towne JB, Bandyk DF, Hussey CV, et al: Abnormal plasminogen: A genetically determined cause of hypercoagulability. J Vasc Surg 1984;*1*:896–902.

42. Lottenberg R, Dolly FR, Kitchens CS: Pulmonary hypertension and recurrent thromboembolic phenomena associated with hypoplasminogenemia. [abstr]. Clin Res 1983;*31*:318A.

43. Nilsson IM, Ljungneer H, Tengborn L: Two different mechanisms in patients with venous thrombosis and defective fibrinolysis: Low concentration of plasminogen activator inhibitor. Br Med J 1985;*290*:1453–1456.

44. Carrell N, Gabriel DA, Blatt PM, et al: Hereditary dysfibrinogenemia in a patient with thrombottic disease. Blood 1983;*62*:439–447.

45. Muller-Berghause G: Pathophysiologic and biochemical events in disseminated intravascular coagulation: Dysregulation of procoagulant and anticoagulant pathways. Semin Thromb Hemost 1989;*15*:58–87.

46. Feinstein DI: Treatment of disseminated intravascular coagulation. Semin Thromb Hemost 1988;*14*:351–362.

47. Kapsch DN, Silver D: Complications and failures of anticoagulatn therapy. *In* Complications in Vascular Surgery. New York, Grune & Stratton, 1985;405–419.

48. Ofusu FA, Fernandez F, Gauthier D, et al: Heparin cofactor II and other endogenous factors in the mediation of the antithrombotic and anticoagulant effects of heparin and dermatan sulfate. Semin Thromb Hemost 1985;*11*:133–137.

49. Clagett GP, Reisch JS: Prevention of venous thromboembolism in general surgical patients. Ann Surg 1988;*208*:227–240.

50. Ware JA, Lewis J, Salzman EW: Antithrombotic therapy. *In* Rutherford RB, et al, eds: Vascular Surgery. Philadelphia, WB Saunders Company, 1989.

51. Hull R, Raskob G, Hirsch J, et al: Continuous intravenous heparin compared with intermittent subcutaneous heparin in the initial treatment of proximal-vein thrombosis. N Engl J Med 1986;*315*:1109–1114.

52. Mohr DN, Ryu JH, Litin SC, et al: Recent advances in the management of venous thromboembolism. Mayo Clin Proc 1988;*63*:281–290.

53. Gallus A, Jackman J, Tillet J, et al: Safety and efficacy of warfarin started early after submassive venous thrombosis or pulmonary embolism. Lancet 1986;*2*:1293–1296.

54. Sevitt S: Venous thrombosis and pulmonary embolism: Their prevention by oral anticoagulants. Am J Med 1967;*33*:703–716.

55. Hull R, Hirsch J, Jay R, et al: Different intensities of oral anticoagulation therapy in the treatment of proximal vein thrombosis. N Engl J Med 1982;*307*:1676–1681.

56. Abers M, Hedner U, Bergentz SE: The antithrombotic effect of dextran. Scand J Haematol 1979;*34* (suppl):61–68.

57. Ring J, Messmer K: Incidence and severity of anaphylactoid reactions to colloid volume substitutes. Lancet 1977;*1*:466–469.
58. Cole CW, Bormanis J: Ancrod: A practical alternative to heparin. J Vasc Surg 1988;*8*:59–63.
59. Zulys V, Teasdale S, Michel E, et al: Ancrod anticoagulation for cardiopulmonary bypass [abstr]. Clin Invest Med 1987;*10*:C44.

3

CURRENT VIEWS ON THE PATHOGENESIS OF VENOUS ULCERATION

P. D. Coleridge Smith and John H. Scurr

There is now general agreement that venous ulceration results from a failure to lower the venous pressure on exercise in the veins of the lower limb. This may be due to disease of the deep veins, the superficial veins, or the communicating veins (1). Some controversy remains about the mechanisms of failure of the calf muscle pump, but the resulting pressure abnormalities are easy to observe and measure. During ambulation the dorsal foot vein pressure falls to low values in subjects with normal veins (2). The resting level of 80 to 100 mm Hg falls to 0 to 20 mm Hg. The pressure then returns to the resting level when the subject stands still. This usually takes in excess of 20 sec. Patients with "venous insufficiency" may fail to reduce the foot vein pressure to a low value, or may show a rapid return of venous pressure to resting levels at the end of exercise, or, usually, may show a combination of both factors (3). While foot vein pressures are not necessarily the same as those in the ankle region, where ulcers commonly occur, it is generally accepted that they reflect pressure abnormalities in the supramalleolar region (4).

The foot vein pressures reflect the severity of the venous abnormality, but do not predict the magnitude of the associated disease. There appears to be a substantial overlap in pressure measurements between patients with normal limbs, those with lipodermatosclerotic changes, and those with frank ulceration (5) (Fig. 3–1). This is true whether pressure fall, refilling time, or an index comprising both is used. This finding has been observed by a number of different authors, including ourselves (6–8). It is clear from these studies that in some patients gross abnormalities of venous function may be tolerated with little or no evidence of skin damage. In other patients, severe ulceration may be associated with minor degrees of venous functional impairment.

From these data we conclude that either existing means of venous functional assessment are inadequate in defining the important factors in the disease, or the tissue response to raised venous pressure is variable. The events that intervene between raised venous pressure and venous ulceration are unclear. Hypotheses have been proposed since the Middle Ages, but more recently have revolved around the proposal that ulceration is attributable to skin hypoxia (9).

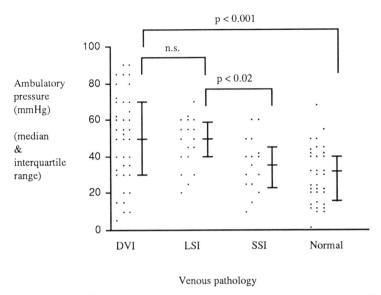

Figure 3–1. The results of ambulatory venous pressure measurements in patients with differing degrees of venous disease. There is substantial overlap between the groups. Group labels are: *DVI*, deep venous insuficiency; *LSI*, long saphenous insufficiency; *SSI*, short saphenous insufficiency.

OLD THEORIES

The association of venous disease and ulceration of the leg has been understood since the time of Hippocrates (10). Wiseman, in the 17th century, thought that ulceration was due to varicose veins (11). In 1914 Homans suggested that ulceration of the skin overlying large varicosities was caused by low oxygen levels in the stagnant blood of the varicosities causing hypoxia of the skin (12). The oxygenation of blood in varicose veins has been the subject of several studies since that time (13,14). It is now clear that with the patient lying supine the hemoglobin saturation with oxygen of blood in varicose veins is greater than that in the veins of normal limbs. When the patient stands, there is no difference between normal subjects and patients with varicose veins. So even if venous blood was responsible for nutrition of the skin, there would be no difference between normal subjects and those with varicose veins (15).

The raised oxygen levels in veins of patients with venous disease led to the suggestion by some that arteriovenous fistulas were present, which might deprive the skin of oxygen (16,17). Research using microspheres and macroaggregates has failed to demonstrate an increase in arteriovenous shunting in the skin of patients with venous disease (18,19).

The Fibrin Cuff Theory

In 1982 Browse and Burnand proposed that oxygen diffusion into the tissues of the skin was restricted by a pericapillary fibrin cuff that they had observed histologically (20). They suggested that increased capillary pressure as a consequence of the raised venous pressure resulted in an increased loss of plasma proteins through the capillary wall. This included fibrinogen, which polymerized to provide the "fibrin cuff" that may be seen around capillaries in the skin, using both histochemical and immunohistochemical methods. Measurements of protein loss from capillaries showed that fibrinogen was quantitatively the most import plasma protein leaking into the tissues in patients with venous disease. Subsequent measurements of fibrinolysis have shown that patients with venous disease have reduced fibrinolytic activity in the blood and veins, which might explain why the fibrin cuff persists (21). It has also been shown in a dog model that it is possible to provoke the appearance of the typical convoluted capillaries of venous disease, fibrin cuffs, and reduced fibrinolysis by raising the venous pressure using an arteriovenous fistula between the femoral artery and vein (22).

In this theory of ulceration, the role of the fibrin cuff in restricting the supply of oxygen to the tissues is central. There is no published evidence to prove that fibrin provides a barrier to oxygen diffusion. It seems probable from the composition of other human connective tissues that such a fibrin gel would comprise much water with a small amount of fibrin. Diffusion of small molecules through such a cuff might be expected to be very similar to that through water and other human tissues. If the assumption is made that the fibrin layer contains 0.5% fibrin, similar to that of a fibrin blood clot, calculations reveal no impairment of oxygen delivery to the tissues. Even a cuff consisting of 100 times more fibrin than this would result in a reduction of oxygen delivery of only 50 per cent (Professor Charles Michel, personal communication). The results of these calculations have not been confirmed by measurement, at the time of writing. Browse and Burnand employed a piece of commercial fibrin from a suture manufacturer in order to assess the permeability of fibrin. They found that this material significantly impeded the passage of oxygen. It is unlikely that fibrin cuffs seen in man are of this composition.

Is Tissue Oxygenation Reduced in Venous Disease?

Accepting these imperfect aspects to the theory, what evidence is there that tissue oxygenation is reduced in venous disease? We have been unable to discover any published data in which direct measurements of skin oxygen have been made in patients with venous disease. This would necessitate inserting a microelectrode into the skin, a potentially difficult exercise requiring skill and patients as well as accurate measuring equipment, but one not outside the capabilities of current technology. There is a much larger literature in which transcutaneous oxygen measurements have been made (23,24). In these a Clark-type electrode equipped with an integral heater is applied to the skin. These devices were originally developed for neonatal monitoring, in which skin heating was used so that the resulting vasodilation would ensure that the measurement accurately reflected the arterial oxygen tension. In venous disease, different findings have been obtained depending on whether the transducer is heated to 43 or 37°C. At the higher temperatures, used by most authors, it has been found that patients with venous disease tend to have lower transcutaneous oxygen pressure ($tcPO_2$) readings than normal subjects (23,24) (Fig. 3–2). Once again there is a substantial overlap between patients with normal limbs and those with differing severity of venous disease. Measurements in our own laboratory have mirrored those of other authors, and it is clear that this assessment does not explain the range of findings in venous disease. Measurements made with an electrode temperature of 37°C

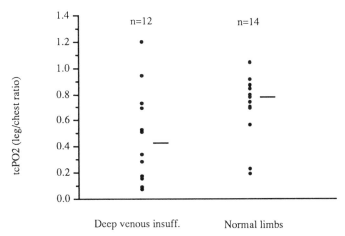

Figure 3–2. The results of transcutaneous oxygen measurements in the lower limbs of patients with normal limbs and those with liposclerotic skin. There is substantial overlap between groups. Readings are expressed as the $tcPO_2$ ratio of leg to chest measurements, to remove any error due to differences in pulmonary function.

are even more paradoxical (25). Under these circumstances, the oxygenation of the skin is greater in patients with venous disease than in normal subjects! This technique has a number of limitations and may be assessing factors other than skin oxygenation.

One important factor is clearly the skin heating. What is known of the response of skin to heating? This has been studied by Tooke and colleagues in patients with diabetes (26). They used a transcutaneous oxygen electrode in which the sensing element had been replaced by a laser Doppler flowmeter optode. Using this device they were able to show that normal subjects could increase skin blood flow 40-fold in response to heating at 43°C, whereas diabetic patients could only increase the flow 20 times. It is possible that similar abnormalities are present in patients with venous disease to explain the reduced $tcPO_2$ in this condition. Therefore, the abnormality detected by this technique may simply be that the microcirculation is unable to increase its flow by the same extent normal skin can and thus the technique does not reflect the basal conditions that might be more accurately assessed by measurement at 37°C.

Hopkins and coworkers used positron emission tomography techniques to assess blood flow and oxygen extraction in the skin and subcutaneous tissues of patients with venous disease (27). They were able to show that there was a reduced oxygen extraction ratio in such tissues, but that skin flow was increased by a substantial amount, so it is not possible to be certain of the oxygen delivery consequences from these measurements.

In view of the difficulties of measuring oxygen delivery, we have measured the clearance of xenon from the skin as an assessment of the efficiency of the circulation in handling a molecule of a size similar to oxygen. We used xenon-133 gas, which has a molecular weight four times that of oxygen and would be expected to diffuse at half the speed of oxygen were there no other restriction on its progress, assuming similar water solubility for oxygen and xenon. We used the technique of Sjerson (28) (Fig. 3–3), in which the xenon gas is applied topically to the skin, avoiding the necessity for injections, which might alter the flow char-

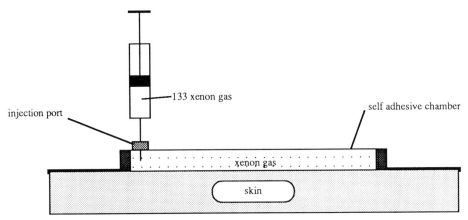

Figure 3–3. Application of gaseous xenon to the skin by the method of Sjerson. Diffusion of gas into the skin is used to avoid the effects that might be produced by injection.

acteristics of the skin. Xenon diffuses out of the skin once in the dermis, so we then covered the skin with an impermeable layer of Saranwrap held in place with a gentle compression dressing. Measurements were made in the supramalleolar region of patients with venous disease causing lipodermatosclerosis, and patients of similar age distribution without venous or arterial disease. In order to stand-ardize blood flow conditions we measured the xenon clearance from the limbs after a 3-min period of ischemia produced by a cuff applied to the limb and inflated above arterial pressure. The skin blood flow response was monitored using laser Doppler flowmetry. The results are shown in Figure 3–4. There was a substantial overlap between the subjects with venous disease and controls when comparing the half-clearance time for xenon from the skin. The hyperemic response was similar, with both groups increasing the flow by two to three times resting levels, as measured by laser Doppler flowmetry (Fig. 3–5). These results demonstrate

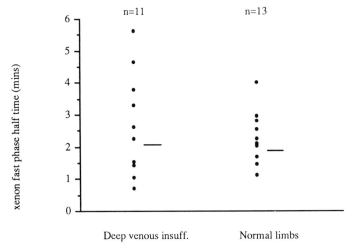

Figure 3–4. Results of hyperemic xenon clearance from the skin in patients with lipodermatosclerosis and with normal skin. No substantial difference is found between these groups. The parameter plotted is the time taken to clear half the xenon from the skin.

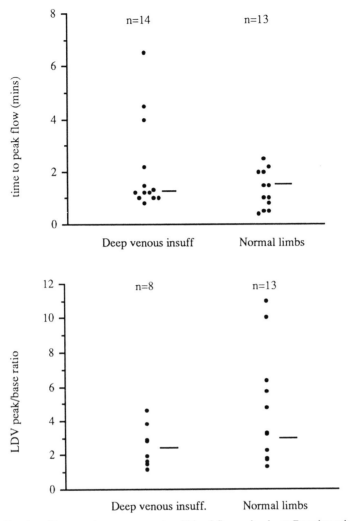

Figure 3–5. Results of hyperemic measurements of blood flow using laser Doppler velocimetry in normal and liposclerotic skin. There is an increase in flow compared with basal levels, and in time to reach peak flow. Again, no substantial difference is seen. *Top*, The time taken to reach peak flow following ischemia. *Bottom*, The increase in flow compared with baseline.

no abnormality of the microcirculation in venous disease in handling a molecule of the size of xenon, and therefore make it unlikely that there is any abnormality in the delivery of oxygen to the tissues in patients with lipodermatosclerosis.

Effects of Profibrinolytic Agents and Pneumatic Compression

One therapeutic possibility in the management of venous disease is the use of profibrinolytic agents to promote absorption of the fibrin cuff. In a preliminary study Browse et al. were able to demonstrate histologic evidence that such an approach was effective, using the profibrinolytic anabolic steroid stanozolol (29). Layer et al. then undertook a study to establish whether stanozolol was useful in the management of venous ulceration. This was a prospective, double-blind, placebo-controlled study, in which patients received up to 60 weeks of treatment with stanozolol or placebo as adjunctive therapy in the management of their ulcers (30). The stanozolol did not influence healing after 75 patients had been studied for a period of 28 months. In a preliminary investigation of stanozolol in the management of patients with lipodermatosclerosis it was claimed that there was a significant effect in reducing the area of affected skin (29). The number of patients in this study was rather small and the crossover design did not include a washout interval between placebo and active treatment periods. We have recently completed a study of a randomized, placebo-controlled, double-blind design in which stanozolol was compared with placebo for the management of lipodermatosclerosis (31). The duration of treatment was 6 months, during which there was a 28 per cent reduction in area of lipodermatosclerosis in the stanozolol groups and 14 per cent in the placebo group (Fig. 3–6). Both groups received compression stockings exerting 30 mm Hg pressure at the ankle (Hohenstein). Transcutaneous oxygen measurements were also made, but this parameter was not influenced by stanozolol or placebo (Fig. 3–7). It is interesting that there should be a reduction in area of lipodermatosclerosis without influence on the $tcPO_2$. This suggests to us that the fibrin cuff is not responsible for the reduction in $tcPO_2$ in venous disease that has been observed by several authors.

In a study on ulcer healing undertaken to investigate the efficacy of pneumatic compression in this disease, we used an SCD (Kendall Healthcare Products Company, Mansfield, MA) intermittent gradient pneumatic compression device to apply 50 mm Hg compression to the lower limbs once per minute for a 4-hr period each day (32). Two groups of patients were studied, a control group that received our standard treatment of wound débriding and compression stockings (30 mm Hg, Hohenstein) and an SCD group who received the pneumatic compression in addition to standard therapy. All patients had ulcers that, were considered difficult to heal, and had been present for at least 3 months. This study was carried out on an outpatient basis, in which patients were given the SCD to use in their own

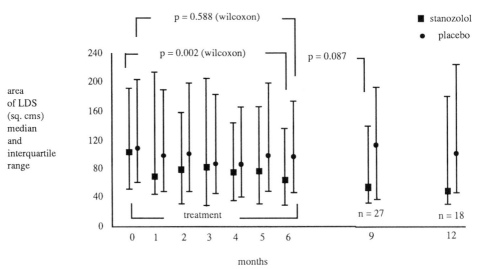

Figure 3–6. Findings in patients with lipdermatosclerotic skin treated with stanozolol or placebo. The graph shows the change in area of lipodermatosclerosis during the 6-month treatment period. Parameters shown are the median and interquartile range of the lipsclerotic area.

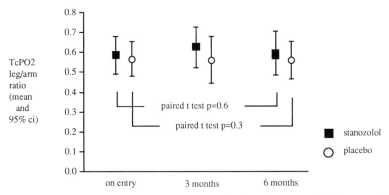

Figure 3–7. Transcutaneous oxygen measurements made in patient treated with stanozolol or placebo. No change was observed in either group. The parameters shown are the mean and standard deviation of the tcPO₂ leg to arm ratio.

home, having been instructed in its use. The pneumatic compression group showed substantially better healing than the control group (Fig. 3–8). The reasons for the efficacy of this device are not easily explained by the fibrin cuff theory. It has been shown that intermittent pneumatic compression may benefit fibrinolysis (33,34) but, as we have pointed out earlier, this alone does not seem to alter ulcer healing. The SCD reduces lower limb edema, but it is uncertain what role this factor plays in venous ulceration, and it is not considered by Browse and Burnand in their hypothesis. Perhaps some other factor not addressed by these authors is influenced by intermittent pneumatic compression. Subsequently, we have shown that some of the microcirculatory parameters we measured in liposclerotic skin are influenced by the SCD. Xenon clearance from the subcu-

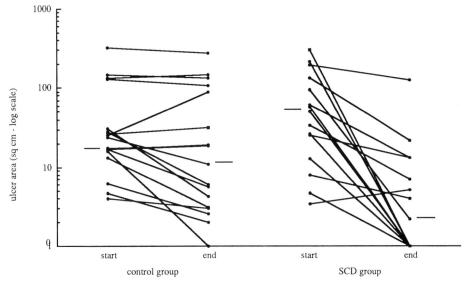

Figure 3–8. Change in ulcer area of patients treated with no additional thrapy or the SCD (Kendall Healthcare Products Company, Mansfield, MA). The SCD group healed more rapidly than the control group. The horizontal bars show the median ulcer areas in the two groups of patients at the start and end of the study.

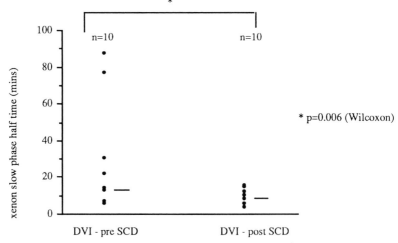

Figure 3–9. Clearance of xenon from the subcutaneous fat before and after 4 weeks of treatment with the SCD sequential gradient pneumatic compression device. More rapid clearance is observed after treatment.

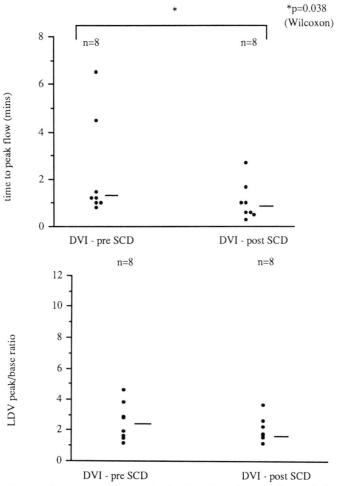

Figure 3–10. Hyperamic response measured using laser Doppler velocimetry before and after 4 weeks' treatment with the SCD sequential gradient pneumatic compression device. An increased hyperemic response is observed after treatment, as measured by the shorter time to reach peak flow. No change in the size of the hyperemic response was detected.

taneous fat is enhanced and the hyperemic response measured by laser Doppler flowmetry as described previously were improved (Figs. 3–9 and 3–10).

A NEW THEORY

The arguments discussed thus far suggest that tissue hypoxia may not be important in the etiology of venous ulceration. Moyses and colleagues studied the limbs of normal subjects in response to raised venous pressure, and measured hematologic parameters as an index of the effect of venous hypertension (35). Their subjects sat on a bicycle saddle with the limbs dependent for a period of 40 min, without moving. Blood samples were taken from the long saphenous vein at the ankle. Moyses et al. found that the hematocrit and red cell count increased in parallel, as would be expected, but that the white cell count remained unchanged despite the increased hematocrit. White cells were being "lost" from the circulation; after 40 min this "loss" accounted for a 25 per cent change in the white cell count. Thomas and colleagues performed a similar study in which they compared patients with normal lower limbs with patients with venous disease resulting in lipodermatosclerosis and ulceration (36). Their patients were permitted to sit with their legs dependent, a less stringent requirement than that of Moyses et al. Blood sampling was again from the long saphenous vein at the ankle. After 60 min patients with venous disease were "trapping" 30 per cent of the white cells and normal subjects were trapping 7 per cent. The white cells were "released" when the patients were permitted to lie supine (Fig. 3–11). This led us to examine the microcirculation using capillary microscopy, employing the technique described by Fagrell (37). Patients were examined in the supine position after sitting for 30 min, then after a period of lying for 30 min, and finally after sitting for a further period of 30 min. The number of visible capillary loops per unit area was determined in patients with normal limbs, varicose veins, and lipodermatosclerosis. Only in the patients with lipodermatosclerosis were there significant alterations in capillary counts. There appeared to be fewer capillary loops in these patients (Fig. 3–12), and the number of loops increased with decreased venous

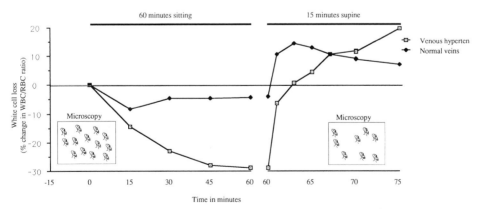

Figure 3–11.   White cell "trapping" observed during dependency in a study by Thomas and Dormandy (36). After a period of 60 min of dependency the patients with venous insufficiency were trapping 30 per cent of the white cells entering their lower limbs, compared with 7 per cent in the control group. The inset diagrams show the implications for the number of visible capillary loops, as deduced from the data in Figure 3–12.

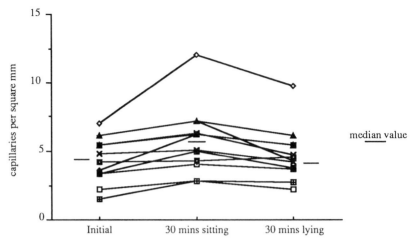

Figure 3–12. The number of capillary loops observed in response to raised venous pressure. There were fewer loops in patients with deep venous insufficiency, shown in this graph. The graph shows that this number increased after a 30-min period of recumbency, and decreased again with increased venous pressure. No change was seen in patients with varicose veins or normal limbs. All capillary loop counting was done with the patients lying supine.

pressure. We suspected that this was a consequence of the white cell trapping observed by Thomas et al. (36).

Bollinger and coworkers have investigated the events in venous disease using fluorescence video capillary microscopy (38). They measured the rate of diffusion of fluorescein out of capillaries after an intravenous injection. They were able to show that capillaries in venous disease are much more permeable than normal to this molecule, contrary to the suggestions made in the fibrin cuff hypothesis. Using simultaneous fluorescence and light capillary microscopy Franzeck and colleagues have described the appearances of capillary loops that are filled with red blood cells, but do not appear to be perfused (39). They suggested that this may be due to capillary "thrombosis." Bollinger et al. have also investigated the lymphatic channels using fluorescence capillary lymphangiograpy (40). There are substantial abnormalities of the small lymphatic channels in this disease, including obliteration of parts of the superficial capillary network and reflux in the cutaneous vessels.

White cell margination is well recognized by microcirculationists. In reperfusion injury it is thought to be important in the mechanism that results in tissue injury following ischemia. White blood cells are substantially larger than red cells and are responsible for many of the rheologic properties of blood. White cells take 1000 times longer than red cells to deform on entering a capillary bed, and are responsible for about half the peripheral vascular resistance despite their small numbers in the circulation compared with red cells (41). In myocardial infarction it has been shown that they cause capillary occlusion, which can be prevented in experimental animals by first rendering the animal leukopenic (42,43). White blood cells have been implicated as the mediators of ischemia in many tissues, including myocardium, brain, lung, and kidneys (44–47). Polymorphonuclear leukocytes, particularly those attached to capillary endothelium, may become "activated," in which case cytoplasmic granules containing proteolytic enzymes are released (48). In addition, a nonmitochondrial "respiratory burst" permits these cells to release free radicals, most notably the superoxide radical, that have non-specific destructive effects on lipid membranes, proteins, and many connective tissue compounds (49). The chemotactic leukotrienes are also released, attracting more polymorphonuclear cells.

We published a hypothesis suggesting that white cell trapping resulted in such processes being triggered, causing degradation of tissues (50). In keeping with the literature on myocardium in critical ischemia, we proposed that white cells might cause occlusion of capillaries, a suggestion originally made by Moyses et al. (35). If some of the capillaries were occluded this might result in heterogenous perfusion and therefore tissue hypoxia and ischemia. From the data presented here it can be seen that we have not been able to support the assertion that venous ulceration is due to tissue hypoxia.

The second part of the theory suggested that white cell activation was part of the process, resulting in release of proteolytic enzymes, superoxide radicals, and chemotactic substances. All classes of white cells appear to become trapped, so a wide range of phenomena is possible. Monocytes might become activated, releasing the cytokines interleukin-1 (IL-1) and tumor necrosis factor α (TNF$_\alpha$) (51). These may achieve many effects. Endothelial cell activation may be one, in which these metabolically active cells permit the passage of much larger molecules than would normally be the case (52). As Burnand and coworkers discovered, the capillaries of patients with venous disease are much more permeable to fibrinogen than normal (53). In addition, they also noticed that fibrinolysis is decreased in patients with venous disease (21). IL-1 acts on endothelial cells to stimulate production of the fibrinolytic inhibitor plasminogen activator inhibitor-1 (PAI-1), and decreases the production of tissue plasminogen activator (tPA), producing the effect on fibrinolysis that is observed (54).

Further Issues in the White Cell Theory

To what extent are white cells implicated in venous disease? While the inflammatory cells are described in dermatology texts on venous disease, they have not previously been implicated in the ulcer process. In order to investigate this we took biopsies of the skin of the supramalleolar region of patients undergoing varicose vein surgery. Three distinct groups of patients were studied. The first were patients with no evidence of skin changes as a consequence of their venous disease. The next group exhibited lipodermatosclerosis, but there had never been ulceration of the limb. Finally, there was a group of patients who had ulceration, but were left with lipodermatosclerosis after healing of the ulcer (55).

Skin biopsies were taken from the liposclerotic area and histologic slides made. Nineteen patients were studied in all, from which a total of 2880 slides were prepared. The number of white blood cells visible in the upper 0.5 mm of the skin in each section was estimated by an observer who was unaware of the diagnosis. The results are shown in Figure 3–13. Patients with normal skin had a low number of white blood cells visible (4/sq mm). There were eight times as many in patients with liposclerotic skin and 40 times as many in patients with healed venous ulcers. The graph shows a distinct separation between these groups, although the total numbers of patients are small. We have subsequently undertaken an immunohistologic study to determine the types of white cell present in this infiltrate. The majority of cells are macrophages in the small numbers of

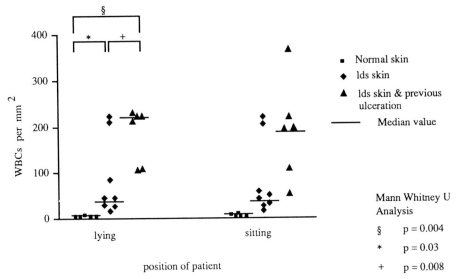

Figure 3–13. Results from a histologic study in which punch biopsies of skin from the gaiter region were examined quantitatively using conventional histologic techniques. All patients had varicose veins, some uncomplicated, some with lipodermatosclerosis, and some with a previous history of ulceration. The graph shows the numbers of white cells visible in the skin of these patients per square millimeter. Repeat biopsy after the patients had sat for 30 min showed no change in the white cell count.

patients studied to date. In addition, there is a T lymphocyte component, but no excess of neutrophils compared with control sections taken from normal limbs. So this infiltrate is a reflection of a chronic inflammatory process, and suggests that an investigation of the cell products of these leukocytes might indicate the mechanisms involved in venous ulceration.

Are the mechanisms we have suggested earlier sufficient to result in skin necrosis? This is certainly the case when an inflammatory response is produced in the skin, to be followed later by an additional stimulus that activates the cells present in the tissues. This produces rapid necrosis of the skin, and is known as the Schwarzmann reaction (56). In the skin of patients with venous disease conditions are set that might permit such a reaction to progress. The inflammatory infiltrate is already present, requiring some minor trigger to precipitate tissue destruction. This might explain why parents with lipodermatosclerosis are at high risk of ulceration in response to minor trauma to the leg.

Are other mechanisms involved in the processes observed in venous disease? This might involve reabsorption of connective tissue, a task normally controlled by a group of enzymes that are regulators of the connective tissue struture, the tissue metalloproteinases. These are widely implicated as mediators of the final pathway in a variety of diseases. It has been shown that IL-1 can stimulate chondrocytes to produce metalloproteinases that remove articular cartilage (57), which mght be important in arthritic conditions. In soft connective tissues, IL-1 exerts effects of fibroblasts that result in the reabsorption of collagen and proteoglycans (58). As suggested previously, it seems likely that IL-1 is released as a consequence of the white cell trapping seen in venous disease, so this mechanism of tissue resorption is not inconceivable as part of the ulceration process.

White blood cells encountering activated endothelial cells produce growth factors, resulting (hypothetically) in angiogenesis, which may be responsible for the apparent proliferation of capillaries described in capillary microscopy studies.

The proof of these mechanisms has yet to be obtained. We are currently investigating these mechanisms and their relation to venous disease.

TREATMENT IN THE FUTURE

The events that surround venous ulceration may seem complex and obscure, and yet without a full understanding of these it will not be possible to design new regimens of therapy. At present the only means by which a new treatment can be evaluated is to design a venous ulcer study. This is not only complex and expensive, but may be confounded by the "noise" that other factors responsible for healing an ulcer bring to such a study. It would be far better to measure a set of tissue parameters and decide whether the new treatment is likely to be effective before investing heavily in an ulcer healing study.

Many of the processes we have described above may be influenced by modern pharmacologic agents. One cytokine antagonist, pentoxifylline, has already been evaluated in this respect. Pentoxifylline antagonizes the effect of TNF_α and IL-1 on polymorphonuclear neutrophils, resulting in much lower likelihood of adhesion and activation (59). In a multicenter study in which 82 patients were entered, pentoxifylline has been shown to result in much better healing rates of ulcers than placebo (60).

A large number of other pharmacologic manipulations is possible. Prostaglandin E_1 inhibits the respiratory burst of neutrophils, preventing the release of superoxide radicals. A preliminary study has suggested that this too is effective in healing venous ulcers (61). A number of other treatments await evaluation, and we think that adjuvant pharmacologic treatments will become commonplace within the next decade for the treatment of this disease.

Even the design of stockings may benefit from a full knowledge of the subcellular mechanisms resulting in ulceration. The hemodynamic effects of stockings have been documented (62), but a complete knowledge of their mechanism of action remains unclear. This is despite the fact that bandaging and compression treatments have been known to be effective in the management of venous disease for over 2000 years!

A full understanding of the mechanisms leading to venous ulceration at present eludes us, but the details will soon become better defined as research is directed at the appropriate pathologic processes.

ACKNOWLEDGMENTS: Our grateful thanks go to the following members of the Department of Surgery of University College and Middlesex School of Medicine, who have undertaken much of the work described in this chapter and made substantial intellectual contribution to our understanding of venous disease: Mr. T. R. Cheatle, Dr. S. Chittenden, Mr. J. Farrah, Ms. G. M. McMullin, and Mr. H. J. Scott.

REFERENCES

1. Nicolaides AN, Zukowski A, Lewis R, Kyprianou P, Malouf GM: Venous pressure measurements in venous problems. *In* Bergan JJ, Yao JST, eds: Surgery of the Veins. Orlando, FL, Grune & Stratton Inc, 1985;111–118.

2. Pollack AA, Wood EH: Venous pressure in the saphenous vein at the ankle in man during exercise and during changes of posture. J Appl Physiol 1949;*1*:649–662.

3. Pollack AA, Taylor BE, Myers TT, Wood EH: The effect of exercise and body position on the venous pressure at the ankle in patients having venous valvular defects. J Clin Invest 1949;*28*:559–563.

4. Højensgård IC, Stürup H: Static and dynamic pressures in superficial and deep veins of the lower extremity in man. Acta Physiol Scand 1952;*27*:49–67.

5. Schanzer H, Converse Pierce E: Pathophysiologic evaluation of chronic venous stasis witth ambulatory venous pressure studies. Angiology 1982;*33*:183–191.

6. Randhawa GK, Dhillon JS, Kistner RL, Ferris EB: Assessment of chronic venous insufficiency using dynamic venous pressure studies. Am J Surg 1984;*148*:203–209.

7. Hoare MC, Nicolaides AN, Miles CR, Shull K, Jury RP, Needham T, Dudley HAF: The role of primary varicose veins in venous ulceration. Surgery 1982;*92*:450–453.

8. Lewis JD, Parsons DCS, Needham TN, Douglas JN, Lawson J, Hobbs JT, Nicolaides AN: The use of venous pressure measurements and directional Doppler recording in distinguishing between superficial and deep valvular incompetence in patients with venous insufficiency. Br J Surg 1973;*60*:312.

9. Browse NL: Venous ulceration: Br Med J 1984;*286*:1920–1922.

10. Adams EF (transl): The Genuine Works of Hippocrates. London, Sydenham Press, 1849.

11. Wiseman R: Severall Chirurgical Treatises. London, Rogston and Took, 1676.

12. Homans J: The aetiology and treatment of varicose ulcers of the leg. Surg Gynecol Obstet 1917;*24*:300–311.

13. Fontaine R: Remarks concerning venous thrombosis and sequelae. Surgery 1957;*41*:6–24.

14. Blumhoff RL, Johnson G: Saphenous vein PO_2 in patients with varicose veins. J Surg Res 1977;*23*:35–36.

15. Scott HJ, Cheatle TR, McMullin GM, Coleridge Smith PD, Scurr JH: A reappraisal of the oxygenation of the venous blood of varicose veins. Br J Surg 1990;*77*:934–936.

16. Pratt GH: Arterial varices. A syndrome. Am J Surg 1949;*77*:456–460.

17. Brewer AC: Arteriovenous shunts. Br Med J 1950;*2*:270.

18. Hehne HJ, Locher JT, Waibel PP, Friedrich R: Zur Bedentung arteriovenoeser anastomosen bei dem primaeren Varicosis und der chronischvenoesen insuffizienz. Vasa 1974;*3*:396–398.

19. Lindmayr W, Lofferer O, Mostbeck A, Partsch H: Arteriovenous shunts in primary varicosis: A critical essay. Vasc Surg 1972;*6*:9–14.

20. Browse NL, Burnand KG: The cause of venous ulceration. Lancet 1982;*2*:243–245.

21. Browse NL, Gray L, Jarrett PEM, Morland M: Blood and vein-wall fibrinolytic activity in health and vascular disease. Br Med J 1977;*1*:478–481.

22. Leach RD: Venous ulceration, fibrinogen and fibrinolysis. Ann R Coll Surg Engl 1984;*66*:258–263.

23. Stacey MC, Burnand KG, Layer GT, Pattison M: Transcutaneous oxygen tensions as a prognostic indicator and measure of treatment of recurrent ulceration. Br J Surg 1987;*74*:545.

24. Clyne CAC, Ramsden WH, Chant ADB, Wenster JHH: Oxygen tension in the skin of the gaiter area of limbs with venous ulceration. Br J Surg 1985;*72*:644–647.

25. Dodd HJ, Gaylarde PM, Sarkany I: Skin oxygen tension in venous insufficiency of the lower leg. J R Soc Med 1985;*78*:373–376.

26. Rayman G, Williams SA, Spencer PD, Smaje LH, Tooke JE: Impaired microvascular response to minor skin trauma in type I diabetes. Br Med J 1986;*292*:1295–1298.

27. Hopkins NFG, Spinks TJ, Rhodes CG, Ranicar ASOA, Jamieson CW: Positron emission tomography in venous ulceration and liposclerosis. Br Med J 1982;*286*:333–336.

28. Sjerson P: Blood flow in cutaneous tissue in man studied by washout of radioactive xenon. Circ Res 1969;*25*:215–229.

29. Browse NL, Jarrett PEM, Morland M, Burnand KG: Treatment of liposclerosis of the leg by fibrinolytic enhancement: A preliminary report. Br Med J 1977;*2*:434–435.

30. Layer GT, Stacey MC, Burnand KG: Stanozolol and the treatment of venous ulceration—an interim report. Phlebology 1986;*1*:197–203.

31. McMullin GM, Watkin GT, Coleridge Smith PD, Scurr JH: The efficacy of fibrinolytic enhancement with stanozolol in the treatment of venous insufficiency. Br J Surg 1990;*77*:A700.

32. Coleridge Smith PD, Sarin S, Hasty JH, Scurr JH: Sequential gradient intermittent pneumatic compression enhances venous ulcer healing—a randomized trial. Surgery 1990 (in press).

33. Caprini JA, Chucker JL, Zuckerman L, Vagher JP, Franck CA, Cullen JE: Thrombosis prophylaxis using external compression. Surg Gynecol Obstet 1983;*156*:599–604.

34. Allenby F, Boardman L, Pflug JJ, Calnan JS: Effects of external pneumatic intermittent compression on fibrinolysis in man. Lancet 1973;*2*:1412–1414.

35. Moyses C, Cederholm-Williams SA, Michel CC: Haemoconcentration and the accumulation of white cells in the feet during venous stasis. Int J Microcirc Clin Exp 1987;*5*:311–320.

36. Thomas PRS, Nash GB, Dormandy JA: White cell accumulation in the dependent legs of patients

with venous hypertension: A possible mechanism for trophic changes in the skin. Br Med J 1988;*296*:1693–1695.

37. Fagrell B: Local microcirculation in chronic venous incompetence and leg ulcers. Vasc Surg 1979;*13*:217–225.
38. Bollingr A, Haselbach P, Schnewlin G, Junger M: Microangiopathy due to chronic venous incompetence evaluated by fluorescence videomicroscopy. *In* Negus D, Jantet G, eds: Phlebologie '85. London, John Libbey & Co. 1986;751–753.
39. Franzeck UK, Speiser D, Haselbach P, Bollinger A: Morphologic and dynamic microvascular abnormalities in chronic venous incompetence (CVI). *In* Davy A, Stemmer R, eds: Phlebologie '89. Montrouge, France, John Libbey Eurotext Ltd, 1989;104–107.
40. Bollinger A, Isenring G, Franzeck UK: Lymphatic microangiopathy: A complication of severe chronic venous incompetence. Lymphology 1982;*15*:60–65.
41. Braide M, Amundson B, Chien S, Bagge U: Quantitative studies of leukocytes on the vascular resistance in a skeletal muscle preparation. Microvasc Res 1984;*27*:331–352.
42. Engler RL, Dahlgren MD, Peterson MA, Dobbs A, Schmidt-Schonbein GW: Accumulation of polymophonuclear leukocytes during three hour myocardial ischemia. Am J Physiol 1986;*251*:H93–H100.
43. Romson JL, Hook BG, Kunkel SL, Abrams GD, Schork MA, Lucchesi BR: Reduction of the extent of ischemic myocardial injury by neutrophil depletion in the dog. Circulation 1983;*67*:1016–1023.
44. Wilson JW: Leucocyte sequestration and morphologic augmentation in the pulmonary network following haemorrhagic shock and related forms of stress. Adv Microcirc 1972;197–232.
45. Linas SL, Shanley PF, Whittenburg D, Berger E, Repine JE: Neutrophils accentuate ischemia-reperfusion injury in isolated perfused rat kidneys. Am J Physiol 1988;*255*:F728–F735.
46. Yamakawa T, Suguyama I, Niimi H: Behaviour of white blood cells in microcirculation of the cat brain cortex during hemorrhagic shock. Intravital micrscopic study. Int J Microcirc Clin Exp 1984;*3*:554.
47. Braide M, Blixt A, Bagge U: Leukocyte effects on the vascular resistance and glomerular filtration of the isolated rat kidney at normal and low flow rates. Circ Shock 1986;*20*:71–80.
48. Weissman G, Smolen JE, Korchak HM: Release of inflammatory mediators from stimulated neutrophils. N Engl J Med 1980;*303*:27–34.
49. Babior BM: Oxidants from phagocytes: Agents of defense and destruction. Blood 1984;*64*:959–966.
50. Coleridge Smith PD, Thomas P, Scurr JH, Dormandy JA: Causes of venous ulceration: A new hypothesis. Br Med J 1988;*296*:1726–1772.
51. Adams DO, Hamilton TA: The cell biology of macrophage activation. Annu Rev Immunol 1984;*2*:283–318.
52. Pober JS: Cytokine-mediated activation of vascular endothelium. Am J Pathol 1988;*133*:426–433.
53. Burnand KC, Clemenson G, Whimster I, Grant J, Browse NL: The effect of sustained venous hypertension on the skin capillaries of the canine hind limb. Br J Surg 1982;*69*:51–54.
54. Schleef RR, Bevilaqua MP, Sawdey M, Gimbrone MA, Loskutoff DJ: Cytokine activation of vascular endothelium: Effects on tissue-type plasminogen activator and type 1 plasminogen activator inhibitor. J Biol Chem 1988;*263*:5797–5803.
55. Scott HJ, Coleridge Smith PD, Scurr JH: White cells and venous disease—a histological study. Ann R Coll Surg Engl (in press).
56. Movat HZ, Burrowes CE: Local Schwarzman reaction. Endotoxin-mediated inflammatory and thrombo-haemorrhagic lesions. *In* Berry G, ed: Handbook of Endotoxins, vol 3: Cellular Biology of Endotoxin. Amsterdam, Elsevier, 1984;260–302.
57. van den Berg WB, van de Loo FAJ, Zwarts WA, Otterness IG: Effects of murine interleukin 1 on intact homologous articular cartilage: A quantitative and autoradiographic study. Ann Rheum Dis 1988;*47*:855–863.
58. Postlethwaite AE, Lachman LB, Mainardi CL, Kang AH: TI: Interleukin 1 stimulation of collagenase production by fibroblasts. J Exp Med 1983;*157*:801–806.
59. Sullivan GW, Carper HT, Novick WJ, Mandell GL: Inhibition of the inflammatory action of interleukin-1 and tumor necrosis factor (alpha) on neutrophil function of pentoxifylline. Infect Immun 1988;*56*:1722–1729.
60. Colgan M-P, Dormandy JA, Jones PW, Schraibman IG, Shanik DG: Oxpentifyline treatment of venous ulcers of the leg. Br Med J 1990;*300*:972–975.
61. Rudovsky G: Intravenous prostaglandin E_1 in the treatment of venous ulcers—a double-bind, placebo-controlled trial. Vasa 1989⊂ppl 28:39–43.
62. Sigel B, Edelstein AL, Savitch L, Hasty JH, Felix WR Jr: Type of compression for reducing venous stasis. Arch Surg 1975;*110*:171–175.

III

DIAGNOSTIC STUDIES

4

CURRENT STATUS OF DUPLEX ULTRASONOGRAPHY IN THE DIAGNOSIS OF ACUTE DEEP VENOUS THROMBOSIS

Robert W. Hobson II, Bruce L. Mintz, Zafar Jamil, and Gary B. Breitbart

Duplex ultrasonography has been applied to the diagnosis of acute deep venous thrombosis (DVT) with increasing frequency. High-resolution, real-time B-mode ultrasound has added a new dimension to the identification of acute and chronic thrombi in the lower extremities, and ultimately may replace phlebography as the anatomic test of choice because of its noninvasive character and recognized lack of morbidity. As with any ultrasonographic technique, the expertise of the examining technologist or clinician is of great importance. Although much of the current equipment includes the capability for the analysis of the Doppler audio output, most clinicians have emphasized the use of B-mode ultrasonography, employing the Doppler examination qualitatively in areas of poor venous imaging. Assessment of variations in venous flow with respiration as well as augmentation of flow with distal compression are used to confirm patency, or with abnormalities to suggest local thrombosis, as originally recommended in use of the hand-held continuous-wave Doppler (1–5).

B-mode imaging of the deep venous system provides a three-dimensional presentation of the deep veins below the level of the iliac crest. These veins can be visualized with a 7.5- or 8.0-MHz transducer, while a 3.0- or 4.0-MHz transducer has been recommended for accurate imaging of the iliac system as well as the deep veins in obese patients. Inaccuracies regarding the visualization of the iliac vein undoubtedly will be overcome with the application of deeper duplex ultrasonographic techniques. However, in some laboratories this has constituted an indication for continued use of hemodynamic studies such as impedance plethysmography (IPG).

The purpose of this chapter is to reveiw the current status of duplex ultrasonography in the diagnosis of DVT in the ambulatory patient and to comment on a continued role for IPG.

PERFORMANCE OF DUPLEX ULTRASONOGRAPHY

The duplex examination is performed with the patient in a supine position with the lower extremities lowered at about 20 degrees with moderate external rotation (5). The common femoral and superficial femoral veins are visualized in both the longitudinal and transverse presentations and gentle pressure is applied with the transducer. In the normal venous segment, this causes coaptation of the walls of the veins (Fig. 4–1) without interposition of echogenic thrombi. This complete coaptation of the walls of the vein constitutes the important confirmation

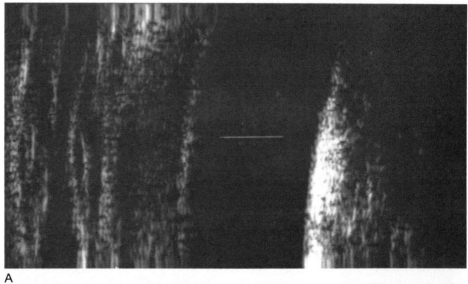

A

B

Figure 4–1.   *A*, Ultrasound marker demonstrates normal iliofemoral venous segment. *B*, Coaptation of the venous walls (ultrasound marker) confirms normalcy.

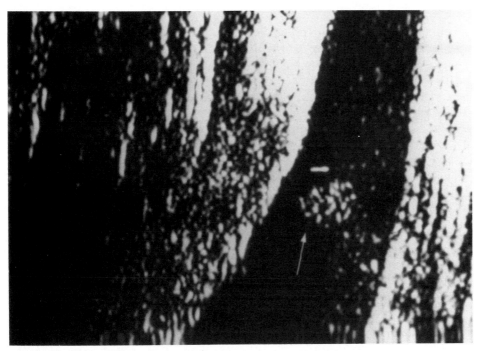

Figure 4–2. Ultrasonogram demonstrating acute intraluminal thrombus with free-floating component (arrow). (From Hobson RW, Mintz BL, Jamil Z, et al: Diagnosis of acute deep venous thrombosis. Surg Clin North Am 1990;*70*:143–157.

of normalcy. Other features include presence of normal Doppler flow signals, visualized normal valve motion, and absence of visualized thrombi. The ultrasonic scanning is continued to the medial thigh; however, visualization of the superficial femoral vein at the adductor hiatus is obscured in some cases by the local fascial planes.

Echogenicity of venous thrombi changes with the passage of time, and this becomes an important feature in the differentiation of acute (Fig. 4–2) and chronic (Table 4–1) thrombi (6). In areas where compressibility of the deep veins is difficult, analysis of the Doppler signals improves diagnostic accuracy (6,7). Valsalva maneuvers can also be used to evaluate changes in venous diameter as well as function of the deep venous valves at the level of the common femoral, superficial femoral, or popliteal veins.

TABLE 4–1. Differential Criteria: Acute Versus Chronic Thrombus[a]

PARAMETER	ACUTE THROMBUS	CHRONIC THROMBUS
Compressibility	Medium	None
Echogenicity	Homogeneous	Heterogeneous
Surface characteristics	Smooth, regular	Irregular
Attachment	Free floating	Firm
Size of vein	Dilated	Normal to moderately contracted with collaterals

[a] Modified from Fronek A: The venous system of the lower extremities. *In* Fronek A (ed): Noninvasive Diagnostics in Vascular Surgery. New York, McGraw-Hill Book Co, 1989.

The popliteal vein is interrogated with the patient in the supine position or by placing the patient in the prone position with 20 to 30 degrees of flexion at the knees (Fig. 4–3). In the ambulatory patient referred for the diagnosis of suspected DVT, visualization of intraluminal thrombus is diagnostic. However, in the hospitalized intensive care unit setting or in the postoperative obese patient, this positioning may be difficult. Under those circumstances, flexing the knees and externally rotating the hips usually allows a satisfactory visualization of the popliteal fossa, but this is one of the recognized deficiencies of the technique. Visualization of the infrapopliteal veins also can be accomplished, (7,8), although Flanagan and colleagues have reported only a 30 per cent success rate with the examination (9). The anterior and posterior tibial veins can generally be visualized in the proximal calf and midcalf, whereas the peroneal veins are more difficult to visualize because of their depth within the posterior compartment. Furthermore, compression of the tibial veins may not be as reliable a study for the presence of DVT. Under circumstances when the vein cannot be compressed and/or visualization is obscured, use of the Doppler spectral analysis for identification of presence or absence of flow and absence of luminal echogenic thrombi should exclude the diagnosis of DVT.

Recent reports have suggested that color Doppler flow imaging (Fig. 4–4) may improve these results. Polak and associates (10) positioned ultrasound probes in the middle third of the calf using an anteriolateral projection for visualization of the anterior tibial and peroneal veins and a posterolateral projection for the posterior tibial and peroneal veins. Compressibility was not a feature of the abnormal examination, and these clinicians used determination of flow at rest and with augmentation by distal compression as the criterion for patency. Visualization and demonstration of augmentation was achieved in 90 per cent of the peroneal veins and 96 per cent of the posterior tibial veins, whereas the anterior tibial vein was demonstrated in only 65 per cent of the legs. While this degree of

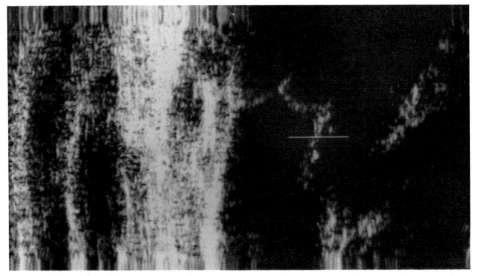

Figure 4–3. Normal popliteal venous segment demonstrating competency of the venous valve (ultrasound marker).

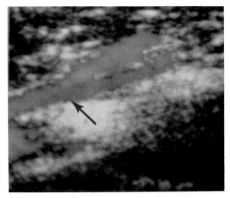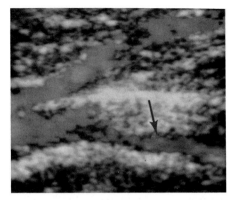

Figure 4–4. Color Doppler flow imaging was used in this case to confirm presence of a normal tibioperoneal venous segment (*left*, arrow, blue in color). The adjacent posterior tibial artery (*right*, arrow, red in color) is also visualized.

visualization can also be achieved with gray-scale instrumentation, the ease with which the veins were localized suggested the clinical applicability of this color imaging technique. Our initial evaluation suggests an enhanced role for color imaging, which will require prospective analysis for determination of its accuracy and potential advantages.

DISCUSSION/CLINICAL APPLICATION

The wide availability of duplex ultrasonography and its lack of morbidity on examination makes this technique particularly applicable in the ambulatory patient suspected of DVT. Since it is apparent that the clinical diagnosis of DVT is accurate in only about 50 per cent of cases (11,12), it becomes of obvious importance to supplement the clinical examination with more objective assessments. Duplex ultrasonography has become the preferred technique in many laboratories. As greater experience with the methodology has developed since the original reports by Talbot (13), accuracy has improved (Table 4–2) and the limitations (17) have been well defined in the literature. Compressibility of the venous segment in the diagnosis of venous thrombosis remains the salient feature of a positive examination. Lensing and colleagues (18) recently documented prospectively the accuracy of this observation for B-mode ultrasonography, with reported sensitivity of 100 per cent and specificity of 99 per cent for above-knee thrombus. A review of recently reported accuracy data suggests comparable results for the diagnosis of above-knee thrombi by several investigators (Table 4–2). The advantages of duplex ultrasound in specialized patient groups, including pregnant females and patients with unusual etiology of DVT (Fig. 4–5), is also obvious.

However, Lensing et al. (18) also reported that direct visualization of the tibial veins was not sufficiently reliable to allow accurate diagnosis of below-knee thrombi. Other investigators (7,9) have achieved a higher degree of accuracy with the technique; however, diagnosis of calf DVT awaits further clinical trials because the reported number of segments examined with phlebographic confirmation has been small and has not allowed prospective assessment in single centers. The clinical significance of below-knee thrombus continues to be the focus of

TABLE 4–2.   Comparison of Venous Duplex Ultrasonography and Phlebography

REFERENCE	SENSITIVITY (%)	SPECIFICITY (%)	POSITIVE PREDICTIVE VALUE (%)	NEGATIVE PREDICTIVE VALUE (%)
Wright et al. (7)	91	95	94	92
Oliver (14)	88	95	95	88
Sullivan et al. (15)	100	92	92	100
Patterson et al. (16)	88	92	89	92
Montefusco et al. (17)	100	99	—	—

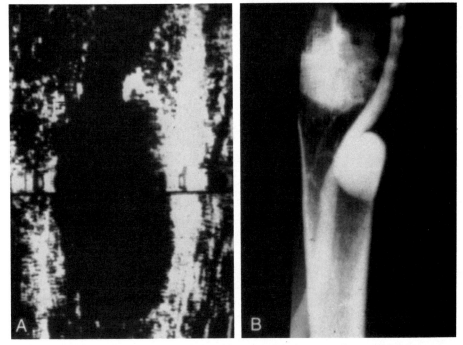

Figure 4–5.   B-mode ultrasonogram (A) and phlebogram (B) demonstrating a popliteal venous aneurysm, the source of venous thromboembolism in this patient. (From Hobson RW, Mintz BL, Jamil Z, et al: Diagnosis of acute deep venous thrombosis. Surg Clin North Am 1990;70:143–157.)

considerable discussion. Although reports in the literature have documented the potential for pulmonary embolus from calf thrombi, recommendations for clinical management have frequently been conservative, avoiding hospitalization and systemic heparinization while conducting a program of surveillance to identify propagation of thrombus into the popliteal or superficial femoral venous systems.

APPLICATION OF NONINVASIVE VASCULAR TESTING

The availability of duplex ultrasonography and the technical ease of its clinical application have made it the preferred examination in many laboratories. An algorithm currently utilized by our group (Fig. 4–6) presents initial use of IPG or

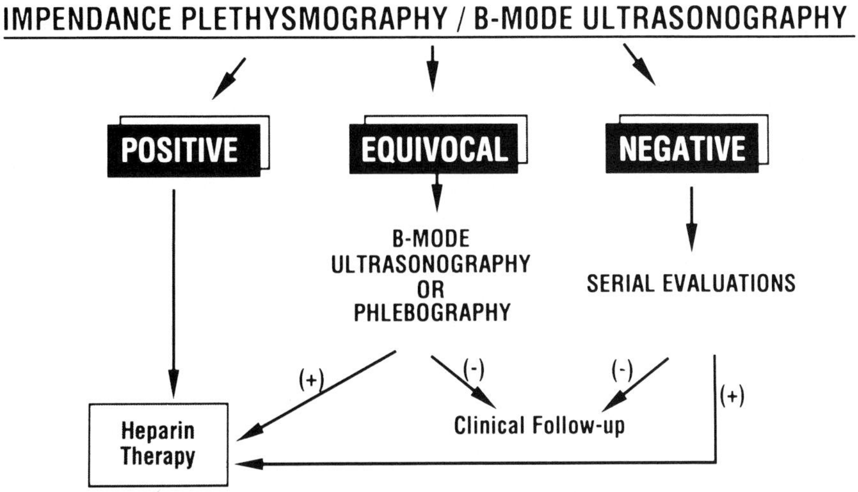

IMPENDANCE PLETHYSMOGRAPHY / B-MODE ULTRASONOGRAPHY

Figure 4–6. Clinical algorithm for noninvasive diagnosis of acute deep venous thrombosis. (From Hobson RW, Mintz BL, Jamil Z, et al: Diagnosis of acute deep venous thrombosis. Surg Clin North Am 1990;70:143–157.)

duplex ultrasonography. Our performance of IPG and serial follow-up has been sufficiently accurate for the diagnosis of above-knee thrombi (19,20) to justify anticoagulant therapy and to avoid treatment in patients with negative studies. Furthermore, in a 6-month clinical follow-up of patients with negative IPGs as reported by Huisman et al. (21), no patient died of thromboembolism. Evidence of recurrent venous thrombosis was rare, and evidence of pulmonary embolus was not detected. These data confirm prospective analyses performed by Hull and associates (22) and Wheeler and colleagues (23). Consequently, phlebography would not be indicated in the presence of a positive IPG, unless the presence of conditions known to give false-positive results, such as congestive failure or venous obstruction due to extrinsic compression, were suspected.

The final role of B-mode ultrasonography in replacing phlethysmographic testing will await further clinical trials. However, Patterson and colleagues (16) have reported an enhanced sensitivity and specificity for duplex ultrasonography (Table 4–2) as compared with IPG. Availability of a dedicated and skilled ultrasonographer is required to achieve reproducible results of comparable accuracy. Acknowledged accuracy in the diagnosis of above-knee thrombi, including confirmation of iliac vein thrombus, will maintain a role for IPG, particularly in institutions in which ultrasonographers represent a limited clinical resource. As we have expanded our use of B-mode ultrasonography, those patients with equivocal IPG results undergo B-mode ultrasonography rather than being referred for phlebography. It is also possible that, with further refinements in the technique and with expanded use of color imaging as noted earlier, the diagnosis of below-knee thrombi may be improved, ultimately allowing B-mode ultrasonography to replace plethysmographic techniques as well as phlebography as the primary diagnostic modality. The results of prospective studies, including an evalaution of the technique's cost effectiveness (taking into account the decreasing expense of basic ultrasonographic equipment), will influence future application of B-mode ultrasonography in clinical practice.

REFERENCES

1. Yao JST, Gourmos C, Hobbs JT: Detection of proximal vein thrombosis by Doppler ultrasound flow-detection method. Lancet 1972;*1*:1–4.
2. Strandness DE Jr, Sumner DS: Ultrasonic velocity detector in the diagnosis of thrombophlebitis. Arch Surg 1972;*104*:180–183.
3. Sumner DS, Lambeth A: Reliability of Doppler ultrasound in the diagnosis of acute venous thrombosis both above and below the knee. Am J Surg 1979;*138*:205–210.
4. Evans DS: The early diagnosis of deep vein thrombosis by ultrasound. Br J Surg 1970;*57*:726–728.
5. Hobson RW, Mintz BL, Jamil Z, Breitbart GB: Diagnosis of acute deep venous thrombosis. Surg Clin North Am 1990;*70*:143–157.
6. Fronek A: The venous system of the lower extremities. *In* Fronek A, ed: Noninvasive Diagnostics in Vascular Surgery. New York, McGraw-Hill Book Co, 1989.
7. Wright DJ, Shepard AD, McPharlin M, Ernst CB: Pitfalls in lower extremity venous duplex scanning. J Vasc Surg 1990;*11*:675–679.
8. Rollins DL, Semrow CM, Friedell ML, Calligaro KD, Buchbinder D: Progress in the diagnosis of deep venous thrombosis: The efficacy of real-time B-mode ultrasonic imaging. J Vasc Surg 1988;*7*:638–641.
9. Flanagan LD, Sullivan ED, Cranley JJ: Venous imaging of the extremeties using real-time B-mode ultrasound. *In* Bergan JJ, Yao JST, eds: Surgery of the Veins. Orlando, FL, Grune & Stratton, 1985;89–98.
10. Polak JF, Cutler SS, O'Leary DH: Deep veins of the calf: Assessment with color Doppler flow imaging. Radiology 1989;*171*:481–485.
11. McLachlin JA, Richards T, Paterson JC: An evaluation of clinical signs in the diagnosis of venous thrombosis. Arch Surg 1962;*85*:738–744.
12. Cranley JJ, Canos AJ, Sull WJ: The diagnosis of deep venous thrombosis: Fallibility of clinical signs and symptoms. Arch Surg 1976;*111*:34–36.
13. Talbot SR: Use of real-time imaging in identifying deep venous obstruction: A preliminary report. Bruit 1982;*6*:41–46.
14. Oliver MA: Duplex scanning in venous disease. Bruit 1985;*9*:206–209.
15. Sullivan ED, Peter DJ, Cranley JJ: Real-time B-mode venous ultrasound. J Vasc Surg 1984;*1*:465–471.
16. Patterson RB, Fowl RJ, Keller JD, Schomaker W, Kempczinski RF: The limitations of impedance plethysmography in the diagnosis of acute deep venous thrombosis. J Vasc Surg 1990;*11*:675–679.
17. Montefusco CM, Bakal CW, Sprayregan S, Rhodes B, Veith FJ: Duplex ultrasonographic venography: The definitive diagnostic tool for thrombophlebitis. Current Critical Problems in Vascular Surgery. St. Louis Quality Medical Publishing Inc, 1989;145–150.
18. Lensing AWA, Prandoni P, Brandjes D: Detection of deep vein thrombosis by real-time B-mode ultrasonography. N Engl J Med 1989;*320*:342–345.
19. Hobson RW, Lynch TG, Jamil Z: Role of the vascular laboratory in the diagnosis of venous disease. *In* DeWeese JA, ed: Operative Surgery. London, Butterworths, 1985;253–263.
20. O'Donnell JA, Hobson RW, Lynch TG, et al: Impedance plethysmography: Noninvasive diagnosis of deep venous thrombosis and arterial insufficiency. Am Surg 1983;*49*:26–30.
21. Huisman MV, Buller HR, TenCate JW, et al: Serial impedance plethysmography for suspected deep venous thrombosis in out patients. N Engl J Med 1986;*314*:823–828.
22. Hull R, Van Aken WG, Hirsch J, et al: Impedance plethysmography using the occlusive cuff technique in the diagnosis of venous thrombosis. Circulation 1976;*53*:696–700.
23. Wheeler HB, O'Donnel JA, Anderson FA, et al: Occlusive impedance phlebography: A diagnostic procedure for venous thrombosis and pulmonary embolism. Prog Cardiovasc Dis 1974;*17*:199–205.

5

STUDY OF DEEP VENOUS THROMBOSIS IN HIGH-RISK PATIENTS USING COLOR FLOW DOPPLER

David S. Sumner, Gregg L. Londrey,
Donald P. Spadone, Kim J. Hodgson, Darr W. Leutz,
and E. Shannon Stauffer

Although the use of prophylactic measures has decreased the incidence of postoperative thromboembolism, deep venous thrombosis (DVT) and pulmonary embolism remain leading causes of morbidity and mortality in patients undergoing high-risk operations. Ideally, these thrombi should be identified and treated before they become symptomatic. Despite the efforts of numerous investigators, no completely satisfactory method has emerged for surveying patients at risk for perioperative DVT. Plebography, which is acknowledged to be highly sensitive and specific, is invasive and has a number of other drawbacks that preclude its routine use. ^{125}I-labeled fibrinogen uptake tests are sensitive to developing calf vein thrombi but fail to detect many of the more dangerous proximal clots. Impedance plethysmography and phleborheography are much less accurate when they are used for surveillance purposes than they are when used to diagnose symptomatic DVT (1). Moreover, these tests are totally insensitive to thrombosis of the below-knee veins.

The accuracy of duplex scanning for diagnosing clinically suspected DVT is well documented and is superior to that of other noninvasive methods (2–4). Recent reports suggest that a high level of accuracy is maintained when duplex scanning is employed for surveillance of high-risk patients (5,6). In this most challenging group of patients, the results with duplex scanning are also far better than those obtained with other noninvasive techniques (4). Duplex imaging, however, is not without its problems. Errors continue to be made in the detection of thrombi in the calf veins, adductor canal region, and iliac veins (7).

Color flow Doppler imaging may obviate some of these problems (8–11). This significant technological advance superimposes a real-time Doppler flow map on the B-mode image. Advantages include the immediate identification of vascular structures and the differentiation of vein from artery. Visualization of flow over a wide range of vessels reduces the need to assess flow patterns by direct Doppler interrogation. Venous compression is less often necessary, since the absence of flow clearly identifies most echolucent clots.

Because color flow imaging has only recently been applied to the study of venous disease, there are few reports documenting its accuracy for detecting clinically suspected DVT and none relating to its accuracy for surveillance of high-risk patients (12,13). At present, no information confirms that the potential advantages of color flow imaging result in an improved accuracy compared to that of conventional duplex scanning or, for that matter, to that of other noninvasive modalities.

In this chapter, we discuss the use of color flow imaging to detect DVT and present our preliminary experience with this modality in patients with clinically suspected venous thrombi and in patients at high risk for developing the disease.

INSTRUMENTATION

The probes of most color flow instruments contain a linear array of crystals that are serially activated to produce a rectangular field of view. Along each scan line, stationary reflectors are displayed as a B-mode gray scale image while moving particles generate Doppler shift frequencies. Flow is color coded (red or blue) according to its direction relative to the orientation of the sound beam. Color is assigned by the operator so that blue coincides with centrally directed flow (predominantly venous) and red with flow directed peripherally (predominantly arterial). Color saturation or hue depends on the magnitude of the frequency shift, which in turn depends on the velocity of blood flow and the angle at which the beam intersects the velocity vector. Thus, provided the angle remains constant, deeper or more intense colors represent slow flow and lighter colors more rapid flow. Total lack of color (a black image) indicates the absence of flow, flow velocities too low to be detected, or flow vectors at a right angle to the sound beam. With "slow flow" software (Quantum Medical Systems, Inc, Issaquah, WA), velocities as low as 0.3 cm/sec can be detected. As with conventional duplex scanning, flow patterns may be evaluated audibly or by real-time spectral analysis by placing the pulsed Doppler sample volume in the flow stream. All parts of the study may be recorded on videotape for review.

While a 7.5-MHz probe can be used to study the superficial veins, a 5-MHz probe is required for those situated more deeply. Both of these probes have relatively large footprints, making them somewhat difficult to use in tight spots. Smaller, less bulky, linear array and sector scanning probes, which allow increased maneuverability and more freedom in orienting the image, have recently become available. These innovations may permit the interrogation of previously inaccessible areas.

SCANNING TECHNIQUE

The technique is similar to that used for conventional duplex scanning. Patients lie supine, with their legs slightly externally rotated, on a bed or examination table that is placed in a reverse Trendelenburg position. Dependency of the legs is necessary to ensure venous filling. Studies begin at the groin, where the common femoral vein and its tributaries are imaged, and proceed distally along the anterior medial thigh to the region of the adductor canal, at which point the superficial femoral vein disappears from view. Popliteal veins are examined with the patients lying prone with their knees flexed to about 30 degrees. Alternatively, in patients who cannot assume the prone position, the popliteal vein may be examined with the patient lying on his or her side. Infrapopliteal veins are first located near the ankle and are then followed up the leg, again with the patient supine and in reverse Trendelenburg. Slight flexion of the knee, by relaxing the calf muscles, avoids venous compression and makes application of the probe easier. In some cases, this examination is best conducted with the patient sitting, the foot resting on a stool or on the examiner's lap. To visualize the anterior tibial vein, the probe is placed over the anterior compartment and directed posteriorly and medially. In this position, the peroneal veins may be seen deep to the anterior tibial vessels, with the interosseous membrane lying between. The posterior tibial vein is studied with the probe applied to the medial calf behind the tibia. This view also permits visualization of the peroneal veins, which lie beyond the posterior tibial vessels. Because the venae comitantes may not lie in the same plane, it is often necessary to reorient the probe to see both of these vessels.

At each level of the leg, the artery is first located and then the probe is shifted slightly to optimize the corresponding venous image. Color not only expedites the identification of vascular structures but also helps distinguish arteries from veins. The velocity of blood flow in the femoral and popliteal veins is sufficiently high to ensure that flow in these veins will be visible without having to be augmented. Below the knee, spontaneous venous flow is less often observed; consequently, in order to see the infrapopliteal veins it is usually necessary to augment flow by compressing the leg, either above or below the probe. Flow in the tibial and peroneal arteries, however, is almost always visible, thus ensuring that the proper area is being examined. To clarify the flow pattern, it may be necessary to listen to the audible signal or record a frequency spectrum.

Longitudinal tracking of veins, which may be difficult with conventional B-mode or duplex scanning, is greatly facilitated by color, permitting the operator to use the long axis view during most of the examination. At selected sites, transverse views are also obtained.

INTERPRETATION

Vessels are defined by both the gray scale and the color flow image. In the absence of color, the lumen is normally blank (black) and the blood–vessel wall interface is sharply delineated. In normal femoral and popliteal veins, the lumen is completely filled with blue pixels (signifying antegrade flow), and the phasic flow pattern induced by respiration is clearly evident. A shift in the color from blue to red in response to a Valsalva maneuver or limb compression is indicative of venous valvular incompetence (retrograde flow). Moderate pressure of the probe on the skin causes normal veins to collapse. This is best observed in the transverse view and with the color off. In the longitudinal axis, prssure on the probe may displace the vein from the field of view, leading to erroneous interpretations.

At the groin, the common femoral vein, lying just medial to the common femoral artery, is easily seen. By manipulating the probe angle, the operator can bring the profunda femoris, superficial femoral, and saphenous veins into the field of view and demonstrate their communication with the common femoral vein (Fig. 5–1). Not infrequently, all three veins may be visualized simultaneously. In a thin, well-prepared patient, it may be possible to examine the distal iliac vein. Between the groin and the adductor canal, the superficial femoral vein is easily imaged. Because this vein is frequently duplicated, a transverse veiw is required to avoid overlooking one of the channels. The popliteal vein and the lesser saphenous vein are also not difficult to image (Fig. 5–2). Again, a transverse view must be obtained, since this vein—like the superficial femoral vein—is often duplicated.

Although the infrapopliteal veins may be "spontaneously" visible, it is usually necessary to augment flow in order to identify their lumina. Because these vessels are so small, the gray scale image is difficult to interpret. Color, therefore, is extremely valuable in this area. Both venae comitantes may be visible simultaneously, and—depending on the approach—the anterior tibial or the posterior tibial vein may appear in the same plane as the peroneal vein (Fig. 5–3).

Absence of color in the lumen of the vein is the hallmark of venous thrombosis. If the venous lumen remains without color after augmentation, it is safe to assume that the vein is clotted (Fig. 5–4). Because fresh thrombi are hypoechoic, they may not be apparent on the gray scale image and can be detected with B-mode scanning only by the absence of compression or, less convincingly, by expansion of the lumen. With conventional duplex scanning the diagnosis may be confirmed by the absence of Doppler signals, but this requires an additional step. In most cases, color flow obviates the need for these additional maneuvers.

As the clot matures, it may become apparent on the gray scale. Even then the absence of color is helpful, particularly in reference to the small infrapopliteal veins, which may be difficult to identify on the gray scale. Provided the adjacent artery is identified, failure to detect the blue color of venous flow in the sur-

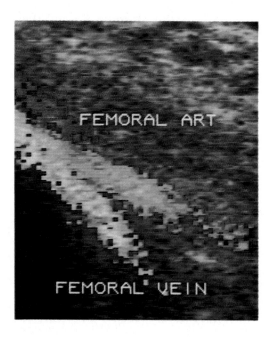

Figure 5–1. Color flow scan of normal groin veins, showing the superficial femoral vein (*above*) as it joins the profunda femoris vein (*below*) to form the common femoral vein. A short segment of the common femoral artery is also visible. This and the following figures are oriented with the cephalic direction being to the left and the tissues closest to the skin at the top.

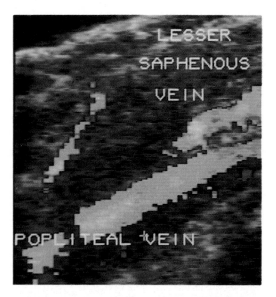

Figure 5–2. A normal lesser saphenous vein is shown joining the popliteal vein. A few red pixels are seen in the popliteal artery, which is captured during diastole.

rounding tissue after augmentation signifies the presence of a clot (Fig. 5–5). (Because of their diminutive diameter, compression studies of tibioperoneal veins are exceedingly hard to interpret.)

Thrombi that partially occlude the venous lumen encroach on the normally smooth color flow image, producing a filling defect (Figs 5–6 and 5–7). The clot, depending on its echogenicity, may or may not be visible on the B-mode image.

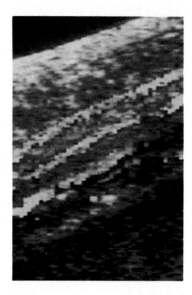

Figure 5–3. Posterior tibial artery (*above*) and peroneal artery (*below*) with their associated venae comitants (blue). Scan was obtained in the lower third of the calf. Venous flow was augmented by calf compression.

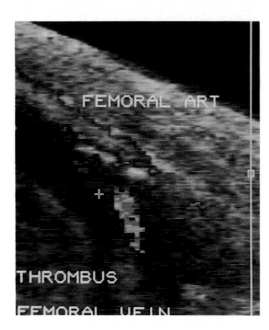

Figure 5–4. Thrombosis of the common, superficial femoral, and profunda femoris veins. The venous lumen is predominantly echolucent (black) but shows a few blue pixels indicating an area of incomplete thrombosis.

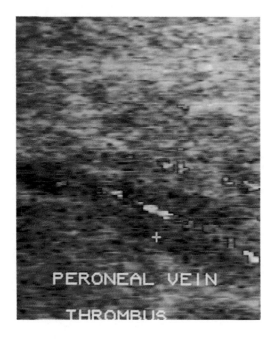

Figure 5–5. Thrombosis of both peroneal venae comitantes. The red pixels define the peroneal artery. Echoes are seen in the peroneal veins, the deeper of which is identified by the green cross.

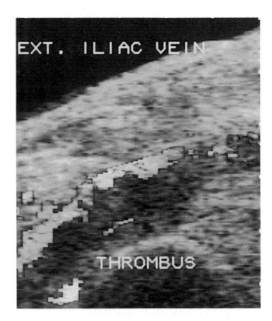

Figure 5–6. Incomplete thrombosis of the external iliac vein. Echogenic thrombus is seen occupying a portion of the venous lumen. A phlebogram of this same area showed an identical picture.

With conventional B-mode scanning, confirmation of the presence of a hypo-echogenic clot can only be obtained by demonstrating incomplete compressibility of the vein. Many of these thrombi will have a tail that remains unattached to the venous wall and, in real time, can be seen to wave about in the flow stream (Fig. 5–8). Flashes of blue interspersed in an echogenic clot are indicative of an old thrombus with recanalization.

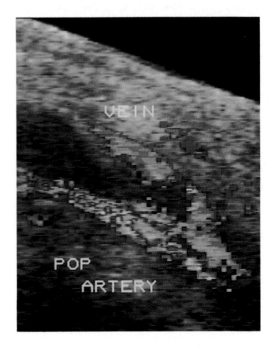

Figure 5–7. Thrombosis of the popliteal vein. There is still flow in the popliteal vein distal to the thrombus.

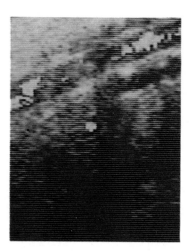

Figure 5–8. A partially occluded superficial femoral vein showing an unattached "tail" that can be seen to fluctuate in the flow stream on the real-time image.

There are several problem areas where visualization is inadequate to confirm the presence or absence of a clot. The external iliac vein is often difficult or impossible to image. Patency can be confirmed indirectly by demonstrating normal phasic flow patterns in the common femoral artery. Continuous flow (or reduced flow) in this vessel strongly suggests the presence of a proximal occlusion. Because observation of the color flow image may not be sufficiently discriminating in this circumstance, spectral analysis or audible interpretation of the Doppler flow signal is usually required. The second problem area is the region of the adductor canal, where the vein is not only imbedded in muscle but abruptly changes direction as it plunges deep into the popliteal space. Indirect confirmation of patency or occlusion can be obtained only by observing the flow pattern just above and below the canal. A normal lumen and free flow of blood suggest patency. Compression maneuvers are uninformative, since the normal vein in this region (owing to its depth) resists compression (7). The third problem area is that of the distal popliteal vein and proximal tibial and peroneal veins. Not only are these veins located deep within the calf, but also their anatomy is complicated at the point where they coalesce. Finally, the veins of the middle and lower thirds of the calf remain a problem area. Even though it is usually possible in normal limbs to identify and follow the six tibial and peroneal veins over most of their course, their small size, multiplicity, and relative depth make diagnosis of venous thrombosis uncertain at best (10,11).

CURRENT EXPERIENCE

During a recent 6-month period, 29 patients (30 limbs) with suspected deep venous thrombosis underwent both color flow imaging (Quad-1, Quantum Medical Systems, Inc, Issaquah, WA) and phlebography. This represents only a small sample of the patients studied by the two techniques. As shown in Table 5–1, the overall sensitivity was 92 per cent. All thrombi above the popliteal vein were

TABLE 5–1.   Accuracy of Color Flow Imaging in Patients with Clinically Suspected Deep Venous Thrombosis[a]

| | | PHLEBOGRAPHY | | | |
| | | Positive | | | |
COLOR FLOW	Negative	Calf	SF-Pop[b]	CF[c]	Total
Negative	12	1			13
Equivocal					
Calf	3				3
Pop	1				1
Positive					
Calf	1	2			3
SF-Pop			2		2
CF				8	8
Total	17	3	2	8	30

[a] Excluding equivocal results: Sensitivity = 12/13 (92 per cent), specificity = 12/13 (92 per cent), predictive value, positive = 12/13 (92 percent), predictive value, negative = 12/13 (92 per cent); including equivocal with positive results: Specificity = 12/17 (71 per cent), positive predictive value = 12/17 (71 per cent).
[b] SF-Pop, superficial femoral and popliteal veins.
[c] CF, common femoral vein.

detected with color flow imaging, for a sensitivity of 100 per cent, but clots in the calf veins were identified in only two of the three limbs (67 per cent) in which they were present on phlebography. There were four equivocal studies (studies with abnormal flow patterns but no visible clot). Three of these involved the calf veins, and one the popliteal vein. Phelbography was normal in all limbs with equivocal findings. There was one false-positive calf study. Excluding the equivocal results, the specificity was 92 per cent (12 of 13 correctly identified). However, if the equivocal and positive studies were grouped together, the specificity dropped to 71 per cent. The negative and positive predictive values (excluding the equivocal studies) were both 92 per cent. When the equivocal results were included in the postive group, the positive predictive value dropped to 71 per cent.

In July of 1989, a prospective study of high-risk patients undergoing total joint replacement was organized by the division of orthopedic surgery in conjunction with the vascular surgical service. All patients admitted to this study underwent bilateral phlebography and color flow imaging on the third to the sixth postoperative day. No preoperative examinations were performed. Pneumatic compression boots were applied to the contralateral limbs of patients undergoing knee replacement and to both limbs of those undergoing hip replacement. Aspirin and coumadin were also administered to some of the patients at the discretion of the operating surgeon. Because the study is ongoing, only preliminary results are currently available.

Phlebographic examinations disclosed deep venous thrombosis in 14 (61 per cent) of 23 knee-replacement patients. Thrombi were found in 13 (57 per cent) of the ipsilateral limbs and in three (13 per cent) of the contralateral limbs (two patients had bilateral involvement). Clots were confined to the proximal infra-popliteal veins in 15 limbs and to the distal popliteal vein in one limb. Most of these clots involved a single vein and were less than 4 cm in length. No thrombi were found proximal to the midpopliteal vein. Color flow imaging correctly identified all negative limbs for a specificity of 100 per cent. None of the color flow images was read as positive (sensitivity of 0 per cent), but four studies in limbs with calf vein thrombosis were read as equivocally positive. If equivocal studies were considered to be positive, the sensitivity would be 25 per cent and the positive predictive value would be 100 per cent. The negative predictive value was 71 per cent (30/42).

Postoperative phlebograms of the 20 patients undergoing total hip replacement demonstrated thrombi in three limbs (15 per cent of the patients and 7.5 per cent of the limbs). Two of the involved limbs were contralateral to the hip replacement. In these limbs the clots were confined to the proximal infrapopliteal veins. The one ipsilateral thrombosis was localized to the superficial femoral vein in the adductor canal region. None of these clots was detected by color flow imaging, and there were no equivocally positive studies (sensitivity of 0 per cent). The specificity was 100 per cent and the negative predictive value was 93 per cent (37/40 limbs).

For the combined hip and knee replacement groups, the negative predictive value of color flow imaging was 82 per cent (67/82 limbs) or 67 per cent (23/39 patients). If only those clots involving the popliteal or more proximal veins are included, the combined negative predictive value was 98 per cent (80/82 limbs) or 95 per cent (37/39 patients).

LITERATURE REVIEW

Few reports are available concerning the accuracy of color flow imaging for detected deep venous thrombosis, and none that address the use of color flow imaging for surveillance of high-risk patients.

Color Flow Doppler in Symptomatic Patients

Foley and associates correlated color flow imaging with phlebography in 47 patients with suspected DVT (9). At the femoral level, there was complete agreement in 12 positive and 35 negative studies. Two of seven isolated popliteal thrombi were not recognized. Both techniques agreed in all 16 patients in whom the tibioperoneal veins were evaluated (12 negative and four positive studies), but in none of the positive cases was the thrombus isolated to the calf. The overall sensitivity and specificity were not provided.

Persson and colleages reported 100 per cent sensitivity and specificity of color flow imaging compared to phlebography in 30 patients with suspected DVT (12). Of the 24 leg studies, 16 were abnormal, 15 of which involved the popliteal or more proximal veins. In only one patient were the clots isolated to the calf veins. Five of six arm studies were abnormal, three of which were in patients in whom a subclavian catheter was in place. Knudson and coworkers, using color flow imaging, correctly identified seven of nine deep venous thromboses of the upper extremity (sensitivity 78 per cent) (13). Absence of clot was correctly predicted in 12 of 13 cases (specificity 92 per cent). Again all of the upper extremities subjected to both color flow imaging and phlebography were symptomatic.

According to a manufacturer's newsletter, Knighton and colleagues from the University of Utah found that the sensitivity of color flow imaging compared to phlebography in 75 limbs with suspected DVT was 79 per cent and its specificity was 88 per cent (regardless of clot size or location or quality of the examination) (14). The sensitivity and specificity for detecting iliofemoropopliteal thrombosis were 96 and 100 per cent, respectively. Almost identical results were quoted for detecting tibioperoneal thrombi (sensitivity 95 per cent, specificity 100 per cent). Presumably, these latter figures relate to studies conducted under ideal conditions.

In a study emphasizing the examination of calf veins, Polak and associates noted that augmenting venous flow by calf compression produced color flow images in 55 per cent of normal anterior tibial veins and in all normal posterior tibial and peroneal veins (10). Augmentation was only slightly less successful in producing a color image of these veins in limbs with suspected deep venous thrombosis. Sixteen thrombi were identified in 49 patients. Two of these were confined to the calf, and both were confirmed by phlebography. The sensitivity and specificity were not reported. Van Bemmelen and coworkers examined 30 normal subjects and found that all paired calf veins could be visualized from the ankle to the popliteal fossa (11). No symptomatic patients were included in their study and no phlebograms were obtained.

Surveillance with Duplex Scanning

Conventional duplex scanning has been employed in several surveillance studies of high-risk patients. Flinn and colleagues from Northwestern University performed preoperative and postoperative duplex scans on 361 consecutive patients undergoing major neurosurgical procedures (6). Scans positive for perioperative DVT were obtained in 17 patients (4.7 per cent). Femoral veins were implicated in 11 cases, popliteal veins in three, and iliac veins in two. Routine scanning of calf veins was not performed. Phlebography confirmed the diagnosis and location of DVT in eight of 10 cases with positive scans (positive predictive value 80 per cent) and the absence of thrombi in four of four patients with negative scans. Because the vast majority of patients were not subjected to phlebography, the true incidence of perioperative DVT remains uncertain. It is likely that many patients developed clots confined to the calf veins. Therefore, the sensitivity of duplex scanning in respect to calf vein thrombi cannot be determined from this study.

Barnes and associates compared the results of pre- and postoperative duplex scanning and phlebography in 78 patients undergoing total hip or knee arthroplasty (5). Duplex scanning was confined to the popliteal and more proximal veins. During the postoperative period, duplex scans were positive in 10 of 12 legs in which phlebograms disclosed proximal DVT (sensitivity 83 per cent). Negative scans were obtained in 135 of 141 limbs in which the phlebograms were negative for proximal venous thrombosis (specificity 96 per cent). Phlebography also demonstrated clots in the infrapopliteal calf veins of 13 patients (17 limbs). Thus, in 52 per cent of the 25 patients with postoperative DVT, clots were confined to the calf veins and were not detected by the scan.

Comerota and coworkers evaluated the accuracy of duplex scanning for detecting postoperative DVT in 38 legs of patients undergoing total joint replacement (4). Noninvasive studies and phlebography were performed on the sixth or seventh postoperative day. Phlebography demonstrated thrombi in the popliteal or femoral veins in seven limbs. All of these thrombi were detected by duplex scanning (sensitivity 100 per cent). Clots confined to the infrapopliteal veins were found in two limbs, but only one of these was detected by duplex scanning (sensitivity 50 per cent). The specificity was 100 per cent.

COMMENTS AND CONCLUSION

Compared with conventional duplex scanning, color flow imaging has some obvious advantages. Color facilities the recognition of arteries and veins, greatly simplifies the task of following vascular structures up and down the limb, graphically displays flow patterns, confirms the absence of blood flow, and demonstrates partial occlusions by displaying defects in the flow image. With color, there is less need to assess venous compressibility [a manuever that, in any case, has been shown to be of questionable accuracy (7)]. Color also reduces, but does not eliminate, the need to evaluate audible or recorded Doppler flow signals. These advantages translate into a less demanding and less time-consuming examination—a feature of considerable importance when surveillance studies are conducted.

Although relatively little information is available concerning the ability of color flow imaging to detect or rule out deep venous thrombosis, there is no reason to suspect that adding color detracts from the accuracy of conventional duplex scanning; in fact, the opposite assumption is more logical. The accuracy of conventional duplex scanning for diagnosing clinically suspected DVT of the popliteal or more proximal veins appears to be well established. Cumulative data from 12 independent laboratories in which 1835 conventional duplex examinations were compared with phlebography indicate an overall sensitivity and specificity of 96 per cent for detecting thrombi in this area (2). More problematic is its ability to detect clots confined to the infrapopliteal veins. That duplex scanning can identify thrombi in the tibioperoneal veins with a remarkable degree of accuracy is supported by the work of Rollins, Elias, and their associates (15,16). These studies, however, are difficult, time consuming, and require the services of skilled technologists. Without exception, all reports identify the infrapopliteal veins as the site where most errors are made. Because thrombi isolated to the tibioperoneal veins are seldom responsible for pulmonary emboli, the tendency has been to downgrade the significance of false-negative results in this area. Propagation of the clot into the popliteal and femoral veins occurs in about 20 per cent of cases, but these potentially dangerous extensions can be detected by serial scanning. Nonetheless, there is a growing suspicion that thrombosis of the infrapopliteal veins may be responsible for chronic venous insufficiency (17,18). If this conjecture ultimately proves to be valid, the importance of detecting tibioperoneal thrombi will have to be reassessed.

Although infrapopliteal veins are more readily identified and followed with color flow imaging than with conventional duplex scanning (10,11), this advantage has not definitely been shown to improve accuracy—although perhaps future studies will. In our study, the most difficult veins to examine (the proximal tibioperoneal and the distal popliteal veins) were also, unfortunately, the most common sites of postoperative thrombosis.

Surveillance of high-risk patients with conventional duplex scanning has produced encouraging results, at least in regard to the detection of thrombi developing in the major proximal veins during the perioperative period (5,6). Indeed, the accuracy of surveillance in the femoral and popliteal veins appears to be comparable to that achieved by duplex studies of symptomatic patients (4). Because the tendency has been to avoid examining the infrapopliteal veins, there is little information concerning the accuracy of surveillance in this area. Our preliminary results suggest that surveillance with color flow imaging fails to detect the vast majority of thrombi developing in the calf veins (although, admittedly, most of these were of limited extent and were confined to a single vein). Nothing can be said regarding the accuracy of color flow surveillance of the proximal veins since only one of our 43 patients developed a clot above the popliteal fossa.

Should routine duplex or color flow screening of high-risk patients be advocated? This issue is generally skirted in the conclusions of most articles. It is generally acknowledged that many tibioperoneal clots will be overlooked by surveillance techniques that neglect the calf or even those that include the calf, as our results show. In our experience, this means that most thrombi developing in the perioperative period would be missed. Again the argument is advanced that infrapopliteal clots have little significance. Yet the only three pulmonary emboli in the study of Flinn and associates occurred in patients with negative scans (6), and the only two patients to develop pulmonary emboli in the study of Barnes and colleagues had clots confined to the calf veins (5). Patients discovered to have proximal thrombi, however, were anticoagulated, and the incidence of pulmonary emboli in those with thrombi confined to the calf veins must have been extremely low. Therefore, these observations do not contradict the generally held opinion that calf vein thrombi pose little immediate threat to the patient provided they do not extend into the proximal veins.

However, even if all hazardous thrombi are detected, can routine perioperative scanning of high-risk patients be considered cost-effective or cost-beneficial? The answer depends on the efficacy of the prophylactic measures employed. Duplex scanning is a time-consuming, labor intensive, moderately expensive study. Although preoperative examinations may not be necessary, serial postoperative studies will be required if the goal is to rule out the propagation of undetected calf vein thrombi in patients with negative scans. The cost of routine duplex scanning is high and must, therefore, be balanced against the incidence, cost, morbidity, and mortality associated with undetected postoperative venous thrombosis. Clearly, our preliminary results do not support the use of color flow imaging for the routine surveillance of high-risk patients.

ACKNOWLEDGMENTS: The authors wish to express their appreciation to Gaynell Romanas and Diane Raymond, who performed the color Doppler studies included in this chapter.

REFERENCES

1. Comerota AJ, Katz ML, Grossi RJ, White JV, Czeredarczuk M, Bowman G, DeSai S, Vujic I: The comparative value of noninvasive testing for diagnosis and surveillance of deep vein thrombosis. J Vasc Surg 1988;7:40–49.
2. Sumner DS: Diagnosis of deep venous thrombosis. In Rutherford RB, ed: Vascular Surgery, 3rd ed. Philadelphia, WB Saunders Company, 1989;1520–1560.
3. Patterson RB, Fowl RJ, Keller JD, Shomaker W, Kempczinski RF: The limitations of impedence

plethysmography in the diagnosis of acute deep venous thrombosis. J Vasc Surg 1989;*9*:725–730.

4. Comerota AJ, Katz ML, Greenwald LL, Leefmans E, Czeredarczuk M, White JV: Venous duplex imaging: Should it replace hemodynamic tests for deep venous thrombosis. J Vasc Surg 1990;*11*:53–61.

5. Barnes RW, Nix ML, Barnes CL, Lavender RC, Golden WE, Harmon BH, Ferris EJ, Nelson CL: Perioperative aymptomattic venous thrombosis: Role of duplex scanning versus venography. J Vasc Surg 1989;*99*:251–260.

6. Flinn WR, Sandager GP, Cerullo LJ, Havey RJ, Yao JST: Duplex venous scanning for the prospective surveillance of perioperative venous thrombosis. Arch Surg 1989;*124*:901–905.

7. Killewich LA, Bedford GR, Beach KW, Strandness DE: Diagnosis of deep venous thrombosis: A prospective study comparing duplex scanning to contrast venography. Circulation 1989;*79*:810–814.

8. Lewis BD, James M, Welch TJ: Current applications of duplex and color Doppler ultrasound imaging: Carotid and peripheral vascular system. Mayo Clin Proc 1989;*64*:1147–1157.

9. Foley WD, Middleton WD, Lawson TL, Erickson S, Quiroz FA, Macrander S: Color Doppler ultrasound imaging of lower-extremity venous disease. AJR 1989;*152*:371–376.

10. Polak JF, Culter SS, O'Leary DH: Deep veins of the calf: Assessment with color Doppler flow imaging. Radiology 1989;*171*:481–485.

11. van Bemmelen PS, Bedford G, Strandness DE: Visualization of calf veins by color flow imaging. Ultrasound Med Biol 1990;*16*:15–17.

12. Persson AV, Jones C, Zide R, Jewell ER: Use of triplex scanner in diagnosis of deep venous thrombosis. Arch Surg 1989;*124*:593–596.

13. Knudson GJ, Wiedmeyer DA, Erickson SJ, Foley WD, Lawson TL, Mewissen MW, Lipchik EO: Color Doppler sonographic imaging in the assessment of upper-extremity deep venous thrombosis. AJR 1990;*154*:399–403.

14. Knighton R, Priest D, Miller F, Lawrence P, Zwiebel W, Brown J: Lower extremity venous examination with color Doppler flow. AngioDynogram (Quantum Medical Systems Inc, Issaquah, WA) 1990;Winter.

15. Rollins DL, Semrow CM, Friedell ML, Calligaro KD, Buchbinder D: Progress in the diagnosis of deep venous thrombosis: The efficacy of real-time B-mode ultrasonic scanning. J Vasc Surg 1988;*7*:638–641.

16. Elias A, Le Corff G, Bouvier JL, Benichou M, Serradimigni A: Value of real time B mode ultrasound imaging in the diagnosis of deep vein thrombosis of the lower limbs. Int Angiol 1987;*6*:175–182.

17. Strandness DE, Langlois Y, Cramer M, Randlett A, Thiele BL: Long-term sequelae of acute venous thrombosis. JAMA 1983;*250*:1289–1292.

18. Moore DJ, Himmel PD, Sumner DS: Distribution of venous valvular incompetence in patients with the postphlebitic syndrome. J Vasc Surg 1986;*3*:49–57.

6

METHODS OF QUANTITATION OF CHRONIC VENOUS INSUFFICIENCY

Andrew N. Nicolaides and Dimitris C. Christopoulos

The symptoms of chronic venous insufficiency are produced by venous hypertension, which is itself the result of obstruction, reflux, or a combination of the two. Venous hypertension results in dilatation of the capillaries with an increased leakage of plasma, plasma proteins, and even red cells. Pericapillary fibrin deposits impair oxygen transport, with eventual hypoxia, ischemia, fat necrosis, skin pigmentation, and ulceration.

Outflow obstruction is found in patients who had deep venous thrombosis without adequate subsequent recanalization and poor development of a collateral circulation. Less frequently it is the result of extramural venous compression. Reflux is found when the valves are damaged either because of venous thromboses followed by recanalization or by dilatation of the vein so that the valve cusps can no longer come in contact with each other.

Varicose veins are often associated with deep-to-superficial reflux because of valvular incompetence of the superficial or communicating system, usually from venous dilatation without previous thrombosis (primary varicose veins). Less often, this association results from valvular damage by thrombosis and recanalization, giving rise to incompetent deep and perforating veins (secondary varicose veins).

Reflux in the deep veins is usually the result of venous thrombosis and recanalization with destruction of the venous valves; more rarely, it is idiopathic. However, recent studies using descending venography have indicated that idiopathic reflux due to "floppy" valve cusps can be found in as many as 30 per cent of cases. This is important because such valves are amenable to valvuloplasty.

Two compensatory physiologic mechanisms exist that tend to ameliorate the effects of venous hypertension. These are the lymphatic drainage and the body's natural fibrinolytic activity. It has been demonstrated that the rate of lymphatic drainage in postthrombotic limbs may be increased up to 10 times, and the fibrinolytic activity that removes the pericapillary fibrin markedly varies between individuals. It is now believed that the development of edema, skin changes, and ulceration is the result of a delicate balance between the severity of venous hypertension and the compensatory mechanisms.

Clinical examination with the classic Trendelenburg and Perthes tourniquet tests can be misleading or impossible when varicose veins are not prominent and can offer relatively little information about the state of the deep veins (obstruction or reflux), although in extreme conditions with a history of pain on walking (venous claudication), severe swelling, and prominent veins over the lower abdominal wall, the diagnosis is obvious. The authors have seen patients whose symptoms became worse after an operation on varicose veins that were acting as collaterals in the presence of undiagnosed and unsuspected deep venous obstruction (often in the superficial femoral vein). Also, we have observed a large number of "recurrent" varicose veins after operation on varicose veins that did not deal with an unsuspected incompetent short saphenous vein.

For these reasons a number of diagnostic investigations have been developed during the last few years. They provide qualitative and quantitative information and can offer answers to most questions posed in a clinical practice. The difficulty is in deciding when to use these methods and how to interpret the results. The aim of this chapter is to provide a brief account of these investigations, outlining their usefulness and limitations and indicating which patients should be subjected to them.

ASCENDING VENOGRAPHY

Ascending venography displays the anatomy and can give an indication of the basic abnormality. Unfortuntely it cannot provide quantitative measurements of any abnormality. The main reason for doing venograms is to confirm the presence and extent of outflow obstruction with visualization of the extent of collateral circulation and sites of reflux.

Until recently venography had been considered to be the "gold standard" for anatomic visualization. However, the development of high-resolution, real-time ultrasonographic imaging equiqment combined with Doppler ultrasound (see "Duplex Scanning" later in this chapter) is now producing a new noninvasive gold standard. The availability of a number of noninvasive techniques that can provide quantitative measurements of the severity of obstruction and reflux and that can be used in combination with duplex scanning answer almost all the questions posed, so that venography tends to be performed in an increasingly smaller number of patients. In the authors' practice it is performed in only 3 to 4 per cent of all patients with venous problems.

DESCENDING VENOGRAPHY

The aim of descending venography is to assess the extent of reflux and by inference the degree of valvular damage in the deep veins of the lower limb. The patient is placed in the 60 degree semi-upright position (1). An 18-gauge end-hole venous catheter is positioned in the common femoral vein at the level of the pubic bone. Repeated boluses of isoosmolar contrast are injected. The competence of the common femoral, superficial femoral, profunda femoris, and popliteal veins as well as the saphenofemoral junction is assessed by determing the extent of distal reflux of the contrast material. Initially the examiner looks for spontaneous

TABLE 6–1.   Grades of Reflux in the Deep Veins on Descending Venography[a]

Grade 0:	No reflux below the confluence of the superficial and profunda femoris veins, i.e., the uppermost valve of the superficial femoral vein is competent.
Grade 1:	Reflux beyond the uppermost valve of the superficial femoral vein, but not below the middle of the thigh.
Grade 2:	Reflux into the superficial femoral vein to the level of the knee. Popliteal valves competent.
Grade 3:	Reflux to a level just below the knee. Incompetent popliteal valves but competent valves in the axial calf veins.
Grade 4:	Reflux through the axial veins (femoral, popliteal and calf veins) to the level of the ankle.

[a] From Herman RJ, Neiman HL, Yao JST, Egan TJ, Bergan JJ, Malave SR: Descending venography: A method of evaluating lower extremity valvular function. Radiology 1980: *137*:63.

reflux; subsequently the patient is asked to do a Valsalva maneuver and then plantarflex the foot gently and not against resistance.

Grades of Reflux

Five grades of reflux (0 through 4) have been described (1,2) (Table 6–1). Although pathologic reflux through the popliteal vein has been shown to be associated with symptoms, the association is not clear cut. For example, in one study reflux through the popliteal vein was found in one in five limbs with skin changes or ulceration and in only 31 per cent of postphlebitic limbs (2). The poor association between popliteal reflux and symptoms is probably due to the following two reasons, in addition to technical errors. It is now well established that skin changes and ulceration can often occur in the presence of reflux in the superficial veins only, provided the retrograde flow at peak reflux exceeds 7 ml/sec (3) (see later in chapter). It has also been demonstrated that competent popliteal valves do not exclude postphlebitic changes, which may be the result of reflux in the tibial veins and incompetent calf perforating veins (4). Unfortunately, the technique of descending venography as described previously will fail to demonstrate reflux in the tibial veins in the presence of competent popliteal or more proximal valves.

The development of duplex scanning ultrasonographic equipment (see "Doppler Ultrasound" later in this chapter) has now provided us with a noninvasive method that can not only detect, but also quantitate reflux in individual veins, so that in the authors' practice descending venography is no longer necessary unless one is looking for floppy valves with a view to valvuloplasty.

AMBULATORY VENOUS PRESSURE MEASUREMENTS

The original observation made in the 1940s of a decrease in venous pressure in the foot during walking (5), and the gradual recovery of venous pressure to the resting value when walking stopped, became the basis of ambulatory venous pressure (AVP) measurements used to supplement the anatomic information provided by venography. In recent years, AVP measurements became the hemodynamic gold standard used in the development of noninvasive methods for screening and

TABLE 6–2. The Incidence of Ulceration (Active or Healed) in Relation to Ambulatory Venous Pressure (AVP) in 251 Limbs[a]

NO. OF LIMBS	AVP (mm Hg)	INCIDENCE OF ULCERATION (%)
34	<30	0
44	31–40	12
51	41–50	20
45	51–60	38
34	61–70	57
28	71–80	68
15	>80	73

[a] From Pollack AA, Wood EH: Venous pressure in the saphenous vein in ankle in man during exercise and changes in posture. J Appl Physiol 1949; *1*:649.

diagnostic evaluation (6). The correlation of AVP with the incidence of ulceration is shown in Table 6–2.

In the presence of severe outflow obstruction and deep venous reflux (including reflux in the popliteal vein) the value of AVP may actually increase during exercise because of the increased blood flow as a result of the exercise hyperemia. This is the group of patients who complain of ''bursting'' pain on walking (venous claudication) despite the presence of competent popliteal valves.

Because the measurement of AVP is invasive, it cannot be repeated frequently nor can it be used as a screening test. It is for this reason that noninvasive screening tests such as plethysmography, Doppler ultrasound, calf volume plethysmography, foot volumetry, and duplex scanning have been developed.

NONINVASIVE VENOUS INVESTIGATIONS

Doppler Ultrasound

Continuous-wave Doppler ultrasound is a useful test for the detection of reflux at the saphenofemoral and saphenopopliteal junctions. It has become an established technique used as a routine in the outpatient clinic because it provides a quick and inexpensive noninvasive method of assessment of the veins of the leg. However, expectations that it would be useful in the detection and localization of incompetent thigh and calf perforating veins were proved false by several studies in the 1970s (7–9).

One of the limitations of continuous-wave Doppler ultrasound is that it cannot insonate an individual vessel selectively; rather, it detects velocity from any artery or vein lying in the path of the ultrasonic beam. For example, at the level of the groin reflux can be in a tributary of the long saphenous vein, the long saphenous vein itself, or the common femoral vein. In these cases Doppler ultrasound cannot identify the exact site of reflux nor can it detect a double long saphenous or femoral vein. In the popliteal fossa, although Doppler ultrasound can detect reflux it cannot detect the level of termination of the short saphenous vein (10,11). Reflux in the gastrocnemius or the Giacomini vein can give false-positive results, indicating deep venous reflux despite the presence of competent popliteal valves. These deficiencies have now been overcome by duplex scanning.

Photoplethysmography

Photoplethysmography is a noninvasive technique that can detect changes in the blood content of tissues and has found its principal use in the study of blood flow and blood volume changes in the skin. Although the skin is essentially opaque to light, slight light transmission and backscattering in the range of the visible and infrared spectrum does occur. In practice, a probe consisting of a light source and a light-sensitive diode is positioned on the skin. Changes in the number of red cells in the dermis affect the backscatter of light and are detected by the light-sensitive probe. Such changes are produced by alterations in venous pressure caused by changes in limb position or by proximal venous occlusion. Photoplethysmography has found relatively little application because of the inability to calibrate the signal, unless one is using time measurements such as the postexercise refilling time. When the refilling time was measured using both photoplethysmography and venous pressure simultaneously in two studies (12,13) a high degree of linear correlation was found (R = .93 and R = .88, respectively).

It should be pointed out that, although the refilling time without and with occlusion of the superficial veins can provide a means of distinguishing between normal limbs, limbs with superficial venous incompetence, and limbs with deep venous incompetence (Table 6–3 and Fig. 6–1), it is not a quantitative index of the severity of deep venous insufficiency. This is demonstrated by Figure 6–2, in which the refilling time is plotted against AVP (venous pressure at the end of exercise). Although the AVP may be from 45 to 100 mm Hg, the refilling time is short (2 to 10 sec) and has no relationship to the AVP.

Duplex Scanning

Duplex scanning, used in the early 1980s for the diagnosis of deep venous thrombosis (14–16), has now been extended to the study of venous valve function (17–19) and venous reflux (20). It has proven to be more accurate than continuous-wave Doppler ultrasound because it not only can detect the presence or absence of reflux at anatomically identified sites but can also provide a quantitative measurement of the severity of such reflux.

Duplex scanning allows the examiner to visualize the venous system in real

TABLE 6–3. Photoplethysmographic Refilling Time (RT) without and with an Ankle Cuff to Occlude Superficial Veins[a]

	REFILLING TIME (sec) (PATIENT STANDING)	
	No Cuff	**Cuff Inflated**
Normal limbs	18–80[b]	18–80
Primary varicose veins[c]	5–18	18–50
Deep venous incompetence	3–12	6–18[d]

[a] From Szendro G, Nicolaides AN, Zukowski AJ, Christopoulos D, Malouf GM, Christodoulou D, Myers A: Duplex scanning in the assessment of deep venous incompetence. J Vasc Surg 1986; 4:237.
[b] RT greater than 18 sec without cuff identifies normal limbs.
[c] Limbs with primary varicose veins have RT less than 18 sec without cuff and RT greater than 18 sec with ankle cuff inflated.
[d] RT less than 18 sec with cuff identifies limbs with deep venous incompetence.

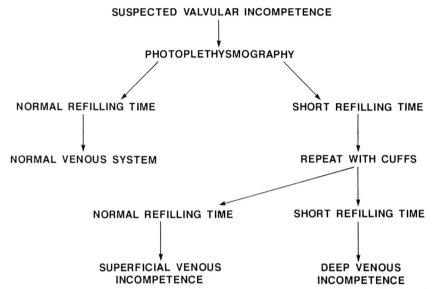

Figure 6–1. Algorithm showing how the refilling time and its changes with the application of cuffs to occlude the superficial veins is a practical diagnostic tool.

time, identify individual veins, position the sample volume of gated Doppler in them, and test for reflux by calf compression and release. Reflux is the effect of gravity, and therefore the patient is examined standing. The ability of duplex scanning to detect reflux in individual veins has demonstrated, for the first time, that reflux can be regional or involve the whole deep venous system. Reflux may

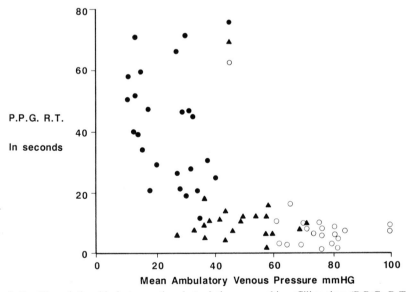

Figure 6–2. The relationship between the photoplethysmographic refilling time (P.P.G. R.T.) and the mean ambulatory venous pressure obtained in the standing position after 10 tiptoes. ● = normal limbs; ▲ = superficial venous incompetence; ○ = deep venous incompetence. Note that for AVP ranging between 45 and 100 mm Hg, the PPG refilling time remains in the same abnormal range (1–10 sec) (20).

be localized in the femoral vein. In the presence of competent popliteal valves such reflux consists of blood flowing down the femoral vein and out to the superficial system through thigh perforating veins. Also, regional reflux can be confined to the tibial veins, usually in the presence of large and multiple incompetent calf perforating veins.

Duplex scanning has made it possible to quantify reflux in individual veins. In a recent study (21), the measurement of retrograde flow (milliliters per second) at peak reflux in the axial veins (long saphenous, short saphenous, and femoropopliteal) has been made in 47 limbs of patients who presented with chronic venous problems (varicose veins, skin changes, and/or ulceration). The results indicate that skin changes or ulceration do not occur when the sum of peak reflux in all the veins is less than 10 ml/sec. The incidence of skin changes and/or ulceration is high when peak reflux exceeds 10 ml/sec irrespective of whether such reflux is in the superficial or the deep veins.

Air Plethysmography

Air plethysmography was used in the early 1960s to study relative volume changes in the lower limb in response to postural alterations and muscular exercise (22). Recent interest in reconstructive surgery of the deep veins has created a need for noninvasive quantitative assessment of venous reflux and calf muscle pump ejection. By calibrating air plethysmography it has become possible to detect whole leg volume changes as a result of exercise in absolute (milliliters) as well as relative units, overcoming the limitations of segmental devices and water plethysmography (3). Segmental volume changes measured with a strain gauge do not necessarily represent changes in the whole leg, and although water plethysmography can provide information on the whole leg, it cannot be used with exercise such as tiptoeing or walking. In addition, gravitationally induced tissue shifts in response to postural changes that interefere with segmental devices on the calf are less likely to occur with air plethysmography because the latter includes all the tissues between the knee and ankle.

The air plethysmograph consists of a 35-cm long tubular polyvinyl chloride air chamber (capacity 5 liters) that surrounds the whole leg from knee to ankle (Fig. 6–3). This is inflated to a pressure of 6 mm Hg and connected to a pressure transducer, amplifier, and recorder. The pressure of 6 mm Hg is the lowest that ensures good contact between the air chamber and the leg. Calibration is performed by depressing the plunger of the syringe (Fig. 6–3), compressing the air in the system (reducing its volume by 100 ml), and observing the corresponding pressure change. The plunger is then pulled back to its original position when the pressure in the air chamber returns to 6 mm Hg.

Initially, the patient is in the supine position with the leg elevated (45 degrees) to empty the veins and the heel resting on a support. After a stable baseline recording is obtained, the subject is asked to stand with the weight on the opposite leg, holding onto an orthopedic frame. An increase in the leg venous volume is observed as a result of the venous filling (Fig. 6–4). This increase is 100 to 150 ml in normal limbs and 100 to 350 ml in limbs with chronic venous insufficiency. The venous filling index (VFI) is defined as the ratio of 90 per cent of the venous volume (VV) divided by the time taken to achieve 90 per cent of filling (VFT_{90}) ($VFI = 90\% \ VV/VFT_{90}$). This is a measure of the average filling rate and is ex-

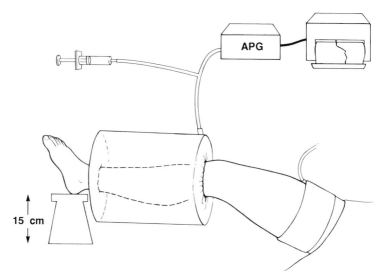

Figure 6–3. Air plethysmograph (APG) consists of a polyvinyl chloride air chamber (5-liter capacity) and a calibration syringe connected to a pressure transducer, amplifier, and recorder.

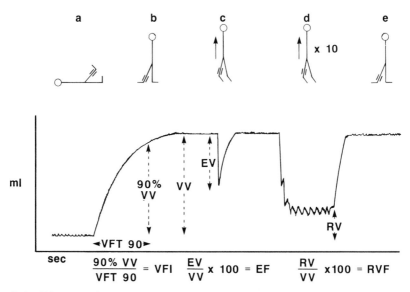

Figure 6–4. Diagrammatic representation of typical recording of volume changes during standard sequence of postural changes and exercise. Patient in supine position with leg elevated 45 degrees (*a*); patient standing with weight on nonexamined leg (*b*); single tiptoe movement (*c*); 10 tiptoe movements (*d*); return to resting standing position as in *b* (*e*). *VV*, functional venous volume; *VFT*, venous filling time; *VFI*, venous filling index; *EV*, ejected volume; *RV*, residual volume; *EF*, ejection fraction; *RVF*, residual volume fraction. (From Christopoulos DC, Nicolaides AN, Szendro G, Irvine AT, Bull M, Eastcott HHG: Air-plethysmography and the effect of elastic compression on venous haemodynamics of the leg. J Vasc Surg 1987;5:148)

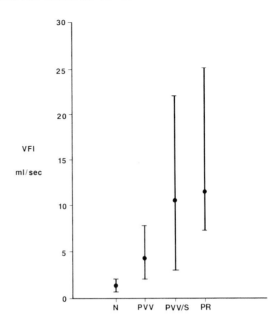

Figure 6–5. Venous filling index (*VFI*) (median and 90 per cent range) in normal (*N*) limbs, limbs with primary varicose veins without sequelae of chronic venous disease (liposclerosis and ulceration) (*PVV*), limbs with primary varicose veins with sequelae of chronic venous disease (*PVV/S*), and limbs with popliteal reflux (*PR*). (From Christopoulos DC, et al: Br J Surg 1988;75:352.)

pressed in milliliters per second. The range of VFI in normal limbs, limbs with superficial venous incompetence, and limbs with deep venous disease is shown in Figure 6–5. A VFI of 2 ml/sec or less indicates absence of significant venous reflux and that the veins are filling slowly from the arterial circulation. A VFI greater than 7 ml/sec is associated with a high incidence of skin changes, chronic swelling, and ulceration irrespective of whether the reflux is in the superficial venous system only or in the deep system. The application of a narrow pneumatic tourniquet (2.5 cm wide) that occludes the superficial veins at the knee (long and short saphenous) will reduce the VFI to less than 5 ml/sec in limbs with primary varicose veins and competent popliteal valves but not in limbs with incompetent popliteal valves on duplex scan (23). Also, measurements before and after conventional surgery for superficial venous incompetence have shown that air pleth-

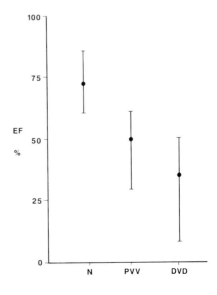

Figure 6–6. Ejection fraction (*EF*) (median and 90 per cent range) in normal limbs (*N*), limbs with primary varicose veins (*PVV*), and limbs with deep venous disease (*DVD*).

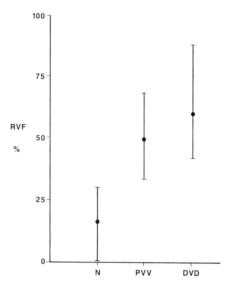

Figure 6–7. Residual volume fraction (*RVF*) (mean and 90 per cent range) in normal limbs (*N*), limbs with primary varicose veins (*PVV*), and limbs with deep venous disease.

ysmography is an effective method for demonstrating the abolition of venous reflux (23).

By asking the patient to do one tiptoe movement with the weight on both legs and then return to the initial position, one can measure the ejected volume (EV) (Fig. 6–4) and ejection fraction (EF) [=(EV/VV)×100] as a result of the calf muscle contraction. The range of EF in normal limbs, limbs with primary varicose veins, and limbs with deep venous disease is shown in Figure 6–6. Also, by asking the patient to do 10 tiptoe movements one can measure the residual volume (RV) and calculate the residual volume fraction (RVF) [=(RV/VV)×100] (Fig. 6–4). The range of RVF in different limbs is shown in Figure 6–7. It has been demonstrated that there is a good linear correlation between RVF and AVP at the end of exercise (Fig. 6–8). This is hardly surprising because, at any time, it is the amount of blood in the veins that determines the venous pressure. Table 6–4 shows how the incidence of ulceration increases in relation to the RVF.

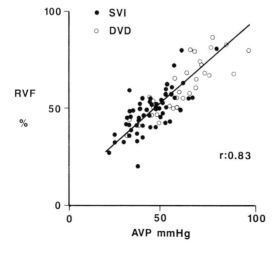

Figure 6–8. Relationship between residual volume fraction (*RVF*) and ambulatory venous pressure (*AVP*) at the end of 10 tiptoe movements. *SVI*, limbs with superficial venous incompetence; *DVD*, limbs with deep venous disease. (From Christopoulos DC, Nicolaides AN, Szendro G, Irvine AT, Bull M, Eastcott HHG: Air-plethysmography and the effect of elastic compression on venous haemodynamics of the leg. J Vasc Surg 1987;5:148.)

TABLE 6–4. Incidence of Ulceration in Relation to Residual Volume Fraction (RVF) of Calf Muscle Pump in 175 Limbs with Venous Disease[a]

RVF (%)	NO. OF LIMBS	INCIDENCE OF ULCERATION (%)
<30	20	0
31–40	24	8
41–50	48	27
51–60	43	42
61–80	32	72
>80	8	88

[a] From Christopoulos D, Nicholaides AN, Cook A, Irving A, Galloway JMD, Wilkinson A: Pathogenesis venous alteration in relation to the cuff muscle pump function. J Surg 1989;*106*:829.

These volume measurements have been used to study the efficacy of the calf muscle pump and quantitatively assess the effect of therapeutic measures such as compression and surgical intervention. They should be used not only to assess the effects of deep venous reconstruction, but also to select the patients who are most suitable for such reconstruction.

PATIENT EVALUATION

The evaluation of patients with chronic venous problems consists first of determining the presence or absence of outflow obstruction and/or reflux in the venous system. The history and clinical examination will indicate the patient's problems and clinical picture. The use of Doppler ultrasound in outpatients by the physician will confirm the presence of obstruction and/or reflux, indicating the site (obstruction: femoropopliteal or iliofemoral; reflux: saphenofemoral junction, saphenopopliteal junction, thigh incompetent perforating veins, or popliteal) in 90 per cent of patients. The remaining 10 per cent will consist of complicated cases many of whom had previous operations on their veins or cases in which the results of Doppler ultrasound are not clear; also, there may be a small group in whom incompetent calf perforating veins are suspected and their presence needs to be confirmed.

Outflow Obstruction

Outflow obstruction may be suspected because swelling is the predominant symptom; the swelling may be associated with a history of deep venous thrombosis and the finding of prominent collateral venous channels in the groin above the pubis or the anterior abdominal wall. Outflow obstruction should always be suspected and investigated in patients with postthrombotic limbs.

Simple leg elevation with the patient supine can provide an estimated of the resting venous pressure by observing the height (in centimeters) of the heel from the heart-level at which the prominent veins collapse.

Doppler Ultrasound

Doppler ultrasound examination with the legs horizontal and the trunk of the patient semisupine (45 degrees), as for deep venous thrombosis, may indicate occlusion of the deep veins by the absence of flow that is phasic with respiration, the absence of augmented flow on calf compression, or the presence of suprapubic collateral flow that is abolished by manual compression of the femoral vein in the opposite groin.

Assessment of Functional Severity of Obstruction

Confirmation of deep venous obstruction and the extent of collateral circulation is obtained by venography. However, the functional severity of the obstruction is difficult to assess from the venogram. Quantitative measurements [maximum venous outflow (MVO)] can be obtained using strain-gauge plethysmography or air plethysmography, and also by measuring the foot-to-arm pressure differential.

In order to measure MVO a thigh cuff is inflated with the limb elevated 10 degrees and the veins are allowed to fill. The cuff is suddenly deflated and measurements are made from the outflow curve. The authors have used strain-gauge plethysmography and the 1-sec outflow method. In our hands normal limbs have an MVO greater than 45 ml/100 ml/min. Measurements of MVO with strain-gauge plethysmography are useful not only in determining the severity of outflow obstruction, but also in following up the development of collateral circulation. In approximately 90 per cent of patients who have an abnormally low MVO soon after deep venous thrombosis, values close to the lower limit of normal will be found 1 year later, presumably because of recanalization and development of collateral channels. However, in 10 per cent of patients the MVO will remain grossly abnormal, and it is these patients who are severely incapacitated, often from persisting venous claudication.

More recently the 1-sec venous outflow has been measured using air plethysmography. It has been found that this is more than 40 per cent of the venous volume in normal limbs. It is 30 to 40 per cent in limbs with mild to moderate obstruction and less than 30 per cent in limbs with severe obstruction.

The arm-foot pressure differential has been used by Raju as another method of assessing the severity of outflow obstruction (24). This method consists of recording the venous pressure in the foot and hand simultaneously with the patient in the supine position at rest. The measurements are repeated after inducing reactive hyperemia. In normal limbs the arm-foot pressure differential (ΔP) is less than 5 mm Hg; a rise of up to 6 mm Hg is observed during reactive hyperemia. Patients with venographic evidence of obstruction and ΔP<5 mm Hg at rest and an increment of less than 6 mm Hg during reactive hyperemia is considered to be fully compensated (grade I). Using such measurements Raju has classified limbs with outflow obstruction into four grades (Table 6–5).

The measurement of MVO (by plethysmography) or arm-foot pressure differential can provide a quantitative indication of the severity of outflow obstruction. The main usefulness may prove to be in the objective study of the natural history and efficacy of surgical reconstructive procedures aiming to improve outflow.

Testing and Patient Management

Accurate localization of venous obstruction because of contemplated surgery will require a venogram, although duplex scanning is proving equally helpful,

TABLE 6–5. Arm-Foot Pressure Differential in Limbs with Outflow Obstruction[a]

GRADE	ΔP (mm Hg) AT REST	PRESSURE INCREMENT DURING HYPEREMIA
I Fully compensated	<5	<6
II Partially compensated	<5	>6
III Partially decompensated	>5	>6 (often 10–15)
IV Fully decompensated	≥5 (often 15–20)	No further increase

[a] From Raju S: New approaches to the diagnosis and treatment of venous obstruction. J Vasc Surg 1986; *4*:42.

particularly for lesions distal to the common femoral vein. Until recently, accurate localization of the sites of deep-to-superficial reflux (saphenofemoral, saphenopopliteal, incompetent thigh perforating veins, calf perforating veins) and reflux in the deep veins (femoral, popliteal, tibial) could only be achieved by venography. Duplex scanning is proving to be a simpler and functionally more accurate test, so that ascending functional or descending venography is now rarely performed. With regard to localization of the site of incompetent perforating veins and the junction of the short saphenous with the popliteal vein, duplex scanning is the method of choice.

These tests and the answers they provide to whether and where obstruction and/or reflux are present are more than sufficient for the rational planning of management. However, quantitative measurements of outflow obstruction and/or reflux are needed for research purposes, particularly for the study of the natural history of patients with different forms of chronic venous insufficiency and for the assessment of established and new methods of treatment. These quantitative measurements have now opened new avenues leading to a better scientific basis for the management of patients.

Until recently, the measurement of AVP had been the only quantitative test available. It was invasive, but it provided an indication of the severity of venous hypertension. It was a measure of the end result of both outflow obstruction and reflux. However, the new tests can separate and dissect out the relative contribution of different abnormalities such as venous obstruction, reflux in the superficial veins, and/or reflux in the deep veins. Also, these tests can assess the function of the calf muscle pump, and determine whether poor function is the result of intrinsic venous disease, a musculoskeletal problem, or both.

REFERENCES

1. Herman RJ, Neiman HL, Yao JST, Egan TJ, Bergan JJ, Malave SR: Descending venography: A method of evaluating lower extremity valvular function. Radiology 1980;*137*:63.
2. Ackroyd JS, Lea Thomas M, Browse NL: Deep vein reflux: An assessment by descending venography. Br J Surg 1986;*73*:31.
3. Christopoulos DC, Nicolaides AN, Szendro G, Irvine AT, Bull M, Eastcott HHG: Air-plethysmography and the effect of elastic compression on venous haemodynamics of the leg. J Vasc Surg 1987;*5*:148.
4. Moore DJ, Himmel PD, Sumner DS: Distribution of venous valvular incompetence in patients with post-phlebitic syndrome. J Vasc Surg 1986;*3*:49.
5. Pollack AA, Wood EH: Venous pressure in the saphenous vein in ankle in man during exercise and changes in posture. J Appl Physiol 1949;*1*:649.

6. Nicolaides AN, Zukowski AJ: The value of dynamic venous pressure measurements. World J Surg 1986;*10*:919.

7. Folse R, Alexander RH: Directional flow detection for localising venous valvular incompetence. Surgery 1970;*67*:114.

8. Miller SS, Foote AV: The ultrasonic detection of incompetent perforating veins. Br J Surg, 1974;*58*:872.

9. O'Donnell J, Burnand KG, Clemenson G, Lea Thomas M, Browse NL: Doppler examination vs clinical and phlebographic detection of the location of incompetent perforating veins. Arch Surg 1977;*112*:31.

10. Hoare MC, Royle JP: Doppler ultrasound detection of saphenofemoral and sapheno-popliteal incompetence and operative venography to ensure precise sapheno-popliteal ligation. Aust NZ J Surg 1984;*54*:49.

11. Vasdekis S, Tonnison H, Hobbs JT, Nicolaides AN: A comparison of duplex scanning, Doppler ultrasound and perioperative venography in assessing the termination of the short saphenous vein. European-American Symposium on Venous Diseases, Washington DC, 31 March–2 April, 1987 (abstr 25ii.).

12. Abramowitz HB, Queral LA, Flinn WR, Nora PF, Peterson LK, Bergan JJ, Yao JST: The use of photoplethysmography in the assessment of venous insufficiency. A comparison to venous pressure measurements. Surgery 1979;*86*:434.

13. Nicolaides AN, Miles C: Photoplethysmography in the assessment of venous insufficiency. J Vasc Surg 1987;*5*:405.

14. Flanigan LD, Sullivan ED, Cranley JJ: Venous imaging of the extremities using real-time B-mode ultrasound. *In* Bergan JJ, Yao JST, eds: Surgery of the Veins. Orlando, FL. Grune & Stratton Inc, 1984;89–98.

15. Hannan LJ, Stedje KJ, Skorez MJ, Karkow WS, Flanigan LD, Cranley JJ: Venous imaging of the extremities: Our twenty-five hundred cases. Bruit 1986;*10*:29.

16. Sullivan ED, David JP, Cranley JJ: Real-time B-mode venous ultrasound. J Vasc Surg 1984;*1*:465.

17. Jaeger K, Bollinger A: Evaluation of venous wall and valve motion. *In* Negus D, Jantet G, eds: Phlebology '85. London, John Libbey and Co, 1986;320–323.

18. Rollins DS, Ryan TJ, Semrow C, Buchbinder D: Characterisation of lower extremity chronic disease using real-time ultrasound imaging. *In* Negus D, Jantet G, eds: Phlebology '85. London, John Libbey and Co, 1986;576–579.

19. Semrow C, Ryan TJ, Buchbinder D, Rollins DL: Assessment of valve function using real-time B-mode ultrasound. *In* Negus D, Jantet G, eds: Phlebology '85. London, John Libby and Co, 1986;352–355.

20. Szendro G, Nicholaides AN, Zukowski AJ, Christopoulos D, Malouf GM, Christodoulou D, Myers A: Duplex scanning in the assessment of deep venous incompetence. J Vasc Surg 1986;*4*:237.

21. Vasdekis S: Quantification of venous reflux by means of duplex scanning. J Vasc Surg 1989;*10*:670.

22. Allan JC: Volume changes in the lower limb in response to postural alterations and muscular exercise. S Afr J Surg 1964;*2*:75–90.

23. Christopoulos D, Nicolaides ANN, Galloway JMD, Wilkinson A: Objective noninvasive evaluation of venous surgical results. J Vasc Surg 1988;*8*:683.

24. Raju S: New approaches to the diagnosis and treatment of venous obstruction. J Vasc Surg 1986;*4*:42.

25. Christopoulos D, Nicholaides AN, Cook A, Irving A, Galloway JMD, Wilkinson A: Pathogenesis venous alteration in relation to the cuff muscle pump function. J Surg 1989;*106*:829–835.

7

COMPUTED TOMOGRAPHY AND MAGNETIC RESONANCE IMAGING OF VENOUS DISORDERS

Robert L. Vogelzang

Most pathologic processes affect veins by compression or occlusion. The diagnostic hallmark of venous occlusion is the presence of thrombosis; other important findings on venography include the presence of collateral veins and features that allow differentiation between acute and chronic thrombosis. The ideal imaging technique for venous disease should differentiate between flowing and clotted blood, be able to judge the chronicity of an occlusion, and be able to identify the etiology of the process originally causing the occlusion, specifically whether or not the occluding thrombus is bland or tumorous in nature.

The imaging of large central veins usually relies upon the injection of contrast material through a catheter placed within the vessel lumen. Venography of these veins is invasive and carries with it the known risks of hemorrhage, hematoma, and thrombosis. Additionally, experienced angiographers and vascular surgeons have always recognized that the venous circulation is much more difficult to image well, primarily because inflow of unopacified blood and the relative distensibility and collapsibility of the veins make artifacts and flow defects a constant problem (Fig. 7–1).

The mesenteric venous circulation presents a different problem because it must be viewed by indirect means—arterial portography, the injection of large boluses of contrast material into the arteries supplying the venous circulation—further leading to problems of inadequate detail due to contrast dilution and flow defects. However, modern digital subtraction angiography can considerably reduce this problem by improving both spatial and contrast resolution (Fig. 7–2).

Other imaging techniques, such as radionuclide venography and gray-scale and Doppler ultrasound of peripheral and central veins, have improved the diagnosis of primary and secondary venous disorders, but in the abdomen these techniques have limitations imposed on them by bowel gas in the case of ultrasound and inadequate spatial resolution in the case of radionuclide scanning.

The cross-sectional imaging techniques of computed tomography (CT) and magnetic resonance imaging (MRI) have contributed greatly to our diagnostic ability as it relates to the central veins of the chest and abdomen. CT of the body,

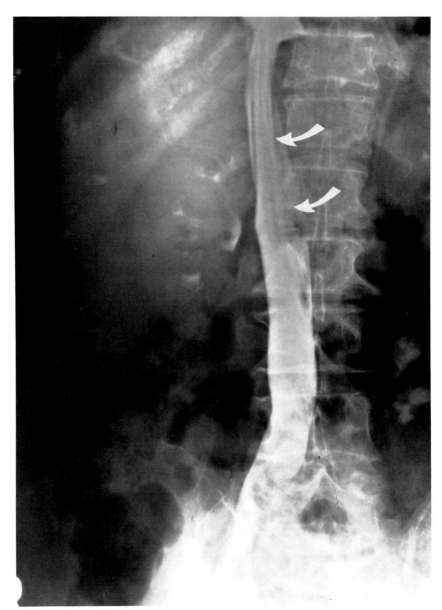

Figure 7–1. Inferior venacavogram demonstrating flow defects from renal veins (arrows) and non-uniform contrast opacification due to unpacified iliac venous blood.

introduced as a practical tool about 12 years ago, has reached a point in its evolution where it is the central diagnostic tool in most processes affecting the visceral organs, although MRI currently participates in the imaging diagnosis of many disorders. MRI, introduced about 6 years ago, has achieved phenomenal success in the field of neuroimaging, where it has largely supplanted CT as the primary imaging technique for most intracranial and intraspinal disease processes. MRI has also proven remarkably effective in the field of bone and joint imaging, where it is now also the preferred technique in many orthopedic and rheumatologic problems. The ability of the tool to detect flow and differentiate between recent

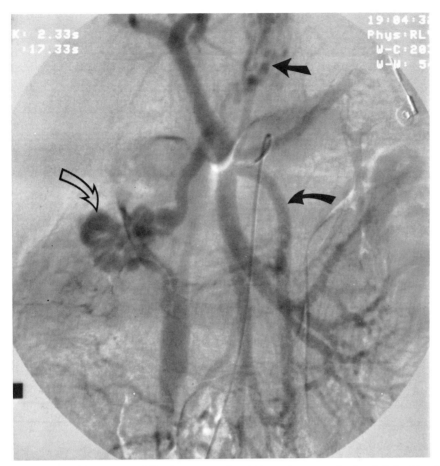

Figure 7–2. Arterial portogram following mesenteric arteriography reported using digital subtraction angiography. Note outstanding visualization of mesenteric and portal veins as well as excellent visualization of a large duodenal varix (curved open arrow) and gastric varices (arrow). Retrograde filling of inferior mesenteric vein (curved closed arrow) is also seen.

and older clots has also implied a larger role in the diagnosis of vascular disorders. This chapter will attempt to highlight the relative contributions of CT and MRI to the diagnosis of disorders that primarily and secondarily affect the large veins of the abdomen and chest.

COMPUTED TOMOGRAPHY

Since its introduction, CT of the body has revolutionized the way medicine is practiced. From the beginning the advantages of the modality in identifying vascular anatomy and pathologic processes affecting it were evident. Early observations about the utility of CT in aortic aneurysm, for example, led to its rapid acceptance as the primary entity for diagnosis of this common disorder (1,2). Descriptions of the appearance of venous thrombosis in the vena cava and mesenteric venous circulation soon followed, along with expositions of variants in caval anatomy and the superiority of CT over arteriography in detecting involvement of the renal veins and inferior cava in renal cell carcinoma (3–7). We have come to rely upon the technique whenever angiographic or venographic findings are confusing or are unclear, and in many vascular disorders have come to rely on it as the sole imaging tool.

Technique

When CT is being performed in a specific search for venous pathology, images obtained both before and after the intravenous administration of contrast are preferred since the diagnosis of some disorders, such as the Budd-Chiari syndrome, is aided by the inclusion of nonenhanced images for reasons discussed later in this chapter. In reality, however, most venous disorders and the processes that cause them are imaged extremely well by contrast-enhanced images alone. We also prefer the use of thin (5-mm) sections when primarily examining vascular structures since this maximizes resolution of the vessel wall and helps avoid some of the problems associated with partial volume averaging.

CT Appearance of Venous Thrombosis

Fresh hemorrhage or clot can be readily distinguished on CT because of its high density on non–contrast-enhanced scans (Fig. 7–3). The higher attenuation of fresh, extravasated, or clotted blood can generally be seen for several days, after which the density gradually diminishes to that of normal soft tissue structures like the aorta. A variety of processes affect the relative density of clot. Age is the most important factor, but clotted blood also is of higher density than unclotted

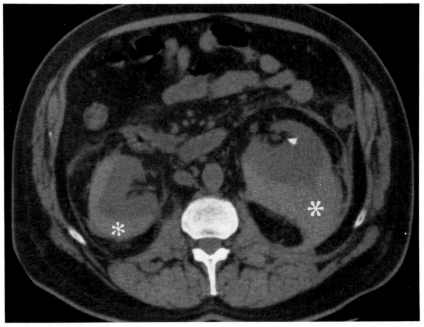

Figure 7–3.   Fresh hemorrhage in subcapsular renal hematoma. Note high-density subcapsular blood characteristic of fresh hemorrhage on noncontrast images.

blood because the higher density components are the cellular elements (8,9). This fact can best be appreciated in a patient who experiences hemorrhage while anticoagulated; the more dependent cellular elements of blood are of higher density (Fig. 7–4). The differences in attenuation values between hemorrhage or clot and other soft tissues, however, are not large, typically on the order of 30 Hounsfield units or less. Thus, the most important determinant in the perceived density of blood is the density of structures surrounding it. This is why the age of thrombotic or hemorrhagic events cannot be accurately judged on contrast-enhanced images; the presence of adjacent, brightly enhancing organs such as the spleen or kidney minimizes the apparent small increase in density in these fluid collections (Fig. 7–5). If the age of an event is an important diagnostic consideration, nonenhanced images should be obtained.

The appearance of vessels that have been enhanced with contrast is readily appreciated. The vessel itself should show uniform contrast enhancement (with a few exceptions). In cases in which contrast enhancement is not as intense as is normally desired, the use of narrow window widths can better demonstrate the vessel. In general, the smallest vessel that can be optimally imaged is about 5 mm in diameter.

Intravascular thrombosis has a highly characteristic appearance on enhanced scans: low-density, intraluminal clot surrounded by the enhancing vessel wall (3) (Fig. 7–6). The appearance is seen in both arterial and venous thrombosis. As indicated, the age of the thrombus usually cannot be determined after intravenous contrast has been given, but some other characteristic signs of chronicity, such as the presence of collaterals and clot retraction, may be seen. Older thrombi may occasionally calcify, and this finding is, of course, readily demonstrable on

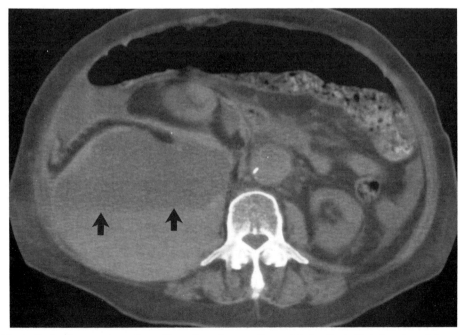

Figure 7–4. Large retroperitoneal hematoma in an anticoagulated patient. Note layering of denser cellular elements posteriorly (arrow).

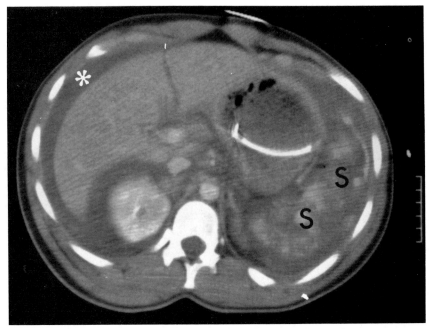

Figure 7–5. Effect of contrast enhancement on perceived density of blood. Fresh hemorrhage was present in this abdomen at the time of surgery. The contrast-enhanced CT, however, shows fluid that appears to be the same density as ascites. Had a precontrast scan been done, this fluid would have appeared much denser.

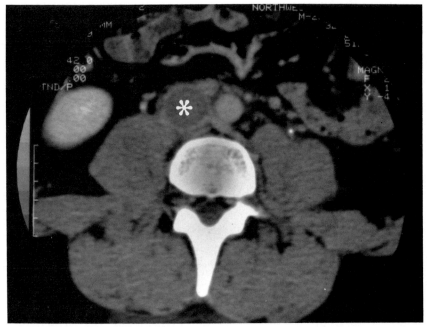

Figure 7–6. Characteristic appearance of inferior vena cava thrombosis on CT. Note enlarged cava with low-density clot and enhanced caval wall (arrow).

CT (10). Other signs of venous occlusion include absent visualization of the vessel itself or replacement by a mass or a lesion in such diseases as renal cell carcinoma or hepatocellular carcinoma. This is particularly true in the large central veins of the chest and abdomen. In the remainder of this section, we will concentrate on the uses of CT in various areas and disease states.

Chest

CT is widely used in diagnosis, staging, and follow-up of benign and malignant diseases of the chest. Some of these disorders affect the mediastinal veins, such as the superior vena cava and its tributaries, the subclavian, and the innominate veins.

Normal Anatomy

While vascular structures are readily seen without the use of intravenous contrast, the diagnosis of thrombosis is quite difficult to make without contrast enhancement. Additionally, differentiation of veins from closely adherent or apposed masses may be virtually impossible without it. Contrast enhancement can, however, introduce some artifacts, particularly since the current trend is to rapidly inject large amounts of contrast via an upper extremity vein. These infusions can cause difficulties in interpretation for the inexperienced observer, but an awareness of the problem and knowledge of techniques for resolving conflicts generally allow accurate diagnoses to be made.

The brachiocephalic veins are anteriorly located vascular structures. The longer left brachiocephalic vein is seen immediately behind the sternum. It joins the right innominate vein to form the superior vena cava, which is well visualized over its vertical course until its termination in the right atrium (Fig. 7–7). The other tributary of the cava, the azygos vein, joins the cava at about the level of the carina (Fig. 7–8). It is this confluence of brachiocephalic veins that causes mixing of contrast-laden blood from the extremity that is being infused and non-opacified blood from the opposite extremity. At their confluence a "pseudo-thrombus" may occur that can be mistaken for caval clot or obstruction, but the very specific appearance and location of the filling defects (in the vena cava just below the venous confluence) usually does not cause confusion. In the rare case in which there is concern about the presence of a clot, delayed scanning after termination of the infusion can resolve the difficulty (11).

Obstruction of the superior vena cava by malignant or benign causes is best imaged with CT. In fact, we recommend that CT be the first test performed when a patient is suspected of having caval occlusion. Not only does CT accurately depict the blockage, but it generally identifies the causative lesion in the form of a tumor or other process (12–14). In our experience, CT accurately depicts both the site of superior vena caval obstruction and important collaterals, and clearly distinguishes between caval thrombosis and external compression. The CT diagnosis of superior vena cava obstruction requires that three criteria be met: 1) intraluminal caval filling defect or extrinsic compression or encasement of major thoracic venous channels is present; 2) collateral venous routes, usually in or around the chest wall, are densely opacified; and 3) there is diminished or absent opacification of central venous structures, such as the innominate vein or superior

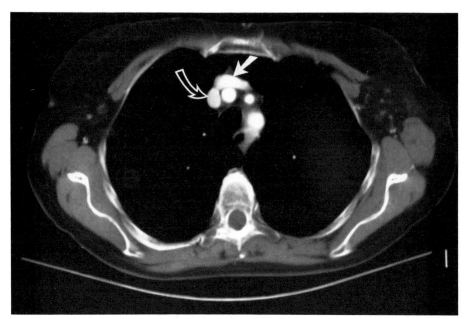

Figure 7–7.   Normal mediastinal anatomy. Note anteriorly located left innominate vein (arrow) joining vena cava (curved arrow). Great vessels are seen posteriorly.

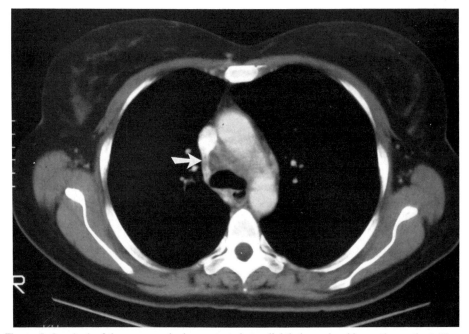

Figure 7–8.   Arch of the azygos vein demonstrated at a slightly lower level in another patient. There is mediastinal tumor, but azygos vein (arrow) is well demonstrated, curving anteriorly to join the cava.

vena cava inferior to the site of obstruction. The azygos vein may also enhance more intensely than usual if the level of obstruction is between the right atrium and the entrance of the azygos vein into the superior vena cava (Fig. 7–9). Similar findings may be seen in obstruction of the innominate or subclavian veins, although thrombus in the vein may not be visualized because of the plane of section through the vein. In situations in which there is unilateral upper extremity swelling, it may be advantageous to infuse contrast material into the affected extremity to better demonstrate collateral vessels.

Moncada and his coworkers have described the superior vena cava syndrome in detail and conclude that CT is the procedure of choice in this condition (14). Yedlicka and colleagues, in a recent review article, stated that superior vena caval obstruction is usually malignant, with 80 to 95 per cent of such cases related to primary or metastatic compression and occlusion (15). They stated that venography is now considered to be of limited value in this entity and that properly performed CT can almost always adequately characterize the abnormalities, particularly since the obstructing mass is shown to optimal advantage. We hold a similar view; at Northwestern Memorial Hospital CT is the procedure of first choice in cases of superior vena cava obstruction. Conventional venography is rarely utilized at our institution.

Pulmonary Embolus

Although CT is not the modality that should be used to investigate pulmonary thromboembolic disorders, central emboli can be seen on enhanced images of the chest (16) (Fig. 7–10). Since CT is frequently ordered when nonspecific chest complaints are encountered, an astute observer may make an important diagnosis. In our experience, we have observed eight cases of pulmonary emboli on CT in the last 5 years. In each case, the event was not suspected clinically.

Cardiac Tumors

CT has been useful for investigation of cardiac tumors. Although two-dimensional echocardiography is the technique of choice in almost every circum-

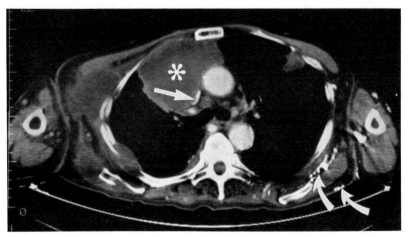

Figure 7–9. Superior vena cava obstruction. Large mediastinal mass compresses and virtually occludes the superior vena cava (arrow). Note extensive filling of chest wall collaterals (curved arrows).

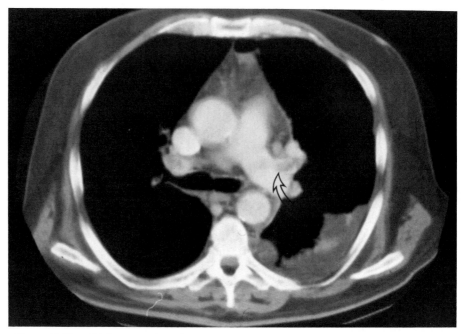

Figure 7–10.   CT demonstration of pulmonary emboli. Note central filling defects (arrows).

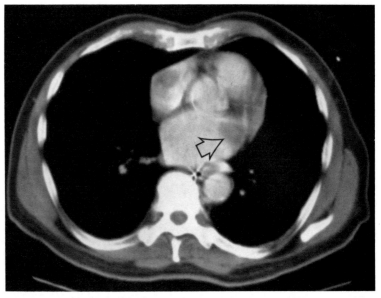

Figure 7–11.   Left atrial thrombus. These thrombi (arrows) were not demonstrated on echocardiography and were a source of repetitive peripheral emboli.

stance, we have had experience with atrial neoplasms and thrombi that have eluded echocardiographic detection and been demonstrated on CT (Fig. 7–11). Other investigators have described similar experiences (17,18).

Anomalies of Mediastinal Veins

CT has proven useful in the detection of congenital abnormalities of the mediastinal veins (19,20). The majority of these anomalies are found incidentally. The most common congenital abnormalities of the unpaired azygos system are azygos and hemiazygos continuation of the inferior vena cava, in which the cava is interrupted by failure of the right subcardinal veins to anastomose with the hepatic veins during fetal development. In these cases, blood from the abdomen returns to the heart via an enlarged azygos vein alone, through a persistent left vena cava, or preferentially into a markedly enlarged accessory hemiazygos system on the right (21–23) (Fig. 7–12). Of course, congenital variants must be distinguished from acquired problems such as thrombosis or compression of the cava, which can also result in azygos system enlargement and flow through alternate pathways. Congenital abnormalities of the superior vena cava including double superior vena cava (the most common anomaly) and absence of the normal right-sided cava with a variety of connections of a left cava to the right atrium (6,7,21,22,24) (Fig. 7–13). Aneurysms of the superior vena cava have also been rarely seen (25).

Abdomen

Primary and secondary pathology of intraabdominal veins is, in general, extremely well detected by CT. In fact, most radiologists prefer CT over venography in the investigation of mesenteric, renal, or ileocaval obstructions. Numerous scientific publications in the last 5 years attest to the efficacy and accuracy of this approach. Each of these three major venous structures will be dealt with here in separate subsections.

Mesenteric and Splanchnic Venous Problems

The diagnosis of splanchnic venous thrombosis is a difficult one because of the protean clinical manifestations and diverse causes of this disorder. Prompt detection is important because portal and mesenteric venous thrombosis accounts for 15 per cent of all cases of mesenteric vascular ischemia, with an estimated mortality rate of 20 per cent (26,27). The definitive nonsurgical diagnosis of portal, splenic, and superior mesenteric venous thrombosis traditionally has been established by arterial portography, splenoportography, and/or transhepatic portography (28–30). In the past 5 years, however, it has become apparent that CT is a very accurate technique for determining the patency of the splanchnic venous circulation. The basic findings are similar to those described elsewhere in the venous and arterial circulation and consist of low-attenuation, intramural clot sharply outlined by an enhanced venous wall (Fig. 7–14). Other signs include enlargement of the affected vein, bowel wall thickening, and mesenteric edema in cases of superior mesenteric venous occlusion with infarction or impending

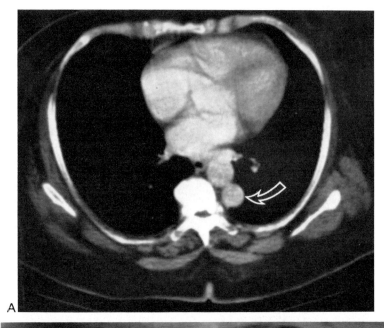

A

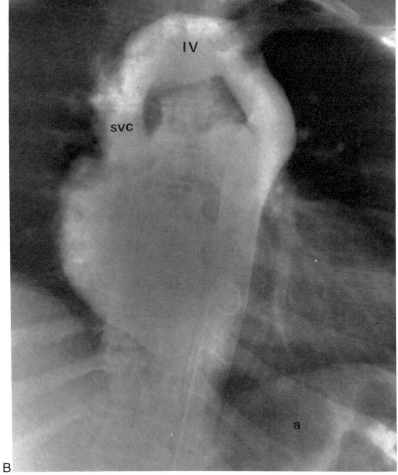

IV

svc

a

B

Figure 7–12. See legend on opposite page.

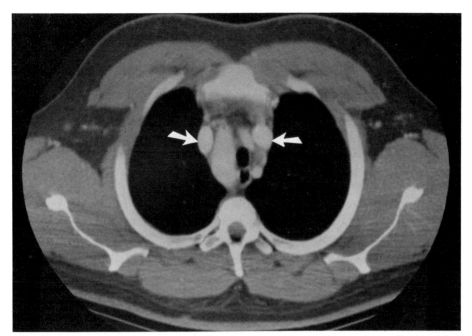

Figure 7–13. Double superior vena cava. Contrast enhanced scan in the superior mediastinum shows double superior vena cavae (arrows). There is mediastinal adenopathy as well.

infarction. Occasionally, the presence of venous collaterals has been noted, particularly in long-standing cases of splenic vein occlusion (31–33).

We have described our experience in CT identification of splanchnic venous occlusion (31). In 14 patients there were diverse etiologies, including coagulopathy, pancreatic carcinoma, cirrhosis, portal hypertension, and hepatocellular carcinoma. We were easily able to identify the thrombosis, which frequently involved more than one vein. When compared to arterial portography in those patients in whom both tests were done, we generally found CT to be more obvious in its detection of the thrombosis and typically more definitive in its identification of extent, primarily because the presence of occlusion frequently made arterial portography more difficult to interpret because of reduced venous opacification. Furthermore, CT was less invasive and allowed longitudinal evaluation of the progress of the disease. Of interest to us was that none of these patients had typical clinical evidence of their visceral venous occlusion and none died primarily of that disease. Most of the major morbidity suffered by these patients did, however, stem from complications of the venous occlusion, with many patients ultimately requiring sclerotherapy, splenectomy, and portal decompression.

In hepatocellular carcinoma portal vein invasion is a common accompaniment, and detection of this finding generally indicates a worse prognosis since most of these patients have unresectable tumors. There has been extensive work by the Japanese in this area, predominantly because of the prevalence of the disease in that country. In addition to the expected finding of a hepatic mass with

Figure 7–12. Accessory hemiazygos continuation of inferior vena cava. *A*, Chest scan shows the accessory hemiazygos vein (arrow) continuing superiorly. *B*, Venogram shows the left system flowing into the innominate vein (IV) and then into the superior vena cava (SVC).

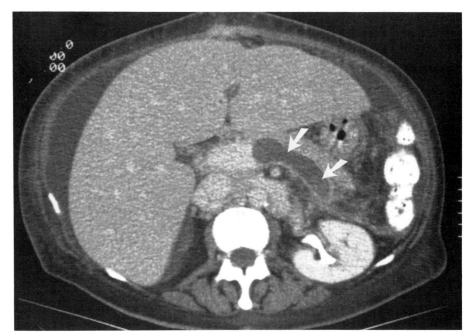

Figure 7–14.   Extensive splenic vein thrombosis (arrows).

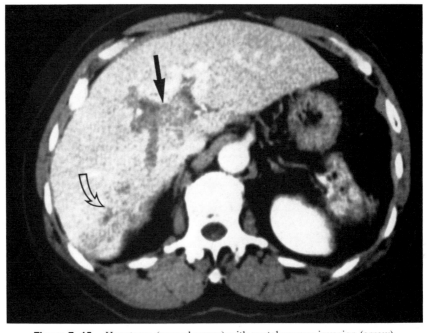

Figure 7–15.   Hepatoma (curved arrow) with portal venous invasion (arrow).

associated low-density portal thrombosis (Fig. 7–15), other reports detail the secondary signs of portal clot, such as decreased contrast enhancement in the segments supplied by the occluded portal vein branch (34,35). Itai and coworkers demonstrated the presence of arterial portal shunts on dynamic CT in 42 patients, consisting of early high-density filling of the portal vein with associated wedge-shaped areas of decreased attenuation in the areas supplied by the involved vein (36). We have noted similar findings in such fistulas from both benign and malignant causes. Other authors have reported similar findings. In chronic obstruction of the portal vein filling defects are not seen, but so-called cavernous transformation of the portal vein can easily be identified on CT as small and medium-sized vessels replacing or surrounding the portal vein (37) (Fig. 7–16). Other features of portal hypertension and cirrhosis include morphologic changes of the liver, such as caudate lobe enlargement with atrophy of the right and left lobes. Ascites and multiple collateral venous channels can also be seen, including esophageal varices, umbilical collaterals, and mesenteric and retroperitoneal varicosities (38) (Fig. 7–17).

Hepatic Venous Thrombosis (Budd-Chiari Syndrome)

Budd-Chiari syndrome, or obstruction of hepatic venous outflow, is an uncommon disease that is associated with a variety of causes, including polycythemia vera, hypercoagulable states, congenital webs, and pregnancy, as well as malignant obstruction due to primary and metastatic neoplasm. Until recently, the diagnosis of Budd-Chiari syndrome could only reliably be made with

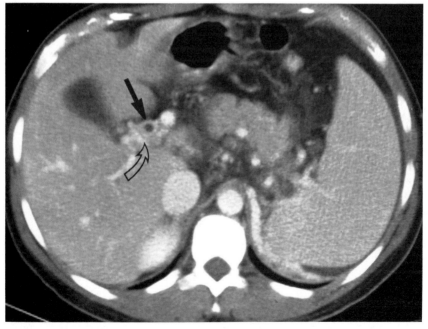

Figure 7–16. Cavernous transformation of the portal vein. Chronic obstruction of the portal vein is demonstrated. The portal vein itself is thrombosed (arrow). The periportal region is filled with numerous enhancing collaterals (curved arrow).

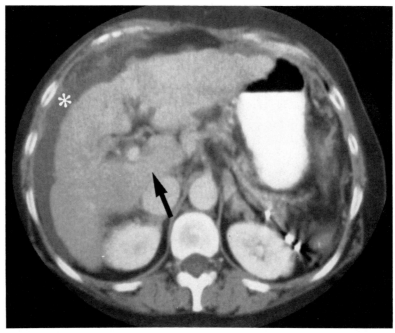

Figure 7–17. Portal hypertension and cirrhosis. Note nodular liver, enlargement of the left lobe and caudate lobe (arrow) and relative atrophy of the right lobe. Ascites is also demonstrated (asterisk).

angiography or venography, but in the past 5 years the Doppler ultrasound and CT features of this distinctive disease have allowed definitive diagnosis in a large percentage of cases. The CT features of the disease relate to the effects of persistent outflow obstruction on the liver. Thus, one sees significant alterations in hepatic contrast enhancement, as well as the venous obstruction so characteristic of other venous thromboses. CT features include: 1) ascites; 2) hepatomegaly; 3) patchy enhancement of the central areas of the hepatic parenchyma, including the caudate lobe, and poor enhancement of the peripheral zones of the liver; 4) nonvisualization or thrombosis of hepatic veins; 5) inferior vena cava thrombosis; and 6) portal vein thrombosis (39–41) (Fig. 7–18). All these changes can be predicted on the basis of the physiologic alterations in portal flow. Since the central portions of the liver, particularly the caudate lobe, frequently have separate and/or shorter hepatic venous drainage, those segments are less likely to be involved by the process. Additionally, portal thrombosis usually occurs secondarily as a result of slowed flow through the congested liver; late changes consistent with cirrhosis are also seen because of portal vein obstruction. High-attenuation caval and hepatic vein thrombi may also allow dating of the processes, as recently discussed by Mori et al. (40). We and others have also described the characteristic findings in some detail (39,42,43).

Conditions Affecting the Inferior Vena Cava and Its Branches

CONGENITAL ANOMALIES. The inferior vena cava, forming as it does from multiple embryonic venous segments, is commonly affected by developmental anomalies, most of which can be seen on CT. Although knowledge of these venous

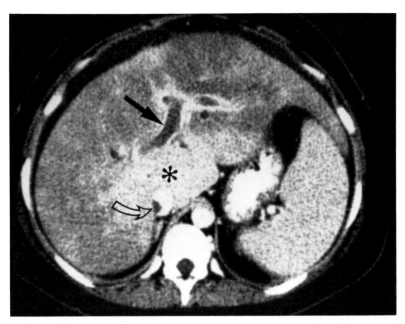

Figure 7–18. Budd-Chiari syndrome. CT demonstrates dense central enhancement of the liver (asterisk) along with hepatomegaly and portal venous thrombosis (arrow). The decreased peripheral enhancement is also characteristic. Caval clot is seen as well (curved arrow).

anomalies was well developed prior to the modern era, CT has allowed even more complete understanding and detailing of the incidence of these variants. The most common abnormalities are:

1.   Transposition of the inferior vena cava (left-sided inferior vena cava). In this variant, the cava is seen on the left side and usually crosses over to the right at the level of the left renal vein, except in extremely rare cases of accessory hemiazygos continuation.

2.   Inferior vena cava duplication. Two cavas are seen below the renal veins. Generally the left cava does not continue above that level. This variant must be distinguished from adenopathy or retroperitoneal masses (Fig. 7–19).

3.   Circumaortic left renal vein. This relatively common anomaly can be easily identified on CT and should be particularly sought when surgery upon the aorta or cava is contemplated. Other types of this "venous collar" include retroaortic left renal vein.

4.   Azygos continuation of the inferior vena cava. This anomaly is frequently associated with congenital heart disease, polysplenia, and abnormal cardiac situs. CT reveals enlarged azygos and hemiazygos veins that should not be mistaken for retrocrural adenopathy (6,7,22,23,24).

ILEOCAVAL THROMBOSIS.   Vena cava thrombosis can be caused by a variety of conditions, but it generally is associated with extension from lower extremity or pelvic vein thrombosis. While ultrasound is extremely helpful in making or suggesting the diagnosis, we have also found CT to be consistent, reliable, and reproducible in the detection of caval thrombosis. We prefer it to venography because of difficulty in obtaining venograms in patients with diffuse lower extremity swelling and femoral venous thrombosis (44–46). Other uses for CT of

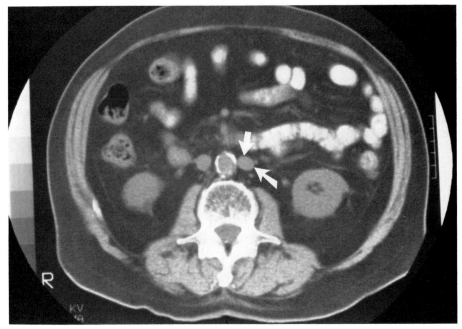

A

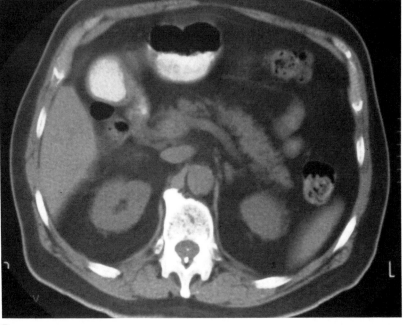

B

Figure 7–19. Vena cava duplication. *A*, Note vena cava on the left side of the abdomen (arrow). *B*, Above the level of the renal veins the cava is right-sided. *C*, Cavogram shows course of the duplicated cava (arrows) into the left renal vein.

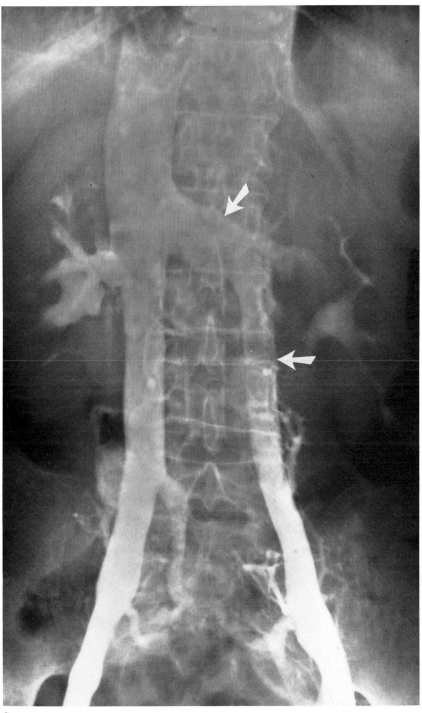

C

Figure 7–19. (*continued*)

the cava include follow-up of vena caval filters, since we have not found trans-abdominal ultrasound to be as reliable in the detection of partially occluding clot and do not wish to subject patients to the potential morbidity of cavography. CT can and does reliably image the presence of thrombus above caval filters (Fig. 7–20) and can show filter malposition, including penetration of the caval wall by the hooks of the Greenfield filter (47).

There are pitfalls in the diagnosis of caval thrombosis. Two common problems have been described, both related to the technique of intravenous infusion. Foot vein infusion of contrast can give misleading artifacts as a result of laminar flow and streaming of contrast; this technique should be avoided whenever possible in favor of arm vein infusion (48). Rapid arm vein infusion can also cause a "pseu-dothrombus," which is characteristically seen in the suprarenal cava and is related to differential caval opacification by more densely enhanced renal venous effluent mixing incompletely with less enhanced infrarenal caval contents (Fig. 7–21). The artifact is seen early during rapid infusion of contrast and can be distinguished from real thrombus by virtue of its relative lack of definition and typical location (49).

Renal Vein Thrombosis

Most occlusion of the renal vein is caused by extension from renal cell car-cinoma. CT has been widely recognized as an accurate technique for the detection of renal venous and caval involvement from renal neoplasms (50). It has been shown to be of similar accuracy to venography in the detection of these problems. The thrombus may extend as far cranially as the right atrium (Fig. 7–22). Benign causes of renal vein thrombosis can also be seen with CT (Fig. 7–23).

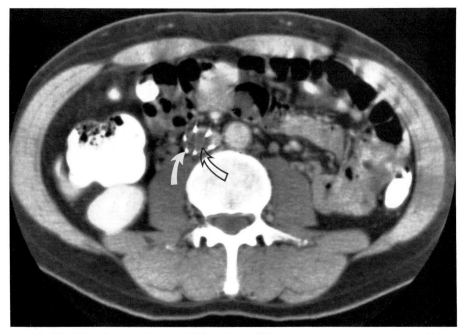

Figure 7–20.   Thrombus in a Greenfield filter. Caval filling defect (open arrow) is noted within the Greenfield filter (closed arrow).

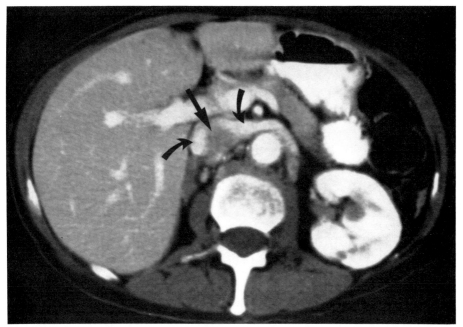

Figure 7–21. Inferior vena cava "pseudothrombus." Low-density caval contents (arrow) are seen in the suprarenal area. Note higher density renal venous blood (curved arrows). Layering of this higher density blood is responsible for the artifact, which is characteristically located in the suprarenal cava.

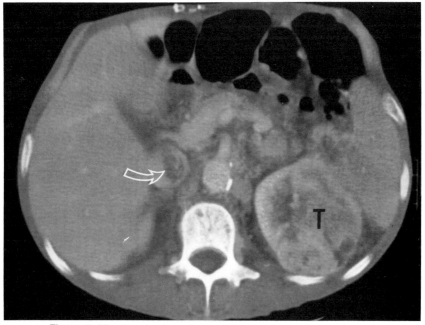

Figure 7–22. Renal cell carcinoma (T) with intracaval tumor (arrow).

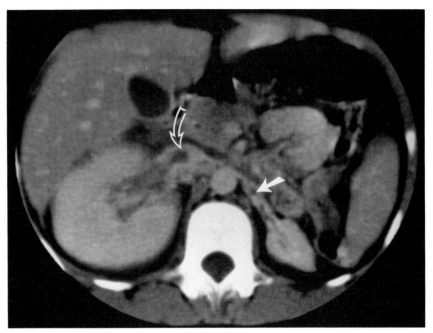

Figure 7–23.   Idiopathic renal vein thrombosis in a child. Right renal vein thrombosis (curved arrow). Chronic thrombosis of the atrophic left kidney is also demonstrated (arrow).

Conclusion

Computed tomography has demonstrated wide applicability and reliability in the detection and accurate depiction of a variety of venous occlusive processes in the chest and abdomen. In many cases, CT is superior to venography in specific disease states and should be the first test ordered when the problems indicated above are suspected.

MAGNETIC RESONANCE IMAGING

MRI has revolutionized our understanding and awareness of neurologic disease; the procedure has supplanted many other imaging techniques, such as CT and angiography, for a wide variety of conditions in the central nervous system in the few short years that have elapsed since the introduction of the technique as a practical reality. In the body, MRI has had major impact in disease processes affecting the musculoskeletal system, and a great deal of research has been devoted to the investigation of the utility of the tool in the chest and abdomen. In theory, MRI has considerable advantages over other techniques like CT since it does not use ionizing radiation, is capable of producing multiplanar sections of any body part, and has inherently greater contrast resolution without the use of potentially nephrotoxic and allergenic intravenous contrast material. Limitations of the technique include long examination times producing a myriad of artifcats related to respiration, and the presence of a strong magnetic field that does not permit ferromagnetic objects to be in the scan room with the patient, thus effectively limiting the scan's utility in the critically ill. Some of these problems have been addressed—for example, the use of pulse sequences that permit rapid scanning in the case of liver MRI, as pioneered by Stark et al. (51–53), and the use of low-field-strength magnets that can be used in critical care applications. MRI has shown promise in imaging of pelvic neoplasms, including detection and staging of tumors of the bladder, rectum, prostate, and female reproductive tract, by virtue of its multiplanar imaging capability, but it should be pointed out that as of yet, MRI has not shown sufficient advantage over CT that it has significantly replaced that modality to any great extent in the chest and abdomen, with the exception of cardiac disorders.

The most heralded aspect of MRI in the body has been the potential of the tool to demonstrate vascular structures to an extent not heretofore appreciated. It was immediately apparent upon the introduction of MRI that flowing blood provided natural contrast for vessels; furthermore, the ability to perform multiple planes of section and to gate the acquisition of images to the cardiac cycle allowed a spectacular look at cardiac chambers and complex cardiac and aortic problems, including disorders such as aortic coarctation, in which the technique has virtually replaced CT and angiography (54).

Any appreciation of MRI and vascular pathology requires at least some understanding of the variable appearance of flowing blood that can be obtained with this tool. The effect of motion on MRI images is one of the most confusing aspects of the technique, and the amount of theoretical and applied research that has been undertaken on this subject in the last 5 years requires book-length synopses and is clearly beyond the small scope of this chapter. It is possible, however, to appreciate the production of an MRI image and how flow can be manipulated to optimize or suppress visualization of structures that contain flowing fluid, such as blood and cerebrospinal fluid. As a gross generalization, flowing blood can appear dark or bright, depending on its velocity, with rapidly flowing arterial blood appearing dark and slower flowing venous blood generating a bright or white signal. The imaging sequence used, however, can greatly alter this basic appearance. For example, in fast scanning techniques with short repetition times and short flip angles the appearances of rapidly and slowly flowing blood may be reversed. Additionally, other factors such as the position of the slice containing the vessel relative to the rest of the multislice imaging volume and the slice thickness are also important. In short, what one sees on MRI when imaging blood vessels can be extremely varied. Judgments made on the basis of a simple understanding (''arteries are dark and veins are bright'') may be woefully inadequate. I recommend that vascular specialists interested in exploring the significant advantages of this modality work closely with a radiologist skilled in production and interpretation of MRI images.

Various factors result in both decreased and increased signal in vessels. Three independent factors that give decreased signal in a vessel are high velocity, turbulence, and odd-echo dephasing. These three factors lead to the flow void phenomenon in arteries, aneurysms, and arteriovenous malformations (Fig. 7–24). Most of this signal loss is related to a basic concept of MRI imaging: in order to give off a signal, protons in the body must be exposed to both a 90 and a 180 degree radiofrequency pulse. Signal loss related to high velocity, or so-called time-of-flight loss, occurs when protons do not remain in the slice of tissue being imaged long enough to acquire both of these radiofrequency excitations. Signal loss therefore results. Three different factors can produce increased signal in flowing blood:

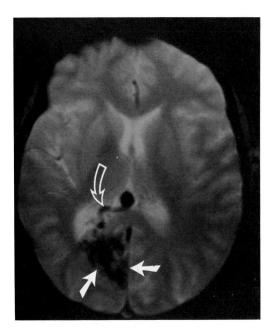

Figure 7–24. Flow void phenomenon in intracranial arteriovenous malformation. Loss of signal within AVM (arrows) and large draining vein (open arrow) results from time of flight signal loss.

flow-related enhancement, even-echo rephasing, and diastolic pseudogating. These three typically cause the most difficulty when attempting to distinguish a normal vessel from a thrombosed one. In general, qualitative criteria of image interpretation are usually sufficient to make the decision. Dark rims around the central zone of the signal on first-echo images that are replaced by signal throughout the vessel on second-echo images, signal on the first-echo images and absence of signal on the second-echo images, and changes of intravascular signal with changes of the imaging plane are only seen in flowing vessels (55–57) (Fig. 7–25).

The appearance of thrombosis on MRI is somewhat more specific and straightforward than that of flowing blood, with venous thrombi almost always appearing hyperintense or bright on both T_1 and T_2 imaging (Figs. 7–26, 7–27). The brightness of thrombus is usually present regardless of the age, as illustrated experimentally by Erdman and his coworkers (58). The main difficulty in the MRI imaging of thrombosis is in differentiation of clot from artifacts created by flowing blood, as discussed previously. This problem is most apparent in the venous circulation, where venous blood is normally bright and the presence of venous thrombosis must be distinguished from this background signal intensity. The techniques noted earlier, as well as a clear understanding of the normal appearance of these vessels, are usually the most helpful in distinguishing thrombus from flowing blood.

Chest

MRI of the chest has been widely used in the imaging of cardiac abnormalities, in which it has obvious advantages over CT because of the ability to obtain multiplanar slices and to gate image acquisition during the cardiac cycle for the detection of cardiac tumors, cardiac thrombi, and pericardial abnormalities (59).

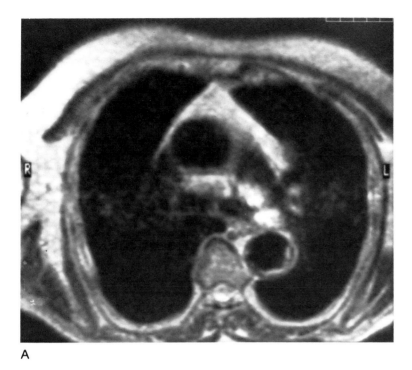

A

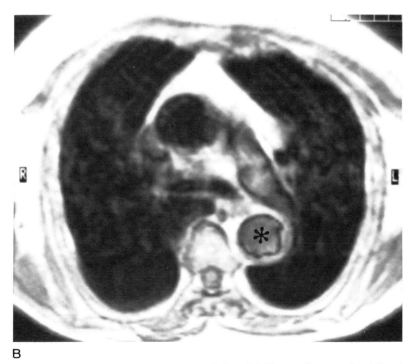

B

Figure 7–25.   Effect of imaging parameters on aortic blood. Difference between first (*A*) and second (*B*) echo of T_1 images shows significant change in intensity of descending thoracic aortic contents. This is characteristic of many of the changes seen in MRI.

Specific disease processes that affect the mediastinal veins include occlusion of the vena cava by benign or malignant causes. MRI has been useful here and generally compares favorably with the depiction afforded by CT. Weinreb and colleagues compared CT and MRI in 14 patients and found them comparable in all regards; in two patients MRI was able to better delineate the presence of residual flow in the cava (60,61). Additionally, MRI can differentiate fibrosis from tumor in many cases.

MRI has also depicted anomalies of the superior and inferior vena cavae, such as azygos continuation (62).

Pulmonary emboli can also be seen with MRI (62,63). The pulmonary hila are readily imaged with MRI. We have found that MRI is particularly well suited to the job of distinguishing tumor from normal vascular structures (Fig. 7–28).

Cardiac Tumors

MRI has proven to be superior to CT for the investigation of cardiac lesions that may be the cause of embolic events. Most investigators prefer it to CT for this use (60,62).

Abdomen

MRI has been very useful in the abdomen, where its accuracy in diseases affecting large veins compares favorably with CT. In specific areas, some investigators believe that MRI may be superior to CT, including in the detection of renal vein thrombosis in renal cell carcinoma and detection of some of the mesenteric venous problems in patients with portal hypertension and cirrhosis (64–68).

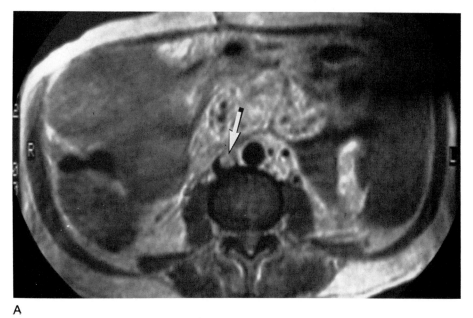

A

Figure 7–26. Inferior vena cava thrombosis. *A*, MR image shows high intensity clot adherent to caval wall (arrow). *B*, Cavogram confirms the finding (arrows).

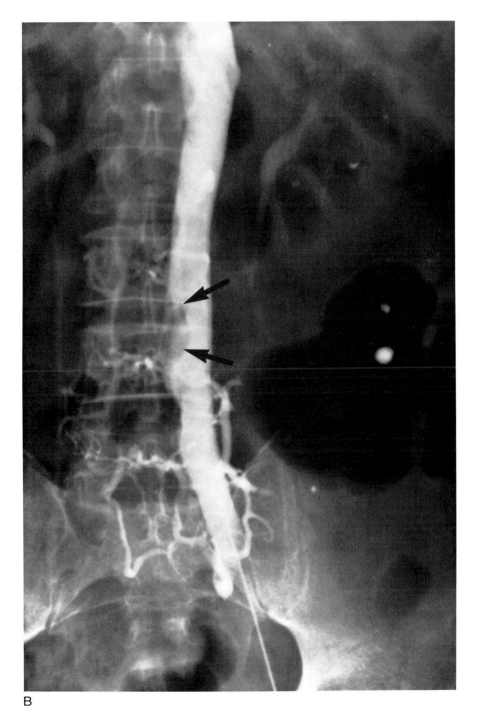

B

Figure 7–26. (*continued*)

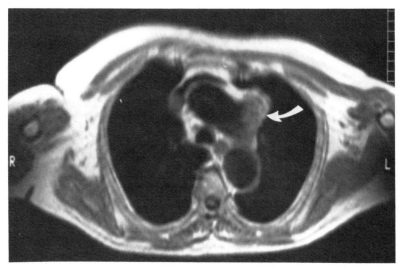

Figure 7–27. Thrombosis within a thoracic aneurysm (arrow) shows markedly increased signal from normally flowing intraaortic blood.

Mesenteric and Splanchnic Thrombosis

MRI has been used for the detection of splanchnic vein thrombosis, including that in the portal vein, in which a study by Levy and Newhouse found that portal vein occlusion is seen as well on MRI as on CT or Doppler ultrasound (69). Others have had similar experiences (64). Our experience is that MRI is accurate in this

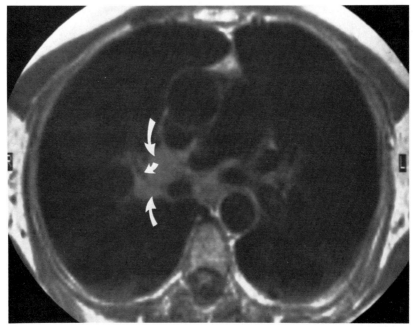

Figure 7–28. Hilar tumor (curved arrows) is readily distinguished from normal vascular structures which do not demonstrate signal (small arrow).

situation and is occasionally extremely useful because of its ability to image in multiple planes. In patients who have had mesenteric venous bypass surgery, surveillance of the patency of the anastomosis has been nicely accomplished by MRI. In hepatoma and other focal liver diseases, MRI provides good depiction of the primary tumor as well as the associated portal vein obstruction.

Hepatic Vein Occlusion

In this entity MRI, like CT, provides a characteristic picture of the Budd-Chiari syndrome, usually consisting of higher signal intensity in the central portion of the liver with lower signal intensity in the peripheral portion as a result of the relative congestion and slow blood flow there (40,51). MRI may also show the absent or thrombosed hepatic veins, particularly in the coronal and sagittal planes. Conversely, since MRI can depict normal hepatic veins well, the presence of well-visualized hepatic veins excludes that diagnosis.

Inferior Vena Cava and Its Branches

MRI is particularly useful in imaging of the vena cava because this structure is readily imaged without the use of contrast material and because the superior extent of caval thrombosis is probably more reliably seen than with CT and ultrasound. Additionally, venous collaterals are more easily separated from enlarged nodes. In the setting of possible renal vein thrombosis, MRI is generally preferred because renal function is usually impaired. In renal cell carcinoma, MRI appears to have a small advantage over CT regarding the staging of the tumor, primarily because MRI can distinguish between extrinsic and intraluminal involvement and can tell the difference between nodal enlargement and enlarged venous collaterals (67).

Imaging of Inferior Vena Cava Filters

MRI is quite useful in the depiction of the status of inferior vena cava filters because of its ability to image in the coronal plane. None of the commercially available filters have shown sufficient ferromagnetic properties so as to tilt or torque, but most are associated with some degree of magnetic artifact that may obscure the cava in the vicinity of the device. The Simon-Nitinol filter is free of such artifact, and the Greenfield filter produces the largest artifact (70,71).

Ileocaval Thrombosis

MRI depicts thrombosis of the ileocaval system well; it is essentially equivalent to CT in its depiction of the thrombosis, which is seen as a characteristically high-intensity abnormality within the vein.

Conclusion

In most cases of venous pathology, MRI appears to have similar accuracy when compared to CT and, in some cases, superior ability to detect abnormality, as in renal cell carcinoma. In an individual institution, the choice of whether to use CT or MRI is one that should be made depending on the local experience with MRI or CT, as well as physician preferences. Certainly, MRI should be investigated and always kept in mind when difficult problems arise or when other imaging modalities fail to adequately answer the question.

REFERENCES

1. Dixon AK, et al: Computed tomography (CT) of abdominal aortic aneurysms: Determination of longitudinal extent. Br J Surg 1981;*68*:47–50.
2. Andersen PE Jr, Lorentzen JE: Comparison of computed tomography and aortography in abdominal aortic aneurysms. J Comput Assist Tomogr 1983;*7*:670–673.
3. Zerhouni EA, Barth KH, Siegelman SS: Demonstration of venous thrombosis by computed tomography. Am J Roentgenol 1980;*134*:753–756.
4. Marks WM, Korobkin M, Callen PW, et al: CT diagnosis of tumor thrombus in the inferior vena cava. Am J Roentgenol 1978;*131*:843.
5. Weyman PJ, McClennan BL, Stanley RJ, et al: Comparison of computed tomography and angiography in the evaluation of renal call carcinoma. Radiology 1980;*137*:417.
6. Royal SA, Callen PW: CT evaluation of anomalies of the inferior vena cava and left renal vein. Am J Roentgenol 1979;*132*:759.
7. Faer MJ, Lynch RD, Evans HO, et al: Inferior vena cava duplication: Demonstration by computed tomography. Radiology 1979;*130*:707.
8. New PFJ, Aronow S: Attenuation measurement of whole blood and blood flow fractions in computed tomography. Radiology 1976;*121*:635–638.
9. Wolverson MK, Crepps LF, Sundaram M, et al: Hyperdensity of recent hemorrhage at body computed tomography: Incidence and morphologic variation. Radiology 1983;*148*:779.
10. Feldberg MAM, Staverman JH: CT demonstration of calcified post-thrombotic inferior vena cava. Diagn Imag Clin Med 1986;*55*:164–167.
11. Godwin JD, Webb WR: Contrast-related flow phenomena mimicking pathology on thoracic computed tomography. J Comput Assist Tomogr 1982;*6*:460–462.
12. Engel IA, Auh YH, Rubenstein WA, et al: CT diagnosis of mediastinal and thoracic inlet venous obstruction. Am J Roentgenol 1983;*14*:521–526.
13. Yedlicka JW Jr, Cormier MG, Gray R, et al: Computed tomography of superior vena cava obstruction. J Thorac Imag 1987;*2*:72–77.
14. Moncada R, Cardella R, Demos TC: Evaluation of superior vena cava syndrome by axial CT and CT phlebography. Am J Roentgenol 1984;*143*:731–736.
15. Yedlicka JW, Schultz K, Moncada R, et al: CT findings in superior vena cava obstruction. Semin Roentgenol 1989;*14*:84–90.
16. Sinner WN: Computed tomography of pulmonary thromboembolism. Eur J Radiol 1982;*2*:8–13.
17. Godwin JD, Herfkens RJ, Skioldebrand CG, et al: Detection of intraventricular thrombi by computed tomography. Radiology 1981;*138*:717.
18. Churchill RJ: CT of the heart. *In* Haaga JR, Alfidi RJ, eds: Computed Tomography of the Whole Body. St. Louis, CV Mosby Company, 1988;649–685.
19. Webb WR, Gamsu G, Speckman JM, et al: Computed tomographic demonstration of mediastinal venous anomalies. Am J Roentgenol 1982;*139*:157–161.
20. Comier MG, Yedlicka JW, Gray RJ, et al: Congenital anomalies of the superior vena cava: A CT study. Semin Roentgenol 1989;*24*:77–83.
21. Dudiak CM, Olson MC, Posniak HV: Abnormalities of the azygos system: CT evaluation. Semin Roentgenol 1989;*24*:47–55.
22. Munechika H, Cohan RH, Baker ME, et al: Hemiazygos continuation of a left inferior vena cava: CT appearance. J Comput Assist Tomogr 1988;*12*:328–330.
23. Cohen MI, Gore RM, Vogelzang RL, et al: Accessory hemiazygos continuation of left inferior vena cava: CT demonstration. J Comput Assist Tomogr 1984;*8*:777–779.
24. Coscina WF, Arger PH, Mintz MC, et al: Concurrent duplication and azygos continuation of the inferior vena cava. J Comput Tomogr 1986;*10*:287–290.
25. Moncada R, Demos TC, Marsan R, et al: CT diagnosis of idiopathic aneurysms of the thoracic systemic veins. J Comput Assist Tomogr 1985;*9*:305–309.
26. Grendell JH, Ockner RK: Mesenteric venous thrombosis. AJR 1982;*82*:358–372.
27. Naitove A, Weisman RE: Primary mesenteric venous thrombosis. Ann Surg 1965;*161*:516–523.
28. Clemett AJ, Chang J: The radiologic diagnosis of spontaneous mesenteric venous thrombosis. Am J Gastroenterol 1975;*63*:209–215.
29. Tey PH, Sprayregen S, Ahmed A, et al: Mesenteric vein thrombosis: Angiography in two cases. AJR 1984;*136*:809–811.

30. Clark RA, Gallant TE: Acute mesenteric ischemia: Angiographic spectrum. AJR 1984;*142*:555–562.

31. Vogelzang RL, Gore RM, Anschuetz SL, et al: Thrombosis of the splanchnic veins: CT diagnosis. AJR 1988;*150*:93–96.

32. Mathieu D, Vasile N, Grenier P: Portal thrombosis: Dynamic CT features and course. Radiology 1985;*154*:737–741.

33. Subramanyam BR, Balthazar EM, Lefleur RS, et al: Portal venous thrombosis: Correlative analysis of sonography, CT, and angiography. Am J Gastroenterol 1984;*79*:773–776.

34. Inamoto K, Sugiki K, Yamasaki H, et al: CT of hepatoma: Effects of portal vein obstruction. Am J Roentgenol 1981;*136*:349–353.

35. Imaeda T, Yamawaki Y, Hirota K, et al: Tumor thrombus in the branches of the distal portal vein: CT demonstration. J Comput Assist Tomogr 1989;*13*:262–269.

36. Itai Y, Furui S, Ohtomo K, et al: Dynamic CT features of arterioportal shunts in hepatocellular carcinoma. AJR 1986;*146*:723.

37. Mathieu D, Vasile N, Dibie C, et al: Portal cavernoma: Dynamic CT features and transient differences in hepatic attenuation. Radiology 1985;*154*:743.

38. Ishikawa T, Tsukune Y, Ohyama Y, et al: Venous abnormalities in portal hypertension demonstrated by CT. Am J Roentgenol 1980;*134*:271–276.

39. Vogelzang RL, Anschuetz SL, Gore RM: Budd-Chiari syndrome: CT observations. Radiology 1987;*163*:329–333.

40. Mori H, Maeda H, Fukuda T, et al: Acute thrombosis of the inferior vena cava and hepatic veins in patients with Budd-Chiari syndrome: CT demonstration. Am J Roentgenol 1989;*153*:987–991.

41. Mathieu D, Vasile N, Menu Y, et al: Budd-Chiari syndrome: Dynamic CT. Radiology 1987;*165*:409.

42. Murphy FB, Steinberg HV, Shires GT, et al: The Budd-Chiari syndrome: A review. AJR 1986;*147*:9–15.

43. Rossi P, Sposito M, Simonetti G, et al: CT diagnosis of Budd-Chiari syndrome. J Comput Assist Tomogr 1981;*5*:366–369.

44. Vujic I, Stanley J, Tyminski LJ: Computed tomography of suspected caval thrombosis secondary to proximal extension of phlebitis from the leg. Radiology 1981;*140*:437–441.

45. Castillo M, Nunez D, Morello G: Review of computed tomography findings in thrombosis of the major abdominal venous pathways. J Comput Tomogr 1986;*10*:205–208.

46. Vujic I, Stanley JH, Tyminski LJ: Computed tomography of suspected caval thrombosis secondary to proximal extension of phlebitis from the leg. Radiology 1981;*140*:437.

47. Miller CL, Wechsler RJ: CT evaluation of Kimray-Greenfield filter complications. AJR 1986;*147*:45–49.

48. Glazer GM, Callen PW, Parker JJ: CT diagnosis of tumor thrombus in the inferior vena cava: Avoiding the false-positive diagnosis. AJR 1981;*137*:1265–1267.

49. Vogelzang RL, Gore RM, Neiman HL, et al: Inferior vena cava: CT pseudothrombus produced by rapid arm-vein contrast infusion. AJR 1985;*144*:843–846.

50. Zeman RK, Cronan JJ, Rosenfield AT, et al: Renal cell carcinoma: Dynamic thin-section CT assessment of vascular invasion and tumor vascularity. Radiology 1988;*167*:393–396.

51. Stark DD: Liver. *In* Stark DD, Bradley WG Jr, eds: Magnetic Resonance Imaging. St. Louis, CV Mosby Company, 1988;934–1059.

52. Stark DD, Hendrick RE, Hahn PF, et al: Motion artifact suppression by fast spin echo imaging. Radiology 1987;*164*:183–191.

53. Stark DD, Wittenberg J, Middelton MS, et al: Liver metastases: Detection by phase-contrast MR imaging. Radiology 1986;*158*:327–332.

54. von Schulthess GK, et al: Coarctation of the aorta: MR imaging. Radiology 1986;*158*:469.

55. White EM, Edelman RR, Wedeen VJ, et al: Intravascular signal in MR imaging: Use of phase display for differentiation of blood-flow signal from intraluminal disease. Radiology 1986;*161*:245–249.

56. von Schulthess GK, Augustiny N: Calculation of T2 values versus phase imaging for the distinction between flow and thrombus in MR imaging. Radiology 1987;*164*:549–554.

57. Bradley WG Jr: Flow phenomena. *In* Stark DD, Bradley WG Jr, eds: Magnetic Resonance Imaging. St. Louis, CV Mosby Company, 1988;108–137.

58. Erdman WA, Weinreb JC, Cohen JM, et al: Venous thrombosis: Clinical and experimental MR imaging. Radiology 1986;*161*:233–238.

59. Peshock RM: Heart and great vessels. *In* Stark DD, Bradley WG Jr, eds: Magnetic Resonance Imaging. St. Louis, CV Mosby Company, 1988;887–920.

60. Weinreb JC, Mootz A, Cohen JM: MRI evaluation of mediastinal and thoracic inlet venous obstruction. AJR 1986;*146*:679–684.

61. McMurdo KK, de Geer G, Webb WR, et al: Normal and occluded mediastinal veins: MR imaging. Radiology 1986;*159*:33.

62. Gefter WB: Chest applications of magnetic resonance imaging: An update. Radiol Clin North Am 1988;*26*:573–588.
63. Fisher MR, Higgins CB: Central thrombi in pulmonary arterial hypertension detected by MR imaging. Radiology 1986;*158*:223–226.
64. Tamada T, Moriyasu F, Ono S, et al: Portal blood flow: Measurement with MR imaging. Radiology 1989;*173*:639–644.
65. Honda H, Yuh WT, Lu CC: Magnetic resonance imaging of renal vein and inferior vena cava thrombosis in a patient with glomerulonephritis: A case report. J Comput Tomogr 1988;*12*:147–149.
66. Itai Y:, Ohtomo K, Kokubo T, et al: Segmental intensity differences in the liver on MR images: A sign of intrahepatic portal flow stoppage. Radiology 1988;*167*:17–19.
67. Choyke PL, Pollack HM: The role of MRI in diseases of the kidney. Radiol Clin North Am 1988;*26*:617–631.
68. Hricak H, Demas BE, Williams RD, et al: Magnetic resonance imaging in the diagnosis and staging of renal and perirenal neoplasms. Radiology 1985;*154*:704–708.
69. Levy HM, Newhouse JH: MR imaging of portal vein thrombosis. Am J Roentgenol 1988;*151*:283–286.
70. Liebman CE, Messersmith RN, Levin DN, et al: MR imaging of inferior vena caval filters: Safety and artifacts. Am J Roentgenol 1988;*150*:1174.
71. Teitelbaum GP, Ortega HV, Vinitski S, et al: Low-artifact intravascular devices: MR imaging evaluation. Radiology 1988;*168*:713.

8

ROUTINE AND SPECIAL PHLEBOGRAPHY IN THE EVALUATION OF VENOUS PROBLEMS

M. Lea Thomas

While contrast phlebography remains the standard against which all other methods of investigation of venous diseases are judged, in many clinical situations it has been partly replaced by other complementary procedures, notably duplex scanning. The advantage of phlebography is that the image resolution obtained by the film-screen combination is far superior to that of other imaging techniques, and phlebography is therefore still necessary when detailed anatomic information is required. Its two main disadvantages are that it is invasive, because a venipuncture is required, and that truly physiologic studies cannot be obtained because of the different properties of contrast medium compared with blood.

Nevertheless, contrast phlebography, with its extreme sensitivity and specificity (1), will retain, for the forseeable future, an important role in the management of venous problems (2).

CONTRAST MEDIA

Using modern low-osmolar contrast media, phlebography has become a very safe procedure with virtually no contraindications or complications (3). Thrombosis due to endothelial damage (4–6), detected in about a third of legs with the ^{125}I-labeled fibrinogen uptake test (7), has been virtually eliminated (8,9). Accidental extravasation of contrast medium, which may lead to tissue necrosis with hyperosmolar agents (10–12), now gives rise to no serious sequelae.

It is now recommended that low-osmolar contrast media should always be used for phelbography (3). If because of financial constraints, or because the newer agents have not received official approval, conventional media are used, they should be diluted to bring their osmolality closer to that of plasma (13). Iopamidol 300 or 370 (14), iohexol 300 or 350 (15), sodium/meglumine ioxaglate 320 (16), or iopromide (17) are suggested media. Ioxaglate, although cheaper, has more minor side effects. The higher iodine concentrations may be needed for the larger proximal veins.

The amount of contrast medium needed for a particular examination varies but, as an approximate guide, about 50 ml is usually sufficient for ascending phlebography of one leg; however, four times this amount may be required for examination of both legs and the lower inferior vena cava, or when repeat studies are necessary.

The poor quality of phlebograms in the past was due to the inability to inject sufficient contrast because of its toxicity. This constraint does not apply to low-osmolar media.

ASCENDING PHLEBOGRAPHY

The term "ascending phlebography" indicates that contrast medium is injected peripherally into a foot vein and passes centrally toward the heart in the venous bloodstream. No special radiographic apparatus is required; a tilting fluoroscopy table with automatic exposure and television monitoring is sufficient. A small (21- or 23-gauge) butterfly needle is introduced into a vein on the dorsum of the foot. The digital vein on the medial aspect of the great toe is useful in edematous legs. A rubber tourniquet is applied above the ankle to assist deep venous filling, and another tourniquet above the knee delays escape of the contrast medium from the calf.

Ideally the patient should be examined vertically to show the deep veins, but this is often unacceptable to the patient. A 30 to 45 degree foot-down position is sufficient, and it is easier to relax the calf muscles, producing better filling of the muscle veins. The use of tourniquets is not universally recommended (1) because of minor discomfort and artifacts, but if the erect posture alone is used the simultaneous filling of both superficial and deep veins can make interpretation difficult. The contrast medium is injected slowly by hand under fluoroscopic control and films are taken from the foot to the lower inferior vena cava. Calf compression just before the film is taken is helpful to fill the proximal veins. If venous thrombosis is suspected, lateral views of the calf are taken to exclude thrombus in the muscle veins. The iliofemoral segments and the inferior vena cava must also be shown fully, if necessary by femoral vein injection on the same side or on the contralateral side (18).

Phlebographic Appearances of Thrombus

Thrombus is seen as a constant filling defect in an opacified vein that is of the same size and shape in at least two films taken with a brief interval between them (18). For accurate diagnosis it is important to try to outline the thrombus itself and not rely solely on nonfilling of veins, which may be the result of technique. A fresh thrombus has a slightly opalescent appearance, with a thin film, or line, of contrast medium surrounding it (Fig. 8–1A–C). Obliteration of this line indicates adherence of the thrombus, and when the thrombus completely occludes a vein there is no contrast medium around it but contrast above and below it and in the collaterals beside it. As thrombus ages it becomes smaller, a thicker layer of contrast medium surrounds it, and its surface is more clearly defined (Fig. 8–1D). The processes of adherence and retraction occur simultaneously. In this way the likelihood of embolism may be estimated (19). Furthermore, a loose thrombus

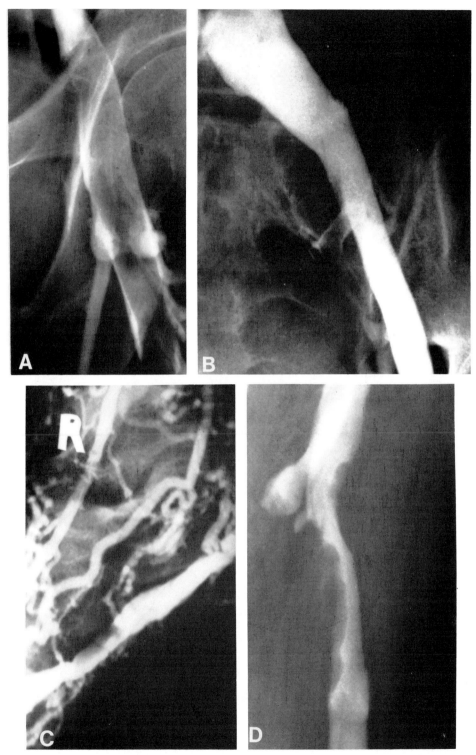

Figure 8–1. *A*, A loose thrombus in the common femoral vein. The thrombus is surrounded by a thin coating of contrast medium, giving a slightly opalescent appearance. The "square cut" appearance at the top of the thrombus indicates that a piece has already embolized. *B* and *C*, unusual sites for recurrent small emboli missed by other techniques: in the internal iliac vein (*B*) and in the medial plantar vein (*C*). *D*, This thrombus, in the upper part of the superficial femoral vein, is adherent to the wall because contrast does not surround it on the medial side. It is unlikely to embolize.

may be "locked in" by adherent thrombus proximal to it, an important feature when planning treatment. The vein may remain totally occluded following thrombosis, return to normal, or recanalize with destruction of valves. Recanalized or postthrombotic veins are narrowed and irregular, with filling defects in the lumen representing organized thrombus, and the valves are deformed and destroyed (Fig. 8–2).

Artifacts

Artifacts are common in phlebograms and results from streaming of contrast medium along the vein wall and uneven mixing of the hyperbaric medium with blood entering from nonopacified tributaries. These may resemble thrombus or postthrombotic changes (20). They can be minimized by using sufficient contrast medium, fluoroscopy, and repeat films in the same projection because, unlike anatomic or pathologic images, they are inconstant in appearance.

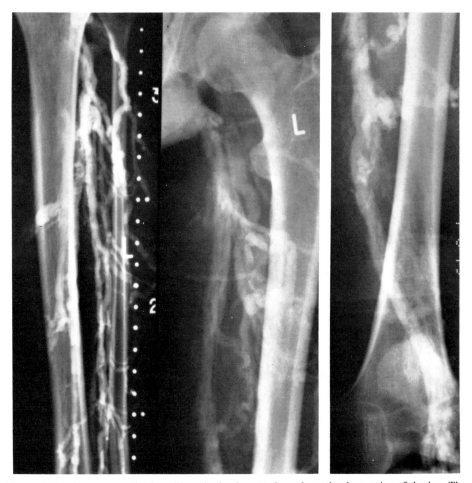

Figure 8–2. Gross generalized postthrombotic changes throughout the deep veins of the leg. The lumen is irregular and no normal valves are present.

VENOUS ULCERATION AND VARICOSE VEINS

Varicose veins are conventionally divided into two groups, primary and secondary. In the former the deep venous system is normal and in the latter it is abnormal, most frequently as a result of past venous thrombosis. Ascending phlebography to show the status of the deep venous system of the leg is important in the prognosis for treatment of both varicose veins and venous ulceration. In the presence of normal deep veins, ligation and stripping of the long or short saphenous vein, localized ablation, sclerotherapy, and ligation of incompetent communicating veins usually have good results. In the presence of an abnormal deep venous system these procedures are likely to have only temporary effects (18,21).

Incompetent Communicating Veins

The standard technique for ascending phlebography is modified because the ankle tourniquet must be sufficiently tight to prevent contrast medium passing into the superficial veins, so that the direction of flow from the deep to the superficial veins can be appreciated, indicating incompetence (22). A ruler with radiopaque markers at 1-cm intervals placed beneath the leg is helpful in relating the position of incompetent communicating veins to bony landmarks such as the malleoli or knee joint (23). If a low, submalleolar communicating vein is suspected the tourniquet should be placed around the forefoot, and if ulceration is present tourniquets above and below the ulcer help to isolate a local incompetent communicating vein. A typical incompetent communicating vein is dilated (more than 3 mm in diameter), particularly at its outer end, is valveless, and connects directly or indirectly to a varicose vein (Fig. 8–3A). Communicating veins can also be shown by direct injection of draining varices (see "Varicography") but because flow of contrast medium is in the normal direction, from superficial to deep veins, secondary characteristics are required to suggest incompetence (Fig. 8–3B).

Varicography

When managing varicose veins, notably recurrences, varicography is very useful if the anatomy of the superficial veins is in doubt or abnormal superficial-to-deep communications are suspected, and for planning short saphenous vein surgery (Fig. 8–4). The technique involves direct injection of varicose veins with contrast medium. With the patient standing, a varicose vein in the group of which the patient complains is punctured. The patient lies on a fluroscopy table, prone or supine, and contrast is injected as the table is tilted from a steep foot-down position, through the horizontal, into a steep head-down position. A lateral view around the upper calf and knee is required to show the short saphenous vein, which lies superficially and must be distinguished from the gastrocnemius veins, which lies more deeply.

Because of the complex connections of the superficial venous system, particularly following surgery, multiple injections into different groups of varicose veins may be required, and the contrast medium may need to be followed by fluoroscopy in straight, oblique, and lateral positions. Because of the hyperbaric nature of contrast medium, prone and supine projections may also be required; for example, a recurrence at the groin is better shown prone (Fig. 8–5). Incom-

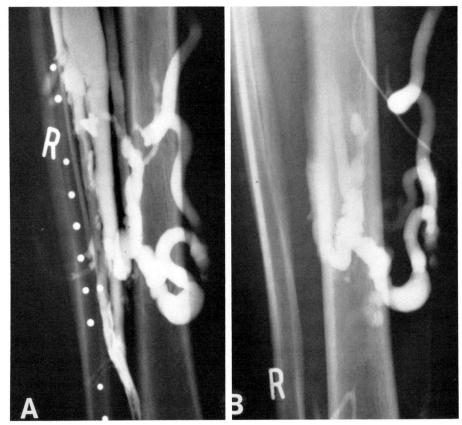

Figure 8–3. *A*, A typical incompetent communicating vein arising from a posterior tibial vein and joining a varicose vein. The communicating vein is irregular, dilated, and valveless. *B*, The same communicating vein shown by varicography.

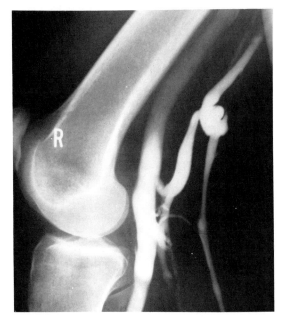

Figure 8–4. The varicogram shows that the short saphenous vein has two connections, one at the usual site in the popliteal fossa and another high in the thigh. This information is required for successful surgery.

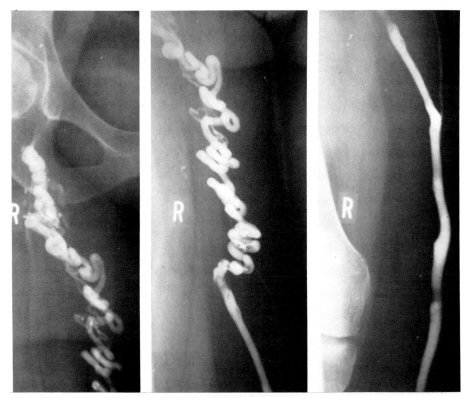

Figure 8–5. A varicogram showing an extensive long saphenous vein recurrence in the groin and upper thigh. Groin recurrences are better shown with the patient prone.

petent communicating veins in the midthigh region are a common cause of recurrence because of failure to ablate these veins during the initial surgery (2,24–27) (Fig. 8–6).

While these communicating veins usually occur in the adductor canal region, their site is inconstant, and although they usually connect with the superficial femoral vein, they may also connect with the deep femoral vein. Other useful information obtained from varicography is the presence of multiple long saphenous veins, which occur in up to 25 per cent of limbs (28), important if surgical stripping of varicose veins is contemplated and to show the termination of the short saphenous vein, which is very variable (29,30). Varicography is less useful in the management of primary varicose veins than recurrences, although varicose veins at unusual sites where there may be unusual connections with the deep venous systems, such as those on the posterolateral aspect of the thigh (31) (Fig. 8–7), can be shown.

Saphenography

The purpose of this investigation is to demonstrate the long saphenous vein to assess its suitability for bypass surgery, such as a saphenofemoral crossover procedure [Palma's operation (32)] for the postphlebitic leg. The long saphenous vein is injected at the ankle and films are taken from the ankle to the groin while

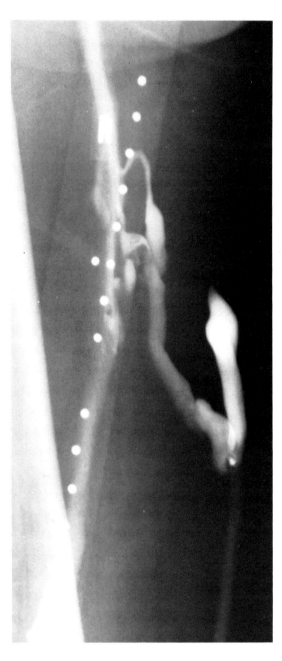

Figure 8–6. There is a large, incompetent-looking communicating vein in Hunter's canal joining the remnant of the long saphenous vein in the upper part of the thigh. The communicating vein is dilated and irregular and shows no valves. The direction of flow of the contrast medium is not a sign of incompetence in varicography.

rotating the tilt of the fluoroscopy table from the foot-down to the head-down position. Radiopaque ball bearings of known size placed on the course of the long saphenous vein enable a more accurate guide to the true diameter of the vein to be made. Brief hand compression of the popliteal vein in the popliteal fossa or the femoral vein at the groin just before filming directs contrast medium into the long saphenous vein, which may be bypassed by communicating veins (28).

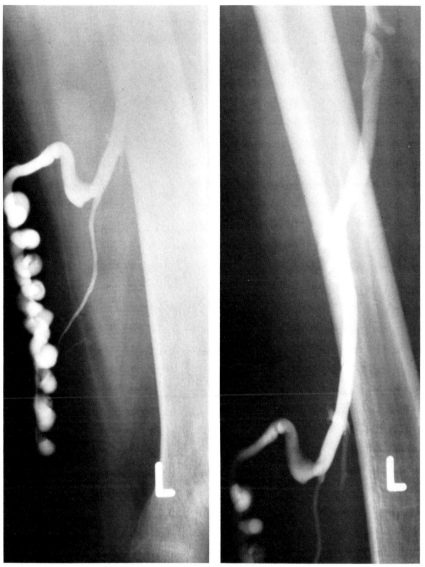

Figure 8–7.   These varicose veins on the lateral aspect of the thigh join the profunda femoris vein.

DESCENDING PHLEBOGRAPHY

Descending phlebography is performed to grade deep vein reflux and valvular function (33–35) (Fig. 8–8). It is also useful to show long saphenous vein reflux (36) (Fig. 8–9) and groin recurrent varicose veins following surgery (27). With the patient supine on the fluoroscopy table the femoral vein is punctured at the groin with an 18-gauge needle with obturator, which is threaded a short distance into the vein. A controlled Valsalva maneuver is performed by the patient that entails maintaining a column of mercury at 40 mm for at least 12 sec by blowing into the barrel of a syringe attached to a manometer. The supine horizontal position is

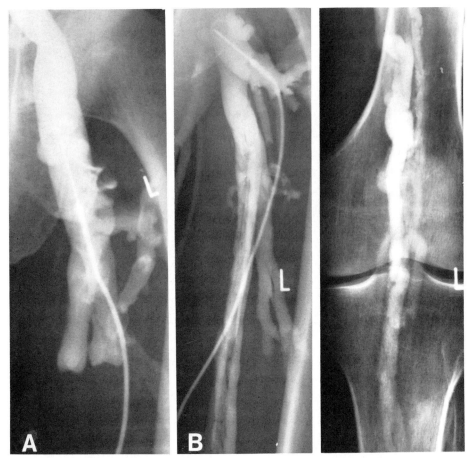

Figure 8–8. *A*, This descending phlebogram shows that there is grade 1 deep vein reflux. Note the clear cutoff of competent valves in the upper part of the superficial femoral vein when the controlled Valsalva maneuver is used. *B*, There is at least grade 3 deep vein reflux. The veins show gross changes of past venous thrombosis.

preferred by patients, and the standard Valsalva maneuver closes normal valve cusps tightly and minimizes the hyperbaric effect of contrast medium, avoiding false-positive degrees of deep vein reflux (34).

VENOUS DYSPLASIAS

Apart from minor anatomic variations, venous dysplasias include aplasia, hypoplasia, venous aneurysms, localized venous angiomas, and extensive rami-fying angiomas extending throughout the tissues of the limb and producing secondary effects in soft tissues and bones (2). The commonest complex venous angiodysplasia is the Klippel-Trenaunay syndrome (37). A feature of the syndrome is persistence of the primitive lateral limb bud vein of the leg, present in about

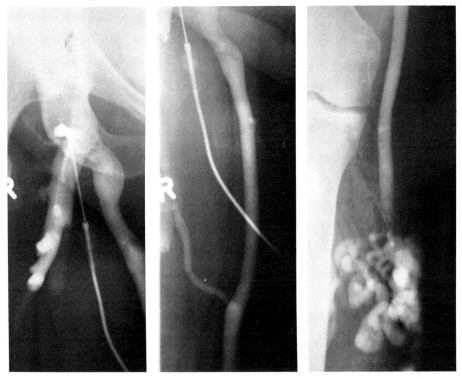

Figure 8–9.   There is grade 1 deep vein reflux shown on this descending phlebogram. There is gross long saphenous vein reflux. The long saphenous vein is dilated and joins a group of varicose veins in the calf.

70 per cent of patients (38,39). This appears on varicography as a valveless, dilated, tortuous channel that may join the profunda femoris vein, the superficial femoral vein, the iliac veins, or the inferior vena cava, frequently with multiple connections.

The most important aspect of investigating this complex venous dysplasia and similar lesions is to demonstrate the normality or abnormality of the deep veins. If the deep veins are absent or hypoplastic, a feature found in about 20 per cent of patients (39), ligation of the superficial veins will aggravate the situation and increase the size and number of varicose veins and the edema (Fig. 8–10).

Phlebographic techniques required to investigate the Klippel-Trenaunay syndrome include ascending phlebography to show the deep venous system and any incompetent communicating veins, varicography, direct contrast injection of the lesions to indicate their connections, and arteriography with follow-through to the venous phase to show the full extent of the dysplasis (18,39) Arteriography may be necessary to exclude arteriovenous fistulas, which are not a feature of the Klippel-Trenaunay syndrome but are part of the Parkes-Weber syndrome (40). Computed tomography is useful in showing the extent of the lesion, particularly whether it has extended into surrounding structures, which would influence its operability.

The most commonly found venous abnormalities in the Klippel-Trenaunay syndrome are shown in Table 8–1.

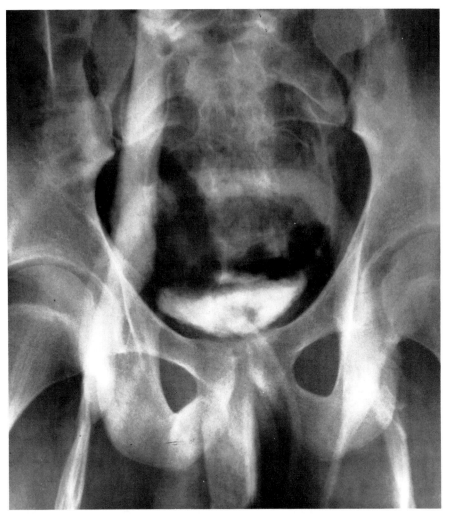

Figure 8–10. Bilateral ascending phelbograms showing the iliac veins in a patient with the Klippel-Trenaunay syndrome. The left common iliac vein is totally absent, with contrast medium passing from left to right through a very large suprapubic collateral. Ligation of this large collateral would lead to edema of the left leg because of its absence of normal deep venous drainage. The iliac veins on the right are normal.

TABLE 8–1. Results of Phlebographic Investigations in Klippel-Trenaunay Syndrome[a]

PHLEBOGRAPHIC FINDINGS	NUMBER	PERCENTAGE
1. Deep veins		
Normal	29	60
Dilatation or reduplication	11	22
Atresia	9	18
2. Incompetent communicating veins	22	45
3. Lateral venous channel draining into:	36	68
(i) Main stem veins	19	53[b]
Popliteal vein	4	11[b]
Superficial femoral vein	6	17[b]
Profunda femoris vein	7	20[b]
External iliac vein	2	5[b]
(ii) Internal iliac veins via gluteals	12	33[b]
(iii) Long saphenous vein	5	14[b]

[a] Results in 49 limbs in 46 patients. From Baskerville PA, Ackroyd JS, Lea Thomas M, Browse NL: The Klippel-Trenaunay syndrome: Clinical, radiological and haemodynamic features and management. Br J Surg 1985;72:232–236, by permission of the publishers, Butterworth & Co (Publishers).
[b] Percentage of 36 limbs with lateral venous channel.

DIGITAL SUBTRACTION PHLEBOGRAPHY

Digital subtraction phlebography has no special place other than to reduce the cost by using less contrast medium. The degregation of the image inherent in the method makes such phlebograms less informative.

REFERENCES

1. Neiman HL: Venography in acute and chronic venous diseases. *In* Bergan JJ, Yao JST, eds: Surgery of the Veins. Orlando, FL, Grune & Stratton Inc, 1985;73–87.
2. Browse NL, Burnand KG, Lea Thomas M: Diseases of the Veins. London, Edward Arnold, 1985.
3. Lea Thomas M: Contrast media in phlebography. *In* Carr DH, ed: Contrast Media. Edinburgh, Churchill Livingstone, 1988;89–96.
4. Meserau WA, Robertson HR: Observations on venous endothelial injury following the injection of venous radiographic contrast media in the rat. J Neurosurg 1961;*18*:289–294.
5. Ritchie WGM, Lynch RR, Stewart GJ: The effect of contrast media on normal and inflamed canine veins. Invest Radiol 1974;*9*:444–455.
6. Zinner G, Gottlob R: Morphologic changes in vessel endothelia caused by contrast media. Angiology 1959;*10*:207–213.
7. Albrechtsson U, Olsson CG: Thrombotic side effects of lower limb phlebography. Lancet 1976;*1*:723–724.
8. Walters HL, Clemenson J, Browse NL, Lea Thomas M: 125 I fibrinogen uptake following phlebography of the leg. Radiology 1980;*135*:619–621.
9. Lea Thomas M, Briggs GM: Low osmolality contrast media for phlebography. Int Angiol 1984;*3*:73–76.
10. Spigos DG, Thane TT, Capek V: Skin necrosis following extravasation during peripheral phlebography. Radiology 1977;*123*:605–606.
11. Berge T, Berquist D, Efsing HO, Hallbook T: Local complications of ascending phlebography. Clin Radiol 1978;*29*:691–696.
12. Lea Thomas M: Phlebography. *In* Ansell G, Wilkins RA, eds: Complications of Diagnostic Imaging, 2nd ed. Oxford, England, Blackwell Scientific Publications, 1987;288–299.
13. Bettman MA, Salzman EW, Rosenthal D, Clagett P, Davies G, Nebesar R, Rabinov K, Ploetz J, Skillman J: Reduction of venous thrombosis complicating phlebography. AJR 1980;*134*:1169–1172.
14. Lea Thomas M, Keeling FB, Piaggio RB, Treweeke PS: Contrast agent induced thrombophlebitis following leg phlebography; iopamidol versus meglumine iothalamate. Br J Radiol 1984;*57*:205–207.
15. Lea Thomas M, Bowles JN, Piaggio RB, Price J, Treweeke PS: Contrast induced thrombophlebitis following leg phlebography: Iohexol compared with meglumine iothalamate. Vasa 1985;*14*:81–83.
16. Lea Thomas M, Briggs GM, Kaun BB: Contrast agent induced thrombophlebitis following leg phlebography: Meglumine ioxaglate versus meglumine iothalamate. Radiology 1985;*147*:399–400.
17. Lea Thomas M, Creagh MF, Mahraj RPM, Tung KT: A comparative trial of the tolerance and diagnostic quality of iopromide and iopamidol when used for leg phlebography. Vasa 1988;*17*:273–274.
18. Lea Thomas M: Phlebography of the Lower Limb. Edinburgh, Churchill Livingstone, 1982.
19. Lea Thomas M, McAllister V: The radiological progression of deep vein thrombosis. Radiology 1971:99:37–40.
20. Lea Thomas M, Caty H: The appearances of artifacts on lower limb phlebograms. Clin Radiol 1975;*26*:527–533.
21. Lofgren EP: Long saphenous vein varicosities. *In* Bergen JJ, Yao JST, eds: Surgery of the Veins. Orlando, FL, Grune & Stratton Inc, 1985;285–299.
22. Lea Thomas M, McAllister V, Rose DH, Tonge K: A simplified technique for the localization of incompetent perforating veins of the legs. Clin Radiol 1972;*23*:486–491.
23. Lea Thomas M, Bowles JN: Incompetent perforating veins. Comparison of varicography and ascending phlebography. Radiology 1985;*154*:619–624
24. Lea Thomas M, Posniak HV: Varicography. Int Angiol 1985;*4*:475–482.
25. Lea Thomas M, Keeling FP: Varicography in the management of recurrent varicose veins. Angiology 1986;*37*:570–575.

26. Corbett CR, McIrvine AJ, Aston NO, Jamieson CW, Lea Thomas M: The use of varicography to identify the sources of incompetence in current varicose veins. Ann R Coll Surg Engl 1984;*66*:412–415.

27. Lea Thomas M, Mahraj RPM: A comparison of varicography and descending phlebography in clinically suspected recurrent groin and upper thigh varicose veins. Phlebology 1988;*3*:155–162.

28. Lea Thomas M, Posniak HV: Saphenography. AJR 1983;*141*:812–814.

29. Lea Thomas M, Chan O: Anatomical variations of the short saphenous vein: A phlebographic study. Vasa 1988;*17*:51–55.

30. Hobbs H: A new approach to short saphenous vein varicosities. *In* Bergan JJ, Yao JST, eds: Surgery of the Veins. Orlando, FL, Grune & Stratton Inc, 1985;301–321.

31. Lea Thomas M, Chan O: Lateral thigh varicose veins: A phlebographic study. Br J Radiol 1988;*61*:372–373.

32. Palma EC: Vein transplants and grafts in the surgical treatment of the post-phleobtic syndrome. J Cardiovasc Surg 1960;*1*:94–107.

33. Herman RJ, Neiman HL, Yao JST, Egan TJ, Bergan JJ, Malave SR: Descending venography: A method of evaluating lower extremity venous valvular function. Radiology 1980;*137*:63–69.

34. Lea Thomas M, Keeling FP, Ackroyd JS: Descending phlebography: A comparison of three methods and an assessment of the normal range of deep vein reflux. J Cardiovasc Surg 1986;*22*:27–30.

35. Ackroyd JS, Lea Thomas M, Browse NL: Deep vein reflux: An assessment by descending phlebography. Br J Surg 1986;*73*:31–33.

36. Lea Thomas M, Bowles JN: Descending phlebography in the assessment of long saphenous vein incompetence. Am J Roentgenol 1985;*145*:1255–1257.

37. Klippel M, Trenaunay P: Du naevus variqueux osteo-hypertrophiques. Arch Gen Med (Paris) 1900;*185*:641–672.

38. Baskerville PA, Ackroyd JS, Lea Thomas M, Browse NL: The Klippel-Trenaunay syndrome: Clinical, radiological and haemodynamic features and management. Br J Surg 1985;*72*:232–236.

39. Lea Thomas M, MacFie GB: Phlebography in the Klippel-Trenaunay syndrome. Acta Radiol 1974;*15*:43–56.

40. Parkes Weber F: Angioma formation in connection with hypertrophy of limbs and hemi-hypertrophy. Br J Dermatol 1907;*19*:231–235.

9

QUANTITATION OF VENOUS REFLUX USING DUPLEX SCANNING

D. E. Strandness, Jr., and Paul van Bemmelen

During its development, deep vein thrombosis most commonly results in total occlusion of the involved venous segments. Recanalization secondary to fibrinolysis will often occur, and happens rapidly with a variable end result (1). While there is no doubt that restoration of patency by this mechanism is a desirable end point, valve function is not often preserved, and its loss is the most serious complication of this common disorder (2–4).

When venous valves become incompetent, the normal directional patterns of flow within the venous system may be drastically altered (2). Normally when the calf muscle pump is activated, the compressing force of the contracting muscle propels blood only in an antegrade direction. During the relaxation phase venous refilling will occur through transcapillary inflow and from the superficial veins via the perforators.

The location and numbers of valves appear to be determined by the function required of them at that level. For example, in areas not subjected to muscular compression, valves are uncommon or absent (5). This is the case for the inferior vena cava and the iliac veins. Below the inguinal ligament, the numbers of valves increase steadily to below the knee, where hundreds of valves can be found. In addition, the communicating veins also have valves that permit only unidirectional flow from the superficial to the deep veins, regardless of the state of muscular activity. The two most constant and largest perforating veins are the greater and lesser saphenous, both of which normally have valves at their point of termination and connection with the deep venous system. Those communicating veins commonly associated with the postthrombotic syndrome are located along the medial side of the lower leg (6).

While the presence of valvular incompetence can be inferred by the presence of postthrombotic changes in the lower limb, it has only been recently that attempts have been made to localize and quantitate this problem. If the documentation and importance of valvular incompetence is to be appreciated, it will be necessary to evaluate the entire venous system from the level of the foot to the abdomen. It will not be possible to fully understand the pathophysiology of the postthrombotic syndrome until this has been accomplished. Any physiologic event that reverses the normal transvalvular pressure gradient will tend to promote reverse flow (reflux). With contraction of the calf muscle pump, the normal gradient will be immediately reversed for the segments distal (toward the foot) to the activated muscle groups. This would include not only the deep veins but the communicating segments as well.

All levels of the venous system must be evaluated to permit an accurate description of the role of valvular incompetence in the production of clinical events. For example, continuous-wave Doppler is perhaps the most common method that is used. This can monitor the direction of flow as modified by either compression proximal to the transducer or a Valsalva maneuver (7). This method has two major problems: first, the magnitude of the force exerted cannot be controlled, and, second, a competent valve at a proximal site may make the evaluation of distal valves difficult if not impossible.

To develop a better method of documenting valvular reflux at all levels of the limb, a set of experiments were carried out using ultrasonic duplex scanning as the method of documenting reflux.

MATERIALS AND METHODS

The study population consisted of 15 men (seven left limbs, eight right limbs) and 17 women (nine left limbs, eight right limbs). They ranged in age from 18 to 35 years. None had a previous history of varicose veins, episodes of venous thrombosis, fractures, surgery, or immobilization of their limbs.

In the first part of the study, the subject was placed in the supine position but tilted to a 10 degree reverse Trendelenburg position. The methods used to induce reverse flow were Valsalva's maneuver, manual compression of the limb, and proximal compression by a pneumatic cuff that could be inflated automatically. The pressure level within the cuff was set to 40 mm Hg to reverse the pressure gradient.

For the second part of the study, the subject stood on a platform while holding onto a frame with the weight supported by the contralateral limb. An automatic cuff inflator was used to rapidly inflate and deflate the cuffs at different levels of the limb. The pressure chosen varied by that part of the limb being examined. For the thigh 80 mm Hg was used, for the calf 100 mm Hg, and for the foot 120 mm Hg. The cuffs varied in width for each segment of the limb. For the thigh a 24-cm wide cuff was used, for the calf a 12-cm cuff, and for the foot a 7-cm cuff. The cuffs were inflated for approximately 3 sec, with the deflation requiring only 0.3 sec.

The velocity and direction of flow was monitored using an Ultramark 8 duplex scanner (Advanced Technology Laboratories, Bothell, WA). The measurements were recorded distal to the cuff when rapid cuff inflation was used and proximal to the cuff when rapid deflation was used. The distance between the cuff and the transducer was always less than 5 cm. The venous segments examined by this approach included the common femoral, deep femoral, superficial femoral, popliteal, posterior tibial at midcalf, and posterior tibial at the level of the ankle.

RESULTS

For the common femoral vein, the duration of reverse flow, (i.e., reflux) with a Valsalva maneuver before the valves closed was 0.69 ± 0.83 sec in the upright position and 1.77 ± 0.96 sec in the supine position. This difference was significant at the $p < .01$ level by the Wilcoxon signed rank test.

Manual compression at literally all levels of the limb was not adequate to obtain reliable and reproducible results. (Fig. 9–1). This pointed out the problems associated with this commonly used method of testing reflux. While there are situations in patients with valvular incompetence in which such a maneuver will induce reverse flow, it is not consistent enough to warrant its use for quantitative determination of this phenomenon.

The most consistent and reliable results were obtained with the patient in the standing position. As noted in Figures 9–2 and 9–3, the reflux duration in 95 per cent of the subjects tested was less than 0.5 sec. In the eight instances with values above that level, those recorded from adjacent venous segments were less than 0.5 sec. An example of how these recordings compare in a normal subject versus a patient with valvular incompetence is shown in Figure 9–4.

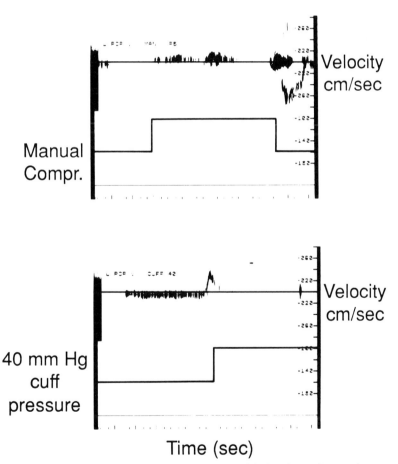

Figure 9–1. When the the thigh is manually compressed with the ultrasonic transducer over the popliteal vein, there is no discernible peak demonstrating valve closure. The subject is in reverse Trendelenburg (− 10 degrees). When a cuff on the thigh is inflated to 40 mm Hg pressure, there is prompt valve closure in 0.37 sec. (From van Bemmelen PS, Bedford G, Beach K, Strandness DE Jr: Quantitative segmental evaluation of venous valvular reflux with duplex ultrasound scanning. J. Vasc Surg 1989;*10*:425–431.)

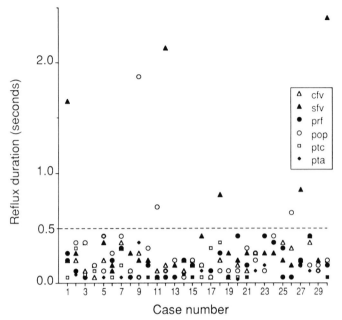

Figure 9–2. Scattergram of reflux durations in 30 normal legs. These data were obtained by deflating cuffs distal to the transducer in the standing position. Ninety-five per cent of the values are below 0.5 sec. *cfv*, Common femoral vein; *sfv*, superficial femoral vein; *prf*, profunda femoris vein; *pop*, popliteal vein; *ptc*, posterior tibial vein at midcalf; *pta*, posterior tibial vein at the ankle. (From van Bemmelen PS, Bedford G, Beach K, Strandness DE Jr: Quantitative segmental evaluation of venous valvular reflux with duplex ultrasound scanning. J Vasc Surg 1989;*10*:425–431.)

DISCUSSION

As noted in this study, the Valsalva maneuver was adequate for only the more proximal venous segments, such as the common femoral vein. However, if there is one competent valve in the iliac vein, this method will be of little use for valves distal to that point. More importantly, for testing of valves in the superficial femoral and popliteal veins, the entire venous system proximal to that level would also have to be incompetent for the Valsalva maneuver to work as a method of testing reflux. Likewise, manual compression is so variable that it cannot be recommended for routine use.

It has been routine to assess the deep venous system with the patient supine or in a 10 degree reverse Trendelenburg position. This position is adequate for documentation of persistent venous obstruction or recanalization of a previously thrombosed venous segment. There are cases in which a valve is found to be competent in the supine position but incompetent in the upright position. This may reflect the extent to which the vein is distended at the time the reverse pressure gradient is generated.

The one test of valvular incompetence that is considered a gold standard is descending phlebography (8). While it is done in the upright position, descending phlebography does have several problems, some of which are:

1. The presence of one competent valve in the superficial femoral vein will prevent the evaluation of more distal venous segments. This might explain why

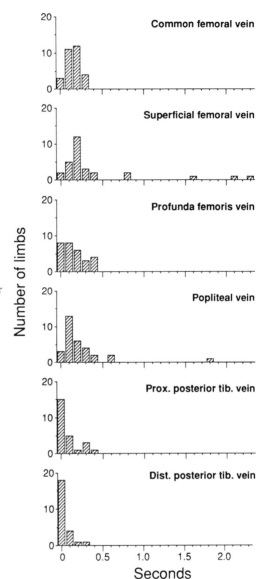

Figure 9–3. Range of reflux duration for each of the venous segments tested.

reflux of contrast was not found in 73 percent of patients with established postthrombotic changes in their limbs.

2.   The higher specific gravity of contrast material to blood (1.28 versus 1.05). Since valves are open in the relaxed vertical leg, contrast material will "trickle" down the normal leg.

3.   Examination is not done after activation of the calf muscle pump. This fails to provide any information as to the amount of diastolic leakage that occurs.

The importance of diastolic leakage in terms of the pathophysiology of the postthrombotic syndrome can best be described by analogy to the valves of the heart. Those valves that close in response to muscular contraction are of the mitral type, and valves that close during relaxation are of the aortic type. While both

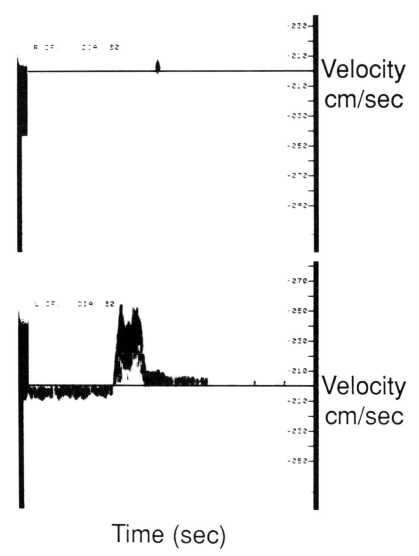

Figure 9–4.   *Top*, Response of a normal valve to deflation of the cuff. The transducer was over the common femoral vein with the cuff about the thigh. *Bottom*, Result of the same test in a patient with a proven recanalized vein. The duration of reflux is 1.33 sec. (From van Bemmelen PS, Bedford G, Beach K, Strandness DE Jr: Quantitative segmental evaluation of venous valvular reflux with duplex ultrasound scanning. J Vasc Surg 1989;*10*:425–431.)

of these functions are important, the prevention of reverse flow during diastole is essential in stopping the reflux that, over time, appears to be most damaging. Compression of the deep venous segments in the absence of competent valves will result in antegrade flow because of the pressure gradient that is produced and the low resistance of draining veins leading to the right heart. During muscular relaxation, flow into the collapsed compressed veins will normally be via the capillary network since the competent valves will prevent reflux.

The methods to test valve function are based upon the systolic-diastolic concepts just presented. As noted, it is important that the transducer be close to the site of compression to be as accurate as possible in defining the exact site of incompetence. The one site where this is not possible is the common femoral vein, where the transducer may have up to three valves between it and the site of pressure generated by the Valsalva maneuver. This would not, of course, apply to the situation in which there are no valves above the inguinal ligament. This is found in about 24 per cent of the population.

How does the current method compare with the results obtained with photoplethysmography and direct venous pressure measurements? While there is no doubt that they can be used to document the hemodynamic response in the presence of incompetent valves, it is not always possible to be sure at what level the problem exists (9).

The cuff deflation method is the most reproducible and useful technique for the documentation of valvular reflux. It also seems to be as close to reality as possible. For example, the short reaction time to valve closure would appear to mimic quite closely the events that occur with activation of the muscle pump. Based upon the results and our current knowledge, it should become the standard method for documenting segmental valvular incompetence.

ACKNOWLEDGMENTS: Supported in part by National Institutes of Health grant No. HL36095-02 and the Netherlands Organization for Scientific Research (NWO), the Hague.

REFERENCES

1. Killewich LA, Bedford G, Beach KW, Strandness DE Jr: Spontaneous lysis of deep venous thrombi: Rate and outcome. J Vasc Surg 1989;9:89–97.
2. Strandness DE Jr, Langlois Y, Cramer M, et al: Long term sequelae of acute venous thrombosis. JAMA 1983;250:1289–1292.
3. Killewich LA, Martin R, Cramer M, et al: An objective assessment of the physiologic changes in the postthrombotic syndrome. Arch Surg 1985;120:424–426.
4. Edwards EA, Edwards JE: The effect of thrombophlebitis on the venous valve. Surg Gynecol Obstet 1937;65:310–320.
5. Basmajian JV: The distribution of valves in the femoral, external iliac and common iliac veins and their relationship to varicose veins. Surg Gynecol Obstet 1952;95:537–542.
6. Haeger K: Leg ulcers, In Hobbs JT, ed: The Treatment of Venous Disorders. Philadelphia, JB Lippincott Co, 1977;273–292.
7. Barnes RW: Doppler ultrasonic diagnosis of venous disease. In Bernstein EF, ed: Noninvasive Diagnostic Techniques in Vascular Disease, 3rd ed. St. Louis, CV Mosby Co, 1985;724–729.
8. Kistner RL, Ferris EB, Randhawa G, Kamida C: A method of performing descending venography. J Vasc Surg 1986;4:464–468.
9. Abramowitz HB, Queral LA, Flinn WR, et al: The use of photoplethysmography in the assessment of venous insufficiency: A comparison to venous pressure measurements. Surgery 1979;86:434–441.

10

DIAGNOSIS OF UPPER EXTREMITY VENOUS THROMBOSIS BY DUPLEX SCANNING

Thomas M. Kerr, Kenneth S. Lutter,
Robert D. Cranley, and John J. Cranley

Duplex scanning has had a revolutionary effect on the vascular laboratory. It has become the standard noninvasive method for examining the carotid arteries (1,2), the veins (3–7), and the arteries and soft tissue of the lower extremity (8), and is showing great promise for examination of the renal (9) and other visceral vessels of the abdomen (10). In the upper extremity it is equally useful, is easier to perform, and affords greater detail because of the decreased tissue mass (11). The number of patients coming to the vascular laboratory for upper extremity problems is much less than those coming for carotid or lower extremity studies. During the period from January 1, 1985 to December 31, 1989 693 duplex scans of the upper extremity were performed (12). Table 10–1 shows the indications or final diagnoses for these upper extremity scans. To put it into a proper perspective, this represents 3 per cent of all tests, 12 per cent of the number of duplex scans of the lower extremity, and 14 per cent of the number of scans done for carotid artery disease.

This report focuses on the 123 instances in which venous thrombosis was diagnosed; 85 of these were axillary-subclavian vein thromboses, eight jugular vein thromboses, and 30 superficial vein thromboses. These 123 instances of thrombosis were found in 693 (18 percent of the upper extremities scanned during this period of time. Axillary-subclavian venous thrombosis was also found in 7 per cent of the patients examined with deep vein thrombosis of the lower extremity. Table 10–2 and Figure 10–1 show numerically and graphically the location of thrombi found.

MATERIALS AND METHODS

All scans were performed with a commercially available, high-resolution duplex instrument (Biosound 2000IIA, Biosound Phase II, or Acuson 128). All scans were graded for quality by the interpreter as follows: poor quality—a portion of the scan was uninterpretable; fair quality—the diagnosis could be made, but the

144

TABLE 10–1. Findings in or Reasons for 693 Consecutive Upper Extremity Scans

	NO.	%
Vein mapping	211	31
Negative scans	201	29
Dialysis graft in place	96	14
Axillary-subclavian venous thrombosis	85	12
Miscellaneous (cysts, hematoma, edema)	36	05
Superficial thrombophlebitis	30	04
Arterial scans	26	04
Internal jugular vein thrombosis	8	01
Total	693	100

entire scan was not well visualized; good quality—all structures well visualized. A standard laboratory protocol was followed in each examination (11) (Figs. 10–2 and 10–3).

All patient hospital charts were reviewed. Medical history, hospital course, demographic information, treatment, and follow-up data were obtained. The variables examined included: symptoms, signs, and their duration; admitting diagnosis; possible hypercoagulable states; presence, type, and extent of existing neoplasia; presence and type of peripheral or central venous access; type of venous line (single or triple lumen); and type of catheter and its site of placement. Also analyzed was the composition of intravenous fluids administered. The diagnostic tests and location of the thrombi were reviewed, as well as the duration and type of anticoagulant or lytic therapy. Follow-up was obtained from the patient's personal physician and/or telephone contact with the patient or his family. Particular attention was given to the incidence of pulmonary embolism and to postthrombotic symptoms and signs, including weakness, heaviness, swelling, and limited motion. We have not seen induration of the subcutaneous tissue or ulceration of the skin, as is seen in the postthrombotic syndrome of the lower extremity.

Accuracy

In a multicenter collaborative study of the accuracy of lower extremity duplex scanning we reported that in extremities with positive phlebograms the scan was

TABLE 10–2. Location of Thrombi in 85 Extremities

Isolated	
Subclavian	61
Axillary	39
Brachial	31
Internal jugular	28
Cephalic	24
Basilic	18
External jugular	11
Internal jugular alone	8
Antecubital	2
Combinations	
Subclavian-axillary	36
Subclavian-axillary-brachial	26
Subclavian-axillary-brachial-internal jugular	9

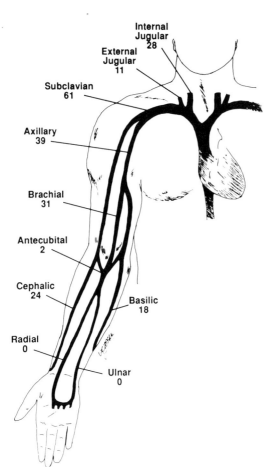

Figure 10–1. Numerical and graphic location of thrombi.

Internal
Jugular
28

External
Jugular
11

Subclavian
61

Axillary
39

Brachial
31

Antecubital
2

Cephalic
24

Basilic
18

Radial
0

Ulnar
0

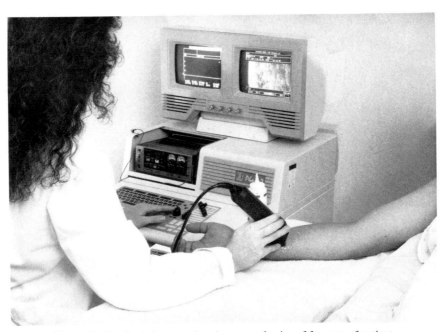

Figure 10–2. Technician performing scan of veins of forearm of patient.

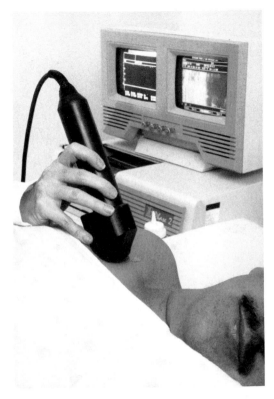

Figure 10–3.   Technician performing scan of subclavian vein of patient.

97 per cent sensitive. (13,14). The phlebogram was negative, however, in 191 extremities and was considered to be incorrect in six instances. Thus it was not a perfect standard when negative, and the duplex scan was slightly more accurate.

We cannot provide similar data in the upper extremity because there is a blind area behind the clavicle. Only six phlebograms were performed in this study. While all were confirmatory, there is the possibility that some subclavian vein thromboses were missed. The jugular, axillary, arm, and forearm veins are more easily seen than the veins of the lower extremity, probably because of the decreased mass in the upper extremity and neck. One would expect the accuracy of the scan to be equal to or better than that in the lower extremity. However, it may not be possible to interrogate the mid- and medial portion of the subclavian vein. The bone prevents visualization of the vein, which cannot be compressed, and the Doppler signal may be unobtainable. Ruling out a thrombus in this area requires a phlebogram.

Figure 10–4 shows a thrombus in the left subclavian vein in a patient in whom the scan was negative. This occurred during the period prior to the initiation of this study. We are unaware of any patients with negative scans during this study who later were found to have subclavian vein thrombosis, but the possibility exists that some were missed.

Signs and Symptoms

As in the lower extremity, the signs and symptoms of deep vein thrombosis are not diagnostic. As indicated in Table 10–1, 201 extremities scanned during

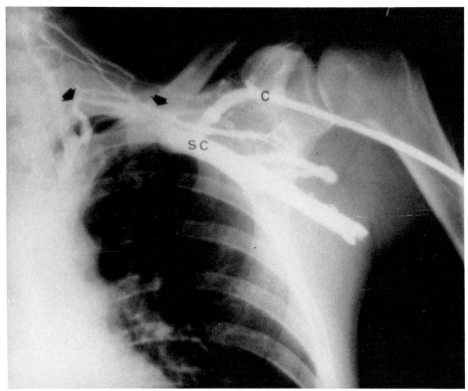

Figure 10–4. Thrombus (arrowheads) in left subclavian vein (SC) diagnosed by phlebogram; the duplex scan was negative. In the mid- and medial portion of the subclavian vein, the clavicle prevents visualization of clot and the cephalic vein (C) cannot be compressed. The Doppler signal may be unobtainable.

the study were found to be negative. All these patients were referred to the laboratory because they were symptomatic. The most common symptoms and signs were pain, tenderness, and swelling. Pain and tenderness were equally common in the extremities that proved to have venous thrombosis and those that proved to be negative. Swelling was more common in the extremities that proved to have thrombosis, but this was not statistically significant.

Superficial Thrombophlebitis

In the past we have considered this diagnosis to be certain on physical examination. While this is still true, we have seen an increasing number that have unexpected, and clinically undiagnosed, extension of the thrombus from the superficial to the deep system in both the lower and upper extremity.

RESULTS

Of 85 patients with axillary or subclavian vein thrombosis, 46 (54 percent) were males. Of all scans performed, the scan quality was judged to be good in 73 per cent of the study population, fair in 24 per cent and poor in 3 per cent.

TABLE 10–3. Axillary-Subclavian Thrombosis: Associated Risk Factors

	NO.	%
Indwelling venous catheter	59/85	69
Excluding indwelling catheter		
Cancer	13/26	50
Physical strain	5/26	19
Hypercoagulability	5/26	19
Drug abuse	3/26	12
Obesity	2/26	08
Pregnancy	1/26	04
Steroid hormones	1/26	04

Tables 10–3 and 10–4 show the associated risk factors. The most common risk factor was a central or peripheral venous catheter (69 per cent of 85 patients with subclavian-axillary venous thrombosis). Table 10–3 also shows the risk factors when the indwelling catheter is excluded. It is of interest that 15 patients with acute cardiac problems developed subclavian-axillary thrombosis but all had central venous lines in place. This may be attributed to the large size of the catheter used in these patients. No cardiac patient who did not have a catheter in place developed subclavian-axillary venous thrombosis.

Of those with a central venous catheter who developed venous thrombosis, 31 were male and 21 female. Twenty-three (42.3 per cent) involved the right side and 29 (57.7 per cent) the left. The average duration of catheter use was 17.3 ± 18.6 days (range 1 to 240). Table 10–5 lists the type of catheters used. Hyperalimentation formula was infused in 27 per cent of the patients with venous thrombosis.

Of the 61 axillary-subclavian vein thrombosis patients available for follow-up, five (8.2 per cent) had a pulmonary embolism. One of these had a negative lower extremity duplex scan and a negative venacavogram. There were five upper extremity venograms and one phleborheogram, all positive. Two of the five patients with a pulmonary embolism died. In each case the cause of death was believed to be pulmonary embolism, although autopsies were not obtained. Two of the five emboli occurred in patients with subclavian-axillary thrombosis with a catheter in place, two in patients without an indwelling catheter, and one from the site of a peripheral venous catheter.

Seven extremities developed axillary-subclavian thrombosis believed to have arisen from a peripheral intravenous site. In five of these extremities thrombus extended from the cephalic or basilic vein into the brachial and the subclavian vein. When the thrombotic process extended into the jugular veins it was included in the axillary-subclavian group. In addition, eight instances of an isolated internal or external jugular vein thrombosis were diagnosed. In six of these it was related

TABLE 10–4. Isolated Jugular Vein Thrombosis: Associated Risk Factors

	NO.	%
Internal jugular venous line	6/8	75
Neck abscess (drug abuse)	1/8	13
Chronic renal failure	1/8	13

TABLE 10–5. Types of Intravenous Line Associated with Thrombosis in 59 Identifiable Catheters

CATHETER TYPE	NUMBER (%)
Swan-Ganz	17 (32)
Triple lumen	13 (24)
Porta-Cath	8 (15)
Peripheral (unspecified)	7 (13)
Dialysis	6 (11)
Pacemaker	2 (4)
Nonspecified	6 (11)

to an indwelling catheter (hyperalimentation). In one instance the thrombosis followed a neck abscess (drug abuse) and in one the patient had chronic renal failure. No pulmonary emboli or postthrombotic sequelae occurred in this group.

At 2 years almost half of all the patients with axillary-subclavian thrombosis were dead, indicating the high risk of this group of patients.

Thirty-six per cent of the patients in this study complained of residual symptoms. It hs been suggested (15) that anticoagulation beyond the acute event may decrease these sequelae. Our experience supports this in the group with a catheter, but not in the noncatheter group. It has also been reported (15,16) that less morbidity results from catheter-associated venous thrombosis as compared to primary venous thrombosis of the axillary-subclavian vein. This was true in this study also.

DISCUSSION

Upper extremity major vein thrombosis is becoming more common because of the frequent use of indwelling catheters, as indicated by Tables 10–2 and 10–3. When the indwelling catheter was excluded malignancy was the commonest predisposing factor. It is of interest that all the cardiac patients with deep vein thrombosis had an indwelling catheter. This is most probably due to the large size of the catheters used. In 27 per cent of the patients with a central line hyperalimentation fluid was infused, making it a high risk factor. Quite unexpectedly, seven instances of a spreading thrombus from a superficial vein to the deep system were encountered.

Duplex scanning of the upper extremity provides a very practical method of diagnosing upper extremity venous thrombosis. The one "blind" area under the clavicle makes it necessary to use phlebography in selected cases.

REFERENCES

1. Barber FE, Baker DW, Strandness DE Jr, et al: Duplex scanner II for simultaneous imaging of artery tissues and flow. IEEE publication 74, CHOop61SU, Ultrasonic Symposium Proceedings. New York, Institute for Electrical and Electronics Engineers, 1974.
2. Comerota AJ, Cranley JJ, Cook SE: Real time B-mode carotid imaging in diagnosis of cerebrovascular disease. Surgery 1981;89:718–729.
3. Talbot SR: Use of real-time imaging in identifying deep venous obstruction: A preliminary report. Bruit 1982;6:41–42.

4. Sullivan ED, Peter DJ, Cranley JJ: Real-time B-mode venous ultrasound. J Vasc Surgery 1984;*1*:465–471.

5. Flanagan LD, Sullivan ED, Cranley JJ: Venous imaging of the extremities using real-time B-mode ultrasound. *In* Bergan JJ, Yao JST, eds: Surgery of the Veins. Orlando, FL, Grune & Stratton, 1984;89–98.

6. Cranley JJ: Seeing is believing. A clot is a clot, on a duplex scan or a phlebogram [editorial]. Echocardiography: A Review of Cardiovascular Ultrasound 1987;*4*:423.

7. Kerr TM, Cranley JJ, Johnson RJ, et al: Analysis of 1084 consecutive lower extremities involved with acute venous thrombosis diagnosed by duplex scanning. Surgery 1990;*108*:520–527.

8. Johnston KW, Kassam M, Cobbold RSC: Relationship between Doppler pulsatility index and direct femoral pressure measurements in the diagnosis of aortoiliac occlusive disease. Ultrasound Med Biol 1083;*9*:271–281.

9. Kohler TR, Zierler RE, Martin RL, et al: Noninvasive diagnosis of renal artery stenosis by ultrasonic duplex scanning. J Vasc Surg 1986;*4*:450–456.

10. Nicholls SC, Kohler TR, Martin RL, et al: Use of hemodynamic parameters in the diagnosis of mesenteric insufficiency. J Vasc Surg 1986;*3*:507–510.

11. Karkow WS, Ruoff BA, Cranley JJ: B-mode venous imaging. *In* Kempczinski RF, Yao JST, eds: Practical Noninvasive Vascular Diagnosis. Chicago, Year Book Medical Publishers; 1987;464–485.

12. Kerr TM, Lutter KS, Moeller DM, et al: Upper extremity venous thromboses diagnosed by duplex scanning. Am J Surg 1990;*160*:202–206.

13. Cranley JJ, Higgins RF, Berry RE, Ford CR, Comerota AJ, Griffin LH: Near parity in the final diagnosis of deep venous thrombosis by duplex scan and phlebography. Phlebology 1989;*4*:71–74.

14. Cranley JJ: Diagnosis of deep venous thrombosis. *In* Bernstein EF, ed: Recent Advances in Noninvasive Diagnostic Techniques in Vascular Disease. St. Louis, CV Mosby Co, 1990;207–221.

15. Donayre CE, White GH, Mehringer SM, Wilson SE: Pathogenesis determines late morbidity of axillosubclavian vein thrombosis. Am J Surg 1986;*152*:179–184.

16. Gloviczki P, Kazmier FJ, Hollier LH: Axillary-subclavian venous occlusion: The morbidity of a nonlethal disease. J Vasc Surg 1986;*4*:333–337.

IV

MANAGEMENT OF ACUTE DEEP VEIN THROMBOSIS

11

PROPHYLAXIS OF DEEP VEIN THROMBOSIS: CURRENT TECHNIQUES

Jack Hirsh

Although effective and safe prophylactic methods are now available for most high-risk surgical patient groups, pulmonary embolism (PE) remains the most common preventable cause of death following major surgical procedures (1–3). Recent studies have reported major PE in between 6 and 13 per cent of autopsies; this corresponds to 0.15 to 0.3 per cent of all adult admissions to hospital (4,5). Most of these emboli arise from venous thrombi in the popliteal or more proximal veins of the legs and pelvis.

Routine screening studies with objective tests in patients undergoing surgical procedures have provided reliable estimates for the incidence of venous thrombosis in patients undergoing a wide variety of surgical procedures. The incidence of venous thrombosis in unprotected patients in these groups is summarized in Table 11–1. For most of these conditions thrombi originate in calf veins; 80 per cent of these thrombi remain limited to the calf and 20 per cent extend into proximal venous segment. In contrast, in hip surgery patients 20 to 30 per cent of thrombi originate in the femoral vein adjacent to the site of surgery and between 30 and 50 per cent of all thrombi following hip surgery are proximal. The patient at high risk for postoperative venous thromboembolism (VTE) can be easily recognized on clinical grounds. The major risk factors are increasing age over 40 years, bed rest for longer than 4 days, extensive surgical procedures, previous venous thrombosis, surgery for malignant disease, major orthopedic procedures, trauma to the legs, postoperative sepsis, and chronic medical illnesses (particularly cardiac disease, pulmonary disease, and recent stroke) (3,4,6). Other risk factors are obesity and the presence of varicose veins.

Safe and effective prophylactic methods have been available to the surgeon for over a decade, yet postoperative VTE remains the most preventable cause of death following major surgical procedures. Why is this? The reason is simple. Prophylaxis is not used routinely in high-risk groups by many general and orthopedic surgeons in North America, and most medical institutions do not have a standardized protocol for prophylaxis in high-risk surgical patients. The attitudes of surgeons toward prophylaxis differ markedly. For example, results of surveys of orthopedic surgeons from different countries revealed marked differences in

TABLE 11–1.   Hospitalized Patients Screened for Venous Thrombosis (VT) with Routine Leg Scanning or Venography

DIAGNOSTIC CATEGORY	SCREENING TEST(S)	VT (%)
Trauma		
Hip fracture	Venogram	40–49
Tibial fracture	Venogram	45
Multiple injuries	Venogram	35
Elective surgery		
General abdominal	Leg scan/venogram	3–51
Splenectomy	Leg scan	6
Thoracic	Leg scan	20–45
Gynecologic	Leg scan	7–45
Prostatectomy (open)	Leg scan	29–51
Prostatectomy (closed)	Leg scan	7–10
Aortofemoral	Leg scan/venogram	4–43
Neurosurgery	Leg scan	29–43
Meniscectomy	Venogram	8
Knee surgery	Venogram	17–57
Knee replacement	Venogram	84
Hip replacement	Venogram	30–65

the frequency of the use of prophylaxis and in the agents used (7–10). In a survey carried out in the United States, the three main reasons given for not using prophylaxis were: 1) VTE is not an important complication of surgery, 2) currently available prophylactic methods are not effective, and 3) the danger of bleeding outweighs the potential benefits of prophylaxis when anticoagulants are used. There is good evidence from clinical trials that challenges these opinions. The results of three separate overview analyses (11–13) confirm that VTE is an important complication of major surgical procedures, that effective prophylactic methods are available, and that if anticoagulant prophylaxis is used the risks of bleeding do not outweigh the benefits of prophylaxis (11–13). Based on these considerations, a recent consensus development conference sponsored by the National Institutes of Health (NIH) recommended the routine use of prophylaxis in high-risk patient groups (14).

PATHOPHYSIOLOGIC BASIS FOR THE PROPHYLACTIC METHODS

The prophylactic methods in current use counteract one or more of the recognized risk factors for venous thrombosis: stasis, increase in blood coagulability, and damage to the vessel wall. It is now clear that these three pathogenetic factors interact closely. Stasis promotes coagulation by limiting the access of activated coagulation factors to thrombomodulin, a powerful thrombin inhibitor bound to endothelial cells and present in greatest density in the capillary circulation. Stasis also produces local hypoxia, which renders endothelial cells thrombogenic by reducing the density of surface-bound thrombomodulin and stimulating the endothelial cells to produce activators of blood coagulation (15). Chronic stasis also reduces local fibrinolytic activity (16). The vascular surface is made thrombogenic by direct injury and by the effects on activated endothelial cells of products of blood coagulation and cytokines (which are released as a result of surgical trauma).

Trauma and surgery result in the production of humoral factors (possibly cyto-kines) that stimulate endothelial cells to synthesize plasminogen activator inhib-itor, thereby impairing postoperative and postraumatic fibrinolytic activity. Fi-nally, activation of blood coagulation by tissue factor is induced by tissue damage and by nondenuding or denuding endothelial injury.

SCREENING FOR POSTOPERATIVE VENOUS THROMBOSIS

The use of screening for venous thrombosis has provided important infor-mation about the indicence of postoperative deep vein thrombosis (DVT) and about the relative effectiveness of prophylactic methods. Routine screening, how-ever, is inefficient and should never replace primary prophylaxis. Clinical diag-nosis is both insensitive and nonspecific and it does not provide a reliable estimate of the incidence of postoperative venous thrombosis. ^{125}I-labeled fibrinogen leg scanning is sensitive and specific for calf vein thrombosis in medical patients and general surgical patients but fails to detect thrombi in the upper third of the su-perficial femoral vein and more proximal leg veins. This is an important limitation in orthopedic patients because many of their thrombi are proximal and, therefore, out of the detection range of ^{125}I-labeled fibrinogen leg scanning. Because of this limitation of leg scanning in orthopedic surgical patients, impedance plethys-mography (IPG) (a test that is sensitive and specific for symptomatic proximal vein thrombosis) and, more recently, B-mode ultrasound imaging have been added to leg scanning as a screen in patients undergoing orthopedic procedures. How-ever, recent studies have demonstrated that approximately 70 per cent of all prox-imal vein thrombi in patients undergoing orthopedic surgical procedures are too small to be detected by IPG (17) and that 40 per cent are not detected by B-mode ultrasound (18). For this reason, the only reliable method for detecting venous thrombosis following hip surgical procedures is routine venography (17,19).

APPROACH TO PROPHYLAXIS

Three approaches have been used to prevent venous thrombosis: 1) reducing venous stasis by intermittent pneumatic compression (IPC), graduated compres-sion stockings, or venoconstriction with dihydroergotamine (DHE); 2) counter-acting increased blood coagulability either with heparin, oral anticoagulants, or more recently low-molecular-weight (LMW) heparins; or 3) rendering the fibrin clot more susceptible to fibrinolysis with dextran polymers that copolymerize with forming fibrin. These prophylactic methods have been applied in a number of ways. Traditionally, venous thrombosis prophylaxis either with anticoagulants or with pneumatic compression has been commenced preoperatively to counteract the effects of the operation on blood coagulability and reduced venous flow. Pro-phylaxis is then continued postoperatively until the patient is fully ambulant. This approach has been modified in recent studies in which prophylaxis was com-menced postoperatively with the aim of preventing microscopic thrombi that form at the time of surgery from growing into clinically important thrombi, and of preventing new thrombi from forming postoperatively. Successful postoperative prophylaxis has been reported with IPC (20), with oral anticoagulants (21), and with LMW heparin (22). Other new approaches have been to commence anticoagulant prophylaxis preoperatively with a very low dose to limit the risk of surgical bleeding and then to increase the dose of anticoagulants postoperatively when the risk of surgical bleeding is reduced. This approach has been used successfully with warfarin prophylaxis and adjusted-dose heparin prophylaxis (23–25). A third approach has been to combine different forms of prophylaxis. This has been achieved most successfully by combining low-dose heparin with graduated compression (26) or DHE (27).

RESULTS OF PROPHYLAXIS

Elective General Surgery

The effects of different prophylactic regimens on the incidence of venous thrombosis detected with ^{125}I-labeled fibrinogen leg scanning after elective general abdominal, thoracic, or pelvic surgery are shown in Table 11–2. The prophylactic regimen was compared with either no treatment or placebo. The results have been pooled to calculate average venous thrombosis rates.

Anticoagulant prophylaxis (low-dose heparin and warfarin) and mechanical methods that counteract stasis reduce venous thrombosis by more than 50 per cent. Most experiences have been obtained with low-dose heparin, in which the risk reduction is greater than 60 per cent. In the pooled analyses performed by Collins and associates (13) and by Clagett and Reisch (12) and in an international trial (28), an excess of wound hematoma, but no increase in major bleeding or fatal bleeding, was found in the low-dose heparin group. Low-dose heparin also reduces the incidence of postoperative proximal vein thrombosis and of fatal PE.

In a study of over 4000 patients comparing low-dose heparin with a control group, low-dose heparin was reported to reduce the incidence of PE and of fatal PE reported at autopsy (29). Fatal embolism was reported in two of 2045 patients in the low-dose heparin group and 16 of 2076 patients in the control group ($p<.005$). In a second large multicenter trial, low-dose heparin was compared with dextran. Fatal PE was reported in six of 1991 patients given low-dose heparin and six of 1993 patients who received dextran (30). Clagett and Reisch (12) ana-

TABLE 11–2. Elective General Surgery Venous Thrombosis (VT) Rates Measured with Leg Scanning in Randomized Comparisons with Placebo Treatment or No Prophylaxis

PREVENTION METHOD	PATIENTS C/T	VT RATE[a] C	VT RATE[a] T	RELATIVE RISK REDUCTION
Low-dose heparin	2748/2668	0.266	0.099	0.63
Full-dose warfarin	85/83	0.256	0.048	0.81
Minidose warfarin	37/32	0.297	0.094	0.68
Dextran	387/379	0.344	0.243	0.29
Graduated compression stockings	571/555	0.260	0.095	0.63
Intermittent pneumatic compression	575/571	0.278	0.112	0.60
Physiotherapy	296/297	0.216	0.185	0.14

[a] C, control group; T, treatment group.

lyzed trials of low-dose heparin in elective abdominal, neurologic, and gynecologic surgery totaling almost 9500 patients and reported that prophylaxis reduced the incidence of fatal PE from 0.7 per cent in the controls to 0.2 per cent ($p<.001$). Collins and associates (13) examined 74 trials that included 14,000 patients who had undergone orthopedic surgery as well as elective abdominal, neurologic, and gynecologic surgery. They reported fatal PE in 0.8 per cent of the controls and 0.26 per cent of patients given heparin ($p<.001$). They also found a small but statistically significant decrease in mortality from 3.3 per cent in the control group to 2.2 per cent in the low-dose heparin group. The review by Clagett and Reisch (12) revealed an average incidence of venous thrombosis of 11.8 per cent in 34 studies in which heparin was given every 12 hr and an incidence of 7.5 per cent in 15 studies in which heparin was given every 8 hr. They found no difference in the incidence of postoperative wound hematoma or major bleeding between the two low-dose regimens, suggesting that the 8-hourly regimen is preferable. In these reviews, there was no difference in the incidence of fatal bleeding between the low-dose heparin group and the control group, but there was a small but statistically significant difference in nonfatal bleeding and in wound hematomas in the heparin group.

Oral Anticoagulants

Oral anticoagulants have been compared with low-dose heparin in patients undergoing gynecologic surgical procedures. Both forms of prophylaxis were equally effective (31). Nicoumalone was given for 5 days preoperatively to achieve a prothrombin time (PT) ratio of 2.0 to 2.5 at the time of surgery (INR = 2.0 to 2.5, equivalent to a PT of 1.3 to 1.4 using a typical North American Prothrombin Time Reagent) and then continued for 14 days, aiming for a PT ratio of 2.0 to 4.0.

More recently, Poller and associates (24) compared the effects of 1 mg/day warfarin with full-dose oral anticoagulants and untreated controls. Venous thrombosis was repeated in 3/32 patients compared with 1/35 given full-dose nicoumalone and 11/37 untreated controls (compared to controls both reductions were statistically significant).

Physical Methods

Both graduated compression stockings and IPC are effective in preventing venous thrombosis in general surgery, urologic surgery, and neurosurgery (11,12).

LMW Heparins and Heparinoids

LMW heparins have been introduced recently as a promising new approach to prophylaxis. Interest in LMW heparins as potential antithrombotic agents was stimulated by two observations in the mid-1970s and early 1980s. The first was the finding that LMW heparin fractions prepared from standard unfractionated (UF) heparin progressively lose their ability to prolong the activated partial thromboplastin time (aPTT) while retaining their ability to inhibit factor Xa (32,33). The second was the observation that LMW heparins produce less bleeding in experimental models for an equivalent antithrombotic effect than the UF heparin from which they are derived (34). The LMW heparins in clinical use are produced from UF heparin by depolymerization. The LMW heparins contain the unique pentasaccharide in approximately the same proportion (i.e., 1:3) as the standard heparin from which they have been derived. Two heparinoids are also being evaluated clinically—dermatan sulfate and ORG 10172, which is a mixture of heparan sulfate, dermatan sulfate, a LMW heparin fraction, and chondroitin sulfate. LMW heparins prolong the aPTT to a lesser extent than UF heparin (35–37).

The antithrombotic effect of LMW heparins, heparin, and heparinoids are effective in inhibiting experimental thrombosis (34,38–40) and are less hemorrhagic than UF heparin for an equivalent antithrombotic activity (34,38,41,42). There is evidence that differences in the effects of UF and of LMW heparins on platelet aggregation or vessel wall permeability may be responsible for the differences in the hemorrhagic properties of these glycosaminoglycans (40,43–46).

A number of different LMW heparins have been approved for use in Europe and some are undergoing clinical evaluation in North America. LMW heparins have a longer half-life than standard heparin and are highly effective and safe when used for thrombosis prophylaxis in general surgical patients.

TABLE 11–3.   Randomized Comparisons between Standard Heparin and LMW Heparins or Heparin Analogues in General Surgery

FIRST DOSE AUTHOR (REF)	DOSE ANTI-XA	DOSE INTERVAL	VT RATE		p VALUE
			LMW Heparin	Heparin	
Fraxiparin (CY 216; Choay/Sanofi)					
Kakkar and Murray (51)	7500 units	Daily	5/196 (.026)	14/199 (.070)	<.05
European Fraxiparin Study Group (28)	7500 units	Daily	27/960 (.028)	42/936 (.043)	<.05
TOTAL			32/1156 (.027)	56/1135 (.049)	RR[a] = 35
Fragmin (Kabi 2165; Kabi)					
Koller et al. (52)	7500 units	Daily	1/23 (.043)	0/20 (.000)	n.s.
	2500 units	Daily	1/74 (.014)	2/72 (.028)	n.s.
Bergqvist et al. (47)	5000 units	Daily	13/217 (.060)	9/215 (.042)	n.s.
Caen (49)	2500 units	Daily	6/195 (.031)	7/189 (.037)	n.s.
Bergqvist et al. (48)	5000 units	Daily	28/505 (.055)	41/497 (.083)	n.s.
Fricker et al. (50)	5000 units	Daily	2/40 (.050)	0/40 (.000)	n.s.
TOTAL			51/1054 (.048)	59/1033 (.057)	RR = 16
Enoxaparin (PK 10169; Pharmuka)					
Samama et al. (53)	60 mg	Daily	4/137 (.029)	5/133 (.038)	n.s.
	40 mg	Daily	3/106 (.029)	3/110 (.027)	n.s.
	20 mg	Daily	6/159 (.038)	12/158 (.076)	n.s.
TOTAL			13/402 (.032)	20/401 (.05)	RR = 36

[a] RR, percentage risk reduction.

There have been at least eight randomized studies in which a LMW heparin has been compared with standard heparin in patients undergoing abdominal surgery (28,47–53). The results are summarized in Table 11–3. A number of the early trials evaluating prophylactic LMW heparin reported excessive bleeding, which, in the light of subsequent experience, was likely due to excessively high doses of LMW heparin. In two large studies reported by Kakkar and Murray (51) and by Breddin and associates [European Fraxiparin Study Group (28)], the incidence of thrombosis was significantly lower in the LMW heparin group but there were no differences detected in the rate of bleeding between the LMW heparin and UF heparin groups. In a recent study in general surgical patients reported by Pezzuoli et al. (54) comparing LMW heparin with no treatment, patients randomized into the LMW heparin group had a significantly lower total mortality and thromboembolic mortality (Table 11–4).

Emergency General or Abdominal-Thoracic Surgery

This very important group of patients has received much less attention than those undergoing elective surgery. There have been no studies comparing low-dose heparin with placebo in this group, although there have been limited studies comparing combined forms of prophylaxis (26).

Neurosurgery, Head Injury, and Spinal Trauma

This group of patients has a high risk of VTE but even small amounts of excessive bleeding are unacceptable. Although low-dose heparin has been shown to be effective and relatively safe in one study of 100 patients (55), it is unlikely to be the prophylactic method of choice, particularly since physical methods that increase blood flow are also very effective in this setting (20,56,57). Low-dose heparin was found to be less effective than adjusted-dose heparin in a small trial of patients with acute spinal cord injury (58). The mean heparin dose in the adjusted-dose heparin group was 26,400 units/24 hr, and this was associated with excessive bleeding.

Elective Hip Replacement and Hip Fracture

Without prophylaxis, approximately 5 per cent of patients having elective hip replacement develop symptomatic PE and up to 0.5 per cent die of this com-

TABLE 11–4. Deaths Recorded during Prophylaxis Trial: Statistical Analysis (One-Tailed Test)[a]

	CY 216 n (%) (N = 2247)	PLACEBO n (%) (N = 2251)	p	% REDUCTION IN ODDS (CI[b] 95%)
General mortality	8 (0.36)	18 (0.80)	<.05	55.7
Fatal PE	2 (0.09)	4 (0.18)	n.s.	50
Thromboembolic mortality	2[c] (0.09)	8[c] (0.36)	<.05	75

[a] Adapted from Pezzuoli G, Serneri GGN, Settembrini P, et al: Prophylaxis of fatal pulmonary embolism in general surgery using double-blind, randomized, controlled clinical trial versus placebo (STEP). Int Surg 1989;74:205–210.
[b] CI, confidence interval.
[c] Including fatal pulmonary embolism.

plication, which remains the major cause of postoperative death (59). The problem is even more serious after hip fracture, when fatal PE occurs in about 4 per cent of patients and accounts for almost 20 per cent of deaths in hospital (59).

Hip Replacement

Prophylaxis against venous thrombosis in patients undergoing major orthopedic surgical procedures is problematic. This is because of the high risk of venous thrombosis and PE in the unprotected patient and because bleeding at the site of operation can jeopardize the success of the joint replacement procedure. The indicence of thromosis in patients undergoing hip and major knee surgery is summarized in Table 11–5. Patients undergoing hip surgery have a 40 to 60 per cent postoperative incidence of calf vein thrombosis and a 20 per cent incidence of proximal vein thrombosis (17,60–63). The anatomic distribution of venous thrombosis after hip surgery differs from that seen after abdominal surgery since in almost 30 per cent of patients the thrombi originate in the femoral vein at the level of the lesser trochanter, often without associated calf vein thrombosis (17,61,62). Thus, it seems likely that there are two separate pathogenic mechanisms for thrombosis following hip surgery—stasis and hypercoagulability, which are largely responsible for calf vein thrombosis, and femoral vein damage induced by surgical manipulation, which is responsible for femoral vein thrombosis (61). Approximately 80 per cent of proximal vein thrombi occur on the operated side, often without associated calf vein thrombosis, whereas calf vein thrombosis occurs with equal frequency in the operated and nonoperated legs (Table 11–6) (17,62). Patients undergoing major knee surgery have a 50 to 70 per cent incidence of calf vein thrombosis and a 20 per cent incidence of proximal vein thrombosis. Most of these proximal vein thrombi occur as extensions of calf vein thrombosis (64).

There is evidence from a number of small randomized trials that the incidence of thrombosis is lower with regional than with general anesthesia (65–68). To date, there is no convincing evidence that the incidence of thrombosis is lowered with a noncemented versus a cemented prosthesis. Results of recent studies indicate that noninvasive tests that are accurate for detecting asymptomatic venous thrombosis in general surgical patients (^{125}I-labeled fibrinogen leg scanning) and for detecting venous thrombosis in symptomatic patients (IPG) are relatively insenstive for detecting venous thrombosis following hip surgery. ^{125}I-labeled fibrinogen leg scanning fails to detect proximal vein thrombosis and IPG fails to detect calf vein thrombi and nonocclusive proximal vein thrombi. Preliminary evidence suggests that B-mode ultrasound imaging is more sensitive than IPG to asymptomatic proximal vein thrombi in patients undergoing hip surgery (18).

TABLE 11–5.   Incidence of Thrombosis in Orthopedic Surgery in Untreated Patients

	HIP (%)	MAJOR KNEE (%)
Calf	40–60	50–70
Proximal	20	20
Fatal PE	1–5	—

TABLE 11–6. Distribution of Thrombi[a]

	CALF ALONE	CALF WITH PROXIMAL EXTENSION	DISCONTINUOUS CALF & PROXIMAL	PROXIMAL ALONE	TOTAL PROXIMAL	TOTAL
OP[b]	66	8	13	28	49	115
NOP[b]	66	5	5	7	17	83

[a] Adapted from Cruikshank MK, Levine MN, Hirsh J, et al; An evaluation of impedance plethysmography and I-125-fibrinogen leg scanning in patients following hip surgery. Thromb Haemost 1989;62(3):830–834.
[b] OP, operated leg; NOP, nonoperated leg.

There is also indirect evidence that methods of prophylaxis that are effective in reducing the incidence of calf vein thrombosis may be less effective in reducing proximal vein thrombosis following hip surgery (19,69). This possibility is plausible since, as discussed earlier, the mechanisms of distal and proximal vein thrombosis after hip surgery may be different (21). For these reasons, the results of studies that have used leg scanning or IPG to assess the incidence of venous thrombosis following hip surgery do not provide reliable estimates of the incidence of venous thrombosis in unprotected patients and may not provide reliable estimates of the effects of prophylaxis on the incidence of venous thrombosis in these patients. Therefore, we have limited our analysis of the effectiveness of prophylaxis in hip surgery to studies that used routine venography to assess the incidence of postoperative venous thrombosis.

The following methods of prophylaxis have been evaluated in patients undergoing hip surgery: aspirin, dextran, low-dose heparin, low-dose heparin combined with DHE, oral anticoagulants, adjusted dose heparin, LMW heparin, and IPC. From Table 11–7 it can be seen that low-dose heparin with or without DHE, oral anticoagulants, dextran, intermittent leg compression, adjusted-dose heparin, and LMW heparins are all found to be effective by routine venography used to detect venous thrombosis postoperatively (19,23,25,60,63,69–82).

The best results have been obtained with adjusted-dose heparin, LMW heparin, and oral anticoagulants. The adjusted-dose heparin regimen popularized by Leyvraz and associates (25) is an 8-hr regimen of subcutaneous heparin that is begun 2 days before surgery. The starting dose of heparin is 3500 international units, with subsequent doses adjusted in steps of 500 to 1000 international units to achieve an aPTT in the upper normal range 6 hr after injection. In their study, the dose of heparin in the adjusted-dose heparin group was increased gradually to an average of 18,900 international units a day by the seventh day after surgery (range 13,500 to 30,000 international units for 24 hr). Compared with fixed low-dose heparin prophylaxis using 3500 international units subcutaneously every 8 hr, the adjusted-dose regimen reduced the overall thrombosis rate as measured by venography of the operated leg on days 7 and 9 after surgery from 39 to 13 per cent ($p<.1$) without increasing blood loss. The adjusted-dose regimen also decreased the incidence of proximal vein thrombosis from 32 to 5 per cent ($p<.003$). A similar protocol was tested in a randomized comparison with LMW heparin in two other studies. The incidence of postoperative venous thrombosis in the adjusted-dose heparin group was similar to that reported in the first study (72–74).

LMW heparin has also proven to be very effective in reducing postoperative

TABLE 11–7. Prophylaxis in Elective Hip Surgery Randomized Controlled Studies

REF.	CONTROL	LOW-DOSE HEPARIN	ADJUSTED-DOSE HEPARIN	LMW HEPARIN	HEPARIN & DHE	ORAL ANTICOAGULANTS	DEXTRAN	ACETYLSALICYLIC ACID	LEG COMPRESSION	ELASTIC STOCKING
81	11/28 (39)[a]	3/32 (9)								
82	19/37 (51)	13/36 (36)								
60	21/50 (42)			6/50 (12)						
63	56/99 (57)			15/97 (15)						
76	30/56 (54)				7/50 (14)					
69	25/47 (53)								15/43 (35)	
79	22/41 (54)									7/35 (20)
25		16/41 (39)	5/38 (13)							
77		11/15 (73)			6/25 (25)	10/51 (20)	14/56 (25)	18/50 (36)		
80		18/25 (72)								
75		27/108 (25)	4/40 (10)	15/120 (13)						
72			28/175 (16)	5/78 (6)						
74				22/174 (13)						
73				25/146 (17)	48/149 (32) 29/49 (59)					
70						8/39 (21)	27/50 (54)			
23						12/72 (17)	11/29 (38)			
19							9/44 (21) 19/97 (20)	55/91 (60)	11/66 (17)	
78				6/103 (6)						
71										
Total incidence[b]	184/358 (51)	88/257 (34)	37/253 (15)	94/768 (12)	90/223 (40)	30/162 (19)	80/276 (29)	73/141 (52)	26/109 (24)	7/35 (20)

[a] Percentage in parentheses.
[b] The totals represent pooled results, but not a formal metaanalysis.

164

venous thrombosis in patients who have undergone elective hip surgery (Table 11–7) (60,63,71,72,74,75,83,84). In most studies using LMW heparin, the agent was commenced preoperatively and then given once daily starting postoperatively. However, in the double-blind placebo control trial reported by Turpie and associates (60), the LMW heparin enoxaparin was given twice daily and prophylaxis was delayed until 12 to 24 hr after the hip replacement. LMW heparin produced a marked reduction of venous thrombosis from 42 per cent in the control group to 12 per cent in the treated group, and the proximal venous thrombosis rate was diminished from 23 to 4 per cent without excessive bleeding. Others using the preoperative regimen and then once-daily LMW heparin reported similar low rates of venous thrombosis after hip replacement in patients given LMW heparins (63,71–75,83,84). Leyvraz and associates reported in a recent study that LMW heparin was significantly more effective than antidiuretic hormone in reducing the incidence of proximal vein thrombosis (74).

Hip Fracture

Clinical trials based on routine venography suggest that oral anticoagulants reduce the rate of DVT after hip fracture by almost 40 per cent, confirming the pioneering studies of Sevitt and Gallagher (85), who found a marked reduction in the incidence of VTE at autopsy in patients given phenindione from the start of their hospital admission. However, oral anticoagulants are associated with a substantial increase in the rate of bleeding in hip surgery patients (86–90) (Table 11–8). Dextran 70 has a similar prophylactic effect on the incidence of DVT. Surprisingly, when the analysis is performed only on studies in which venography was used routinely, there is no evidence that low-dose heparin given alone or with DHE is particularly effective in reducing the incidence of venous thrombosis. The most impressive results have been obtained with LMW heparins, although this information derives from one dose ranging study (91) and one study comparing LMW heparin to dextran (92).

Knee Surgery

There have only been two randomized trials using objective outcome measures in patients undergoing major knee surgery (Table 11–9). In a study reported by Hull and associates (64), patients treated with IPC were compared with an untreated control group. The incidence of venous thrombosis was reduced from 66 per cent in the control group to 6 per cent in patients treated with IPC, a risk reduction of 90 per cent. In the second study, low-dose warfarin was compared

TABLE 11–8. Bleeding with Oral Anticoagulants in Hip Surgery: Pooled Analysis of Seven Studies (17, 19, 21, 23, 26, 27, 29, 61)

	ORAL ANTICOAGULANT	CONTROL
No. of patients	505	505
Total bleeds (%)	101 (20)[a]	49 (9.7)

[a] Confidence interval 16.5 to 23.5.

TABLE 11–9.   Knee Surgery—Prophylactic Approaches

AUTHOR (REF.)	NUMBER OF PATIENTS/THROMBI (%)		RISK REDUCTION
	IPC	Control	
Hull et al. (64)	32/3 (6)	29/19 (66)	90% (CI[a] 84–98%)
	Low-Dose Warfarin	**Dextran**	
Francis et al. (23)	14/3 (21)	8/8 (100)	79% (CI 71–87%)

[a] CI, 95% confidence interval.

with dextran in 22 patients undergoing major knee surgery (23). The incidence of venous thrombosis was 100 per cent in the dextran group compared with 21 per cent in the low-dose warfarin group, a risk reduction of 79 per cent. These differences were statistically significant ($p<.05$) for both studies.

REFERENCES

1. Morrell MT, Dunnill MS: The post-mortem incidence of pulmonary embolism in a hospital population. Br J Surg 1968;55:347–352.
2. Coon WW: The spectrum of pulmonary embolism. Arch Surg 1976;111:398–402.
3. Havig O: Deep vein thrombosis and pulmonary embolism. Acta Chir Scand 1977;478(suppl):1–120.
4. Bergqvist D, Lindblad B: A 30 year survey of pulmonary embolism verified at autopsy: An analysis of 1274 surgical patients. Br J Surg 1985;72:105–108.
5. Dismuke SE, Wagner EH: Pulmonary embolism as a cause of death: The changing mortality in hospitalized patients. JAMA 1986;255:2039–2042.
6. Salzman EW, Hirsh J: Prevention of venous thromboembolism. In Colman RW, Hirsh J, Marder VJ, Salzman EW, eds: Hemostasis and Thrombosis: Basic Principles and Clinical Practice, 2nd ed. Philadelphia, JB Lippincott Co, 1987;1252–1265.
7. Simon T, Stengle J: Antithrombin practice in orthopaedic surgery. Results of a survey. Clin Orthop 1974;102:181–187.
8. Morris GK: Prevention of venous thromboembolism: A survey of methods used by orthopaedic and general surgeons. Lancet 1980;2:572–574.
9. Bergqvist D: Prevention of postoperative deep vein thrombosis in Sweden. Results of a survey. World J Surg 1980;4:489–495.
10. Paiement GD, Wessinger SJ, Harris WH: Survey of prophylaxis against venous thromboembolism in adults undergoing hip surgery. Clin Orthop 1987;223:188–193.
11. Colditz GA, Tuden RL, Oster G: Rates of venous thrombosis after general surgery: Combined results of randomised clinical trials. Lancet 1986;2:143–146.
12. Clagett GP, Reisch JS: Prevention of venous thromboembolism in general surgical patients. Ann Surg 1988;208:227–240.
13. Collins R, Scrimgeour A, Yusuf S, et al: Reduction in fatal pulmonary embolism and venous thrombosis by perioperative administration of subcutaneous heparin. N Engl J Med 1988;318:1162–1173.
14. Conference: Prevention of deep venous thrombosis and pulmonary embolism. Lancet 1986;1:1202–1203.
15. Ogawa S, Gerlach H, Esposito C, et al: Hypoxia modulates the barrier and coagulant function of cultured bovine endothelium: Increased monolayer permeability and induction of procoagulant properties. J Clin Invest 1990;85:1090–1098.
16. Keber D, Keber I, Stegnar M, Vene N: t-PA and PAI-1 antigen and activity changes in patients with heart failure before and after arm venous occlusion. Unpublished manuscript.
17. Cruickshank MK, Levine MN, Hirsh J, et al: An evaluation of impedance plethysmography and I-125-fibrinogen leg scanning in patients following hip surgery. Thromb Haemost 1989;62:830–834.
18. Borris LC, Christiansen HM, Lassen MR, et al: Comparison of real-time B-mode ultrasonography and bilateral ascending phlebography for detection of postoperative deep vein thrombosis following elective hip surgery. Thromb Haemost 1989;61(3):363–365.

19. Paiement GD, Bell D, Wessinger SJ, et al: New advances in the prevention, diagnosis and cost effectiveness of venous thromboembolic disease in patients with total hip replacement. *In* Brand RA, ed: The Hip. St. Louis: CV Mosby, 1987;94–119.

20. Turpie AGG, Hirsh J, Gent M, et al: Prevention of deep vein thrombosis in potential neurosurgical patients: A randomized trial comparing graduated compression stockings alone or graduated compression stocking plus intermittent pneumatic compression with control. Arch Intern Med 1989;*149*:679–681.

21. Powers PJ, Gent M, Jay R, et al: A randomized trial of less-intense warfarin or acetylsalicylic acid in the prevention of venous thromboembolism after surgery for fractured hip. Arch Intern Med 1989;*149*:771–774.

22. Turpie AGG, Levine MN, Hirsh J, et al: A double-blind randomized trial of ORG 10172 low molecular weight heparinoid in the prevention of deep vein thrombosis in thrombotic stroke. Lancet 1987;*1*:523–526.

23. Francis CW, Marder VJ, Evarts CM, et al: Two-step warfarin therapy: Prevention of postoperative venous thrombosis without excessive bleeding. JAMA 1983;*249*:374–378.

24. Poller L, McKernan A, Thomson JM, et al: Fixed minidose warfarin: A new approach to prophylaxis against venous thrombosis after major surgery. Br Med J 1987;*295*:1309–1312.

25. Leyvraz PF, Richard J, Bachmann F: Adjusted versus fixed-dose subcutaneous heparin in the prevention of deep vein thrombosis after total hip replacement. N Engl J Med 1983;*309*:154–157.

26. Wille-Jorgensen P, et al: Prophylaxis of pulmonary embolism following emergency abdominal surgery [abstr 409]. Thromb Haemost 1989;*62*(1):129.

27. Sasahara AA, DiSerio FJ: Dihydroergotamine-heparin prophylaxis of DVT in total hip replacement patients: A multicentre trial. Thromb Haemost 1987;*58*(suppl):240.

28. European Fraxiparin Study Group: Comparison of a low molecular weight heparin and unfractionated heparin for the prevention of deep vein thrombosis in patients undergoing abdominal surgery. Br J Surg 1988;*75*:1058–1063.

29. Kakkar VV, Corrigan TP, Fossard DP: Prevention of fatal postoperative pulmonary embolism by low doses of heparin. Lancet 1975;*2*:45–51.

30. Gruber UF, Saldeen T, Brokop T, et al: Incidences of fatal postoperative pulmonary embolism after prophylaxis with Dextral 70 and low-dose heparin: An international multicentre study. Br Med J 1980;*1*:69–72.

31. Taberner DA, Poller L, Burslem RW, et al: Oral anticoagulants controlled by the British comparative thromboplastin versus low-dose heparin in prophylaxis of deep vein thrombosis. Br Med J 1978;*1*:272–274.

32. Johnson EA, Kirkwood TBL, Stirling Y, et al: Four heparin preparations: Anti-Xa potentiating effect of heparin after subcutaneous injection. Thromb Haemost 1976;*35*:586–591.

33. Andersson L-O, Barrowcliffe TW, Holmer E, et al: Anticoagulant properties of heparin fractionated by affinity chromatography on matrix-bound antithrombin III and by gel filtration. Thromb Res 1976;*9*:575–583.

34. Carter CJ, Kelton JG, Hirsh J, et al: The relationship between the hemorrhagic and antithrombotic properties of low molecular weight heparins and heparin. Blood 1982;*59*:1239–1245.

35. Barrowcliffe TW, Merton RE, Gray E, Thomas DP: Heparin and bleeding: An association with lipase release. Thromb Haemost 1988;*60*:434–436.

36. Barrowcliffe TW, Thomas DP: Low molecular weight heparins: Antithrombotic and haemorrhagic effects and standardization. Acta Chir Scand [Suppl] 1988;*543*:57–64.

37. Ofosu FA, Smith LM, Anvari N, Blajchman MA: An approach to assigning in vitro potency to unfractionated and low molecular weight heparins based on the inhibition of prothrombin activation and catalysis of thrombin inhibition. Thromb Haemost 1988;*60*:193–198.

38. Cade JF, Buchanan MR, Boneu B, et al: A comparison of the antithrombotic and hemorrhagic effects of low molecular weight heparin fractions. Thromb Res 1984;*35*:613–625.

39. Ockelford PA, Carter CJ, Mitchell L, Hirsh J: Discordance between the anti-Xa activity and antithrombotic activity of an ultra-low molecular weight heparin fraction. Thromb Res 1982;*28*:401–409.

40. Van Ryn-McKenna J, Ofosu FA, Hirsh J, Buchanan M: Antithrombotic and bleeding effects of glycosaminoglycans with different degrees of sulfation. Br J Haematol 1989;*71*:265–269.

41. Andriuolli G, Mastacch R, Barbanti M, Sarret M: Comparison of the antithrombotic and hemorrhagic effects of heparin and a new low molecular weight heparin in rats. Haemostasis 1985;*15*:324–330.

42. Esquivel CO, Bergqvist D, Bjork CG, Nilsson B: Comparison between commercial heparin, low molecular weight heparin and pentosan polysulfate on hemostasis and platelets in vivo. Thromb Res 1982;*28*:389–399.

43. Salzman EW, Rosenberg RD, Smith MH, Lindon JN, Favreau L: Effect of heparin and heparin fractions on platelet aggregation. J Clin Invest 1980;*65*:64–73.

44. Fernandez F, Nguyen P, Van Ryn J, Ofosu FA, Hirsh J, Buchanan MR: Hemorrhagic doses of heparin and other glycosaminoglycans induce a platelet defect. Thromb Res 1986;*43*:491–495.

45. Fernandez F, Van Ryn J, Ofosu FA, Hirsh J, Buchanan MR: The hemorrhagic and antithrombotic effects of dermatan sulfate. Br J Haematol 1986;64:309–317.

46. Blajchman MA, Young E, Ofosu FA: The effects of unfractionated heparin, dermatan sulfate and low molecular weight heparin on vessel wall permeability in rabbits. Ann NY Acad Sci 1989;556:245–254.

47. Bergqvist D, Burmark US, Frisell J, et al: Low molecular weight heparin once daily compared with conventional low dose heparin twice daily. A prospective double blind multicentre trial on prevention of postoperative thrombosis. Br J Surg 1986;73:204–208.

48. Bergqvist D, Matzsch T, Burmark US, et al: Low molecular weight heparin given the evening before surgery compared with conventional low dose heparin in prevention of thrombosis. Br J Surg 1989;75:888–891.

49. Caen JP: A randomized double-blind study between a low molecular weight heparin Kabi 2165 and standard heparin in the prevention of deep vein thrombosis in general surgery. Thromb Haemost 1988;59:216–220.

50. Fricker J-P, Vergnes Y, Schach A, et al: Low dose heparin versus low molecular weight heparin (Kabi 2165, Fragmin^R) in the prophylaxis of thromboembolic complications of abdominal oncological surgery. Eur J Clin Invest 1988;18:561–567.

51. Kakkar VV, Murray WJG: Efficacy and safety of low molecular weight heparin (CY216) in preventing postoperative venous thromboembolism: A co-operative study. Br J Surg 1985;72:786–791.

52. Koller M, Schoch U, Buchmann P, et al: Low molecular weight heparin (KABI 2165) as thromboprophylaxis in elective visceral surgery. A randomized double-blind study versus unfractionated heparin. Thromb Haemost 1986;56:243–246.

53. Samama M, Bernard P, Bonnardot VP, et al: Low molecular weight heparin (enoxaparine) compared with unfractionated heparin thrice a day in prevention of postoperative thrombosis. Br J Surg 1988;75:128–131.

54. Pezzuoli G, Serneri GGN, Settembrini P, et al: Prophylaxis of fatal pulmonary embolism in general surgery using double-blind, randomized, controlled, clinical trial versus placebo (STEP). Int Surg 1989;74:205–210.

55. Cerrato D, Ariano C, Fiacchino F: Deep vein thrombosis and low-dose heparin prophylaxis in neurosurgical patients. J Neurosurg 1978;49:378–381.

56. Turpie AGG, Gallus AS, Beattie WS, et al: Prevention of venous thrombosis in patients with intracranial disease by intermittent pneumatic compression of the calf. Neurology 1977;27:435–438.

57. Turpie AGG, Delmore T, Hirsh J, et al: Prevention of venous thrombosis by intermittent sequential calf compression in patients with intracranial disease. Thromb Res 1979;15:611–616.

58. Green D, Lee MY, Ito VT, et al: Fixed vs adjusted-dose heparin in the prophylaxis of thromboembolism in spinal cord injury. JAMA 1988;260:1255–1258.

59. Sheppeard H, Henson J, Ward DJ, et al: A clinic-pathological study of fatal pulmonary embolism in a specialist orthopaedic hospital. Arch Orthop Traumatic Surg 1981;99:65–71.

60. Turpie AGG, Levine MN, Hirsh J, et al: A randomized controlled trial of low molecular weight heparin (enoxaparine) to prevent deep vein thrombosis in patients undergoing elective hip surgery. N Engl J Med 1986;315:925–929.

61. Stamatakis JD, Kakkar W, Sagar S, et al: Femoral vein thrombosis and total hip replacement. Br Med J 1977;2:223–225.

62. Nillius AS, Nylander G: Deep vein thrombosis after total hip replacement: A clinical and phlebographic study. Br J Surg 1979;66:324–326.

63. Hoek J, Nurmohamed MT, ten Cate H, et al: Prevention of deep vein thrombosis (DVT) following total hip replacement by a low molecular weight heparinoid (ORG 10172) [abstr 1637]. Thromb Haemost 1989;62(1):520.

64. Hull R, Delmore TJ, Hirsh J, et al: Effectiveness of intermittent pulsatile elastic stockings for the prevention of calf and thigh vein thrombosis in patients undergoing elective knee surgery. Thromb Res 1979;16:37–45.

65. McKenzie PJ, Wishart HY, Gray I, Smith G: Effects of anaesthetic technique on deep vein thrombosis: A comparison of subarachnoid and general anaesthesia. Br J Anaesth 1985;57:853–857.

66. Modig J, Borg T, Karlstrom G, et al: Thromboembolism after total hip replacement: Role of epidural and general anesthesia. Anesth Analg 1983;62:174–180.

67. Modig J, Hjelmstedt A, Sahlstedt B, Maripuu E: Comparative influences of epidural and general anaesthesia on deep venous thrombosis and pulmonary embolism after total hip replacement. Acta Chir Scand 1981;147:125–130.

68. Thorburn J, Louden JR, Vallance R: Spinal and general anaesthesia in total hip replacement: Frequency of deep vein thrombosis. Br J Anaesth 1980;52:1117–1121.

69. Gallus AS, Raman K, Darby T: Venous thrombosis after elective hip replacement—the influence of preventive intermittent calf compression and of surgical technique. Br J Surg 1983;70:17–19.

70. Fredin HO, Rosberg B, Arborelium M Jr, et al: On thrombo-embolism after total hip replacement in epidural analgesia: A controlled study of dextran 70 and low-dose heparin combined with dihydroergotamine. Br J Surg 1984;71:58–60.

71. Borris LC, Hauch O, Jorgensen LN, et al: Enoxaparin versus dextran 70 in the prevention of postoperative deep vein thrombosis after total hip replacement—a Danish Multicentre Study. Paper given at Proceedings of the Danish Enoxaparin Symposium, February 3, 1990.

72. Dechavanne M, Ville D, Berruyer M, et al: Randomized trial of a low-molecular weight heparin (Kabi 2165) versus adjusted-dose subcutaneous standard heparin in the prophylaxis of deep-vein thrombosis after elective hip surgery. Haemostasis 1989;19:5–12.

73. Estoppey D, Hochreiter J, Breyer HG, et al: ORG 10172 (Lomoparan) versus heparin-DHE in prevention of thromboembolism in total hip replacement—a multicentre trial [abstr 1107]. Thromb Haemost 1989;62(1):356.

74. Leyvraz PF, et al: Satellite Symposium (Fraxiparine; Tokyo) 1990 (In press).

75. Planes A, Vochelle N, Mazas F, et al: Prevention of postoperative venous thrombosis: A randomized trial comparing unfractionated heparin with low molecular weight heparin in patients undergoing total hip replacement. Thromb Haemost 1988;60:407–410.

76. Evarts CM, Feil EJ: Prevention of thromboembolic disease after elective surgery of the hip. J Bone Joint Surg [Am] 1971;53:1271–1280.

77. Harris WH, Salzman EW, Athanasoulis C, et al: Comparison of warfarin, low-molecular-weight dextran, aspirin, and subcutaneous heparin in prevention of venous thromboembolism following total hip replacement. J Bone Joint Surg [Am] 1974;56:1552–1562.

78. Harris WH, Athanasoulis C, Waltman AC, Salzman EW: Prophylaxis of deep-vein thrombosis after total hip replacement: Dextran and external pneumatic compression compared with 1.2 or 0.3 gram of aspirin daily. J Bone Joint Surg [Am] 1985;67:57–62.

79. Ishak MA, Morley KD: Deep venous thrombosis after total hip arthroplasty: A prospective controlled study to determine the prophylactic effect of graded pressure stockings. Br J Surg 1981;68:429–432.

80. Kakkar VV, Stamatakis JD, Bentley PG, et al: Prophylaxis for postoperative deep-vein thrombosis: Synergistic effect of heparin and dihydroergotamine. JAMA 1979;241:39–42.

81. Moskovitz PA, Ellenberg SS, Feffer HL, et al: Low-dose heparin for prevention of venous thromboembolism in total hip arthroplasty and surgical repair of hip fractures. J Bone Joint Surg [Am] 1978;60:1065–1070.

82. Rogers PH, Walsh PN, Marder VJ, et al: Controlled trial of low dose heparin and sulfinpyrazone to prevent venous thromboembolism after operation on hip. J Bone Joint Surg [Am] 1978; 60:758–762.

83. Bansillon V, Dejour H, Besson L, et al: Prevention des thromboses veneuses profondes en chirurgie orthopedique pour mise en place d'une prothese totale de hanche. Essai randomise de determination de la posologie optimale. Ann Chir 1987;41:377–385.

84. Planes A, Vochelle N, Ferru J, et al: Enoxaparin low molecular weight heparin: Its use in the prevention of deep vein thrombosis following total hip replacement. Haemostasis 1986;15:152–158.

85. Sevitt S, Gallagher NG: Prevention of venous thrombosis and pulmonary embolism in injured patients. A trial of anticoagulant prophylaxis and phenindione in middle-aged and elderly patients with fractured necks of femur. Lancet 1959;2:981–989.

86. Borgstrom G, Greitz T, Vander Linden W, et al: Anticoagulant prophylaxis of venous thrombosis in patients with fractured neck of the femur: A controlled clinical trial using venous phlebography. Acta Chir Scand 1965;129:500.

87. Eskeland G, Solheim K, Skorten F: Anticoagulant prophylaxis, thromboembolism and mortality in elderly patients with hip fractures: A controlled clinical trial. Acta Chir Scand 1966;131:16.

88. Hamilton HW, Crawford JS, Gardiner JH, et al: Venous thrombosis in patients with fracture of the upper end of the femur. J Bone Joint Surg [Br] 1970;52:268.

89. Morris GK, Mitchell JR: Warfarin sodium in the prevention of deep venous thrombosis and pulmonary embolism in patients with fractured neck of femur. Lancet 1976;2:869.

90. Pinto DJ: Controlled trial of an anticoagulant (warfarin sodium) in the prevention of venous thrombosis following hip surgery. Br J Surg 1970;57:349.

91. Barsotti J, Dabo B, Andreu J, et al: Prevention of deep vein thrombosis (DVT) by enoxaparine (Lovenox[R]) after surgery for fracture of femoral neck, one daily injection of 40 mg versus two daily injections of 20 mg. Thromb Haemost 1987;58(suppl):241.

92. Bergqvist D, Kettunen K, Suomalainen O, et al: A prospective randomized comparison between ORG 10172 and dextran 70 in hip fracture patients—thromboprophylaxis and safety [abstr 1105]. Thromb Haemost 1989;62(1):355.

12

THROMBOLYTIC THERAPY FOR DEEP VEIN THROMBOSES AND PULMONARY EMBOLI

Robert A. Graor

The ideal agent for the treatment of deep vein thromboses and pulmonary emboli should reverse the thrombotic process and clear the thrombotic material from the lower extremity veins or pulmonary arteries, thereby preserving anatomic and physiologic hemodynamic integrity of the venous and pulmonary arterial system. The clearance of thrombotic material from valvular structures and the restoration of normal cardiopulmonary hemodynamic function should be rapidly obtainable.

Venous thrombosis and pulmonary embolism usually occur as common and serious complications in medical and surgical patients and on occasion may affect otherwise healthy ambulating patients. The standard therapy for deep vein thrombosis and pulmonary embolism has been anticoagulant therapy. The rationale for heparin therapy was established in 1916 when it was shown to be an effective anticoagulant (1). It was not until 1960 that a controlled trial demonstrated that anticoagulation resulted in a lower incidence of fatal pulmonary emboli following an episode of deep vein thrombosis (2). In this study, treatment after a pulmonary embolus with heparin followed by oral anticoagulation was given to 16 patients with established pulmonary embolism. None suffered a recurrence and none of these patients died. Nineteen patients with pulmonary emboli were given supportive treatment only, which resulted in five deaths from pulmonary emboli and an additional 10 patients with recurrent pulmonary emboli. This prospective study was then halted, and no further studies have been undertaken regarding the need for anticoagulation therapy with heparin for pulmonary emboli patients. In a subsequent study by Kanis of 22 patients with pulmonary embolism, in whom anticoagulant therapy was withheld because these patients were thought to be at too high a risk for bleeding, 17 deaths resulted, most of which occurred within 48 hr (3). All subsequent studies were designed to assess different modes of heparin therapy, to compare heparin therapy alone to use of fibrinolytic agents followed by heparin therapy, and to study the efficacy of heparin therapy in preventing the recurrence of lethal pulmonary embolism. The application of these data to the treatment of deep vein thrombosis (DVT) has focused on the prevention of major fatal pulmonary embolism as a complication of this disease, predicated on the principle that pulmonary embolism resulting from DVT is unpredictable, and therefore all patients should be treated with anticoagulation.

The therapeutic approach to the patient presenting with DVT includes three major principles of management: 1) suppostive care of the patient, 2) prevention of acute embolic complications of the clot, and 3) prevention of the long-term sequelae due to the posthrombotic syndrome. In order to address the third of these principles, the physician must understand the natural history and hemodynamics of acute DVT and identify those patients who are at particular risk. Patients with subsequent venous valvular destruction or chronic venous obstruction must be followed and treated for the remainder of their lives, since the posthrombotic syndrome is persistent and rarely correctable surgically. It is therefore important for the physician to determine whether therapy of the acute condition will influence the long-term outcome.

The frequency of residual venous insufficiency and recurrent thrombosis suggests that heparin does not alter the disease course in situ, and studies have demonstrated that thrombus propagation can occur while the patient is fully anticoagulated (4–8). With proximal extension of calf vein thrombi or preexisting thrombi within the more proximal venous system, nearly two thirds of these patients will have residual thrombus and loss of venous function that produces altered venous hemodynamic return and the signs and symptoms of the postphlebitic syndrome, including leg swelling, pigmentation, and ulceration.

Heparin is the treatment of choice in most patients with venous thromboembolic disease, and the outlook for survival is excellent, although thrombus progression or embolization occurs in less than 5 per cent, of patients on this therapy. In patients with pulmonary embolism treated with heparin, the recurrence rate is also less than 5 per cent, with a very low mortality; even in patients with massive embolization or shock mortality is generally less than 20 per cent. It should be emphasized that safe, effective methods of prophylaxis against the development of DVT and pulmonary emboli are now available and should be used in all hospitalized patients to prevent death and morbidity from venous thromboembolism. Prophylaxis is much more cost-effective than treating the established diseased.

THROMBOLYTIC THERAPY

Available data suggest that anticoagulant therapy is effective for most patients with venous thromboembolic disease, but on theoretical grounds it is not ideal because it acts to prevent thrombus extension and does not promote dissolution of thrombi that have recently formed (1,2). Therefore, although anticoagulation is effective in reducing the important immediate complications of venous thromboembolism, it may be relatively ineffective in preventing some of the late sequelae (4–8).

Thrombolytic therapy has a number of potential advantages over anticoagulant therapy, including promotion of clot dissolution leading to restoration of normal hemodynamic circulation, reduction or prevention of venous valvular damage, and the potential for preventing the postphlebitic syndrome, which represent the most important aspects of this therapy. Specifically, in the pulmonary arterial bed, the advantages include rapid reduction of hemodynamic disturbances and prevention of or reduction in damage to the pulmonary vascular bed, which may reduce the likelihood of chronic thromboembolic pulmonary hypertension. In addition, there is evidence from clinical studies that thrombolytic therapy may be more effective than anticoagulants in patients with acute massive venous thrombosis or massive pulmonary embolism.

Although thrombolytic agents were approved for the treatment of pulmonary emboli in 1977, their use has not become as widespread as initially predicted (9,10). Only three randomized trials of pulmonary embolism therapy have compared thrombolytic agents with heparin (11–13). In these trials, no reduction in mortality from pulmonary embolism was apparent with streptokinase or urokinase, even though clots lysed more frequently when these agents were used. In two of the three studies, bleeding complications occurred more frequently after thrombolysis (11,13). Follow-up of patients treated with streptokinase or urokinase for pulmonary embolism has demonstrated increases in pulmonary capillary blood volume and pulmonary diffusing capacity compared with heparinized patients (14). However, the clinical significance of these improvements in pulmonary parameters remains uncertain.

THROMBOLYTIC THERAPY FOR DEEP VENOUS THROMBOSIS

Streptokinase and Urokinase

Thrombolysis with streptokinase for DVT has been evaluated in a number of small studies, and streptokinase therapy has been shown to produce a greater effect on lysis of the deep vein thrombi than does heparin therapy. However, whether thrombolytic therapy reduces the frequency of the postphlebitic syndrome in these patients has not yet been established.

Six properly designed, randomized trials comparing intravenous streptokinase to heparin in the treatment of DVT using repeat venography as the major end point have been reported (15–20). None of these trials was large enough to adequately determine both the efficacy and the safety of streptokinase. Goldhaber et al. performed a pooled analysis on these studies and demonstrated that thrombolysis was achieved approximately four times more often among patients treated with streptokinase than among those treated with heparin ($p<.001$) (21). Three of these six trials had sufficient data to allow comparison of bleeding complications, which occurred approximately three times more often in the streptokinase group compared to the heparin group (15,19,20).

There are only a few properly designed trials of urokinase in venous thrombosis. Clinical reports indicate rates of clot lysis similar to those shown with streptokinase but improved safety and shorter durations of infusion with urokinase (22,23).

There have also been only a few reports of the long-term effects of thrombolytic therapy in DVT. Examining the literature and taking into account the requirements for long-term clinical trials, the studies of Elliot et al., Arnesen et al., and Common et al. should be cited (20,24,25). Follow-up in these studies ranged from 7 to 76 months, and the results indicated that 24 of 62 (40 per cent) streptokinase-treated patients had normal veins, compared to only one of 58 (2 per cent) patients treated with heparin (Table 12–1). The clinical evaluation of

TABLE 12–1.   Long-Term Results of Three Prospectively Randomized Studies Comparing Heparin and Streptokinase Treatment of DVT[a]

TREATMENT	# PATIENTS	FOLLOW-UP		NORMAL VENOUS FUNCTION
		Ulceration	Symptom Free	
Streptokinase	62	0	35 (56%)	24 (40%)
Heparin	58	5 (9%)	14 (24%)	1 (2%)

[a] Data from Elliott et al. (20), Arnesen et al. (24), and Common et al. (25).

the aforementioned long-term trials indicates that none of the 62 streptokinase-treated patients had open leg ulcers, compared to five of 58 (9 per cent) patients treated with heparin. In addition, 35 of the 62 (56 per cent) patients treated with streptokinase were free of long-term symptoms, compared to only 14 of the 58 (24 per cent) patients treated with heparin.

Results of a trial reported by Kakkar et al. indicated the frequency of the postphlebitic syndrome was not lower in patients treated with streptokinase compared with heparin after more than 5 years of follow-up (16). However, this has not been the experience in other trials.

A functional evaluation of the veins of patients initially treated with streptokinase for DVT was performed by Johansson et al. (8). Using occlusion plethysmography and a mean follow-up period of 2 years, they found an excellent correlation between anatomically normal phlebograms and normal venous outflow capacity and valvular function. These normal outcomes occurred in 42 per cent of the streptokinase-treated patients in this series, and the authors concluded that an initial complete thrombolysis provides a good opportunity for obtaining lasting restoration of deep venous anatomy and function without signs and symptoms of venous insufficiency.

O'Donnell et al. published the results of a study of a highly selected group of 21 patients with iliofemoral venous thrombosis in whom they found a high frequency of venous insufficiency symptoms leading to ulceration, hospitalization, and surgical procedures (4). The patients with venous insufficiency averaged eight visits to a doctor per year and had extensive disability leading to high frequency of unemployment. The authors calculated that the average medical expenses per patient over 10 years were approximately $38,000 (in 1976).

In a study done at The Cleveland Clinic, we found that when streptokinase and urokinase were compared, both medications produced a high degree of clot lysis (80 per cent) in patients with recent (less than 7-day-old) DVTs (Table 12–2) (23). When comparing complications, urokinase had fewer major complications and was significantly safer ($p < .01$) than streptokinase. When this information was subjected to cost analysis, it was found that, because of the safety advantage and the shorter infusion times seen with urokinase, the significantly higher cost of urokinase was obliterated by the frequent complications of streptokinase and the longer hospital stays.

Complications

The major complication associated with thrombolysis is hemorrhage. This is not an unexpected complication since the choice of this therapy is designed to

**TABLE 12–2.   Streptokinase Versus Urokinase—Efficacy, Complications, and
Cost Differences in a Single Study[a]**

TREATMENT	% COMPLETE LYSIS	COMPLICATIONS	COST/TREATMENT
Streptokinase (N = 30)	24 (80%)	5 (17%)	$0
Urokinase (N = 30)	25 (83%)	0 (0%) $p = .019$	$11.00

[a] From Graor RA, Young JR, Risius B, Ruschhaupt WF: Cost-effective comparison of streptokinase and urokinase in the treatment of deep vein thrombosis. Ann Vasc Surg 1987;*1*:524–528.

produce clot lysis and thereby will lyse any hemostatic fibrin plug irrespective of its pathologic, morphologic, or anatomic characteristics. In addition, coagulation factors such as fibrinogen and factors V, VII, and VIII are degraded, leading to a slightly reduced coagulation potential (26). Finally, there is some clinically undetermined anticoagulation effect from the fibrin(ogen) degradation products formed during fibrinolytic therapy, which interfere with normal clot structure and probably also with normal platelet function (27).

Although it is difficult to determine the exact frequency with which major bleeding occurs, Straub performed a literature review on the frequency of bleeding in patients treated with streptokinase (28). His survey included 549 patients treated for DVT. Fatal bleeding occurred in four (0.73 per cent) and major nonfatal bleeding occurred in 63 (11.5 per cent). In this review the mean duration of treatment was extremely long at 106 hr. Other criticisms of these data would include the lack of a uniform definition of major bleeding. It is apparent that the greatest risk for bleeding while on lytic therapy is when the therapy is continued for a prolonged period of time, perhaps 3 to 4 days as demonstrated in this review.

Interestingly, comparison studies on bleeding complications with heparin demonstrate similar figures. Holm gathered information on 710 patients treated for DVT with standard anticoagulation with heparin (29). Fatal bleeding was found in 0.3 per cent and nonfatal major bleeding complications in 7.3 per cent.

Other nuisance-type complications, including fevers, nausea, vomiting, and other allergic reactions, occur frequently in streptokinase-treated patients (23). These complications occur rarely with urokinase or tissue plasminogen activator (tPA).

Other Thrombolytic Agents

Few data using other experimental thrombolytic agents for the treatment of DVT are available. Initial case reports on the use of recombinant tPA (rtPA) in patients with acute proximal vein thrombosis have demonstrated mixed results. Turpie et al. reported on 24 patients 12 of whom received rtPA and 12 of whom received placebo (30). Of the 12 patients who received rtPA, five (42 per cent) obtained greater than 50 per cent lysis of thrombi, four (33 per cent) obtained significant but less than 50 per cent lysis, and three showed no evidence of lysis. In the heparinized group, two patients had obtained less than 50 per cent lysis and 10 patients showed no clot lysis at all. Two patients in the rtPA group had overt hemorrhage, one had marked bruising, and one developed hemarthrosis 10 days after total hip replacement. An additional two patients had a fall in hemoglobin greater than 20 gm/liter but without overt bleeding. In the heparin group there was one spontaneous hemarthrosis in a shoulder.

In a follow-up study by this same group, rtPA was given concomitantly with heparin in two 8-hr infusion regimens given 24 hr apart. Twenty patients were studied: 10 in the rtPA plus heparin group and 10 in the heparin plus placebo group. Results similar to those of the first study were obtained in terms of thrombolytic and hemorrhagic effects. Six of the 10 patients treated with rtPA showed greater than 50 per cent clot lysis, one showed less than 50 per cent, and three showed no evidence of clot lysis. No patients in the heparin group showed evidence of thrombolysis. Three of the 10 patients in the rtPA-treated group had spontaneous hemorrhages compared to none in the heparin group. In contrast to the first study, there was minimal reduction in the indices of thrombolysis.

Conclusions

Although most patients with thromboembolism are not currently being treated with thrombolytic agents, this practice may change over the next few years as physicians and nurses become more familiar with thrombolytic drugs in the treatment of DVT, pulmonary emboli, and other vascular clinical entities. The data available demonstrate that streptokinase and urokinase can produce clot lysis and probably produce beneficial effects if complete clot lysis occurs. There is some evidence to suggest that urokinase is safer than streptokinase. No prospective trials have been generated to compare tPA with streptokinase or urokinase.

The optimal duration of treatment for DVT is dependent upon the rate and quantity of clot lysis. In all circumstances, the treatment of acute DVT with thrombolytic agents can be effectively undertaken in properly selected patients. Further improvements in therapeutic schedules should focus on the optimal individual doses, improvement in patient selection, and new delivery procedures for the thrombolytic agents.

THROMBOLYTIC THERAPY FOR EMBOLISM

Deep vein thrombosis of the legs is the most common origination site for pulmonary emboli (31,32). Pulmonary embolism is a common cardiovascular disorder that can cause pulmonary hypertension, right ventricular dysfunction, or death. Standard therapy for pulmonary emboli has employed heparin anticoagulation followed by warfarin and has not in general included thrombolytic therapy. The reason that the standard therapy for pulmonary emboli has been anticoagulation therapy is that this provides excellent prophylaxis against additional thromboembolic events and death while the natural fibrinolytic mechanisms gradually lyse the previously formed clot (2).

The distinct advantage for choosing thrombolytic therapy is that these agents actively dissolve formed thrombus and thereby quickly restore cardiopulmonary function toward normal (Figs. 12–1 and 12–2). Thrombolysis relieves the obstruction to the pulmonary artery blood flow and thus improves right ventricular function, reduces pulmonary artery pressure, and ameliorates pulmonary tissue perfusion. There is also evidence that thrombolytic therapy may also reduce the

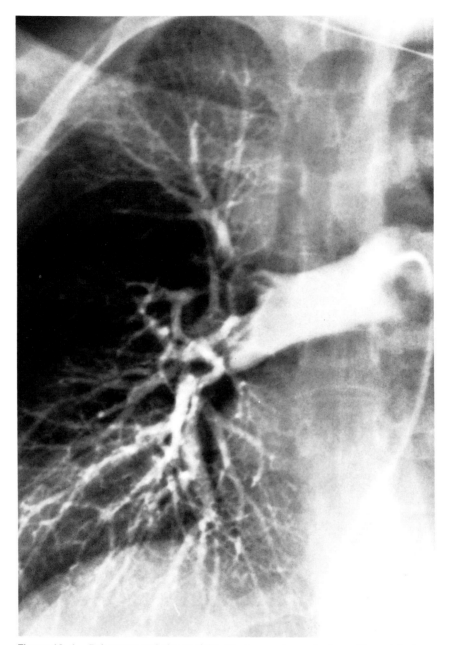

Figure 12–1. Pulmonary embolus to right pulmonary artery prior to urokinase infusion.

frequency of chronic pulmonary hypertension as a result of pulmonary emboli (14).

The cardiopulmonary response to a pulmonary embolism depends upon the size of the embolus, the coexistent cardiopulmonary disease, and the humoral responses caused by the thrombotic material in the pulmonary arteries. In general, when a pulmonary embolism obstructs pulmonary artery blood flow, right ventricular afterload increases and subsequent right ventricular dilatation occurs. In patients without prior cardiopulmonary disease, right ventricular pressure increases when approximately 25 per cent of the pulmonary blood flow is obstructed. Right ventricular systolic pressures continue to rise as the degree of obstruction increases. During the acute event, the previously unstressed normal right ventricle cannot generate a maximum mean pulmonary artery pressure that exceeds 30 to 40 mm Hg. As the afterload continues to increase, the right ventricle begins to

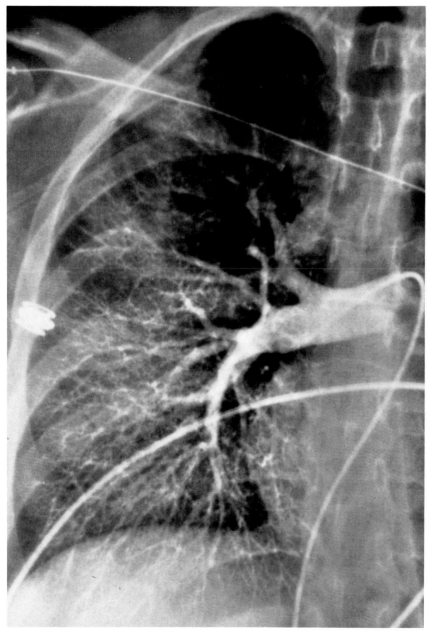

Figure 12–2. Pulmonary angiogram following urokinase infusion showing resolution of pulmonary embolus.

fail as right atrial pressure rises. When forward cardiac output can no longer be sustained, clinical shock ensues. If rapid reversal of the cardiopulmonary hemodynamics does not occur, death will.

Thrombolytic Therapy Versus Anticoagulation

Pathologic data demonstrate that treatment of major pulmonary emboli with anticoagulation therapy alone will result in complete resolution in less than 25 per cent of patients after 1 to 4 weeks and in 50 per cent of patients after 4 months (33). Five clinical studies totaling 210 randomized patients demonstrated more rapid anatomic or physiologic improvement among patients treated with thrombolytic agents than heparin therapy (Table 12–3) (12,13,34–36). However, no studies detected significant differences in mortality, possibly because of the low rate of mortality among control subjects and the small sample sizes.

The well-known, large Phase I portion of the Urokinase Pulmonary Embolism Trial (UPET), sponsored by the National Heart, Lung and Blood Institute, randomized a comparison of heparin and urokinase in 160 patients with angiographically documented pulmonary emboli. All patients received hemodynamic angiographic and nuclear studies (36). Twenty-four hours after the initiation of therapy, the urokinase-treated patients exhibited significantly greater hemodynamic and anatomic improvement than did heparin-treated patients. However, within 5 to 7 days of therapy, no difference between the two groups could be demonstrated by lung scanning. Although 2 weeks following therapy recurrent pulmonary emboli occurred less often in urokinase-treated patients (17 versus 23 per cent), this difference did not achieve statistical significance.

Patients treated with urokinase or streptokinase have been shown to have improved pulmonary capillary blood volume and pulmonary diffusion capacity compared with patients who received standard heparin anticoagulation (14). In addition, one might presume that the lytic therapy may also remove or reduce the source of embolus in the venous system, in addition to lysing the pulmonary emboli, and therefore also reduce the severity or the incidence of venous insufficiency. Thrombolytic therapy, therefore, might hypothetically enable one to

TABLE 12–3.   Summary of Pulmonary Embolus Comparative Trials of Heparin and Thrombolytic Treatment

STUDY	# PATIENTS	TREATMENT ALLOCATION	OUTCOME
Tibbutt et al. (12)	32	Random; 15 heparin, 17 thrombolytic	Improved right heart pressures and anatomy in thrombolytic group
Hirsh et al. (34)	27	Nonrandom; 10 heparin, 17 streptokinase	Hemodynamic & anatomic improvement in thrombolytic group
Miller et al. (35)	23	Nonrandom; 9 heparin, 14 thrombolytic	Anatomic improvement in thrombolytic group
Ly et al. (13)	25	Random/nonrandom; 11 heparin, 14 thrombolytic	Anatomic improvement statistically better in thrombolytic group
Phase I UPET (36)	160	Random; 78 heparin, 82 urokinase	Improved hemodynamic and anatomic response in urokinase group

shorten safely the duration of conventional heparin and warfarin therapy after administering a lytic agent.

The urokinase-treated patients in Phase I of the UPET study had a 27 per cent frequency of severe bleeding (defined as a fall in the hematocrit greater than 10 per cent and/or requiring blood transfusion of more than two units). Urokinase-treated patients in Phase II of the UPET had a 12 per cent rate of severe bleeding (37). The reduction in bleeding in the second trial is an indication of either greater experience with thrombolytic agents by the investigators or perhaps less aggressive transfusion in situations where bleeding may have been previously perceived as severe.

These data convinced the participants at the National Institutes of Health Consensus Development Conference (1980), and they suggested that thrombolytic agents were not being used often enough for patients with pulmonary embolism. They further suggested that thrombolytic agents be used in those patients who have obstruction of blood flow to a lobar or multiple pulmonary segments or those who are hemodynamically compromised, regardless of the size of the pulmonary embolus (9). Despite these recommendations, the use of thrombolytic therapy for pulmonary embolism has continued to progress very slowly, whereas the administration of lytic therapy for acute myocardial infarction and other vascular diseases has occurred with increasing frequency and effectiveness.

The development of tPA for treatment of pulmonary emboli has produced encouraging results. An initial report of tPA-treated pulmonary emboli by Goldhaber et al. showed that 28 of 30 patients had angiographic evidence of clot lysis after treatment with tPA (38). Qualitative improvement as defined in terms of extent of lysis of pulmonary artery thrombus (marked, moderate, slight, or unchanged) showed marked or moderate improvement in 83 per cent of patients. With regard to the quantitative scoring, the pretreatment angiographic score was 6.1 (representing large pulmonary emboli generally involving two or more lobes) with improvement to 4.7 (after 2 hr) and further improvement to 3.2 (after 6 hr) of tPA infusion. This represents a 48 per cent overall improvement in clot lysis.

Average pulmonary artery pressures decrease significantly after tPA therapy from a mean pulmonary artery pressure of 21 to 18 mm Hg ($p = .003$). Among the patients with pulmonary hypertension, whose pulmonary artery pressure exceeded 17 mm Hg, the average mean pressure decreased from 24 to 20 mm Hg ($p = .001$). In a subset of patients, right ventricular dysfunction and tricuspid regurgitation were documented with Doppler echocardiography prior to treatment; this resolved rapidly after tPA therapy.

Conclusion

Pulmonary embolism remains a common illness in the United States, and during the past decade the fatality rate has not improved (39). In part this may be due to use of anticoagulation therapy alone, and the resulting lack of resolution of pulmonary artery clots, which may occur in 75 per cent of patients after 1 to 4 weeks and in 50 per cent of patients after 4 months. In contrast, thrombolysis dissolves any clot that has already formed and can be followed by standard heparin anticoagulation to prevent new clots from forming.

The rationale for employing thrombolysis in pulmonary emboli is that it relieves the obstruction to pulmonary artery blood flow and thus improves right ventricular function, reducing pulmonary artery pressure and ameliorating pulmonary tissue perfusion. By accelerating the reversal of right heart failure, thrombolysis might reduce mortality from pulmonary emboli. In addition, by dissolving deep vein thrombi this treatment might also decrease the frequency of recurrent pulmonary emboli and venous insufficiency. In the urokinase/streptokinase pulmonary embolism trials, urokinase was proven to dissolve thrombi quicker than streptokinase and more completely than heparin therapy.

The development of an optimal thrombotic regimen in pulmonary emboli still leaves unanswered the question of when thrombolytic therapy should be employed, as opposed to standard heparin anticoagulation alone without thrombolysis. A proposed therapeutic strategy might be to use heparin for a single segmental or subsegmental pulmonary embolus without hemodynamic instability and to consider thrombolytic therapy for all other patients with multiple segmental, lobar, or small pulmonary emboli with hemodynamic instability.

REFERENCES

1. McLean J: The thromboplastic action of cephalin. Am J Physiol 1916;*41*:250.
2. Barritt DW, Jordan SC: Anticoagulant drugs in the treatment of pulmonary embolism: A controlled clinical trial. Lancet 1960;*1*:1309–1312.
3. Kanis JA: Heparin in the treatment of pulmonary thromboembolism. Thrombos Diathes Haemorrh 1974;*32*:519–527.
4. O'Donnell TF, Brose NL, Burnand KG, et al: The socioeconomic factors of an iliofemoral thrombosis. J Surg Res 1977;*22*:483.
5. Strandness DE, Langlois Y, Cramer M, Randlett A, Thiele BL: Long-term sequelae of acute venous thrombosis. JAMA 1983;*250*:1289.
6. Moore DJ, Himmell PD, Sumner DS: Distribution of venous valvular incompetence in patients with the postphlebitic syndrome. J Vasc Surg 1986;*3*:49.
7. Comerota AJ: An overview of thrombolytic therapy for venous thromboembolism. *In* Comerota AJ, ed: Thrombolytic Therapy. New York, Grune & Stratton, 1988;65–89.
8. Johansson L, Nylander G, Hedner U, et al: Comparison of streptokinase with heparin: Late results in the treatment of deep vein thrombosis. Acta Med Scand 1979;*206*:93.
9. Thrombolytic therapy in thrombosis: A National Institutes of Health Consensus Development Conference. Ann Intern Med 1980;*93*:141.
10. Marder VJ: Are we using fibrinolytic agents often enough? Ann Intern Med 1980;*93*:136.
11. Sasahara AA, Sharma GVRK, McIntyre KM, et al: A national cooperative trial of thrombolysis in pulmonary embolism: Phase I results of urokinase therapy. J Louisiana State Med Soc 1972; *124*:130.
12. Tibbutt DA, Davies JA, Anderson JA, et al: Comparison by controlled clinical trial of streptokinase and heparin in the treatment of life-threatening pulmonary embolism. Br Med J 1974; *1*:343.
13. Ly B, Arnesen J, Eie H, et al: Controlled clinical trial of streptokinase and heparin in the treatment of major pulmonary embolism. Acta Med Scand 1978;*203*:465.
14. Sharma GVRK, Burleson VA, Sasahara AA: Effective thrombolytic therapy on pulmonary capillary blood volume in patients with pulmonary embolism. N Engl J Med 1980;*303*:842.
15. Robertson BR, Nilsson IM, Nylander G: The value of streptokinase and heparin in the treatment of acute deep venous thrombosis: A coded investigation. Acta Chir Scand 1968;*134*:203.
16. Kakkar VV, Flanc C, Howe CT, et al: Treatment of deep vein thrombosis. A trial of heparin, streptokinase and arvin. Br Med J 1969;*1*:806.
17. Robertson BR, Nilsson IM, Nylander G: Thrombolytic effect of streptokinase as evaluated by phlebography of deep venous thrombi of the leg. Acta Chir Scand 1970;*136*:173.
18. Tsapogas MJ, Peabody RA, Wu KT, et al: Controlled study of thrombolytic therapy in deep vein thrombosis. Surgery 1973;*74*:973.
19. Porter JM, Seaman AJ, Common HH, et al: Comparison of heparin and streptokinase in the treatment of venous thrombosis. Am J Surg 1975;*41*:511.
20. Elliot MS, Immelman EJ, Jeffery P, et al: A comparative randomized trial of heparin versus streptokinase in the treatment of acute proximal venous thrombosis: An interim report of a prospective trial. Br J Surg 1979;*66*:638.

21. Goldhaber SZ, Buring JE, Lipnick RJ, et al: Pooled analyses of randomized trials of streptokinase and heparin and phlebographically documented acute deep vein venous thrombosis. Am J Med 1984;*76*:393.

22. Sharma GVRK, O'Connell DJ, Belko JS, Sasahara AA: Thrombolytic therapy in deep vein thrombosis. *In* Paoletti R, Sherry S, eds: Thrombosis and Urokinase. New York, Academic Press, 1977;181.

23. Graor RA, Young JR, Risius B, Ruschhaupt WF: Cost-effective comparison of streptokinase and urokinase in the treatment of deep vein thrombosis. Ann Vasc Surg 1987;*1*:524–528.

24. Arnesen H, Heilo A, Jakobsen E, Ly B, Skaga E: A prospective study of streptokinase and heparin in the treatment of deep vein thrombosis. Acta Med Scand 1978;*203*:457.

25. Common HH, Seamon AJ, Rosch J, Porter JM, Dotter CT: Deep vein thrombosis treatment with streptokinase or heparin: Follow up of a randomized study. Angiology 1976;*27*:645.

26. Bell WR: Streptokinase and urokinase in the treatment of pulmonary thromboemboli. From a national cooperative study. Thromb Haemost 1976;*25*:57.

27. Fratantoni JC, Ness P, Simon TL: Thrombolytic therapy. Current status. N Engl J Med 1975; *293*:1073.

28. Straub H: Letale komplikationen der fibrinolyse. Munch Med Wochenschr 1982;*124*:17.

29. Holm HA: Trombosebehandling med heparin. *In* Hoechst N, ed: Dyp Venous Trombose og Lungeemboli. Oslo, Publisher, 1981.

30. Turpie AGG, Jay RM, Carter CJ, Hirsch J: A randomized trial of recombinant tissue plasminogen activator for the treatment of proximal deep vein thrombosis [abstr]. Circulation 1985;*72*:III–193.

31. Hume M, Sevitt S, Thomas DP: Venous Thrombosis and Pulmonary Embolism. Cambridge, MA, Harvard University Press, 1970.

32. Hull RD, Hirsh J, Carter CJ, et al: Pulmonary angiography, ventilation lung scanning and venography for clinically suspected pulmonary embolism and abnormal perfusion lung scans. Ann Intern Med 1983;*98*:891.

33. Dalen JE, Alpert JS: Natural history of pulmonary embolism. Prog Cardiovasc Dis 1975;*17*:259.

34. Hirsh J, McDonald IG, Hale GA, et al: Comparison of the effects of streptokinase and heparin in the early rate of resolution of major pulmonary embolism. Can Med Assoc J 1971;*104*:485.

35. Miller GAH, Sutton GC, Kerr IH, et al: Comparison of streptokinase and heparin in the treatment of isolated acute massive pulmonary embolism. Br Med J 1971;*2*:681.

36. Urokinase Pulmonary Embolism Trial. Phase 1 results. JAMA 1970;*214*:2163.

37. Urokinase Pulmonary Embolism Trial Study Group. Urokinase-Streptokinase Embolism Trial. Phase II results. JAMA 1974;*229*:1606.

38. Goldhaber SZ, Vaughan DE, Markis JE, et al: Acute pulmonary embolism treated with tissue plasminogen activator. Lancet 1986;*2*:886–889.

39. Goldhaber SZ: Pulmonary embolism death rates. Am Heart J 1988;*115*:1342–1343.

13

THROMBECTOMY IN ACUTE DEEP VEIN THROMBOSIS: LONG-TERM FOLLOW-UP

Bernard Hans Nachbur and Hans-Beat Ris

INDICATIONS FOR VENOUS THROMBECTOMY

Before reporting long-term results of venous thrombectomy it is necessary to define the indications for this intervention. Late results depend largely upon whether this intervention is performed with the purpose of salvaging life, a limb, or an organ or simply as a means of preventing postphlebitic sequelae in acute and subacute cases of deep venous thrombosis (DVT). If a patient's life is threatened because of sudden bilateral phlegmasia dolens and consecutive arterial ischemia of both legs (Fig. 13–1), and venous thrombectomy saves the patient's life and both his limbs, then it is fair to consider this a success, irrespective of functional long-term results. Likewise, if a kidney transplant fails because of iliofemoral venous thrombosis and venous thrombectomy can restore renal function, then this on its own merit underlines the value and importance of mastering the technique of thrombectomy, again irrespective of long-term venous function.

Although the main object of this chapter is to report on the long-term outcome of venous thrombectomy as opposed to conservative treatment with anticoagulants, the relevance of thrombectomy for limb or life salvage needs to be illustrated.

Bilateral Phlegmasia Dolens

Case Report 1

B.M. is a 48-year-old farmer who had been operated on for a fracture of the right tibia, which was repaired by intramedullary pin fixation. In the postoperative course he had an event of pulmonary embolism that was subsequently treated by full-dose heparin. In spite of adequate systemic heparinization the patient had recurrent pulmonary embolism and then underwent inferior vena cava (IVC) interruption by percutaneous introduction of a Günther filter. Shortly thereafter the patient developed acute bilateral DVT of the lower extremities involving obstruction of the IVC up to the level of the filter. This was proven by computed tomography with contrast enhancement, showing a Günther filter in an oblique, almost horizontal position (Fig. 13–2). Whether the filter had been dislodged by the

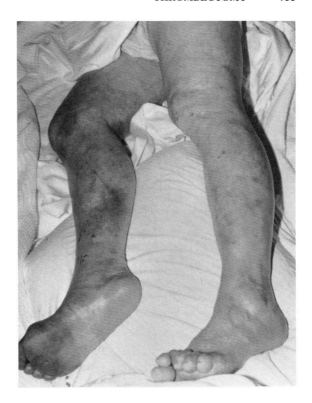

Figure 13–1. A 55-year-old patient with acute thrombosis of the inferior vena cava and the deep iliofemoropopliteal veins of both legs leading to bilateral phlegmasia cerulea dolens, ischemia of both legs, and a life-threatening state of shock.

sheer momentum of a large embolus or whether dislodgement into the oblique position had occurred spontaneously and had thus become the reason for extensive bilateral DVT remains a matter of debate. The patient developed signs of DVT characterized by swelling and cyanosis of both lower limbs. Within less than 4 hr he felt excruciating and intractable pain in both legs with loss of arterial pulsations bilaterally. Following his referral to our hospital the patient was in a state of shock, with massive pain in both legs and in desperate awareness of impending death. Inguinal pulses were barely palpable initially and became inperceptable by the time of simultaneous inguinal incision.

Operative treatment was performed within less than 30 min after referral. Iliofemoral veins were 2.5 cm in diameter and thrombotic, in sharp contrast to the filiform, pulseless femoral arteries. Following iliofemorocaval thrombectomy with a Fogarty balloon catheter, the arterial circulation improved rapidly. Pedal pulses were palpable within a few hours and the patient became hemodynamically stable. The reperfusion syndrome made fasciotomy mandatory. The arteries had only been inspected but otherwise remained untouched.

This patient survived a life-threatening state of acidosis and hemodynamic shock due to sudden sequestration of blood following iliofemorocaval occlusion involving the total venous cross-section of both limbs and causing secondary occlusion of the arteries in both legs. Ischemia was probably due to the fact that the critical closing pressure of the arteries was overcome by the sudden increase of interstitial pressure. Without immediate venous thrombectomy this patient would not have survived, or would at least have lost both legs. Failure to achieve immediate restoration of blood flow by unblocking obstructed veins in similar cases would be hard to forgive.

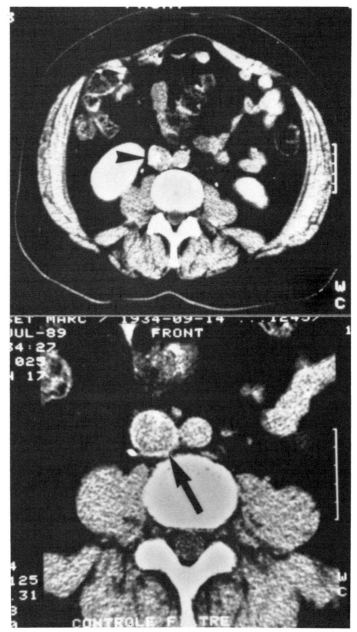

Figure 13–2. Computed tomography scans of patient in Figure 13–1 showing thrombotic occlusion of the inferior vena cava (*arrow*) that is grossly enlarged from a Günther vena cava filter on downward and causing life-threatening phlegmasia cerulea dolens of both legs.

One year following this episode the patient is well, but venous function assessed by phlebodynamic plethysmography is pathological.

Renal Vein Thrombosis in Kidney Transplants

Iliofemoral venous thrombectomy has been applied three times successfully to restore renal function following kidney transplantation. An example for this is presented in the next case report.

Case Report 2

Figure 13–3 shows the phlebographic occlusion of the left iliac vein in a 5-year-old boy with a kidney transplant that stopped functioning on the 10th postoperative day. Following iliofemoral venous thrombectomy the glomerular filtration rate (Fig. 13–4) returned to normal and urine output rose from total renal shutdown to daily levels of around 1 liter.

Exercising the technique of venous thrombectomy was instrumental for salvage of the transplanted organ; the functional venous long-term outcome becomes a secondary importance in such situations, even though in this boy venous function as examined later was normal.

RATIONALE FOR VENOUS THROMBECTOMY

Acute iliofemoral venous thrombosis can cause dramatic or even catastrophic complications, as depicted in the two case reports, or may give rise to late sequelae such as venous claudication, swelling, a feeling of heaviness, ulceration, eczema, and occupational impairment often leading to insurance claims. Heparin and oral anticoagulants are generally regarded as the mainstays in the treatment of acute DVT, not only because they usually control pulmonary embolism but also because this treatment—especially if combined with leg elevation and a few days of bed

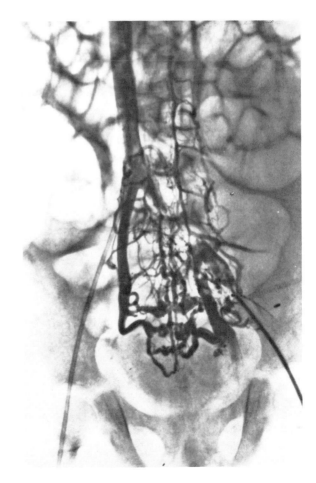

Figure 13–3. Venogram of a 5-year-old boy 10 days after successful renal transplant. Urine output had suddenly ceased totally as a result of iliac vein thrombosis and thrombotic occlusion of the renal vein. The phlebogram shows occlusion of the common iliac vein and a collateral circulation reaching the contralateral side.

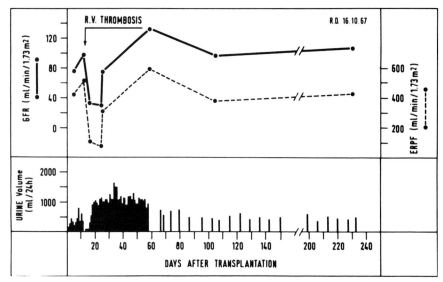

Figure 13–4. Postoperative course of 5-year-old patient shown in Figure 13–3 following initially successful kidney transplantation. Glomerular filtration rate (GFR) and renal plasma flow decreased dramatically on the 10th postoperative day owing to iliac and renal vein thrombosis. Surgical thrombectomy was followed by immediate recovery of all renal parameters.

rest—results in relatively rapid decrease of symptoms. However, the majority of patients will develop late sequelae, especially if there is extensive involvement of the deep veins. Also, patients who have experienced DVT once are prone to have DVT again. The Ad Hoc Committee Reporting Standards in Venous Disease (1) has listed a prior history of lower extremity DVT as the greatest single risk factor for a subsequent episode of DVT. The postthrombotic sequelae are caused by chronic venous hypertension, which results either from venous obstruction or from reflux because of destruction of venous valves.

In spite of the advent of phlebography, noninvasive diagnostic tools, heparin, systemic anticoagulation, and compression hosiery, the outlook for many patients with DVT remains unfavorable, although probably no longer quite so bleak as reported by Browse et al. (2) and Widmer et al. (3,4). Raju and Fredericks (5) have recently reported the actual long-term outcome of medical therapy in a careful hemodynamic study of 29 limbs with proven DVT. Their results emphasize the need to restore venous flow following thrombotic occlusion.

HOW CAN OCCLUDED VEINS BE CLEARED?

Restoration of flow in occluded veins can be achieved either by systemic or regional fibrinolysis or by surgical thrombectomy with or without a protective arteriovenous fistula.

In a prospective trial of heparin, streptokinase, and Arwin (ancrod) for treatment of DVT, Kakkar et al. (6) demonstrated that heparin and Arwin (purified venom of the Malaysian pit viper) do nothing to restore patency and that systemic fibrinolysis with streptokinase can give rise to potentially dangerous hemorrhage or pulmonary embolism, or may be contraindicated in many instances. Olow et al. (7) have also reported disappointing results with fibrinolysis, and Eklof et al. (8,9) reported life-threatening intraabdominal hemorrhage from the liver and spleen. In fact, almost all published series include bleeding complications, intracranial hemorrhage being the most dreaded. Persson, for example, reported a fatal intracranial hemorrhage from an arteriovenous malformation in a series of 15 patients treated by streptokinase or urokinase (10).

In contrast, surgical thrombectomy can be performed without risk of serious complications. Pulmonary embolism, the most likely mishap, can be avoided by proper Trendelenburg positioning of the patient (11).

TECHNIQUE OF VENOUS THROMBECTOMY

The technique of venous thrombectomy has been described (12) and is depicted schematically in Figure 13–5. Surgical thrombectomy is never performed for femorocrural DVT alone; it is performed for iliofemoral thrombosis alone or in combination with femorocrural thrombosis. The operation is performed under local anesthesia. The first and most important step is to clear the venous pathways in the pelvis. This is done by dissecting out the femoral veins at the strategic junction in the groin: the common femoral, the deep femoral, and the circumflex femoral veins are all encircled, as well as the saphenous vein near or at its orifice with the common femoral vein. The patient is then positioned in 20 to 30 degrees of Trendelenburg, whereupon the common femoral vein is incised longitudinally from the saphenous vein 2 cm distal to it. A venous Fogarty catheter with a balloon capacity of 40 ml is passed up into the IVC. The patient is requested to perform the Valsalva maneuver while the dilated balloon is drawn downward. Brisk reflux

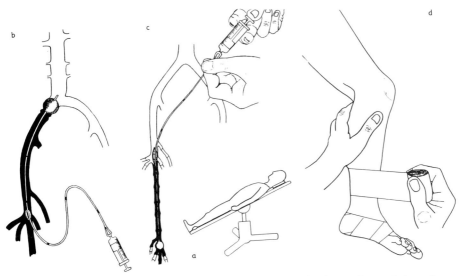

Figure 13–5. Schematic diagram of venous thrombectomy, which is usually carried out from a longitudinal incision in the groin. Details of the technique are given in the text. Trendelenburg's position (a) is necessary for the first stage of the operation, iliofemoral thrombectomy; (b). Thereafter the table is returned to the horizontal position for thrombectomy and expulsion of thrombus in the distal pathways (c). Crural thrombi are dislodged either manually or with Ace bandages as shown here (d).

from above connotes successful thrombectomy. The maneuver is usually repeated two to three times. Surprisingly, more often than not, loosened thrombi can be extracted with a forceps from the iliac vein.

Following copious regional heparinization the operating table is repositioned horizontally. A smaller balloon catheter is passed for extraction of adjacent thrombotic material. It is important to "uncork" the various venous tributaries in the groin in order to increase distal flow. Calf vein thrombi are either dislodged by manual compression or flushed out by rinsing with saline to which 100,000 units of urokinase can be added. In a number of young women with DVT resulting from contraceptives, regional thrombolysis and thrombectomy were combined by isolated perfusion therapy using extracorporeal circulation. We introduced this method in 1980 (13) and demonstrated good fibrinolytic activity in the perfused extremity while fibrinogen levels and euglobulin clot lysis times remained normal systemically. Regional heparinization of the distal venous pathways is not feasible if the valves are competent. Therefore, it is recommended to give a systemic dose of heparin immediately after encircling the veins in the groin and just before venotomy.

Many authors use a temporary protective arteriovenous fistula to increase flow in the venous pathway and thus prevent rethrombosis. This is done by using the saphenous vein, which is anastomosed to the common femoral artery. We have used this adjunctive procedure only occasionally.

EFFICACY OF THROMBECTOMY

Venous thrombosis often advances by stealth. When patients are bedridden or when assessment of an extremity is obscured by a cast, the true age of a thrombus is usually hard to determine. This has been examined and described in detail by Leu (14). Because early in the use of the procedure (i.e., in the 1960s) venous thrombectomy was performed injudiciously and without proper indications, results were disappointing (15). Rethrombosis occurred rather frequently. Moreover, indiscriminate, traumatic instrumentation (with ring strippers and similar devices) caused harm, as demonstrated by early phlebographic control (16). Thus, venous thrombectomy was discredited.

Thrombectomy will be successful only if performed early (i.e., within the very first days following onset of thrombosis) and under the assumption that a reaction between the endothelial lining of the venous wall and the thrombus has not yet taken place. When fibroblasts begin to invade the thrombus, surgical thrombectomy is doomed to failure. Best results are therefore achieved when the thrombus is on the verge of or has only just occluded the vein.

RESULTS OF VENOUS THROMBECTOMY

Short-Term Results

Excellent clearance of occluded veins can be achieved with thrombectomy in properly selecting patients. This has been demonstrated by repeat venograms performed in our patients (Figs. 13–6 through 13–8). Short-term results are func-

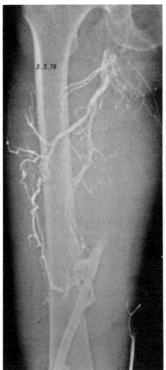
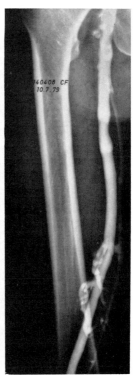

Figure 13-6. Venograms showing iliofemoral DVT of the right leg before thrombectomy (*left*) and 1 year after surgical thrombectomy (*right*). Note complete restoration of valvular morphology.

tionally and radiologically good. These are demonstrably superior to the short-term results of conservative treatment. But how do thrombectomized patients compare with those treated medically with heparin, oral anticoagulants for 4 to 6 months, and prescription of compression stockings after more than 5 years?

Long-Term Results

There are a number of reports in the literature underscoring the merits of venous thrombectomy, but only a few that compare long-term results of surgery with conservative management (8,17,18). Only two studies (8,19) are based on randomized, prospective trials. Eklof et al. (8) reported one in 1985. Their results, shown in Tables 13–1 through 13–3, reveal significant advantages in the surgical cohort. The other prospective study (17) comes from the same group of Swedish authors and relates the 5-year outcome of two randomized study groups. The results of Plate et al. are given in Tables 13–4 and 13–5, and show a tendency toward better long-term results in the surgical groups. However, these authors did not find the benefit to be very striking. This study revealed slightly more asymptomatic patients in the surgical group (37 versus 18 per cent) and less frequent severe postthrombotic sequelae (16 versus 27 per cent) in the surgical group (not statistically significant). The iliac vein was significantly ($p < .05$) more often normal following thrombectomy (71 versus 30 per cent) as demonstrated by radionuclide angiography, but occlusion plethysmography showed an outflow capacity (61 versus 45/min/100 ml) that was not significantly better. Ambulatory venous pressure was significantly ($p < .05$) lower and venous refill time significantly ($p < .05$) more often normal in the surgical group.

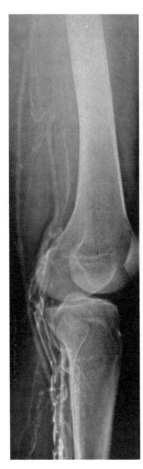
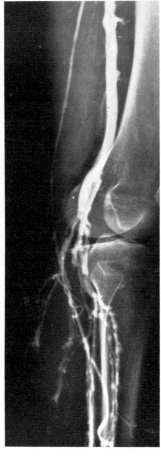

Figure 13–7. Lateral view of venogram of a 26-year-old patient with subacute iliofemoropopliteo-crural DVT associated with oral contraceptives left. *B*, Repeat venogram 11 days following combined surgical iliofemoral thrombectomy and isolated regional perfusion of the peripheral pathways with streptokinase. Patency was obtained over the entire length of the deep venous system. Note restoration of valves after treatment (right).

TABLE 13–1.   Conservative Treatment Versus Thrombectomy with an Adjuvant Temporary Arteriovenous Fistula[a,b]

	CONSERVATIVE TREATMENT	SURGICAL THROMBECTOMY	SIGNIFICANCE LEVEL
Number	32	31	
Age and sex	well stratified		
Duration of swelling in days	1.7	2.3	
Mean duration of hospitalization in days	9	10	
Free of symptoms following treatment	7%	42%	$p < .005$
Radiologic patency	35%	76%	$p < .025$
Dilated collateral veins	62%	24%	$p < .01$
Patent femoropopliteal segment—no reflux	41%	86%	$p < .05$

[a] From Eklof B, Einarsson E, Plate G: Role of thrombectomy and temporary a-v fistula in acute iliofemoral venous thrombosis. *In* Bergan JJ, Yao JST, eds: Surgery of the Veins. Orlando, FL, Grune & Stratton, 1985; 131–145.
[b] $N = 63$; study began July 1, 1979.

TABLE 13–2.   Correlation between Femoral Vein Pressure Increase with Leg Work and Radiologic Patency

PATENCY	PRESSURE INCREASE FOLLOWING LEG WORK	
Very good	3.2 mm Hg	
Moderately good	8.0 mm Hg	$p < .005$
Radiologic rethrombosis	10.0 mm Hg	

[a] From Eklof B, Einarsson E, Plate G: Role of thrombectomy and temporary a-v fistula in acute iliofemoral venous thrombosis. *In* Bergan JJ, Yao JST, eds: Surgery of the Veins. Orlando, FL, Grune & Stratton, 1985; 131–145.

Plate et al.'s study has a few medical flaws that are of sufficient importance to skew the results and obscure tendencies that could possibly gain statistical significance:

1.   Patients developing DVT during pregnancy or in the puerperium were excluded from the study and routinely offered surgery!

2.   The average age of both treatment groups was relatively high—59 (medical) and 55 years (surgical), respectively—and comprised patients up to the age of 80 in the surgical group. It is our conviction that patients older than 60 years and nearing retirement age should not be offered surgery or rather will have no need for it because they are in a position to evade the ill effects of venous hypertension.

3.   In six of a total of 19 surgical patients the extent of thrombosis was unknown before the operation (no venogram).

4.   In the surgical group at least one patient was included who had definite signs of prior DVT. This is a contraindication to surgery or at least merits exclusion from the study.

5.   Maximum venous outflow is not a valid test for examining venous function after 5 years because it is performed on elevated limbs and is unable to distinguish between veins with competent valves and recanalized veins with incompetent valves. That the difference between the two groups for this parameter is not significant is therefore hardly surprising.

Personal Results

We have recently analyzed and compared the long-term functional outcome of two equally large cohorts of patients treated either surgically for restoration of venous patency and valvular function (24 patients) or medically with heparin,

TABLE 13–3.   Rate of Pulmonary Embolism in Patients Treated Conservatively Versus by Thrombectomy as Assessed by Pulmonary Scintigraphy[a]

Pulmonary embolism before treatment[b]	65%
Superimposed pulmonary embolism first week after initial treatment	
Conservative group	23%
Surgical group	15%

[a] From Eklof B, Einarsson E, Plate G: Role of thrombectomy and temporary a-v fistula in acute iliofemoral venous thrombosis. *In* Bergan JJ, Yao JST, eds: Surgery of the Veins. Orlando, FL, Grune & Stratton, 1985; 131–145.
[b] Danger of pulmonary embolism is not increased by the surgical intervention; on the contrary, the authors believe thrombectomy to have a protective effect.

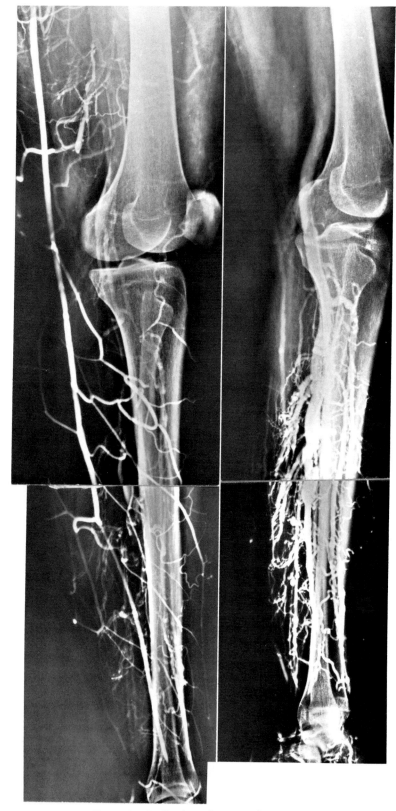

Figure 13–8 See legend on opposite page.

TABLE 13–4. Patient and Thrombus Characteristics in 41 Patients with Acute Iliofemoral Venous Thrombosis Available for Follow-up at 5 Years[a]

	MEDICAL GROUP	SURGICAL GROUP
Patients		
Mean age in years (range)	59 (15–79)	55 (18–80)
Sex (males/females)	9/13	5/14
Thrombus		
Side (right/left)	6/16	3/16
Extension (proximal/entire leg/unknown)	5/15/2	2/11/6
Mean duration in days (range)	2 (1–7)	2 (0–5)

[a] From Akesson H, Brudin L, Dahlstrom JA, Elkof B, Ohlin P, Plate G: Venous function assessed during a 5 year period after acute ilio-femoral venous trombosis treated with anticoagulation. Eur J Vasc Surg 1990;4:43–48.

TABLE 13–5. Five-Year Results in Medical and Surgical Groups[a]

	TREATMENT		p-VALUE (MANN-WHITNEY U-TEST)
	Medical	Surgical	
Occlusion plethysmography	$n = 20$	$n = 17$	
MVO[b] (ml/min/100 ml)	45 (12–87)	61 (24–61)	n.s.
Foot volumetry	$n = 19$	$n = 14$	
EV_{rel}[c] (ml/100 gm/min)	0.9 (0.0–1.8)	1.0 (0.0–1.9)	n.s.
Q/EV_{rel} (min^{-1})	4.7 (0.5–18.3)	3.3 (1.1–7.4)	n.s.
Foot vein pressure	$n = 18$	$n = 10$	
Pressure reduction (%)	36 (6–78)	52 (26–81)	n.s.
Ambulatory venous pressure (mm Hg)	60 (21–95)	43 (18–70)	$p < .05$
90% refill time (sec)	13 (0–71)	14 (4–38)	n.s.

[a] From Akesson H, Brudin L, Dahlstrom JA, Elkof B, Ohlin P, Plate G: Venous function assessed during a 5 year period after acute ilio-femoral venous trombosis treated with anticoagulation. Eur J Vasc Surg 1990;4:43–48.
[b] MVO, maximum venous outflow.
[c] EV, expelled volume.

oral anticoagulants, and compression stockings (25 patients). This retrospective study (18) was also intended to examine the impact of duration and extent of DVT as predictive factors of late outcome: over a follow-up time of 7.6 years for surgically treated and 7.9 years for medically treated patients, operative mortality was nil.

Assessment of venous function was based on clinical observations as well as on measurements of hemodynamic parameters. Nonfatal pulmonary embolism after onset of treatment occurred in both groups with an equal frequency of 13 per cent. The diagnosis of pulmonary embolism was based on radiologic signs, electrocardiographic tracings, and clinical evidence; lung scintigrams were not performed routinely and therefore there is little doubt that a number of silent emboli were missed. Patients operated on for iliofemoral DVT were with few exceptions not using any form of adjunctive hosiery, which was in sharp contrast to the conservatively managed group. If onset of DVT had occurred more than

←

Figure 13–8. *Left,* A 21-year-old female patient with acute iliofemoropopliteocrural DVT following childbirth. *Right,* Repeat phlebogram 12 days following surgical thrombectomy (ileofemoral) and isolated regional perfusion with streptokinase. Before thrombectomy the contrast medium flows through the collateral circulation (i.e., the greater saphenous vein). After clearance of the deep veins centripetal flow to and through the deep venous system is clearly demonstrable.

3 days earlier and extended from the iliofemoral axis to the popliteocrural level, surgery usually failed and patients were not better off than in the comparable medical group. The same pattern of late outcome was found for all other clinical and hemodynamic parameters: clinical signs of venous hypertension as manifested by swelling, pigmentation, trophic changes of the skin, eczema, phlebectatic changes, and distended superficial collaterals; valvular incompetence as judged by sonography; patient's self-assessment; and the expelled volume (EV) and refilling time measured by dynamic plethysmography after standardized leg work. The mean EV was 1.1 ± 0.5 ml/100 gm/min for the surgical group treated early for iliofemoral DVT and 0.7 ± 0.5 ml/100 gm/min for the corresponding medical group ($p = .05$). Recovery or refilling time was 50 ± 26 sec for the surgical group and 28 ± 26 sec for the medical group ($p = .03$. Figure 13–9 shows an example of a computerized phlebodynamic strain-gauge plethysmograph made 8 years after successful venous thrombectomy, illustrating normal EV and normal refilling time! Figure 13–10 shows a pathologic tracing in a leg treated conservatively.

Thus, the clinical and hemodynamic effects of surgical thrombectomy were significantly superior to conservative management in iliofemoral thrombosis treated within 3 days. For extensive thrombosis treated early the advantage of surgical thrombectomy was also evident, but the difference between the two treat-

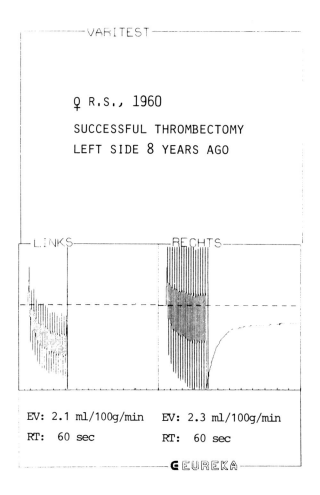

Figure 13–9. Example of dynamic plethysmography in a 29-year-old patient 8 years after successful venous thrombectomy of the left leg. The calf pump function is fully normalized [expelled volume (EV) = 2.1 mg/100 gm/min] and refilling time (RF) of the veins is also normal (60 sec).

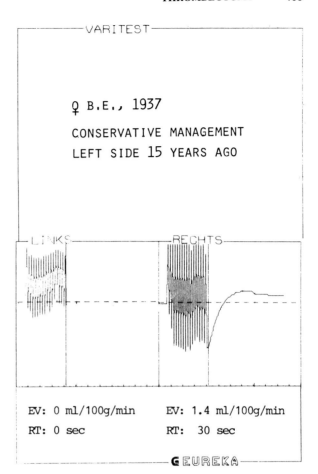

Figure 13–10. Dynamic plethysmography in a 52-year-old patient with iliofemoral thrombosis of the left leg treated conservatively 15 years ago. Expelled volume (EV) and refilling time (RT) are zero.

TABLE 13–6.   Patient and Disease Characteristics in Medical and Surgical Management of DVT[a]

	MEDICAL TREATMENT	THROMBECTOMY
Number of assessed limbs	25	24
Mean age at onset of treatment (years)	30	29
Mean follow-up time (years)	7.9	7.6
Sex (% women)	76	67
Sex (% left side)	64	79
Duration of DVT < 3 days[b]		
I + F	10	8
I + F + P (+ C)	3	9
Duration of DVT > 3 days[b]		
I + F	6	3
I + F + P (+ C)	6	4

[a] From Gänger KH, Nachbur BH, Ris HB, Zurbrügg H: Surgical thrombectomy versus conservative treatment for deep venous thrombosis; functional comparison of long-term results. Eur J Vasc Surg 1989;3:529–538.
[b] I, iliac; F, femoral; P, popliteal; C, crural (thrombosis).

TABLE 13–7. Conservative Treatment Versus Thrombectomy[a]

	TREATMENT		SIGNIFICANCE LEVEL (STUDENT'S *t* TEST)
	Conservative	Surgical	
Total Number	25	24	
Depending on compression stockings[b]			
I + F < 3 days			
I + F + P < 3 days	85%	20%	*p* < .05
I + F > 3 days			
Signs of venous hypertension[b]			
I + F < 3 days			
I + F + P < 3 days	76%	26%	*p* < .05
I + F > 3 days			
Free of symptoms[b]			
I + F < 3 days			
I + F + P < 3 days	26%	76%	*p* < .05
I + F > 3 days			
Mean expelled volume[b]			
(ml/100 gm/min)			
I + F < 3 days	0.7 ± 0.5	1.1 ± 0.5	*p* = .05
Recovery or refilling time (sec)[b]			
I + F < 3 days	50 ± 21	28 ± 26	*p* = .03
No iliofemoral reflux[b]			
I + F < 3 days	30%	100%	*p* < .05
I + F + P < 3 days			
I + F > 3 days	33%	68%	*p* <. 05

[a] From Gänger KH, Nachbur BH, Ris Hb, Zurbrügg H: Surgical thrombectomy versus conservative treatment for deep venous thrombosis; functional comparison of long-term results. Eur J Vasc Surg 1989; 3:529–538.
[b] I, iliac; F, femoral; P, popliteal (thrombosis).

ment groups was not significant owing to the small numbers of these treatment subgroups. The advantage of surgery was totally lost in patients operated on for extensive DVT of long duration (i.e., greater than 3 days). It can be concluded from this study, therefore, that the key to successful surgery is early recognition, involvement of the iliofemoral segment, and treatment within the first 3 days, before the clot has become adherent to the vein wall. Our results are compiled in Tables 13–6 and 13–7.

CONCLUSIONS AND SUMMARY

1. The functional long-term outcome of medically treated iliofemoropopliteal thrombosis is frequently associated with a lasting handicap, regardless of duration and extent of the disease prior to treatment.

2. Successful thrombectomy of iliofemoral thrombosis is possible in the vast majority of patients operated on within 3 to 5 days following onset of disease and allows patients to lead a normal life, without compression stockings or restriction of any form of activity.

3. Early detection and treatment of iliofemoral thrombosis is the key to successful thrombectomy.

4. Iliofemoral thrombosis with involvement of the popliteal and crural segments is not a contraindication to surgery, provided the operation is performed within 3 days of onset of the disease.

REFERENCES

1. Porter JM, Rutherford RB, Clagett GP, et al: Ad Hoc Committee Reporting Standards in Venous Disease. J Vasc Surg 1988;8:172–181.
2. O'Donnell TF, Browse NL, Burnand KG, Thomas ML: The socioeconomic effects of an iliofemoral venous thrombosis. J Surg Res 1977;22:483–488.
3. Widmer LK, Brandenberger E, Schmitt HE, Widmer MT, Voelin R, Zemp E, Madar G: Zum Schicksal des Patienten mit tiefer Venenthrombose. Dtsch Med Wochenschr 1985;110:993.
4. Widmer LK, Brandenberger E, Widmer MT, Schmid HE, Duckert F, Marbet G, Ritz R: Late sequelae of deep venous thrombosis. Int Angiol 1982;1:31–37.
5. Raju S, Fredericks R: Late hemodynamic sequelae of deep venous thrombosis. J Vasc Surg 1986; 4:73–79.
6. Kakkar VV, Flanc C, Howe CT: Treatment of deep vein thrombosis. A trial of heparin, streptokinase and Arwin. Br Med J 1969;1:898–910.
7. Olow B, Anderson J, Eklof B, et al: Deep venous thrombosis treated with a standard dosage of streptokinase. Acta Chir Scand 1970;136:181–189.
8. Eklof B, Einarsson E, Plate G: Role of thrombectomy and temporary a-v fistula in acute iliofemoral venous thrombosis. In Bergan JJ, Yao JST, eds: Surgery of the Veins. Orlando, FL, Grune & Stratton, 1985;131–145.
9. Eklof B, Gjöres JE, Lotti A, et al: Spontaneous rupture of liver and spleen with severe intraabdominal bleeding during streptokinase treatment of deep venous thrombosis. VASA 1977; 6:369–371.
10. Persson AV: Treatment of acute deep venous thrombosis with emphasis on fibrinolytic therapy. In Bergan JJ, Yao JST, eds: Surgery of the Veins. Orlando, FL, Grune & Stratton, 1975;145–151.
11. Nachbur B: Chirurgische Behandlung akuter und subakuter Phlebothrombosen. In Kappert A, ed: Lehrbuch und Atlas der Angiologie. Bern, Hans Huber Verlag, 1985;385–387.
12. Nachbur B: Diagnose und Therapie der tiefen Phlebothrombose der unteren Extremitäten. Helv Chir Acta 1987;54:571–596.
13. Nachbur B, Beck EA, Senn A: Can the results of treatment of deep venous thrombosis be improved by combining surgical thrombectomy with regional fibrinolysis? J Cardiovasc Surg 1980;21:347–352.
14. Leu HJ: Histologische Altersbestimmung von arteriellen und venösen Thromben und Emboli. VASA 1973;2:265–273.
15. De Weese JA: Iliofemoral venous thrombectomy. In Bergan JJ, Yao JST, eds: Venous Problems. Chicago, Year Book Medical Publishers, 1978;421–435.
16. Nachbur B, Senn A, Wälti R: Ergebnisse der chirurgischen Behandlung des akuten Venenverschlusses. Helv Chir Acta 1967;34:123–131.
17. Plate G, Akesson H, Ohlin P, Eklof B: Long-term results of venous thrombectomy combined with a temporary arteriovenous fistula. Eur J Vasc Surg (in press).
18. Gänger KH, Nachbur BH, Ris HB, Zurbrügg H: Surgical thrombectomy versus conservative treatment for deep venous thrombosis; functional comparison of long-term results. Eur J Vasc Surg 1989;3:529–538.
19. Rutherford RB: Role of surgery in iliofemoral venous thrombosis. Chest 1986;89(suppl):434–437.

V

TREATMENT OF SUPERFICIAL VENOUS INSUFFICIENCY

14

SURGICAL PROCEDURES FOR VARICOSE VEINS

John J. Bergan

> . . . as for the veins of the leg, the area involved is so extensive, the anastomoses so free, and the other factors so prejudicial that the problem of surgical treatment is a more difficult one, and the passing years have left a trail of obsolete operations.
>
> W. WAYNE BABCOCK, PHILADELPHIA, 1907 (1)

It is with these words that Babcock reintroduced the subject of intraluminal stripping into treatment of varicose veins at the beginning of this century. Had he been writing 80 years later, he might have added that not only had surgical procedures come and gone, but the entire armamentarium of operations for varicose veins had been virtually abandoned by the majority of the general surgeons and their colleagues in vascular surgery. As a result, in the 1980s, proprietary clinics advertising in newspapers and magazines made their appearance. A surgical vacuum existed in the treatment of varicose veins and this was filled, as is nature's law, by people who could and would intervene to ablate varicosities.

Good reasons had been given by surgeons for abandoning surgical therapy of venous varicosities. The operations inherited from the 1920s and 1930s were too extensive, aesthetically unappealing, and too morbid to justify their performance (Fig. 14–1). Standard greater and lesser saphenous vein stripping with added multiple incisions for the removal of varicose clusters proved cosmetically unsatisfactory even though late healing of the surgical wounds produced fine scars and little disfigurement. A wave of coronary bypass and peripheral bypass surgeons decried removal of saphenous veins that might better be used for arterial reconstruction at another site and time. Third, complications of the varicose vein operations, including superficial dysthesias, paresthesias, and other unwanted sensations, cast doubt on the value of the procedures.

Nevertheless, a small group of interested physiologists, surgeons, and, on the continent of Europe, phlebologists persisted in treatment of patients with primary venous stasis disease. Gradually, guidelines for specific therapy emerged, noninvasive tests of venous function developed, and interventional plans became more patient specific. As a result, operations became more satisfactory from both a physiologic and a cosmetic point of view. It is the purpose of this chapter to summarize these new approaches in order to lay out a pattern of practice that will be satisfactory in treating patients with primary venous stasis (varicose veins).

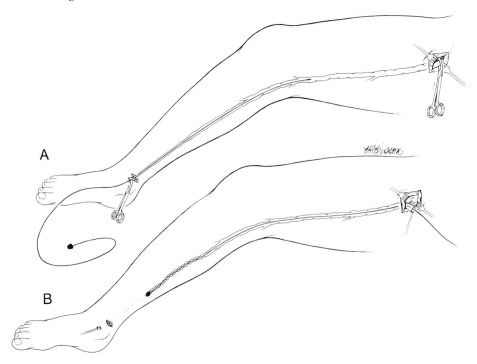

Figure 14–1. Many surgeons in practice today were taught that greater and lesser saphenous vein stripping was the cornerstone of the operation to treat varicose veins. The incisions were placed at ankle and groin, and multiple transverse incisions were made over varicosities, dissecting out the clusters and ligating proximal and distal tributaries. Meticulous surgeons would often spend 4 to 6 hr per extremity and the cosmetic results ranged from merely satisfactory to outrageously disfiguring.

HISTORICAL INTRODUCTION

As indicated, many operations for venous varicosities have come and gone. Highlights in the history of treating venous disorders is the subject of another chapter in this volume. However, the 20th century and present-day treatment of venous varicosities was ushered in with the contribution of Trendelenburg, described in the German literature of 1891 (2). His operation was simply ligation of the saphenous vein at the saphenofemoral junction and in the thigh. It was based on the theoretical principle that reflux of blood into the saphenous vein could be stopped with a simple high ligature. Within 20 years, uncertain results of the procedure and a recurrence of varicosities in a large percentage of cases (from 22 to 72 per cent) (3) led to more radical surgical methods, including total removal of the saphenous system, multiple ligature of perforating veins, and radical excisions as described subsequently (4).

As simple ligation became inadequate, methods of removing varicose veins intraluminally and extraluminally were introduced. In 1905, Keller advocated intraluminal stripping with a twisted wire (5). This was quickly followed by Charles Mayo's description of the extraluminal stripper in 1906 (6), and this, in turn, by Babcock's invention of the relatively stiff intraluminal wire, which contributed the acorn-shaped tip (1). John Homans, another famous name in American surgery, strongly advocated flush saphenofemoral ligation and radical excision of varicosities for extensive venous stasis disease (7). Variations on this general theme emerged sequentially and included various forms of sclerotherapy.

The most outstanding contribution to knowledge of venous anatomy in this era was that of R. S. Sherman, who performed meticulous studies summarized in his 1949 publication (8). This important work set the stage for physiologic testing, which would identify precise methods of surgical therapy in treating symptomatic patients who bore the external stigmata of varicose veins.

INDICATIONS FOR INTERVENTION

This volume is concerned with diagnosis and treatment of venous disorders. Because varicose veins are found in nearly 50 per cent of the adult female population, in theory varicose veins may be thought of by some as being normal. Patients with varices have no such thought. They have, nevertheless, a variety of lower extremity symptoms and present themselves for medical consultation. Many do not like the appearance of their legs. This is a valid reason for seeking medical therapy and may be the only indication for intervention.

Other patients are referred to specialists because of the presence of varicosities. Presumably, the specialist will give good consultation and advice, and whether to intervene or not will be decided upon. Another sizeable group of patients will appear with symptoms that are, in fact, due to degenerative arthritis, arterial occlusive disease, idiopathic or hypoproteinemic edema, neurospinal compression, congestive heart failure, or simply obesity. Certainly, many of these patients, and many others whose only problem is varicose veins, require no treatment. Advice regarding skin hygiene and mild, nonprescription elastic support may prove to be better therapy than intervention.

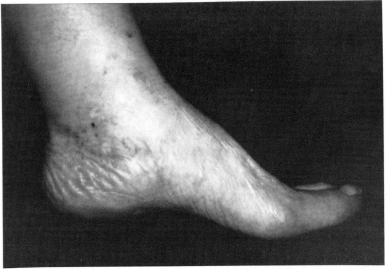

Figure 14–2.   A surprisingly frequent indication for varicose vein treatment is external hemorrhage. This photograph shows the left foot of an elderly woman who experienced a frightening torrent of bleeding from her left ankle. The retromalleolar site is marked by cutaneous hemosiderin pigmentation, indicating long-standing dermal venous hypertension. Residual edema is easily identified, and adjacent, thinly covered venous blebs are seen here and are typical.

Even excluding those patients who have sought only advice, there will remain a large number who deserve interventional care. Appearance or approved cosmesis is an acceptable indication for intervention. However, the mode of therapy chosen should produce a bettering of epidermis, not a worsening of the appearance of the skin. Beyond cosmetic indications, other more solid indications include recurrent superficial thrombophlebitis in varicose veins; external hemorrhage from subcutaneous varicose veins (Fig. 14–2); chronic, cyclic, recurrent pain due to varicose veins; and disabling edema with or without subcutaneous cellulitis, induration, or liposclerosis.

CHOICE OF INTERVENTION

Once indications for intervention have been decided upon, there is need to decide what form of intervention will prove long lasting and most satisfactory in an individual patient (Fig. 14–3). There are essentially four courses of action to be chosen from. The first is nonintervention, and certainly this will be appropriate for many patients with cosmetic complaints and for all others whose complaints are due to conditions other than venous stasis.

Excluding nonintervention as an option, three others remain. The first is *elastic compression* alone, which may be chosen for the very aged with relatively severe problems or for younger and middle-aged individuals whose problems are relatively trivial. Support stockings and especially support pantyhose, woven of nonelastic but synthetic fibers with memory, have provided a great deal of relief of stasis symptomatology to women with standing occupations and those women whose venous stasis symptomatology is exacerbated by the latter half of a men-

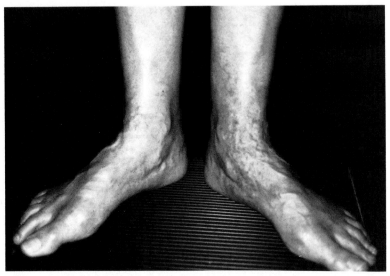

Figure 14–3. The right foot and medial ankle of a 48-year-old woman whose right varicose vein stripping was performed 20 years previously. No treatment was given to the left lower extremity, which now shows the corona phlebectatica, dermal pigmentation, venous hypertension, and varicosities that are the result of her genetic inheritance and hormonal cycling. This dramatically shows the persistence and durability of the surgical result.

strual cycle and the first 2 days of a menstrual period. Similarly, men without obvious external varicosities but with venous stasis symptomatology have profited by below-knee elastic support stockings. Many intercontinental air travelers have also received benefit from the wearing of such stockings. Furthermore, external elastic support is the mainstay of therapy for symptomatology caused by deep venous insufficiency whether due to obstruction or reflux.

The third therapeutic option is *sclerotherapy*. A variety of opinions on this subject exist. However, certain guidelines have emerged. Sclerotherapy can obliterate any vein at any time. However, lasting results of sclerotherapy are best achieved in the smallest veins, in veins below the knee, and in veins not subject to high-pressure reflux. Such reflux may originate in veins that communicate between the deep venous circulation and the superficial circulation at the saphenofemoral junction, the saphenopopliteal junction, and other sites. To be more specific, sclerotherapy is the only treatment for venectatic or telangiectatic blemishes in the thighs and legs. It is of some value in small, abnormal venules in the popliteal space and in the legs below the knee, especially when these vessels are smaller than 2 mm in diameter. Other varicosities may be obliterated by sclerosis but only if proximal venous reflux is abolished by surgical or other techniques. It should be mentioned in this regard that there is a school of thought, especially on the European continent, that saphenous venous reflux can be obliterated by sclerotherapy and that specific communicating veins can be obliterated by sclerotherapy. American surgeons disagree with this concept.

Surgical intervention is best employed when reflux is proven at the saphenofemoral level or saphenopopliteal level and when clusters of varicosities are large and derive from subcutaneous veins superficial to the membranous fascia that may or may not communicate with the greater and lesser saphenous venous system. Surgical intervention is particularly valuable for large varicosities that are present in the thighs and that have origins distinct from the saphenous vein. Such clusters of varicosities make take their origin from pelvic leak, from lateral perforating veins communicating with the profunda femoris venous system, or from anterior or anteromedial communicating veins that communicate directly with the deep venous system. Similarly, large clusters of varicosities that terminate in the greater saphenous vein but originate from reflux through the hunterian perforator and the anteromedial calf perforating vein (Boyd's perforator) can be managed successfully by stab avulsion, thus obviating the need for sclerotherapy.

SCLEROTHERAPY ALONE FOR VARICOSE VEINS

While it is not the object of this chapter to describe the use of sclerotherapy in treatment of venous varicosities, a brief summary of previous studies is in order. Two are relevant and typical of conclusions reached and results achieved. These are the report of Jakobsen (9) and the earlier report of Hobbs (10). Both studies have pointed out that there is essentially no disability experienced by patients treated by sclerotherapy, that normal occupations can be carried out whether these are in the home or in industry. With regard to results, patients receiving sclerotherapy perceive their subjective results as being better than do objective evaluators at all periods of observation following sclerotherapy. As time passes, objective observation of return of varicosities occurs to a larger extent in patients receiving sclerotherapy than in those who have surgical intervention.

In general terms, the most effective treatment of venous varicosities by sclerotherapy is achieved as indicated previously; that is, varicose veins below the knee lend themselves to more complete compression and therefore, more long-lasting results than varicosities of the thigh. Furthermore, the largest varicosities are the most difficult to obliterate, in contrast to the smallest, which are quite easy to erase. Jakobsen's observations in three groups of patients treated and observed for more than 3 years are succinctly summarized in his statement, " A Kruskal-Wallis test showed the results of radical operation at three years after treatment to be significantly better than the results of combined treatment ($P <$ 0.0005) and combined treatment to be significantly better than sclerotherapy alone ($P < 0.0005$)."

SAPHENOFEMORAL LIGATION ALONE

The Trendelenburg operation has been revisited many times in the nearly 100 years since its introduction. Trendelenburg as a surgeon made brilliant observations, and his innovative techniques must have been marvelous even at that time. Unfortunately, regarding proximal ligation, he was simply wrong. It is tempting in these last years of the 20th century to return to the Trendelenburg operation, because it can be performed in a very brief time under local anesthesia in an outpatient surgical unit for minimum cost to the patient and to the economy. These advantages are considerable but not outweighed by repeated observations that this is a totally inadequate operation. Stanley Rivlin pointed out that in 5500 patients personally seen and examined by him, 1453 had been subjected previously to such an operation, unsuccessfully. More than two thirds of his patients had failure of juxtafemoral ligation (11). Many other reports confirm this observation and a host of others attempt to explain this failure on anatomic grounds. Among the latest of these is a mercifully brief report in late 1989 that stated that surgical construction of a barrier of cribriform fascia over the saphenofemoral junction significantly reduced the incidence of recurrent varices (12).

These anatomic explanations, including a detailed diagrammatic description of the variations of the termination of the greater saphenous vein at the fossa ovalis, have appealed to surgeons. Nevertheless, there is no substitute for direct observation rather than anatomic conjecture. Duplex scanning has now revealed the true cause of failure of the Trendelenburg procedure. Many observations with imaging have now been made and confirm the fact that greater saphenous patency is maintained right up to the site of interruption. The reason for such patency may be ascribed to tributary vein flow into the saphenous vein, which, in turn, is incompetent. Flow is maintained by reflux in a distal direction, thus preventing descending thrombosis and obliteration of the greater saphenous lumen while continuing hypertension in the varicosities.

Rutherford's observations on this are typical. His study was actually directed at the amount of residual saphenous vein available for bypass after various forms of surgical interruption (13). In this study, Rutherford et al. had sufficient patients available to examine those with distal partial, proximal partial, and total removal of the saphenous vein, as well as those with high ligation alone. These were compared to normal limbs. In the high-ligation-alone group, the mean length of available saphenous vein was 108.8 cm and all 10 of the subjects (100 per cent) had greater than 60 cm of saphenous vein available for use as bypass. Simply stated, duplex scanning confirms the fact that high ligation alone allows persistence of distal reflux after surgical intervention.

LIGATION AND SCLEROTHERAPY

To the surgeon of the immediate post–World War II era, saphenofemoral interruption with sclerotherapy implied injection of sclerosant solution directly into the exposed saphenous vein at the time of saphenofemoral interruption. Elaborate techniques were developed and included the use of catheters, asepto syringes, and other methods. The sclerosant solutions were frequently quite strong and evaluation of the methods were frequently followed by the phrase, this method "has given uniformly good results" (14); however, the results would be totally undocumented by any data analysis.

LIGATION AND STRIPPING OF SAPHENOUS
AND VARICOSE VEINS

Preoperative evaluations are as important as surgical technique in treating varicose veins. These may include photoplethysmography, varicography, Doppler examination, visual inspection, and skin marking. Of these, only visual inspection, skin marking, and Doppler examination for reflux are essential. Photophlethysmography and light reflection rheography make use of the fact that the subdermal tangle of blood vessels is largely a venous pool. Infrared light beamed through the epidermis into this pool can be reflected back and give a semiquantitative evaluation of the emptying of that pool and its refilling. Refill time as assessed by photophlethysmography and light reflection rheography correlates well with venous pressure refill time. With the examination done with the patient in a comfortable sitting position, legs dependent, in a warm room, and with tourniquets placed at below-knee and then above-knee positions, accurate differentiation between deep and superficial venous reflux can be ascertained. The effect of tourniquets on reflux gives an estimate of the beneficial effects of superficial venous stripping.

Varicography is planned and used whenever the surgical situation is complex. Several indications of are: after previous major vein stripping; in the presence of massive, recurrent varicose veins; in identifying tributaries to the lesser saphenous system; and in identifying popliteal fossa and gastrocnemius veins (described later in this chapter). Furthermore, identification of the termination of the lesser saphenous vein at the popliteal vein is well done with on-table varicography if preoperative duplex imaging has failed to reveal this junction.

Surgery is always preceded by Doppler examination. The patient is examined standing, supported by an adjacent chair or table. The Doppler probe is placed on the greater saphenous vein in the thigh, on the femoral vein, on the lesser saphenous vein, and on the popliteal vein sequentially. The patient is asked to breathe deeply, cough, and Valsalva as each site is examined. Reverse flow during inspiration, coughing, or Valsalva is a reliable index of reflux.

Preoperative marking is done with a felt-tipped, indelible marking pen, with the relative size of the varix indicated by breadth of the line and individual palpable fascial defects marked by circles (Fig. 14–4). Accurate marking is an absolute requisite to successful varicosity removal. Subsequently, during the surgical procedure such markings may dictate the placement of surgical incisions.

At surgery, the greater and lesser saphenous veins are ignored if Doppler studies show their terminations to be competent. This point deserves emphasis because surgical literature contains many descriptions of removal of the saphenous veins and very few details of preservation of these structures.

Surgeons have no difficulty in identifying the greater saphenous termination through a short, oblique groin incision placed at the groin crease in patients who do need removal of this vein. The incision is begun at the medial edge of the femoral pulse and is carried medially as far as is necessary (2 to 3 cm). Distal stripping is carried out only to the distal thigh or upper anteromedial calf, as indicated previously (Fig. 14–5). Removal of the saphenous vein below upper calf level is usually unnecessary and is occasionally associated with damage to the saphenous nerve. Removal of the greater saphenous vein for gross incompetence automatically removes the midthigh communicating veins (Hunterian perforators), which are a source of recurrent venous insufficiency. A short vertical incision in the distal thigh or upper anteromedial calf allows the stripping instrument to be

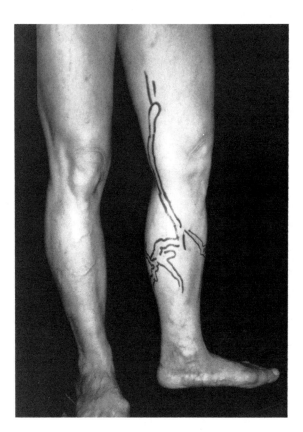

Figure 14–4. The left lower extremity of a patient found to have saphenofemoral reflux, hunterian tributary reflux, and development of varicose clusters from the Boyd perforating vein. Prior greater saphenous sclerotherapy had failed, as had distal sclerotherapy to leg varicosities. Surgical treatment included saphenous vein stripping to the anteromedial calf with clipping of the Boyd perforator and the hunterian perforator, and avulsion of distal varicosities.

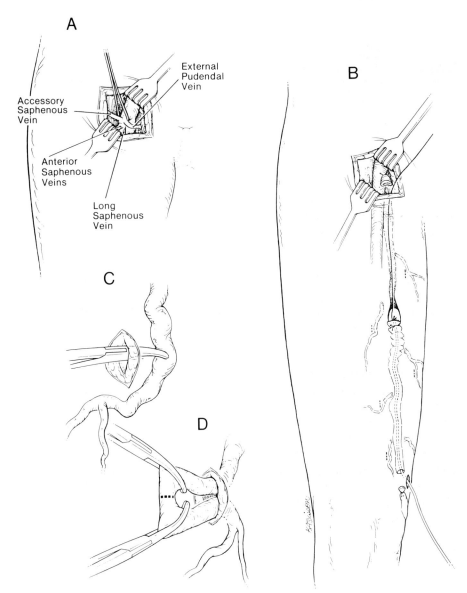

Figure 14–5. Although greater saphenous stripping may vary from one patient to another, the general principles are illustrated here. *A*, The termination of the greater saphenous vein and its multiple tributaries is exposed through a 2- to 3-cm transverse incision in the groin crease. Artistic license has enlarged the incision as depicted here. *B*, The intraluminal stripper is passed distally or proximally, the vein fixed by ligature proximally, and the retrieving ligature secured snugly. Stripping distally minimizes lymphatic and tributary damage and avoids saphenous nerve branch avulsion. When the stripper head reaches the distal incision, the distal vein is fixed to the stripping device by ligature and the entire complex is removed through the proximal incision. *C*, The initial steps in stab avulsion, which consist of a vertical or transverse incision in skin lines, grasping the subcutaneous varicosity, which is superficial to the membranous fascia. *D*, Division of the offending varicosity prior to proximal and distal avulsion.

removed from the lumen of the vein at this point. The stripper head is brought down to that point, the vein fixed to the stripper by ligature, and the stripper, stripper head, and vein retrieved proximally at groin level. This allows the distal incision to be very small and quite cosmetic. The device for retrieving the stripper and vein is a simple heavy ligature or 3-mm umbilical tape.

Lesser saphenous stripping is required in a minority of cases and should always be preceded by identification of the termination of the short saphenous vein by duplex or color flow imaging or intraoperative varicography. The lesser saphenous vein origin is approached at the lateral aspect of the ankle (Fig. 14–6). This is done with great care because the sural nerve is intimately associated with the lesser saphenous vein at this point and may lie within the layers of fascia rather than deep to it. At the termination of the short saphenous vein in the popliteal fossa, the vein should never be ligated until the surgeon has seen the popliteal junction clearly. This dissection may be difficult and complicated by

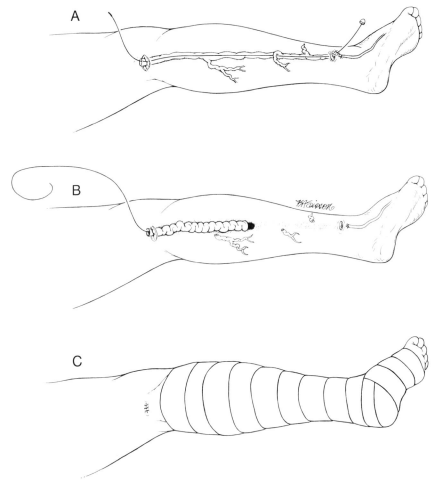

Figure 14–6. Steps in lesser saphenous vein stripping are illustrated in these three diagrams. *A*, Meticulous attention to detail allows preservation of the sural and peroneal nerves while these steps are accomplished. *B*, Traditional stripping is shown; however, the techniques illustrated in Figure 14–5 may be utilized in removing the lesser saphenous system also. *C*, External support is essential after removal of axial veins and clusters of varicosities, and this is maintained for 24 to 48 hr.

large tributaries. Some of these join the lesser saphenous vein from above and some may come from varicosities within the nerve. It is essential that the popliteal vein and peroneal nerve be carefully preserved during this part of the dissection.

STAB AVULSION

When greater and lesser saphenous stripping was abandoned as the cornerstone of the operation for varicosities, it was replaced by the stab avulsion technique of varicosity removal. Because of the meticulous marking that precedes the surgical procedure today, each of the varicose veins, singly or in clusters, can be removed through minimal incisions. Associated incompetent perforating veins are treated simultaneously either by accurate hemostatic clipping or removal of the end organ (the varicosity). The incisions are made with a sharp-pointed blade (#11) directly over the vein and the varicosity is lifted through the wound with fine-pointed forceps. After surrounding fat is cleared away, the loop of vein that appears through the wound is doubly clamped and divided. Each end is teased out through the incision as the areolar tissue on the surface is dissected off. The forceps are always placed close to the skin to prevent the vein from breaking, and traction on the skin itself allows tributaries to be broken and greater lengths of the varicosity removed. Observation has shown that varicosities are divided clinically into two types; those that are white on their surface avulse well, and

Figure 14–7. This perspective drawing illustrates the anatomic facts that clusters of varicosities are frequently placed superficial to the membranous fascia and may be removed by the stab avulsion technique. Axial veins such as the greater and lesser saphenous veins are deep to the membranous fascia and are partially supported by it. They lie superficial to the deep fascia, as in the case of the greater saphenous vein, or penetrate the deep fascia at variable locations, as in the case of the lesser saphenous vein.

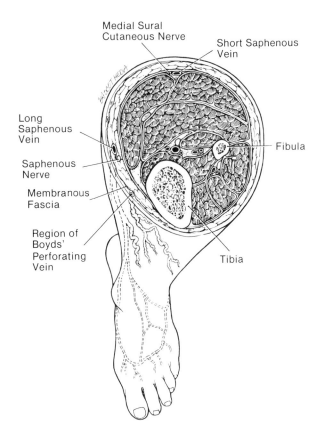

Medial Sural Cutaneous Nerve

Short Saphenous Vein

Long Saphenous Vein

Saphenous Nerve

Membranous Fascia

Region of Boyds' Perforating Vein

Fibula

Tibia

those that are blue in color often tear easily. Distal or proximal incisions are made within the markings in order to ensure that total removal of offending varicosities is accomplished.

Varicosities removed by this technique are inevitably tributaries to axial veins (Fig. 14–7) and do not require ligation except if they terminate in the axial vein and that vein is to be left in place. Perforator veins associated with clusters of varices are clipped or ligated, of course. Incisions made for local varicosity removal are made small enough that sutures are unnecessary and tape closure can be utilized. Should an individual incision be made longer than the average, it can

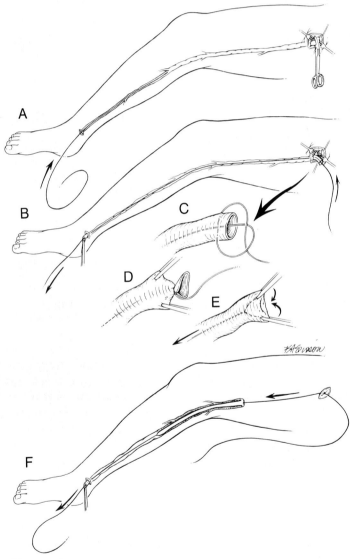

Figure 14–8. The steps in removal of the greater saphenous vein by invagination. In practice, the vein is removed to the hunterian perforator in the thigh or to the Boyd perforator in the anteromedial calf. The essential steps are shown. *A*, Introduction of intraluminal stripper. *B*, Removal of the intraluminal device and substitution of an intraluminal ligature. *C*, *D*, and *E*, Attachment of the ligature to the proximal venous stump and the steps in invagination of this stump within the saphenous lumen. *F*, Removal in a distal direction of the saphenous vein.

be closed by an inverted, absorbable synthetic suture and covered over with the usual tape closure.

ALTERNATIVE TECHNIQUES

Many variations on the technique of vein removal have been offered, used, or abandoned, as indicated by Babcock near the turn of the century. One of the oldest of these has been revived on the European continent by Jean van der Stricht and Paul Ouvry. This is illustrated in Figure 14–8. In essence, the technique consists of invaginating the greater saphenous vein within itself, thus minimizing

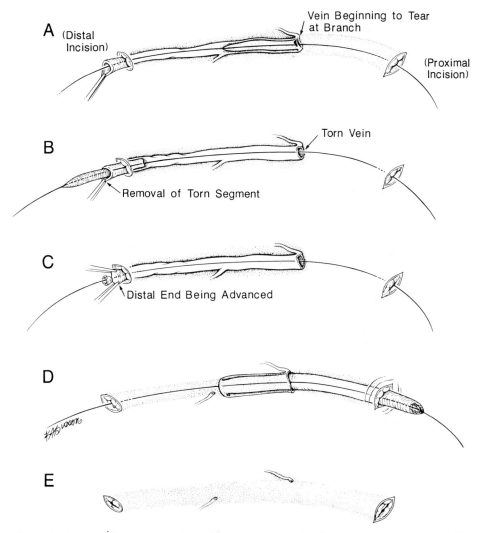

Figure 14–9. Steps in removal of the residual venous segment after proximal vein tearing. *A*, The tearing is seen to begin at a tributary branch. *B*, The removal of the torn segment. *C* and *D*, Attachment of the distal segment of vein to the intraluminal ligature and its invagination as the vein is removed from below upward. *E*, The final completion of removal of the entire venous segment.

the diameter of the tunnel created by vein removal. The method is flawed by tearing of the vein at site of tributary junctures. Also, as is true of all stripping techniques, accumulation of blood within the tunnel may cause postoperative pain and even skin pigmentation. Ouvry has modified the technique by attaching a 5- or 10-cm wide gauze strip to the ligature proximally and drawing this gauze strip within the invaginated vein and the tunnel. The gauze acts as a compressive hemostatic agent within the tunnel and may be removed at any time during the operation. It does, in fact, minimize blood accumulation and aids in preventing tearing of the saphenous vein during the invagination.

While the technique has aesthetic appeal, it is flawed by experience that shows that tearing of the saphenous vein occurs. Because the ligature introduced intraluminally and drawn from above downward is still in place within the lumen of the vein within the patient, even though a stump of vein has been torn free proximally, the distal end of the vein can be attached to the ligature and withdrawn proximally (Fig. 14–9).

Combinations of various stripping and avulsion techniques are applied in individual cases. These may include internal stripping by standard techniques or by intraluminal invagination with or without removal of segments by extraluminal devices.

RECURRENT VARICOSE VEINS

Surgery has a clear place in the late removal of recurrent varicose veins. These may actually be residual following incomplete sclerotherapy, new veins not treated at sclerotherapy or a prior operation, or residual veins left at prior surgery. Possibly, it would be most correct to refer to varicose veins following therapy as being either residual veins missed at the time of original therapy or recurrent veins that were formerly normal and then became varicose because of the underlying genetic or physiologic abnormality, which was not corrected.

Varicography may be very important to accurate removal of residual or recurrent varicosities. Complexities introduced by prior surgery can be unraveled by such direct imaging of offending incompetent veins. At groin level, a number of causes of recurrence have been identified. These include failure to complete flush ligation of the saphenous vein, failure to remove terminal tributaries to the saphenous vein, failure to identify duplicated saphenous veins or their tributaries, and failure to remove the termination of the saphenous vein, thus allowing mid-thigh communicating veins to develop recurrent saphenous incompetence. At the popliteal level, recurrent varicosities frequently develop in scar tissue through transgastrocnemius communicating veins not ligated at the initial operation as well as secondary muscular communicating veins. Isolated, recurrent, superficial varicosities also occupy a major place in failures of primary therapy. These are best managed by careful marking and simple avulsion through small incisions as indicated earlier or by sclerotherapy as described elsewhere in this volume.

It should be emphasized that not all recurrent veins are caused by inadequate primary operations of sclerotherapy. Abnormal veins clearly develop after primary therapy even in the absence of deep venous incompetence. The stab avulsion surgical technique lends itself well to treatment of such veins (15).

GASTROCNEMIUS VEINS

Increasing experience has shown that veins entering the popliteal fossa are not simply the lesser saphenous vein and its contributors. From both the arterial and the venous point of view, the popliteal fossa is complex. Unfortunately, few surgeons are aware of the very important vein of Giacomini, which is a popliteal saphenous connection, and not all surgeons are aware of the gastrocnemius veins. Furthermore, the short saphenous vein itself frequently joins the posteromedial tributary of the long saphenous vein as a continuation of the femoral popliteal vein of Giacomini rather than entering the popliteal vein itself.

In addition to these, there are two other vein systems that must be acknowledged. The first is the vein (veins) of the popliteal fossa, described by Dodd, and the second are the gastrocnemius veins, also described by Dodd (16). Because the gastrocnemius veins are important but are seldom recognized as the cause of symptoms, they are emphasized here. These veins drain the two heads of the gastrocnemius muscle and terminate joining the popliteal vein near the saphenopopliteal junction. Incompetence is most often detected in the medial gastrocnemius veins, which may be grossly dilated as a result of failure of their many valves. When surgery is done in the popliteal fossa, the gastrocnemius complex of veins must be attended to at the same time that the short saphenous vein is operated upon.

When varicography is done on the operating table, a lateral view is utilized, and sometimes an oblique projection is necessary to separate out what appear to be one or two large veins but in truth are six or eight overlapping veins. Such varicography identifies the termination of the short saphenous vein absolutely and supplements preoperative duplex imaging. Fortunately, incisions to explore the gastrocnemius veins and the other veins of the popliteal fossa, in conjunction with interruption of the short saphenous vein, can be transverse, which heal with little residual scarring.

Experienced surgeons have recognized that pain, especially in young women toward the end of a menstrual cycle and for several days of a menstrual period, may be due to insufficiency of the veins of the popliteal fossa (17). Such a syndrome may be associated with lesser saphenous incompetence but with the lesser saphenous vein being deep to the deep fascia and therefore impalpable. Furthermore, in some patients a communicating vein joints the incompetent posterior calf venules to the incompetent proximal long saphenous system, and this communicating vein may be missed unless a very careful examination supplemented by Doppler evaluation is done.

Finally, the gastrocnemius veins may be tributary to the short saphenous vein at a midcalf (gastrocnemius) point, as emphasized by J. Hobbs (personal communication). Young women will note such such cyclic pain in association with difficulty in wearing close-fitting boots as a result of increased calf and ankle circumference. A visual tipoff to this syndrome will be a patch of dilated venules or venous flare at the midcalf point.

CONCLUSIONS

In the absence of deep venous obstruction or reflux, superficial varicosities lend themselves to surgical removal and effective sclerotherapy. Choice of intervention becomes very individual, but decisions regarding therapy are aided by objective clinical observation and use of a simple hand-held Doppler. The surgery and sclerotherapy are not difficult and the results, to patient and surgeon, are most gratifying.

REFERENCES

1. Babcock WW: A new operation for the extirpation of varicose veins of the leg. NY Med J 1907; *86*:153–156.
2. Trendelenburg F: Ueber die Unterbindung der Vena saphena magna bei Unterschenkelvarican. Beitr Klin Chir 1890;*7*:195–210.
3. Bier A, Braun H, Kummel H: Chirurgische Operations Lehre. Leipzig JA Barth 1917;*5*:334.
4. deTakats G: Ambulatory ligation of the saphenous vein. JAMA 1930;*94*:1194–1197.
5. Keller WL: A new methods of extirpating the internal saphenous and similar veins in varicose conditions: A preliminary report. NY Med J 1905;*82*:385–386.
6. Mayo CH: Treatment of varicose veins. Surg Gynecol Obstet 1906;*2*:385–388.
7. Homans J: The operative treatment of varicose veins and ulcers. Surg Gynecol Obstet 1916;*22*:143–158.
8. Sherman RS: Varicose veins: Further findings based on anatomic and surgical dissections. Ann Surg 1949;*130*:218–232.
9. Jakobsen BH: The value of different forms of treatment for varicose veins. Br J Surg 1979;*66*:182–184.
10. Hobbs JT: Surgery and sclerotherapy in the treatment of varicose veins. Arch Surg 1974;*109*:793–796.
11. Rivlin S: The surgical cure of primary varicose veins. Br J Surg 1975;*62*:913–917.
12. Glass GM: Prevention of recurrent saphenofemoral incompetence after surgery for varicose veins. Br J Surg 1989;*76*:1210.
13. Rutherford RB, Sawyer JD, Jones DN: The fate of residual saphenous vein after partial removal or ligation. J Vasc Surg (in press).
14. McPheeters HO: Saphenofemoral ligation with the immediate retrograde injection. Surg Gynecol Obstet 1945;*81*:355–364.
15. Browse NL, Burnand KG, Thomas ML: Disease of the Veins, Pathology, Diagnosis, and Treatment. London, Edward Arnold, 1988.
16. Dodd H: The varicose tributaries of the popliteal vein. Br J Surg 1965;*52*:350–354.
17. Browse N: The painful deep vein syndrome. Lancet 1970;*1*:1251–1253.

15

RECURRENT VARICOSE VEINS AND SHORT SAPHENOUS INSUFFICIENCY: Evaluation and Treatment

Simon G. Darke

Recurrence is defined here as persistence or reemergence of varicosities after previous operative treatment. Because recurrence is almost inevitable following compression sclerotherapy alone without surgery [63 per cent at 3 years (1) and 93 per cent at 6 years (2)], this particular aspect is not considered.

Primary varicose veins affect between 10 and 12 per cent (3,4) of the adult population. Increased demand and expectation have led to an almost doubling in the numbers treated in the United Kingdom in the last decade (5). With this growing workload it is particularly regrettable that recurrence should occur, not only because of the obvious dissatisfaction and distress for the patient but also because it compounds the strain that this form of surgery demands from health care resources. These, then, are but two important reasons why this common problem is worthy of consideration.

CLASSIFICATION AND INCIDENCE

The loose definition of recurrence referred to above can be refined into more specific categories:

Type 1: Recurrence varicosities without associated incompetence in the saphenous systems.

Type 2: "Recurrence" due to the evolution or persistence of varicosities derived from incompetence in a second saphenous system (e.g., in the short saphenous following previous saphenofemoral ligation).

Type 3: Varicosities derived from recurrence of incompetence in either the saphenofemoral or saphenopopliteal junction following apparently adequate previous ligation.

A further group, which for obvious reasons are important to recognize, are recurrent "varicose veins" due to the development of superficial collaterals as a consequence of obstruction of the deep system from previous vein thrombosis. Diagnosis is likely to depend on venography (6). This group is important to recognize because further surgical intervention may be hazardous and prejudice the venous return. However, these problems are outside the remit of this paper and are not considered further.

An ongoing survey by the author addressing this issue is based on a consecutive series of patients with varicose veins referred for treatment. This clinical material is thought to be relatively representative of the situation as it exists within the population. The author serves a geographically "captive community" and in general acts as a secondary referral center, so bias that inevitably results from a refined tertiary referral system is less likely to occur. It must be conceded, however, that a special interest in complex venous problems is well known to primary physicians. Thus unusual cases tend to be directed selectively. It is difficult to estimate the degree to which this might occur.

Preliminary data show that over a 9-month period 184 new patients with primary uncomplicated (no venous ulcer) varicose veins were evaluated. Of these, 135 (73 per cent) had had no previous surgery. There were therefore 49 patients, 27 per cent of the total, who had recurrence as defined above:

> Type 1: Thirteen of these 49 patients (26 per cent) had recurrent varicosities but no evidence clinically, or a Doppler ultrasound (vide infra) of incompetence either primarily or recurrently in either the long or short saphenous systems.
> Type 2: Four patients (8 per cent) presented with incompetence in the short saphenous system after having previously had the saphenofemoral junction ligated. There were no patients in whom the opposite situation had apparently occurred.
> Type 3: Thirty-two patients (65 per cent) had recurrent saphenous incompetence, 27 of these at the saphenofemoral junction and five at the saphenopopliteal junction.

These data are comparable to the findings in a similar study of 501 new patients by Sheppard (7). Recurrence after surgery was present in 28 per cent of the total number of patients. Ninety per cent of these recurrences were attributable to recurrent saphenofemoral incompetence.

These surveys look at the incidence within a population of patients presenting for further management. An alternative analysis of equal relevance is to review the recurrence rate in a series of patients systematically followed up after surgery. The classic study by Hobbs (2) compared surgery with injection sclerotherapy. Patients with saphenous incompetence treated by surgery showed a "failure rate" (unspecified apropos of the above classification) of about 10 per cent at 6 years. In a personal series by Royle (8) at a minimum follow-up of 5 years 18 per cent of 367 patients had sufficiently severe recurrence to warrant further surgery. Lofgren (9) reported an experience from the Mayo Clinic of 278 patients examined at 10 years. Fifteen per cent had recurrent varicosities of sufficient severity to require further surgery. After 20 years the proportion had risen to 32 per cent. Berridge and Makin (10) reported a recurrence rate of 20 per cent 3 to 10 years after surgery in 164 patients. Of these 34 patients, 25 (76 per cent) had developed recurrent saphenous incompetence (saphenofemoral except for one saphenopopliteal). In a study by Jakobsen (1), the patients, most of whom had saphenous incompetence, were prospectively allocated into radical surgery (strip and tie of appropriate saphenous system), saphenous ligation without stripping and subsequent injections, or injections alone. The recurrence rate at 3 years in these three groups of patients were 10, 35, and 63 per cent, respectively.

This data, from a number of different countries, illustrate the following points. Recurrence rate, even after comprehensive surgery is 10 to 20 per cent, and this probably increases with time. Recurrent saphenofemoral incompetence plays a major role in these patients.

DIAGNOSIS, PREVENTION, AND MANAGEMENT

Type 1

Recurrence in this category will be categorized by varicosities without the stigmata of saphenofemoral or saphenopopliteal incompetence either primarily or secondarily (vide infra). Under these circumstances preoperative varicography indicates the presence of incompetent thigh perforating veins as the principal source of recurrence (11). This form of recurrent varicosities was first reported in 1944 by Sherman (12), who found a high recurrence rate in patients he had treated by flush saphenofemoral ligation alone. Dodd (13) studied 52 limbs, 40 of which had recurrent varicose veins after previous surgery. At operation he exposed the subsartorial canal and found one incompetent perforator in 10 patients, two in a further 10 patients, and three in one patient. Wide exposure of this nature would not be appropriate in contemporary practice. Preoperative varicography gives useful information, both in confirming the cause for the recurrence and as anatomic guidance regarding operative strategy for its eradication (11).

The question that must be asked is whether failure to remove the long saphenous trunk at the time of the initial surgery increases the risks of thigh recurrence. Is it more common after simple groin ligation alone? The contention has been studied by the author (14), by means of perioperative descending venography performed down the isolated long saphenous vein after disconnection from its junction with the common femoral vein. This procedure was undertaken in 80 limbs of 60 patients. Twenty-seven had ulceration and the remainder had no skin change; all had normal deep systems on ascending and descending venography. In none of these limbs were competent valves demonstrated in the saphenous trunk to knee level. The mean number of albeit incompetent valves was two. Thigh perforators were present in 87 per cent. These were inferred to be "incompetent" if they were greater than 3 mm in diameter, had no identifiable valves, and were varicose or directly associated with localized varicosities of the long saphenous vein (15). On this basis, 15 of the limbs were thought to have contained incompetent thigh perforating veins, but these rather rigid criteria for incompetent thigh perforators may represent an underestimate. Even if this is not the case, it is possible that a proportion of competent perforators might subsequently become incompetent with time and changing hemodynamics. The data is summarized in Table 15–1.

To leave an incompetent saphenous trunk connected by an incompetent thigh perforator to the deep system would seem to be an inevitable recipe for recurrence. Papadekis et al. (16) reported supportive evidence. Forty-two patients, all of whom had had previous saphenofemoral ligation for varicose veins, predominantly without stripping, were studied by ascending venography for recurrent varicose veins. Fifteen had recurrent saphenofemoral reflux. In 80 per cent at least one incompetent thigh perforating vein was demonstrated and in 20 per cent more than one was seen. There was no consistency as the anatomic site of these incompetent thigh communicating veins; they were seen throughout the thigh. These conclusions are supported by experience that shows an increased recur-

TABLE 15–1. Perioperative Descending Saphenography in Patients with Long Saphenous Incompetence

	NO SKIN CHANGE	SKIN ULCERATION
No. of saphenograms	53	27
Contrast to knee joint	51	24
Contrast to calf	33	17
Varicose long saphenous vein	31	21
Mean length of normal vein seen (mm)	150	160
Mean width of normal vein seen (mm)	6	7
Long saphenous veins with valves	34[a]	9[a]
Mean no. valves present	2	2
Direct thigh perforators	46	24
Thigh perforator "incompetence"	8	7

[a] Statistically significant at $p < .05$.

rence after simple ligation compared with ligation and excision/stripping of the saphenous trunk (1,17,18).

The contrary argument might be put that the vein should be preserved in case of future need for coronary artery or femoropopliteal bypass grafting. Our data showed varicose changes in 65 per cent of the excised veins, which would have rendered them unsuitable for this purpose even if they had been preserved (Table 15–1). Lofgren (9) found in a retrospective inquiry that it was uncommon for a patient who had previously undergone stripping to be denied subsequent bypass surgery for this reason.

On the basis of this data, therefore, it would seem likely that recurrences of this category will be kept to a minimum by accurate saphenofemoral disconnection and excision by whatever means of the saphenous trunk to just below the knee.

Type 2

Varicose veins are an inherent condition with a strong familial predisposition (19,20). It is hardly surprising, therefore, that a second saphenous system should become involved in the same limb. However, this does not appear to occur with sufficient frequency to justify prospective ligation and excision of both long and short saphenous systems, if one remains healthy in the presence of varicose change in the other at the time of the initial evaluation. It is of interest to speculate as to whether synchronous involvement of both systems, in particular the short saphenous system, has been overlooked at the time of the original surgery by an inexperienced clinician. Furthermore, on more than one occasion the author has anecdotal evidence of the wrong system being excised, invariably the long saphenous instead of the short. These, then, are persistent rather than recurrent varicose veins. In order to avoid this error, accurate initial assessment is essential.

This author, in common with a number of other workers, is firmly of the opinion that hand-held unidirectional Doppler ultrasonography is essential in the evaluation of both long and particularly short saphenous incompetence (21–25). The author's experience and the principles and techniques involved have been described in detail elsewhere (26), but the results are now summarized.

Given that the incompetent system most likely to be overlooked is the short saphenous, what is the incidence? In an attempt to answer this question 100 consecutive limbs in 67 new patients with primary and otherwise uncomplicated varicose veins were evaluated by clinical and Doppler examination (20). Reference has already been made to the relatively representative nature of the author's clinical practice. Limbs were assessed in the outpatient clinic at the time of first presentation for involvement of long saphenous and short saphenous systems and the incidence of incompetence. Assessment was by a combination of inspection, standard clinical tests, and Doppler ultrasound. Those patients with Doppler evidence of incompetence in the popliteal vein and by inference the likelihood of significant deep incompetence were excluded (6). On this basis all patients were thought to have primaray varicose veins.

The patient stands immobile facing the examiner and the probe is located over the saphenofemoral junction by moving it medially from the femoral arterial signal until this ceases. Confirmation of correct position is obtained by manual calf compression, which produces an audible signal. On releasing the calf compression, no further signal is heard if both deep and superficial systems are competent. Occasionally a very short refluxing signal (less than 1 sec) may be heard. This is not regarded as significant. If a further signal, similar to that heard on compression, follows release of compression, this is regarded as signifying valvular incompetence. Abolition of the refluxing signal by compression of the long saphenous vein in the thigh (manually or by tourniquet) confirms saphenofemoral incompetence.

A similar procedure is followed for assessing saphenopopliteal incompetence. The patient stands immobile facing away from the examiner with the affected limbs slightly flexed to abolish muscular contraction. The probe is located over the popliteal vein in the popliteal fossa by first finding the arterial signal and moving slightly laterally. Confirmation is again established by calf compression. A refluxing signal of releasing calf compression that is abolished by compression of the short saphenous vein in the upper calf signifies saphenopopliteal incompetence with a competent deep venous system. Continuing reflux in this situation signifies incompetence within the deep venous system.

The localization of varicosities to long or short saphenous veins is achieved by demonstrating sonic continuity from the varicosity to the saphenofemoral or saphenopopliteal junction. With the probe in place over the relevant junction, tapping the varicosities produces a short audible signal. Confirmation has been demonstrated by varicography in a proportion of cases. This is of particular value with calf varicosities. The whole examination can be accomplished in a matter of a few minutes and requires little expertise.

Table 15–2 shows the results of this study. In 27 of these limbs the varicosities were derived from the short saphenous system, in 25 of which the saphenopopliteal junction was incompetent, and in eight patients there had been previous surgery directed toward the saphenopopliteal junction. (This aspect will be considered later in the chapter.) Other workers employing similar Doppler techniques have found the short saphenous to be the source of varicosities in comparable proportions (24,25). Clearly it is mandatory that saphenopopliteal incompetence be specifically and systematically sought and recognized. Otherwise persistent varicosities will inevitably result.

**TABLE 15–2. Outcome of Unidirectional Doppler System Analysis on 100
Consecutive Limbs with Varicose Veins**

	LONG SAPHENOUS	SHORT SAPHENOUS
Total	85	27
Incompetent	60	25
Competent	25 (29%)	2 (7%)
Recurrent	6	8
	(All incompetent)	(All incompetent)
Both systems	6	6

Type 3

Reference has been made previously as to the value of Doppler ultrasonography in the evaluation of varicose veins. In the context of type 3 patients it is particularly relevant, as other workers have demonstrated (11). Recurrent saphenofemoral incompetence can be demonstrated by applying the tests referred to earlier or more simply as a retrograde sonic impulse over a recurrent varix on asking the patient to cough. This implies loss of valvular function between that point and the intraabdominal venous system. Localized pressure over the saphenofemoral junction, or a tourniquet in the upper thigh, should control the reflux. Although strictly speaking this may not imply precisely saphenofemoral recurrence (vide infra), in practical terms this at the outset must be the assumption.

For a more accurate preoperative diagnosis and evaluation venography is required. In its simplest form this consists of varicography alone (11,27), although comprehensive ascending and descending venography (6) adds a complete evaluation of the venous morphology, which may have advantages. By these means four types of recurrent saphenous incompetence can be identified: types 3a through 3d.

Morphology of Recurrent Saphenofemoral Incompetence

TYPE 3A.   In this type it is apparent that an incomplete or inadequate groin ligation has previously been undertaken (17). Either a persistent accessory saphenous vein or a major branch emanating from the saphenofemoral trunk has been missed. These communicate with varicosities further down the leg.

TYPE 3B.   In this type an incompetent thigh perforator communicates with a saphenous trunk and in turn the varicosities in the lower limb. If the valves above this level in the superficial (or more rarely deep) femoral vein are incompetent then this will be indistinguishable clinically on ultrasound from true saphenofemoral incompetence. This situation is not uncommon, particularly if the perforator is high in the thigh. (This is a variation of type 1 as stated earlier, the difference being that the proximal valves in the femoral veins are incompetent or there are none present.)

TYPE 3C.   This is the common source of recurrence, and this important concept has yet to be widely recognized. It is due to a "neovascularization" that establishes a new channel between the femoral and an adjacent vein—either the residual unstripped main saphenous trunk, an accessory saphenous vein, or one of its tributaries. This can be readily demonstrated by both ascending and descending venography (6,28) and is apparent at operation (29). The histologic evolution of this phenomenon has been documented in man and it shows that in the early postoperative period there is organizing thrombus into which numerous small vessels emerge. Within a year these become fewer and those that remain enlarge, and develop muscle and elastin in their walls resembling mature veins (29). This has been duplicated in animal experimentation (30). The author has personal experience that this phenomenon of neovascularization can occur within less than 1 year of surgery, an observation that has been noted by others (28).

TYPE 3D. Recurrences may occasionally occur directly from the pelvic veins, principally the internal iliac vein, or via the internal pudendal. Similar recurrences can be seen down the veins of the round ligament. Although strictly speaking these are not recurrent "saphenofemoral" varicose veins, they are likely to be interpreted as such in the first instance. These fortunately uncommon cases lead to diagnostic and management difficulties, and complex venographic procedures may be required to elucidate the exact morphology.

Prevention of Recurrent Saphenofemoral Incompetence

What then can be undertaken at the time of primary surgery to minimize the incidence of recurrent saphenofemoral incompetence? Type 3a recurrence is due to technical incompetence and should theoretically be comprehensively avoidable by accurate anatomic groin dissection and flush saphenofemoral ligation, including all tributaries of the long saphenous system.

Type 3b recurrence will be minimized by excision of the long saphenous trunk to knee level. It seems likely that it is in part this factor that leads to the improved results when this is employed as opposed to simple groin ligation (1,17,18). It must be conceded, however, that there may be accessory saphenous trunks that are not detected and excised at the time of primary surgery, which might account for this form of recurrence in a proportion of patients. On this basis, therefore, if more than one major trunk is apparent at the time of primary surgery they should all be removed.

Type 3c neovascularization is the most common, the most interesting, and likely to be the most difficult to treat. These patients may come back with repeated problems, with further recurrences in about 15 per cent (31). What might be done to minimize the risk? Certainly it would seem to make sense to remove all trunks of the saphenous system to which this neovascularization process might "attach" itself.

Regarding the saphenofemoral junction itself, Sheppard (7) suggested reflecting a flap of mobilized pectineus fascia over the femoral vein at the site of the ligated saphenous stump. Glass (32) took great care to close the cribriform fascia but noted some recurrences through this. He studied a further group of 268 limbs undergoing surgery for the first time and treated by saphenous ligation. He augmented this with a patch closure of synthetic mesh over the exposed common femoral vein. The recurrence rate was only 1 per cent at a mean follow-up of 5 years.

Surgery for Recurrent Saphenofemoral Incompetence

With regard to the actual reexploration, the principle is to first find the common femoral vein through a fresh surgical field rather than to explore through the old scar. The latter approach leads down to reconstituted veins, which are friable and difficult to dissect.

Initially, the common femoral vein is identified above the recurrence either by a medial approach (33) or, as the author's preference, a lateral approach via the femoral fascia overlying the femoral artery. A vertical incision is made over the medial aspect of the femoral arterial pulsation similar to the standard manner for exposure of this vessel for arterial reconstruction. The medial border of the artery is identified first as it emerges beneath the inguinal ligament. Once this is accomplished the vein is easily identified through what is likely to be a virgin operative field. It is straightforward to follow this down and identify and re-ligate the recurrent (or less frequently persistent) trunks. At this juncture is would seem sensible to employ some form of fascial covering as described above. A prosthetic mesh should certainly be considered.

RECURRENT SAPHENOUS INCOMPETENCE AND VENOUS ULCERATION

What role and relevance does recurrent saphenous incompetence have in venous ulceration? The author has addressed this issue in a series of patients with ulceration that has previously been reported in detail (6). Over a 30-month period a consecutive series of patients referred to the author with chronic venous disorders has been studied. A total of 594 patients have been assessed. Table 15–3 shows the categories into which these patients have been divided. Those who on clinical grounds were thought to have primary varicose veins by skin changes or excessive pain and swelling are not considered further. All those with "ulcer" had current ulceration or lesions that had only healed within the previous 3 months. Those designated as having "pain and swelling" syndrome both had measurable calf edema (and, in some, in the thigh as well) and described pain, often provoked by exercise and in excess of the ache that may be associated with primary and uncomplicated varicose veins. Thus, three groups of patients were identified on clinical grounds and are studied and compared:

1.   There were 42 patients with 48 limbs with ulcer alone. In 14 limbs there was a past history of deep thrombosis and in 16 limbs a family history of similar disorders.

2.   There were 46 patients with 52 limbs with ulcer and pain and swelling as well. In 20 limbs there was a family history of similar disorders and in 15 a past history of deep vein thrombosis.

TABLE 15–3. Clinical Classification of Patients with Chronic Venous Disorders

Total number of patients	594
Patients with primary varicose veins	466
No saphenous incompetence	46
Saphenous incompetence	420
Patients with complex disorders	128 (145 limbs)
48 limbs ulcer	(26 women, mean age = 56)
52 limbs ulcer pain and swelling	(22 women, mean age = 54)
45 limbs pain and swelling alone	(22 women, mean age = 40)

3.   There were 39 patients with 45 limbs with isolated pain and swelling syndrome. They tended to be a little younger than the other groups. In 17 limbs there was a family history of a similar disorder. There was a past history of deep venous thrombosis in 11 legs.

All these patients were assessed clinically and by Doppler ultrasound to determine the presence of saphenous and popliteal incompetence. Ascending venography was employed to detect evidence of previous deep vein thrombosis. Descending venography was used to detect saphenous and deep vein incompetence (6). We looked at the 100 limbs with ulceration and the abnormalities that were found. The findings are summarized in Table 15–4.

How should these different types of patients be treated? Surgical options include the more conventional means of saphenous ligation and ankle perforator interruption, or reconstructive surgery, or a combination of the two. Those patients with isolated calf perforator incompetence and normal deep veins comprised 6 per cent of the total. In these appropriate ligation or interruption can be expected to bring about good results (34,35).

In 29 per cent of limbs with ulcer, saphenous and perforator incompetence were the only abnormalities. Thus, it is important to recognize that ulceration may occur in the presence of normal deep veins and without the evidence of previous thrombosis. Preoperative ambulatory pressure measurements in this group of patients indicated that saphenofemoral ligation and saphenous excision can be expected to reestablish relatively normal venous hemodynamics (36). Furthermore, following this procedure ulcers remain healed, often without the subsequent use of compression stockings. It is concluded,therefore, that in these patients the associated perforator "incompetence" can usually be ignored. This group of patients is the easiest to treat and offer the best chance of a lasting successful outcome.

There were a total of 42 limbs with primary deep incompetence of at least grade II severity [Kistner classification (37)]. Thirty-one per cent of the limbs combined saphenous and perforator and deep incompetence without evidence of previous deep vein thrombosis. What is the value of saphenous excision alone in these patients? Three-year follow-up reveals good clinical results, with ulcer healing in nine out of 10 such patients undergoing saphenous ligation for the first time. What happens to quantifiable venous function studies in these patients? Photoplethysmography and ambulant dorsal foot vein pressure studies were undertaken before and after saphenous ligation and excision. Where appropriate, ankle tour-

TABLE 15–4.   Venous Morphology as Determined by Comprehensive Clinical, Doppler and Phlebographic Assessment in Ulcerated Limbs with or without Pain and Swelling

KISTNER GRADE[a]	
I Perf. alone	6
II Perf. saph.	29
III Perf. saph. DVI	31
Perf. DVI	11
IV Phlebitic ± other	23
Total no. limbs studied	100

[a] Perf., perforator incompetence; Saph., saphenofemoral incompetence; DVI, deep venous incompetence.

niquets were used to minimize the effects of perforator incompetence. The results showed severe continued dysfunction without apparent change or improvement from preoperative readings (38). Others have made similar observations (39–42).

What is the significance of this? The first point is that deep incompetence does have measurable consequences on venous dynamics and by inference is of clinical significance. Thus, it would be justifiable to attempt correction if the clinical situation so demanded. However, clearly this is not the case in those patients in whom the results are, in the short term at least, quite satisfactory by simple saphenous excision alone.

The second point is the apparent paradox between clinical improvement and failure to normalize venous pressure measurements. This has been noted in other studies (41). The inference is that the tests are simply too crude to register subtle improvements and that it is not necessary to "normalize" function to accrue clinical benefit. Nonetheless, it suggests that the improvement may not be maintained in the longer term (42). This is supported by the observation that there are patients within this study with residual primary deep incompetence who have ulceration in spite of saphenous ligation performed several years previously. There were 13 patients in this category (see Table 15–5). In nine there was recurrence of saphenofemoral incompetence. The morphology of this recurrence was the typical type 3c described previously, with neovascularized veins reconnecting with distal superficial varicosities. Further ligation of the recurrence has conferred no apparent benefit in six out of eight of these patients treated so far. However, when subfascial ligation was added the majority of the patients remained healed.

Pathogenesis of Venous Ulceration Associated with Primary Incompetence

What are the wider implications of primary incompetence of saphenous, perforator, and deep systems? It seems likely from these data that any one of these three forms of incompetence may, by itself, lead to ulceration. When these primary forms of incompetence occur in combination they probably have a cumulative effect. They are due to a inherent weakness in the venous wall and are probably progressive, but at a variable rate within one individual. Correction of one lesion when they coexist will bring about improvement, but the duration of this will depend upon the severity and rate of deterioration of those that remain. Thus it seems sensible to undertake the simplest operative procedure first and

TABLE 15–5.   Incidence of Previous Saphenofemoral Ligation and Recurrent Saphenofemoral Incompetence in Venous Ulcer

KISTNER GRADE AND VENOUS ABNORMALITY[a]	NO.	PREVIOUS SAPHENOFEMORAL LIGATION	RECURRENT SAPHENOFEMORAL INCOMPETENCE
I. Perf.	6	0	0
II. Perf. Saph.	29	0	0
III Perf. Saph. DVI	31	9	9
DVI	11	4	0
IV Postphlebitic ± other	23	6	1
TOTAL	100	19	10

[a] Perf., perforator incompetence; Saph., saphenofemoral incompetence; DVI, deep venous incompetence.

only resort to complex reconstructions when the benefits of these are apparently exhausted. This philosophy is fundamental to the management of venous disorders. Whether there is merit in re-ligating the recurrent saphenofemoral incompetence is difficult to say. Certainly on its own this is inadequate. When combined with perforator ligation it produced good results, but whether perforator ligation alone would have achieved the same results is not certain at the moment.

It is interesting to note that recurrent saphenofemoral incompetence in this particular selected group of complex patients was only found in those with associated deep incompetence. Does this same association pertain to recurrence at groin level in patients with varicose veins otherwise uncomplicated by skin changes? Preliminary data from descending venography in 13 out of 24 limbs from the author's series referred to at the outset of this chapter, of recurrent saphenofemoral incompetence presenting without skin problems, have revealed deep incompetence [minimum grade II, Kistner classification (37)]. However, we do not know the incidence of primary deep incompetence in patients with varicose veins uncomplicated by venous ulceration irrespective of whether they have developed recurrence after surgery to the saphenofemoral or popliteal junction.

SHORT SAPHENOUS (SAPHENOPOPLITEAL) INCOMPETENCE

Anatomic Aspects

There are important considerations that distinguish incompetence behind the knee from that presenting in the groin, not least of which is the wide anatomic variation that exists in the veins of the popliteal fossa. In contrast to the femoral vein, the composition of which is relatively consistent, the formation of the popliteal vein shows wide variation. In a classic study by Williams (43) published in 1953, the "conventional" concept of a single popliteal vein at knee joint level was shown to be present in only 26 per cent of limbs studied; in 66 per cent there were two popliteal veins. Furthermore, in the formation of these dual veins there was considerable variation. One was frequently found to be much longer than the other. Essentially the composition depends on a variation of the unification of the six venae comitantes of the anterior and posterior tibial and peroneal arteries. To this high degree of complexity must be added the union with the muscular veins from the soleus and gastrocnemius muscles. These at least appeared to be more constant than the main trunks. The pair of veins from the soleus tend to join the peroneal veins, thus making the latter bigger than the posterior tibial veins. In general this junction was found below the level of the knee join, but the veins that drain the two heads of the gastrocnemius predominantly join the larger popliteal trunk above the level of the knee joint.

To this variation of popliteal vein anatomy, with the inevitable potential for confusion and perioperative misinterpretation, must be added information on the vagaries of the saphenopopliteal junction itself and the other adjacent veins that constitute a potential source for varicosities in the popliteal fossa. For this we turn to a quite outstanding piece of meticulous, personally documented clinical work published in 1965 by Harold Dodd (44). To quote this author, "goaded by recurrences, persistent varices" he utilized, in 444 consecutive cases, a variety of perioperative tests of competence: applying proximal occlusive slings, watching venous filling, and injecting saline and testing for reflux of blood. By these means he identified incompetence not only in the short saphenous vein itself, but also in the medial and lateral gastrocnemius veins and what he described as the "popliteal area" vein—an often large vessel, independent of the short saphenous arising in the superficial fat over the popliteal space and calf.

In 72 per cent of this large number of operations the gastrocnemius veins were found to be incompetent: in 47 per cent the medial, in 19 per cent the lateral, and in 5 per cent both. The termination of these veins was again variable; they may drain directly into the popliteal at or above the level of the knee, singly or as a common trunk, or they may drain into the short saphenous itself. The popliteal area vein was anatomically present in 40 per cent of the cases, of which just under half were incompetent. These veins may enter the popliteal space from any angle; half terminate in the short saphenous, the remainder into the gastrocnemius veins or the popliteal itself. Dodd emphasized the need for flush ligation of these veins rather than limiting dissection to the point at which they penetrate the fascia.

A final crucial anatomic point is the subfascial course of the greater part of the short saphenous vein (45). It is subcutaneous in only the lower aspect of the leg. This in part accounts for the failure to recognize incompetence clinically.

Recurrent Short Saphenous Incompetence

Against this minefield of anatomic variation it is not surprising that relatively little has been published on other aspects of recurrent short saphenous incompetence. Data become fragmented and anecdotal. However, it seems logical to try to follow the sequence of types of recurrence that have applied to the saphenofemoral junction. These are now considered with aspects of how the risks of recurrence can be minimized.

Type 1

My data indicates that recurrent varicosities in the short saphenous system without incompetence in the popliteal fossa are uncommon. All eight patients with short saphenous recurrence had persistent or recurrent incompetence at the popliteal level (see Table 15–2). However, it does seem to be theoretically possible that incompetent ankle perforators might connect with a persistent short saphenous trunk, but I personally have never been able to demonstrate this. On this basis, there would not seem to be such a pressing need to strip the short saphenous vein (see later in this chapter). The failure to demonstrate this form of recurrence may be a function of the predominantly subfascial (deep) course of the short saphenous vein.

Type 2

Recurrence may be due to evolution in the short saphenous system after previous long saphenous surgery. Reference has already been made to the need for scrupulous and systematic initial clinical evaluation of the short saphenous system in assessing patients presenting with varicose veins. The need for unidirectional Doppler assessment is again emphasized.

Type 3a

Because of the significant anatomic variation, recurrence due to incomplete or inadequate primary ligation represents a major source of technical inadequacy. To the wide anatomic uncertainty to which reference has already been made must be added the practical aspect of the site of the saphenopopliteal junction and how can this be best located. Moosman and Hartwell (45) found that in 25 per cent of cases the short saphenous vein did not join the popliteal vein but terminated in the superficial and deep veins of the thigh (17.5 per cent) after coursing through the popliteal area, and in veins below the knee in 8 per cent. In Dodd's series (44) 15 per cent passed through the popliteal space to hamstring muscle veins, the long saphenous vein, and once (out of 444) to the superficial femoral vein. In 4 per cent it ended below the knee in calf muscle veins. In the remainder (80 per cent) it entered the popliteal vein mainly at its upper end. These figures from two big series are remarkably similar.

How, then, can the termination be best identified to allow for an accurate and cosmetic transverse skin incision and rapid localization at exploration? Clinical evaluation alone, even with the knee slightly flexed, is extremely difficult (44). An extension of the Doppler technique to which reference has already been made is helpful. By following the incompetent vein upward and serially squeezing and releasing the calf, a point is reached when reflux is no longer heard. This is because insonation is now focused above the junction onto the competent popliteal vein (although this too can be incompetent, thus confusing the issue further). This has been put to the test and compared with perioperative varicography and operative findings (46). In nine cases out of 10 the Doppler probe was within 2 cm of what proved to be the saphenopopliteal function. [My own doubt about this technique is that there is a constant but variably sized posterior axial vein (44) running down the thigh to join the short saphenous; "reflux" may be demonstrable in this as a function of normal directional flow and cause confusion.] An alternative to this is perioperative varicography with needle markers appropriately inserted. This had its protagonists (47), but many would now agree that it has been superceded by ultrasound (46).

Undoubtedly, the gold standard in evaluation is duplex scanning, preferably color coded (48). This has the capacity to give not only comprehensive anatomic data but also functional information regarding which anatomic modalities are incompetent. In the author's mind there is little doubt that preoperative color duplex scanning will play an increasing role in the resolution of this very difficult area of surgery. This will give valuable inforamtion to assist in the interpretation of the operative findings, regarding not only the saphenopopliteal itself but also the gastrocnemius veins, which are so easily overlooked (49) and become increasingly varicose with age (50).

Type 3c

Little has been written about neovascularization at the saphenopopliteal junction, although the author has anecdotal evidence that this does occur (6) and has demonstrated it by descending venography in patients with coexistent deep incompetence. On this basis a case could be made for wrapping the popliteal veins with mesh and stripping the short saphenous trunk, although the latter runs the risk of injury to the sural and tibial nerves, which lie in close proximity.

SUMMARY

1.   Recurrent varicose veins constitute about 25 per cent of "new" patients referred for assessment.

2.   Recurrence occurs in 20 to 30 per cent of patients followed up after surgery; the rate increases with time.

3.   Various types of recurrence are recognizable:

Type 1: Mainly through incompetent thigh perforating veins.
Type 2: Evolution through a second system, usually the short saphenous; unidirectional Doppler ultrasonography will detect this.
Type 3: Recurrent saphenofemoral incompetence mainly due to "neovascularization" or regrowth of communications.

4.   Types 1 and 3 recurrence will probably be minimized by stripping the long saphenous trunk.

5.   There is wide anatomic variation in the veins of the popliteal fossa. The popliteal "vein" is most often double.

6.   In only 80 per cent of limbs does the short saphenous terminate in the popliteal fossa.

7.   Varicosities also arise from the gastrocnemius veins, usually the medial, and from the "popliteal area" vein.

8.   It is anticipated that color-coded duplex scanning will play an increasing role in the evaluation of popliteal fossa varicosities.

9.   Recurrent saphenofemoral incompetence was studied in patients with venous ulceration, all of whom had coexistent perforator and deep incompetence. Groin re-ligation alone did not heal the ulcers, but when this was combined with subfascial perforator ligation the initial results were favorable.

REFERENCES

1.   Jakobsen BH: The value of different forms of treatment for varicose veins. Br J Surg 1979; 66:182–184.
2.   Hobbs JT: Surgery and sclerotherapy in the treatment of varicose veins. Arch Surg 1974;109:793–796.
3.   Coon WW, Willis PW III, Keller JB: Venous thrombo-embolism and other venous disease in the Tecumseh Community Health Study. Circulation 1973;48:839–846.
4.   Widmer LK, Hall T, Kactin H: Epidemiology and sociomedical importance of peripheral venous disease. In Hobbs JT, ed: The Treatment of Venous Disorders. Lancaster, England, MTP Press Ltd, 1977;3–12.
5.   Campbell WB: Varicose veins. Br Med J 1990;300:763–764.
6.   Darke SG, Andress MR: The value of venography in the management of chronic venous disorders of the lower limbs. In Greenhalgh RM, ed: Diagnostic Techniques and Assessment Procedures in Vascular Surgery. Orlando, FL, Grune & Stratton, 1985;421–446.
7.   Sheppard H: A procedure for the prevention of recurrent sapheno femoral incompetence. Aust NZ J Surg 1978;48:322–326.
8.   Royle JP: Recurrent varicose veins. World J Surg 1986;10:944–958.
9.   Lofgren EP: Treatment of long saphenous varicosities and their recurrence. A long term follow up. In Bergan JJ, Yao JST, eds: Surgery of the Veins. Orlando, FL, Grune & Stratton, 1985; 285–299.

10. Berridge DC, Makin GS: Day case surgery: A variable alternative for surgical treatment of varicose veins. Phlebology 9187;2:103–108.
11. Corbett CR, McIrvine AJ, Aston NO, Jamieson CW, Lea Thomas ML: The use of varicography to identify the sources of incompetence in recurrent varicose veins. Ann R Coll Surg Engl 1982;66:412–415.
12. Sherman RS: Varicose veins: Anatomic findings and an operative procedure based upon them. Ann Surg 1944;120:772–784.
13. Dodd H: The varicose tributaries of the superficial femoral vein passing into the Hunter's canal. Postgrad Med J 1959;35:18–23.
14. Sutton R, Darke SG: Stripping the long saphenous vein: Per-operative retrograde saphenography in patients with and without ulceration. Br J Surg 1986;73:305–307.
15. Thompson H: The surgical anatomy of the superficial and perforating veins of the lower limb. Ann R Coll Surg Engl 1979;61:198–205.
16. Papadakis K, Christodoulou C, Christopoulos D, Hobbs J, Malouf GM, Grigg M, Irvine A, Nicolaides A: The number and anatomical distribution of incompetent thigh perforating veins. Br J Surg 1989;76:581–584.
17. Lofgren EP, Lofgren KA: Recurrence of varicose veins after the stripping operation. Arch Surg 1971;102:111–114.
18. Munn SR, Morton JB, MacBeth WAAG, McLeish AR: To strip or not to strip the long saphenous vein? A varicose veins trial. Br J Surg 1981;68:426–428.
19. Reagan B, Folse R: Lower limb haemodynamics in normal persons and children of patients with varicose veins. Surg Gynecol Obstet 1971;132:15–22.
20. Gunderson J: Hereditary factors in varicose veins. In Hobbs JT, ed: The Treatment of Venous Disorders. Lancaster, England, MTP Press Ltd, 1977;13–17.
21. Nicolaides AN, Miles C, Zimmerman H: The non invasive assessment of venous insufficiency. In Greenhalgh RM, ed: Hormones and Vascular Disease. London, Pitman Medical, 1981;209–237.
22. Chan A, Chisholm J, Royle JP: The use of directional Doppler ultrasound in the assessment of sapheno femoral incompetence. Aust NZ J Surg 1983;53:399–402.
23. McIrvine AJ, Corbett CRR, Aston NO, Sherriff EA, Wiseman PA, Jamieson CW: The demonstration of sapheno femoral incompetence: Doppler ultrasound compared with standard clinical tests. Br J Surg 1984;71:509–510.
24. Hoare MC, Royle JP: Doppler ultrasound detection of sapheno femoral and sapheno popliteal incompetence and operative venography to ensure precise sapheno popliteal ligation. Aust NZ J Surg 1984;54:49–52.
25. Sheppard M: The incidence, diagnosis and management of sapheno femoral incompetence. Phlebology 1986;1:23–32.
26. Mitchell DC, Darke SG: The assessment of primary varicose veins by Doppler ultrasound—the role of sapheno popliteal incompetence and the short saphenous system in calf varicosities. Eur J Vasc Surg 1987;1:113–115.
27. Starnes HF, Vallance R, Hamilton DNH: Recurrent varicose veins: A radiological approach to investigation. Clin Radiol 1984;35:95–99.
28. Glass GM: Neovascularisation in recurrent varices of the great saphenous vein in the groin, phlebography. Angiology 1988;39:577–582.
29. Glass RM: Neovascularisation in recurrence of the varicose great saphenous vein following transection. Phlebology 1987;2:81–91.
30. Glass RM: Neovascularisation in restoration of continuity of the rat femoral vein following surgical interruption. Phlebology 1987;2:1–6.
31. Greaney MG, Makin GS: Operation for recurrent sapheno femoral incompetence using a medial approach to the sapheno femoral junction. Br J Surg 1985;72:910–911.
32. Glass GM: Prevention of recurrent sapheno femoral incompetence after surgery for varicose veins. Br J Surg 1989;76:1210.
33. Li AKC: A technique for re-exploration of the sapheno femoral junction for recurrent varicose veins. Br J Surg 1975;62:745–746.
34. Negus D, Friegood A: The effective management of venous ulceration. Br J Surg 1983;70:623–627.
35. Thomas AMC, Tomlinson PJ, Boggan RP: Incompetent perforating vein ligation in the treatment of venous ulceration. Ann R Coll Surg Engl 1986;68:214–215.
36. Sethia KK, Darke SG: Long saphenous incompetence as a cause of venous ulceration. Br J Surg 1984;71:754–755.
37. Kistner RL: Transvenous repair of the incompetent femoral vein valve. In Bergan JJ, Yao JST, eds: Venous Problems. Chicago, Year Book Medical Publishers, 1978;492–509.
38. Darke SG, Lamont PL, Lansdown M, Hadley J, McMullen KW: The value of saphenous and perforator ligation in the presence of co-existent primary deep incompetence. Eur J Vas Surg 1991 (in press).

39. Queral LA, Whitehouse WM, Flinn WR, Neiman NL, Yao JST, Bergan JJ: Surgical correction of chronic deep venous insufficiency by valvular transposition. Surgery 1980;87:688–695.

40. Nicolaides AN, Miles CM: Photoplethysmography in the assessment of venous insufficiency. J Vasc Surg 1987;5:405–412.

41. O'Donnel TF, Mackey WC, Shepard AD, Callow AD: Clinical phlebographic and haemodynamic assessment of the popliteal valve transplant. *In* Proceedings of the 2nd International Vascular Symposium, 1986, London. Abstract S22.6.

42. Eriksson I, Almgren B: The influence of the profunda femoris vein and venous haemodynamics of the limb. J Vasc Surg 1986;4:390–395.

43. Williams AF: The formation of the popliteal vein. Surg Gynecol Obstet 1953;97:769–772.

44. Dodd H: The varicose tributaries of the popliteal vein. Br J Surg 1965;52:350–354.

45. Moosman DA, Hartwell SW: The surgical significance of the subfascial course of the lesser saphenous vein.Surg Gynecol Obstet 1964;113:761–766.

46. Gilliland EL, Gerber CJ,Lewis JD: Short saphenous surgery, preoperative Doppler ultrasound marking compared with on table venography and operative findings. Phlebology 1987;2:109–114.

47. Hobbs JT: Per-operative venography to ensure accurate sapheno popliteal vein ligation. Br Med J 1980;223:1578–1579.

48. Vasdekis SN, Clarke GH, Hobbs JT, Nicolaides AN: Evaluation of non invasive and invasive methods in the assessment of short saphenous vein termination. Br J Surg 1989;76:929–932.

49. Hobbs JT: The enigma of the gastrocnemius vein. Phlebology 1988;3:19–30.

50. May R, Nissl R: Varizen der vena gastrocnemia. Fortschr Rontgenstr 1965;105:229–234.

16

COMPRESSION SCLEROTHERAPY AND ITS COMPLICATIONS

Mitchel P. Goldman

Rarely does the physician have the luxury of administering a totally benign therapy in the treatment of any disease. As with any therapeutic technique, sclerotherapy carries with it a number of potential complications. Fairly common, and often self-limiting, side effects include perivascular cutaneous pigmentation, edema of the injected extremity, a flare of new perivascular telangiectasias, localized urticaria over injected sites, localized hirsutism, and stress-related problems. Relatively rare complications include localized cutaneous necrosis, systemic allergic reactions, thrombophlebitis of the injected vessel, arterial injection with resultant distal necrosis, deep vein thrombosis with pulmonary emboli, and nerve damage. This chapter will address the pathophysiology of these reactions, methods for reducing their incidence, and treatment of their occurrence.

POSTSCLEROTHERAPY HYPERPIGMENTATION

Cutaneous pigmentation to some degree is a relatively common occurrence following sclerotherapy of veins varying in size from varicose to capillary (Fig. 16–1). This complication has been reported in 30 per cent of patients treated with sodium tetradecyl sulfate (STS) (1), 30 per cent of patients treated with hypertonic saline (HS) (2–5), and 10.7 (6) to 30 (3,7) per cent of patients treated with polidocanol (POL).

Despite therapeutic attempts, pigmentation often lasts from 6 to 12 months. Pigmentation has been estimated to last over 1 year in 1 (8) to 10 (3) per cent of patients. It is important to recognize that in certain patients this pigmentation may be present over superficial varicosities and telangiectasias prior to sclerotherapy. Hyperpigmentation as a result of "physiologic" diapedesis of red blood cells through fragile vessels is common in venous stasis or over varicose veins (9). Therefore, preoperative documentation, including photographs, may be beneficial during follow-up patient visits.

Postsclerotherapy pigmentation usually results from hemosiderin deposition either through extravasation of red blood cells or leakage of hemoglobin extravascularly through the damaged endothelium of a sclerosed vein. Goldman et al.

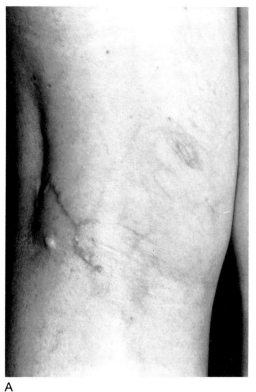

A

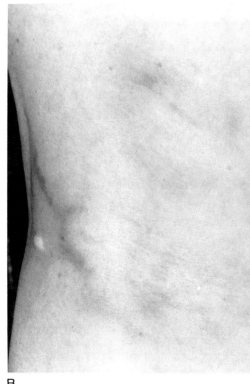

B

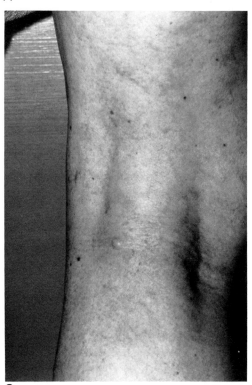

C

Figure 16–1. This series of photographs illustrates the usual evolution and resolution of hyperpigmentation after sclerotherapy. *A*, Presclerotherapy appearance of a reticular varicosity not associated with saphenofemoral or saphenopopliteal reflux. *B*, Four weeks after sclerotherapy treatment. Note mild pigmentation at the distal aspect of the treated vein. An obvious thrombotic coagula is present in the main body of the treated vein. *C*, Two years after initial treatment with complete resolution of the treated vein and hyperpigmentation. Resolution of associated telangiectasia is also apparent. (From Goldman MP: Sclerotherapy Treatment of Varicose and Telangiectatic Leg Veins. St. Louis, Mosby-Yearbook Inc., 1991.)

(10) have microscopically examined this pigmentation in six patients 6 weeks to 6 months after treatment of leg telangiectasia with POL, STS, and HS. There were no apparent histologic differences in the degree of pigmentation between the three sclerosing agents. In each biopsy specimen stained for both hemosiderin and melanin, pigmentation was solely due to hemosiderin. This also occurred in one patient who was Hispanic.

The extent of endothelial destruction with resulting inflammation and extravasation of red blood cells is thought to influence the development of postsclerotherapy hyperpigmentation. Cloutier and Sansoucy (11) and Tournay (1) stated that STS has the highest incidence of pigmentation among sclerosing solutions. Foley (12) claimed that the addition of 100 units/ml of heparin decreases the incidence of pigmentation, but in a large series of patients Duffy (3) and Sadick (13) did not find this to occur. Sclerosing solutions reported to have the lowest incidence of postsclerotherapy pigmentation are chromated glycerin and sodium salicylate (14,15). Norris et al. (16) have observed an increased incidence (60 per cent) of pigmentation in patients treated with 1 per cent POL over that in those treated with 0.5 per cent POL (20 per cent). Therefore, sclerosing solutions of high concentration also have a higher incidence of causing pigmentation.

In addition to utilizing the lowest effective concentration and strength of sclerosing solution, removal of postsclerotherapy coagula may also decrease the incidence of pigmentation. Thrombi are thought to occur to some degree after sclerotherapy of all sizes of veins. This is secondary to the inability to completely occlude the vascular lumen with external pressure (15). Persistent thrombi are thought to produce a subacute perivenulitis that can persist for months. The "perivenulitis" favors extravasation of red blood cells through damage to the endothelium or by increasing its permeability. In addition, intratissue fixation of hemosiderin may occur (11). This provides a rationale for drainage of all foci of trapped blood between 2 and 4 weeks after sclerotherapy.

Thrombi are best removed by gentle expression of the liquefied clot through a small incision made with a 21-gauge needle, #11 blade, or lancet. A rocking action around the clot may aid in its expulsion. This should be continued until all dark blood is removed. The art is to find the right place to puncture. This is best perceived as a soft fluctuating spot. If the thrombosis is in the deep dermis, the area should be marked and 1 per cent lidocaine infiltrated around the area to facilitate a less painful removal. Compression pads and/or stockings are then worn an additional 3 days to prevent further thrombosis formation and to aid in adherence of the opposing endothelial walls to establish effective endosclerosis.

Therefore, to prevent the development of pigmentation, sclerotherapy should produce limited endothelial necrosis without total destruction with its resulting diapedesis of red blood cells. This may be achieved by meticulous technique, avoidance of excessive injection pressures, selection of appropriate solution concentration, and treatment of areas of reflux venous return in a proximal-to-distal manner.

Treatment of pigmentation, once it occurs, is often unsuccessful. Because this pigmentation primarily is due to hemosiderin deposition and not melanin incontinence, bleaching agents that affect melanocytic function are usually ineffective. Exfoliants (trichloroacetic acid or phenolate) may hasten the apparent resolution of this pigmentation by decreasing the overlying cutaneous pigmentation, but carry a risk of scarring, permanent hypopigmentation, and postinflammatory hyperpigmentation. The recommended treatment is "flash-bulb therapy" or "chronotherapy." Since the majority of patients will have a resolution of pigmentation within 1 year, time and photographic documentation tend to be very satisfactory for the understanding patient.

TEMPORARY SWELLING

Multiple factors are responsible for swelling of a treated area. These factors include changes in the pressure differential between the intravascular and perivascular space along with changes in endothelial permeability. Edema is most common when varicose veins or telangiectasia below the ankle are treated. This relates both to the increase in gravitational intravascular pressure in this area and to the relative sparsity of perivascular fascia at the ankle.

The extent of edema is also related to the degree of perivascular inflammation produced by the sclerosing solution. This appears to correlate with the strength of the sclerosing solution. The by-products of inflammation, including histamine, increase endothelial permeability.

Edema may also occur if compression is not given in a graduated manner. This may be produced when one tries to give localized pressure on the thigh over an injected vein with the addition of a tape dressing over or under a graduated compression stocking. If the patient is informed of the possibility of a tourniquet effect from the extra compression, he or she can remove the dressing at the first sign of edema distal to the dressing. Another method of avoiding the tourniquet effect is to only tape halfway around the thigh or calf.

There are two techniques that may limit this complication. First, limit perivascular inflammation. Ankle edema occurs much less frequently if one limits the quantity of sclerosing solution to 1 ml per ankle. Second, apply a graduated pressure stocking after injections in this area. A recent study on the use of compression hosiery in the treatment of leg telangiectasia found a significant decrease in the incidence of ankle edema when a 30- to 40-mm Hg graduated compression stocking was worn for 3 days after sclerotherapy (17).

TELANGIECTATIC MATTING

The new appearance of previously unnoticed fine red telangiectasias occurs in a number of patients following either sclerotherapy or surgical ligation of varicose veins and leg telangiectasia (Fig. 16–2). This has been termed "telangiectatic matting" (TM) by Duffy (3). The reported incidence varies from 5 (7) to 75 (16) per cent. The largest retrospective analysis to date (of 2120 patients with leg telangiectasia) reported a 16 per cent incidence (18). TM may appear anywhere on the leg but appears to occur more frequently on the thighs.

Probable risk factors for the development of TM in patients with leg telangiectasia include obesity, use of estrogen-containing hormones, pregnancy, and a family history of telangiectatic veins. Age and excessive standing do not appear to influence the incidence of TM (18). In addition, Davis and Duffy (18) have reported on the virtual disappearance of leg telangiectasia and TM in a 51-year-old female with estrogen receptor–positive breast carcinoma after initiation of

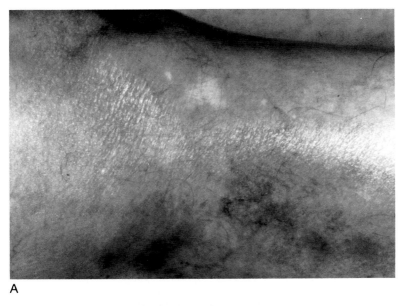

A

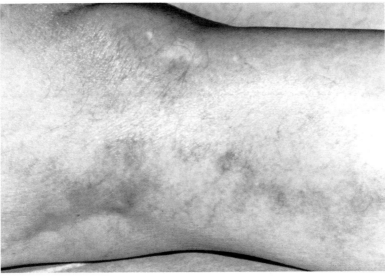

B

Figure 16–2. Typical telangiectatic matting in a 72-year-old female 6 weeks after sclerotherapy. *A,* Before treatment, right lateral knee. *B,* Six weeks after treatment. (From Goldman MP: Sclerotherapy Treatment of Varicose and Telangiectatic Leg Veins. St. Louis, Mosby-Yearbook Inc., 1991.)

antiestrogen therapy with tamoxifen citrate (Nolvadex). Thus, it may be prudent to withhold estrogen therapy during sclerotherapy treatment.

Postsclerosis TM was first described in the 1960s by Ouvry and Davy (19). They observed that the incidence of matting was proportional to the degree of inflammation and thrombus formation. The etiology of TM is unknown, but it has been thought to be related either to angiogenesis or a dilatation of existing subclinical blood vessels by promoting collateral flow through arteriovenous anastomoses. One or both of these mechanisms may occur. Experimentally, there are

TABLE 16–1. Angiogenic Factors[a]

Inflammation
Obstruction of blood flow—thrombosis, anoxia
Disruption of endothelial continuity
Heparin secretion by mast cells
Endothelial leakage of fibrinogen
Estrogen receptors

[a] From Goldman MP: Sclerotherapy Treatment of Varicose and Telangiectatic Leg Veins. St. Louis, Mosby-Yearbook Inc, 1991.

a number of etiologic factors that can initiate or contribute to angiogenesis (Table 16–1).

Sclerotherapy produces most of the etiologic factors responsible for angiogenesis. It is the author's opinion that inflammation is the most important etiologic factor. Inflammation may be considered as a hypermetabolic state with new vessel growth occurring secondary to increased metabolic demand. Mast cells are found in increased numbers in inflammatory states. Since mast cell heparin is one factor responsible for capillary endothelial cell migration, in an attempt to decrease angiogenic stimuli one should try to limit the degree of inflammation as much as possible. Thus it is important to limit the quantity and strength of solution to that amount that will not produce excessive endothelial damage. This was confirmed by Weiss and Weiss (20), who found that in a random sample of 113 sclerotherapy patients, 10 developed TM with injection of 1 per cent POL into vessels less than 1 mm in diameter. When 0.5 per cent POL was utilized for subsequent treatments in these patients, none developed further areas of TM.

LOCALIZED URTICARIA

Localized urticaria occurs after injection of all sclerosing solutions (Fig. 16–3). It is usually transient (lasting about 30 min) and is probably the result of endothelial irritation. Localized urticaria is not likely an allergic response because it occurs even after injection of 23.4 per cent unadulterated HS. It is probably related to the release of endothelial factors after these cells have been destroyed by the sclerosing solution. Alternatively, it may occur as the earliest manifestation of perivascular inflammation, again through release of endothelial or platelet-derived factors.

Approximately 40 per cent of patients studied by Norris et al. (16) described temporary itching after injections with POL regardless of drug dosage. Duffy (3) reported an almost 100 per cent occurrence of urticaria with injection of either POL or HS-heparin-lidocaine solutions. The urtication is usually more intense when more concentrated solutions are used (3,7).

In the author's experience, localized urticaria and itching may be diminished by applying topical steroids immediately after injection and by limiting the injection quantity per injection site. This is particularly helpful in patients who are to wear a graduated support stocking following treatment. Systemic antihistamines may also be useful in limiting urticaria when given prior to sclerotherapy.

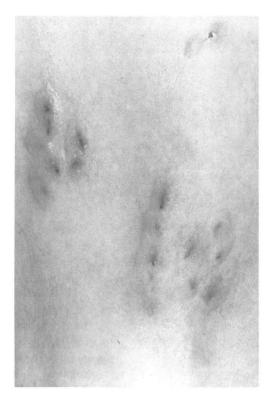

Figure 16–3. Urtication immediately after sclerotherapy with POL 0.5 per cent. (From Goldman MP: Sclerotherapy Treatment of Varicose and Telangiectatic Leg Veins. St. Louis, Mosby-Yearbook Inc., 1991.)

STRESS-RELATED SYMPTOMS

The vasovagal reflex is not an uncommon adverse sequela of any surgical or invasive procedure. It has been estimated to occur in 1 per cent of patients during sclerotherapy (21) and is more frequent when using the techniques of Fegan or Sigg (22). With these latter two techniques, 21- to 25-gauge needles are inserted while the patient it sitting or standing and blood is allowed to flow freely from the punctured vein. Duffy, who performs sclerotherapy with 30-gauge needles in reclining patients, estimated the incidence of vasovagal reactions to be 0.001 per cent (3). Interestingly, the percentage of men who experience this response far exceeds the percentage of women.

Vasovagal reactions have typical clinical findings. The usual symptoms include lightheadedness, nausea, and sweating. The patient may also experience shortness of breath and palpitations. Syncope rarely occurs, but usually provokes the most concern to the physician and staff. Vasovagal reactions are most often preceded by painful injection, but may occur just from the sight of the needle or the smell of the sclerosing solution.

The main concern in a vasovagal reaction is that the patient will fall and be injured. Therefore, both the nurse and physician should watch the patient closely for signs of restlessness and excessive perspiration. All such reactions are easily reversible when the patient assumes the supine or Trendelenburg position. Preventative measures consist of recommending that the patient eat a light meal prior to the appointment, maintaining good ventilation in the treatment room, and communicating with the patient during the procedure.

Another concern with the vasovagal reaction patient is to not assume that an allergic reaction is occurring. If subcutaneous epinephrine is given in the mistaken belief that an anaphylactic reaction is occurring, the symptoms will become both exaggerated and obscured. This only further confuses the clinical situation and adds to patient apprehension regarding further treatment sessions.

More serious stress-induced problems include exacerbation of certain underlying medical diseases. Patients with a history of asthma may experience wheezing, which can be treated with a bronchodilator. Patients with coronary artery disease may develop angina, treatable with sublingual nitroglycerin tablets. Urticaria is easily treated with an oral antihistamine but may be a sign of systemic allergy. Finally, triggering of frequent migraine headaches has also been noted to occur after sclerotherapy (3).

LOCALIZED HIRSUTISM

Localized hypertrichosis developing after sclerotherapy has been described several times with the use of multiple sclerosing agents. The etiology is thought to be secondary to an improved cutaneous oxygen content with localized increase in hair growth, or to a long-standing low-grade inflammatory reaction with stimulation of new hair growth.

CUTANEOUS NECROSIS

Cutaneous necrosis may occur with the injection of any sclerosing agent (Fig. 16–4). Its cause may be secondary to extravasation of a sclerosant into the perivascular tissues, injection into a dermal arteriole or an arteriole feeding into a telangiectatic or varicose vein, or a reactive vasospasm of the vessel. An additional cause is excessive cutaneous pressure by compression techniques.

Extravasation of caustic sclerosing solutions may directly destroy tissue. Even the most adept physician may inadvertently inject a small quantity of sclerosing solution into the perivascular tissue. Sclerosing solutions vary in the degree of cellular necrosis they produce. Goldman et al. (23) examined the effect of intradermal injection of the three most commonly used sclerosing solutions in the United States in rabbit skin and concluded that in the concentrations of the agents studied, POL is less likely to cause necrosis on extravasation into intradermal tissues than is HS or STS. Miyake et al. (24) intradermally injected multiple sclerosants, including POL, STS, and HS. Although the concentrations of POL and STS were not specified, they found significant cutaneous necrosis with all agents except POL. POL appears experimentally to be the least toxic to subcutaneous tissue. However, in sufficient concentration it will cause cutaneous necrosis.

Unfortunately, even when sclerotherapy is performed with expert technique, utlizing the safest sclerosing solutions and concentrations, cutaneous ulceration may occur. Therefore, it appears that extravasation of caustic sclerosing solutions alone is not totally responsible for this complication.

de Faria and Moraes (25) have observed that one in 26 leg telangiectasias are associated with a dermal arteriole. It is the author's opinion that inadvertent

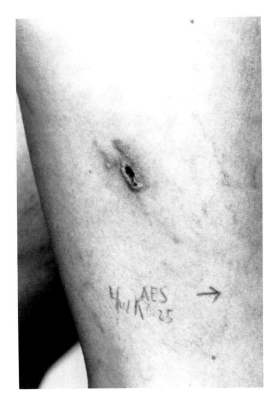

Figure 16–4. Cutaneous necrosis 6 weeks after sclerotherapy with POL 0.25 per cent. Note that 2 ml of solution was injected into a feeder vein approximately 10 cm distal to the necrotic area. (From Goldman MP: Sclerotherapy Treatment of Varicose and Telangiectatic Leg Veins. St. Louis, Mosby-Yearbook Inc., 1991.)

injection into or near this communication is the most common cause of cutaneous ulcerations. The development of 3- to 6-mm diameter ulcerations occurs in the author's practice in approximately 0.0001 per cent of injections with 0.5 per cent POL. Four consecutive ulcerations that appeared over the course of 1 year were excised. In these patients, each cutaneous ulceration occurred as a result of occlusion of the feeding dermal arteriole. This produced a classic wedge-shaped arterial ulceration. Therefore, it appears that this complication may be unavoidable to some extent.

Finally, excessive compression of the skin overlying the treated vein may produce tissue anoxia with the development of localized cutaneous ulceration. Subcutaneous tissue flow on the leg is decreased when cutaneous pressure exceeds 20 mm Hg (26). Therefore, it is recommended that patients not wear a graduated compression stocking producing over 30 to 40 mm Hg pressure when lying down for prolonged periods of time.

Whatever the etiology for the ulceration, it must be dealt with when it occurs. Fortunately, ulcerations when they occur are usually fairly small, averaging 4 mm in diameter in the author's practice. At this size, primary healing usually leaves an acceptable scar (Fig. 16–5). The use of a number of occlusive and/or hydrocolloid dressings has been found by the author to result in an apparent decrease in wound healing time. More importantly, occlusive dressings decrease the pain associated with an open ulcer. However, because an ulcer may take 8 to 12 weeks to completely heal even under ideal conditions, if possible excision and closure of these lesions is recommended at the earliest possible time. This affords the patient the fastest healing with an acceptable scar.

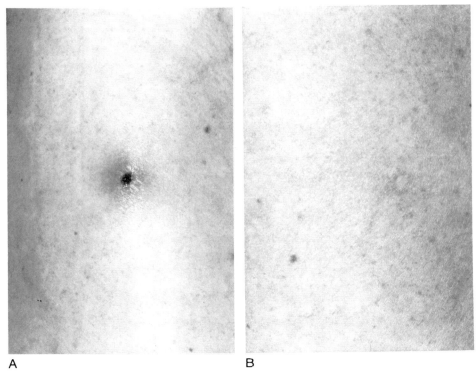

A   B

Figure 16–5.   Cutaneous ulceration on the posterolateral thigh. *A*, Three weeks after treatment with POL 0.5 per cent. *B*, After 6 months. Treatment consisted of a duoderm dressing that was changed every 2 to 4 days until complete healing occurred in 5 weeks. Note the cosmetically acceptable stellate scar. (From Goldman MP: Sclerotherapy Treatment of Varicose and Telangiectatic Leg Veins. St. Louis, Mosby-Yearbook Inc, 1991.)

SYSTEMIC ALLERGIC REACTION/TOXICITY

Fortunately, systemic reactions secondary to sclerotherapy treatment occur very rarely. Minor reactions such as urticaria are easily treated with an oral antihistamine. Because of the possibility of angioedema or bronchospasm, each patient with evidence of an allergic reaction should be examined for stridor and wheezing by auscultating over their neck and chest while they breathe normally. Supine and sitting blood pressure and pulse should be checked to rule out orthostatic changes, hypotension, or tachycardia that might result from the vasodilatation that precedes anaphylactic shock.

Minor degrees of angioedema can again be treated with oral antihistamines; however, if stridor is present an intramuscular injection of diphenhydramine and intravenous corticosteroids should be administered and a laryngoscope and endotracheal tube should be available.

Bronchospasm is estimated to occur after sclerotherapy in 0.001 per cent of patients (3). It usually responds to the addition of an inhaled bronchodilator or intravenous aminophylline (6 mg/kg over 20 min) to the antihistamine-corticosteroid regimen already noted.

Anaphylaxis is a systemic hypersensitivity response caused by exposure, or more commonly reexposure, to a sensitizing substance. Anaphylaxis is usually an immunoglobulin E–mediated, mast cell activated reaction that occurs usually within minutes of antigen exposure. The signs and symptoms of anaphylaxis may initially be subtle and often include anxiety, itching, sneezing, coughing, urticaria, and angioedema. Wheezing may occur with hoarseness of the voice and vomiting. Shortly after these presenting signs breathing becomes more difficult and the patient usually collapses from cardiovascular failure secondary to systemic vaso-dilatation.

The recommended treatment is to give epinephrine 0.2 to 0.5 ml 1:1000 sub-cutaneously. This can be repeated three to four times at 5- to 15-min intervals to maintain a systolic blood pressure above 90 to 100 mm Hg. This should be followed with establishment of an intravenous line of 0.9 per cent sodium chloride. Di-phenhydramine hydrochloride 50 mg is next given along with cimetidine 300 mg, both intravenously, and oxygen is given at 4 to 6 liters/min. An endotracheal tube or tracheostomy is necessary for laryngeal obstruction. For asthma or wheezing intravenous theophylline 4 to 6 mg/kg is infused over 15 min. At this point it is appropriate to transfer the patient to the hospital. Methylprednisolone sodium succinate 60 mg is given intravenously followed with the same dose every 6 hr for four doses. Corticosteroids are not an emergency medication because their effect only appears after 1 to 3 hr. They are given to prevent the recurrence of symptoms 3 to 8 hr after the initial event. The patient should be hospitalized overnight for observation.

Sodium Morrhuate

Sodium morrhuate causes a variety of allergic reactions ranging from mild erythema with pruritus to generalized urticaria to anaphylaxis (13). It has been estimated that "unfavorable reactions" occur in 3 per cent of patients (27). The reason for the high number of allergic reactions with this product may be related to the inability to remove all the fish proteins that are present. In fact, 20.8 per cent of the fatty acid composition of the solution is unknown (28).

Many cases of anaphylaxis have occurred within a few minutes after the drug is injected, or more commonly when therapy is reinstituted after a few weeks (13). Most of these cases occurred before 1950. Rarely, anaphylaxis has resulted in fatalities (27,29,30) many of which have not been reported in the medical literature (31).

Ethanolamine Oleate

Ethanolamine oleate (Ethamolin, Glaxo Pharmaceuticals) is a synthetic mixture of ethanolamine and oleic acid with an empirical formula of $C_{20}H_{41}NO_3$. The minimal lethal intravenous dose in rabbits is 130 mg/kg (32). The oleic acid component is responsible for the inflammatory action. Oleic acid may also activate coagulation in vitro by release of tissue factor and Hageman factor. Ethanolamine is thought to have a decreased risk of allergic reactions compared to sodium morrhuate or STS (33). However, allergic reactions have been associated with this sclerosing agent.

Anaphylactic shock has been reported following injection in three cases by the product manufacturer (34). Another case of a nearly fatal anaphylactic reaction to the fourth treatment of varicose leg veins with 1 ml of solution has also been reported (35). In one additional case a fatal reaction occurred in a male with a known allergic disposition (34). Another episode of a fatal anaphylactic reaction occurred in a women during her third series of injections (31). This represented one reaction in 200 patients from that author's practice. Generalized urticaria occurred in about 1/400 patients, and responded rapidly to an antihistamine (36).

Sodium Tetradecyl Sulfate

A comprehensive review of the medical literature (in multiple specialites and languages) disclosed a total of 47 cases of nonfatal allergic reactions to STS in a review of 14,404 treated patients. This included six case reports (37). A separate review of treatment in 187 patients with 2249 injections disclosed no evidence of allergic or systemic reactions (38). An additional report of 5341 injections given to an unknown number of patients found "no unfavorable reaction" (39). If one were to combine only those reviews of over 1000 patients the incidence of nonfatal allergic reactions would be about 0.3 per cent (13).

Fegan (40) reviewed his experience with STS in 16,000 patients. He reported 15 cases of "serum sickness, with hot stinging pain in the skin, and an erythematous rash developing 30 to 90 minutes after injection." These patients subsequently underwent additional uneventful treatment with STS after premedication with antihistamines. Ten additional patients developed "mild anaphylaxis" that required treatment with epinephrine.

Since all reported cases of allergic reactions are of the immunoglobulin E–mediated immediate hypersensitivity type, it is recommended that patients remain in or near the office for 30 min following sclerotherapy when STS is utilized. However, patients may also develop allergic reactions hours or days after the procedure. For example, urticaria occurred 8 hr after treatment in one patient (41), and 2 weeks after treatment in two other patients (42). Therefore, patients should be warned about the possibility of allergic reactions and how to obtain care should a reaction occur.

Polidocanol

Allergic reactions to POL have only been reported in four patients in a recent review of the world's literature, with an estimated incidence of 0.01 per cent (37). In addition, patients who are allergic to STS or iodine have no allergic manifestations to injections of POL. However, rare allergic reactions have been reported, including a case of nonfatal anaphylactic shock and generalized urticaria (43,44). Jaquier and Loretan (45) believe that the decrease in antigenicity is secondary to the absence of a benzene nucleus and a paramine group, and the presence of a lone free alcohol group. Thus, allergic reactions to POL are much rarer than those reported with STS.

Chromated Glycerin

Scleremo (SCL, 72 per cent chromated glycerin; France) is a sclerosant whose incidence of side effects is very low (15). Hypersensitivity is a very rare complication (19,46). Hematuria accompanied by ureteral colic can occur transiently following injection of large doses. Ocular manifestations, including blurred vision and a partial visual field loss, have been reported by a single author, with resolution in less than 2 hr (47).

Polyiodide Iodine

Polyiodide iodine (Varigloban, Chemische Fabrik Kreussler & Co, Wiesbaden-Biebrich, West Germany; Variglobin, Globopharm, Switzerland) is a stabilized water solution of iodide ions, sodium iodine, and benzyl alcohol. Sigg et al. (48) reported on their experience in over 400,000 injections with Varioglobin. In 1975 they reported an incidence of side effects of 1.25/1000 injections: 0.13/1000 allergic cutaneous reactions, 0.04/1000 localized necrosis, and 1/1000 varicophlebitis. No systemic allergic reactions were observed. Obvious contraindications to the use of variglobin are hyperthyroidism and allergies to iodine and benzyl alcohol.

Iodine solutions may also produce bronchial-mucosal lesions if used in high concentration. Therefore Wenner (49) recommended that a maximum of 5 ml of 12 per cent solution be used in a single sclerosing session.

Hypertonic Saline

Alone, HS has no evidence of allergenicity or toxicity. The only complication from its specific use is hypertension, which may be exacerbated in predisposed patients when an excessive sodium load is given. In addition, hematuria may occur after injection of large quantities of HS into varicose veins. Hematuria probably occurs secondary to hemolysis of red blood cells during sclerotherapy.

However, the addition of heparin and/or lidocaine to HS confers upon it the associated risk of reaction to the adulterants. Fever, urticaria, and anaphylaxis occur occasionally after administration of heparin. Pruritus, local tenderness, and burning sensations associated with large, indurated, erythematous plaques have also been reported to occur 10 to 20 days after beginning prophylactic doses of heparin (13). Therefore, there is a measurable risk of toxicity to heparin.

The addition of lidocaine has also been advoated to minimize patient discomfort during injection of hypertonic saline. Although the most common etiologies for the patient to give in a history of previous allergic reaction to lidocaine are psychogenic or vasovagal reactions, allergic reactions may occur.

SUPERFICIAL THROMBOPHLEBITIS

Before the advent of modern-day sclerotherapy, which employs graduated compression to limit thrombosis, thrombophlebitis, both superficial and deep, occurred in a significant number of sclerotherapy patients. In fact, it was commonly thought that phlebitis was so common a sequela of sclerotherapy that there was doubt over whether this form of therapy was legitimate. Fortunately, with the use of compression and the realization of the adverse effects from thrombus formation in treated veins, the incidence of thrombophlebitis greatly decreased.

Superficial thrombophlebitis appears 1 to 3 weeks after injection as a tender, erythematous induration over the injected vein. It has been estimated to occur in up to 1 per cent of patients (42), although in the author's experience this complication occurs in some degree in approximately 0.01 per cent of patients. Severe cases requiring treatment with compression and antiinflammatory agents occur in less than 0.001 per cent of patients. The etiology of thrombophlebitis may be related in part to treatment technique. An inadequate degree or length of compression results in excessive intravascular thrombosis. Perivenous inflammation usually is observed only at those parts of the limb not covered by a compression dressing. Thus, to avoid this complication one should prevent and/or minimize the development of postsclerosis thrombosis. This is accomplished with compression pads and hosiery.

Thrombophlebitis is not a complication that should be taken lightly. If untreated, the inflammation and clot may spread to perforating veins and the deep venous system, leading to valvular damage and possible pulmonary embolic events. Therefore, when thrombophlebitis occurs the thrombus should be evacuated and adequate compression with frequent ambulation maintained until the pain and inflammation resolve. Aspirin or other nonsteroidal antiinflammatory agents may be helpful in limiting both the inflammation and the pain.

ARTERIAL INJECTION

The most feared complication in sclerotherapy is inadvertent injection into an artery. Fortunately, this complication is very rare (13). The development of an embolus when a sclerosing solution is injected into an artery occurs when the solution denatures blood, producing a sludge embolus that obstructs the microcirculation, causing stagnation, secondary thrombosis, and necrosis. There is little effect on the major vessel (artery) with injection. Spasm does not occur.

The most common location for this to occur is in the posterior or medial malleolar region, specifically in the posterior tibial artery. The patient will usually, but not always, note immediate pain. Cutaneous blanching of the injected area usually occurs in an arterial pattern in association with a loss of pulse and progressive cyanosis of the injected area.

Another area where the artery and veins are in close proximity is at the junction of the femoral and superficial saphenous veins. In this location the external pudendal artery bifurcates and may surround the greater saphenous vein shortly after its connection with the femoral vein. Because of the anatomic variation of these collateral arteries in this location, duplex scanning is recommended to guide needle placement prior to injection of sclerosing solution.

Arterial injection is a true sclerotherapy emergency. The extent of cutaneous necrosis usually is related to the amount of sclerosant injected. Therapeutic efforts to treat this complication are usually unsatisfactory but should be attempted. Browse et al. (22) recommended that upon realization of arterial injection, blood and sclerosant should be aspirated back into the syringe to empty the needle of sclerosant. In addition, aspiration of the injected artery as rapidly and completely as possible may help in removal of injected sclerosant if performed immediately. The needle should not be withdrawn, but the syringe replaced with one containing 10,000 units of heparin, which should be injected slowly into the artery. Periarterially infiltrated 3 per cent procaine 1 ml will complex with STS and render it inactive. The foot should be cooled with ice packs to minimize tissue anoxia. Immediate heparinization for 6 days with administration of intravenous 10 per cent dextran 500 ml/day for 3 days is recommended. Intravenous streptokinase may be considered if there are no other contraindications for its use. Finally, oral prazosin, hydralazine, or nifedipine should be considered for 30 days.

Prevention of this dreaded complication is best accomplished by visualization of the blood emanating from the needle. If it is pulsatile and continues to flow after the leg is horizontal, injection should not be attempted at this site.

PULMONARY EMBOLISM/DEEP VENOUS THROMBOSIS

Fortunately, pulmonary emboli only very rarely occur. In the 1930s and 1940s pulmonary emboli after sclerotherapy of varicose veins occurred in, at most, 0.14 per cent of patients (50,51). More recently, with the onset of compression techniques in combination with sclerotherapy, this complication has become even less common. Sigg (52) reported pulmonary emboli occurring only once in 42,000 injections. Fegan (40) reported that he has never seen conclusive evidence of deep vein thrombosis after injection treatment of 16,000 patients in his clinic.

The etiology of deep vein thrombosis with pulmonary embolism development after sclerotherapy is unclear. The chemical endophlebitis produced by sclerotherapy should anchor the thrombus to the site of injection. Therefore, the most logical explanation for the development of emboli is damage to the deep venous system by migration of sclerosing solution or a partly attached thrombosis into deep veins from superficial veins. This may occur either by injection of large quantities of sclerosing solution or by physical inactivity after injection. In addition, tributary communicating veins, if not compressed, may force early clots into the deep circulation with muscle contraction. Therefore, one must both limit the quantity of sclerosing solution per injection site to assure that the agent will remain within the superficial system and rapidly stimulate blood flow in the deep venous system after sclerotherapy with compression and muscle movement.

NERVE DAMAGE

Because of close proximity, the saphenous and sural nerves may be injected with sclerosant. Injection into a nerve is reported to be very painful, and if continued may cause anesthesia and sometimes a permanent interruption of nerve function (22). Occasionally, a patient may complain of an area of paresthesia in the treated leg. This is probably secondary to perivascular inflammation extending from the sclerosed vein to adjacent superficial nerves. Steps to limit inflammation include the use of nonsteroidal antiinflammatory medications and high-potency topical or systemic steroids. However, this complication may take 3 to 6 months to resolve.

REFERENCES

1. Tournay PR: Traitment sclerosant des tres fines varicosites intra ou saous-dermiques. Soc Franc Phlebo 1966;*19*:235–241.
2. Bodian EL: Techniques of sclerotherapy for sunburst venous blemishes. J Dermatol Surg Oncol 1985;*11*:696–704.

3. Duffy DM: Small vessel sclerotherapy: An overview. *In* Callen J, Dahl M, Golitz L, Schachner L, Stegman S, eds: Advances in Dermatology, vol 3. Chicago, Year Book Medical Publishers, Inc, 1988;221–240.

4. Alderman DB: Surgery and sclerotherapy in the treatment of varicose veins. Conn Med 1975; *39*:467–471.

5. Weiss R, Weiss M: Resolution of pain associated with varicose and telangiectatic leg veins after compression sclerotherapy. J Dermatol Surg Oncol 1990;*16*:333–336.

6. Cacciatore E: Experience of sclerotherapy with aethoxysklerol. Min Cardioang 1979;*27*:255–262.

7. Goldman P: Sclerotherapy of superficial venules and telangiectasias of the lower extremities. Dermatol Clin 1987;*5*:369–379.

8. Georgiev M: Postsclerotherapy hyperpigmentations: A one year follow-up. J Dermatol Surg Oncol 1990;*16*:608–610.

9. Leu HJ, Wenner A, Spycher MA: Erythrocyte diapedesis in venous stasis syndrome. Vasa 1981; *10*:17–23.

10. Goldman MP, Kaplan RP, Duffy DM: Postsclerotherapy hyperpigmentation: A histologic evaluation. Dermatol Surg Oncol 1987;*13*:547–550.

11. Cloutier G, Sansoucy H: Le traitement des varices des membres inferieurs par les injections sclerosantes. Union Med Can 1975;*104*:1854–1863.

12. Foley WT: The eradication of venous blemishes. Cutis 1975;*15*:665–668.

13. Sadick N: Treatment of varicose and telangiectatic leg veins with hypertonic saline: A comparative study of heparin and saline. J Dermatol Surg Oncol 1990;*16*:24–28.

14. Hutinel B: Esthetique dans les scleroses de varices et traitement des varicosites. La Vie Medicale 1978;*20*:1739–1743.

15. Goldman MP: Sclerotherapy Treatment of Varicose and Telangiectatic Leg Veins. St. Louis, Mosby-Yearbook Inc., 1991.

16. Norris MJ, Carlin MC, Ratz JL: Treatment of essential telangiectasia: Effects of increasing concentrations of polidocanol. J Am Acad Dermatol 1989;*20*:643–649.

17. Goldman MP, Beudoing D, Marley W, Lopez L, Butie A: Compression in the treatment of leg telangiectasia. J Dermatol Surg Oncol 1990;*16*:322–325.

18. Davis LT, Duffy DM: Determination of incidence and risk factors for post-sclerotherapy telangiectatic matting of the lower extremity: A retrospective analysis. J Dermatol Surg Oncol 1990;*16*:327–330.

19. Ouvry P, Davy A: Le traitement sclerosant des telangiectasies des membres inferieurs. Phlebologie 1982;*35*:349–359.

20. Weiss RA, Weiss MA: Incidence of side effects in the treatment of telangiectasias by compression sclerotherapy: Hypertonic saline vs. polidocanol. J Dermatol Surg Oncol 1990 (in press).

21. Winstone N: *In* The Treatment of Varicose Veins by Injection and Compression. (Proceedings of the Stoke Mandeville Symposium). Hereford, England, Pharmaceutical Research STD Ltd, 1971;41.

22. Browse NL, Burnard KG, Thomas ML: Diseases of the Veins: Pathology, Diagnosis and Treatment. London, Edward Arnold, 1988;242–243.

23. Goldman MP, Kaplan RP, Oki LN, Bennett RG, Strick A: Extravascular effects of sclerosants in rabbit skin: A clinical and histologic examination. J Dermatol Surg Oncol 1986;*12*:1085–1088.

24. Miyake H, Kauffman P, de Arruda Behmer O, et al: Mechanisms of cutaneous necrosis provoked by sclerosing injections in the treatment of microvarices and telangiectasias: Experimental study. Rev Assoc Med Brazil 1976;*22*:115–120.

25. de Faria JL, Moraes IN: Histopathology of the telangiectasias associated with varicose veins. Dermatologia 1963;*127*:321–329.

26. Chant ADB: The effects of posture, exercise and bandage pressure on the clearance of 24Na from the subcutaneous tissues of the foot. Br J Surg 1972;*59*:552–555.

27. Dick ET: The treatment of varicose veins. NZ Med J 1966;*65*:310–313.

28. Monroe P, Morrow CF Jr, Millen E, Fairman RP, Glauser FL: Acute respiratory failure after sodium morrhuate esophageal sclerotherapy. Gastroenterology 1983;*85*:693–699.

29. Lewis KM: Anaphylaxis due to sodium morrhuate. JAMA 1936;*107*:1298.

30. Dodd H, Oldham JB: Surgical treatment of varicose veins. Lancet 1940;*1*:8–10.

31. Shelley J: Allergic manifestations with injection treatment of varicose veins: Death following injection of monoethanolamine oleate. JAMA 1939;*112*:1792–1794.

32. Meyer NE: Monoethanolamine oleate: A new chemical for obliteration of varicose veins. Am J Surg 1938;*40*:628–629.

33. Hedberg SE, Fowler DL, Ryan LR: Injection sclerotherapy of esophageal varices using ethanolamine oleate: A pilot study. Am J Surg 1982;*143*:426–431.

34. Product insert. Research Triangle Park, NC, Glaxo Pharmaceuticals, 1989.

35. Foote RR: Severe reaction to monoethanolamine oleate. Lancet 1944;*2*:390–391.

36. Reid RG, Rothine NG: Treatment of varicose veins by compression sclerotherapy. Br J Surg 1968;*55*:889–895.

37. Goldman MP, Bennett RG: Treatment of telangiectasia: A review. J Am Acad Dermatol 1987; *17*:167–182.

38. Steinberg MH: Evaluation of sotradecol in sclerotherapy of varicose veins. Angiology 1955; *6*:519–532.

39. Nabatoff RA: Recent trends in the diagnosis and treatment of varicose veins. Surg Gynecol Obstet 1950;*90*:521–528.

40. Fegan G: Varicose Veins: Compression Sclerotherapy. London, William Heinemann Medical Books Ltd, 1967.

41. Fronek H, Fronek A, Saltzbarg G: Allergic reactions to sotradecol. J Dermatol Surg Oncol 1989; *15*:684.

42. Mantse L: The treatment of varicose veins with compression sclerotherapy: Technique, con-traindictions, complications. Am J Cosmetic Surg 1986;*3*:47–53.

43. MacGowan WAL, Holland PDJ, Browne HI, Byrnes DP: The local effects of intra-arterial in-jections of sodium tetradecyl sulphate (S.T.D.) 3 per cent. Br J Surg 1972;*59*:101–104.

44. Ouvry P, Chandet A, Guillerot E: First impressions of aethoxysklerol. Phlebologie 1978;*31*:75–77.

45. Jaquier JJ, Loretan RM: Clinical trials of a new sclerosing agent, aethoxysklerol. Soc Fran Phleb 1969;*22*:383–385.

46. Ouvry P, Arlaud R: Le traitement sclerosant des telangiectasies des membres inferieurs. Phle-bologie 1979;*32*:365–370.

47. Wallois P: Incidents et accidents de la sclerose. *In* Tournay R, ed: La Sclerose des Varices, ed 4. Paris, Expansion Scientifique Francaise, 1985;297–319.

48. Sigg K, Horodegen K, Bernbach H: Varizen-Sklerosierung: Welchos ist das wirUsamste Mittel? Deutsohes Arzteblatt 1986;*34/35*:2294–2298.

49. Wenner L: Anwendung einer mit Athylalkohol modifizierten Polijodidjonenlosung bei sklero-seresistenten Varizen. Vasa 1983;*12*:190–192.

50. Smith L, Johnson MA: Incidence of pulmonary embolism after venous sclerosing therapy. Minn Med 1948;*31*:270–272.

51. Natali J, Marmasse J: Enquete sur le traitement chirugical des varices. Phlebologie 1962;*15*:232–284.

52. Sigg K: Zur Behandlung der Varicen Phlebitis und ihrer Komplikationen. Der Hautarzt 1950;*1–2*:443–450.

17

THE TREATMENT OF VULVAL AND PELVIC VARICES

John T. Hobbs

Varicose veins in the perivulval area are a common, although not frequently recognized, disorder. Vulval varices are reported as being present in between 2 and 10 per cent of pregnancies (1,2). They usually appear suddenly after the second month of a second pregnancy and become more marked and persistent with subsequent pregnancies. After each delivery the veins become less apparent, especially on the vulva. In 4676 patients seen in my Vein Clinic during the period 1964 to 1972, 4 per cent of the women were noted to have varicose veins in the perivulval region (3).

Almost half of perivulval varicose veins arise from an incompetent long saphenous vein via the superficial external pudendal or posteromedial tributaries (Fig. 17–1), and these are cured by treatment involving the saphenofemoral junction and the leg veins. In rare instances veins on the vulva may be associated with venous malformations on the labia, clitoral area, or vagina with or without arteriovenous malformations on the limbs or trunk. Occasionally vulval varices are found in association with cancer of the cervix or uterine body. Rarely they may be associated with crossover collaterals of occluded deep veins following pelvic vein thrombosis. Sometimes the pelvic symptoms are minimal and the veins are seen to arise from the internal iliac veins via the internal pudendal, obturator, or inferior gluteal veins; phleboliths may be present, suggesting the possibility of previous venous thrombosis. Rarely the veins arise from the round ligament, mimicking varicocele in the male.

Often the perivulval veins are asymptomatic, apart from the disfigurement caused by their presence, or symptoms may be related to the leg veins. However, there is an important group of women with troublesome symptoms who need to be identified because treatment is relatively simple and cure is usually permanent, even despite further pregnancies. The symptoms are those of the pelvic congestion syndrome, and this has been shown to be associated with gross dilatation and incompetence of the ovarian veins. Sometimes the communications to veins in the thigh are the reentry routes from reflux down the ovarian veins.

INVESTIGATIONS

When the clinical examination reveals atypical varices on the buttock or upper posteromedial thigh radiating from the perivulval region, further investigations

250

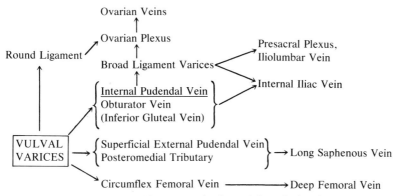

Figure 17–1. The communications of the vulval varices.

are indicated to demonstrate the proximal communications of these veins. Non-invasive investigations are preferred, at least as an initial screening, before invasive methods are used. The methods used include the following.

Pelvic Ultrasound Examination

This simple noninvasive test was used in a series of 50 patients as a potential screening method. It required the patient to drink a liter of water an hour before the examination so that the bladder was full. This fluid-filled "cystic" space created an ultrasonic window and provided a suitable reference. The method could not be used if there were poor renal function or if the patient were unable to retain urine. With the patient lying supine, serial transverse pictures were obtained at 1- to 2-cm intervals. The uterus and ovaries were easily seen but the presence or absence of varices in the broad ligament did not correlate with the venographic studies. In a significant number of patients varices were not seen during the ultrasound examination, but were subsequently demonstrated by other methods.

Laparoscopy and Laparotomy

Laparoscopy is now a routine examination for the investigation of pelvic pain and can identify pelvic inflammatory disease, polycystic ovaries, and endometriosis. Sometimes during this examination dilated veins are seen in the broad ligament and hilum of the ovary, but the ovarian veins cannot be seen because of their retroperitoneal position. Similarly, during laparotomy the broad ligament varices are easily seen but again the ovarian veins are less obvious.

Vulval Varicography

This simple procedure has been used in more than 500 patients presenting with perivulval varices. Initially it was used as an outpatient screening examination but, although distal communications were usually well demonstrated, it sometimes failed to reveal varices in the broad ligaments or dilated ovarian veins, which were later seen on direct venography. The contrast media used initially (Conray 70 per cent; Hypaque 45 per cent) were thrombogenic, and some patients claimed that their symptoms were reduced by this procedure and in some the varices on the upper thigh disappeared. For reasons of safety, nonionic contrast medium (Niopam 300) is now used (4,5). When perivulval varices are not associated with the pelvic congestion syndrome and treatment is confined to the leg veins, per-operative varicography is used to accurately locate the proximal communications.

Per-uterine Venography

This technique was first described in 1925 by Heinen and Siegel (6) and has since been reported by several European and American authors. It involves the injection of 20 ml of contrast medium into the muscular wall of the fundus of the uterus through a special needle. With modern contrast media this examination has become a rapid, safe, and painless outpatient procedure. Although large varices are seen in the broad ligament, the ovarian veins are not always filled, even with unilateral pressure over the iliac fossa. In some patients studied by this method the ovarian veins were not seen, but when these patients were investigated by selective ovarian venography grossly dilated ovarian veins were demonstrated.

Duplex Ultrasound and Color Flow Imaging

Blood flow in peripheral vessels can be demonstrated by examination with Doppler ultrasound and particularly duplex scanning. Furthermore, if color flow imaging is used the direction of flow is clearly demonstrated. Arteries appear as intermittent pulsating red images and the veins as blue conduits. Reflux in the veins appears as red when it is induced. This technique has been shown to be of particular value in the popliteal fossa. G. Richardson, in Wagga Wagga, Australia (personal communication, 1988) has much experience with color flow imaging and has recently demonstrated an ultrasound window in the loin that can be used to visualize the ovarian vein and demonstrate its size and the presence or absence of reflux. This technique may therefore be used as a noninvasive screening test for selecting patients for study by selective ovarian venography.

Selective Ovarian Venography

It is essential to demonstrate the ovarian veins in women suffering from the pelvic congestion syndrome. A Seldinger catheter is introduced into the right femoral vein and passed to the gonadal veins. Both ovarian veins and their proximal valves are demonstrated. Reflux is confirmed by a Valsalva maneuver; on tilting to the erect position contrast may pass down through the pelvic varicosities to the vulval varices and sometimes to the legs.

TREATMENT

Vulval varices are most marked during pregnancy and may cause irritation and discomfort, particularly heaviness when standing. Rarely they rupture spontaneously, resulting in a large vulval hematoma. Occasionally the varices may tear and bleed profusely during delivery.

Since vulval varices rapidly disappear, after delivery treatment should be symptomatic. During pregnancy the symptoms are usually controlled by firm support using stretch pants and localizing the applied pressure with sanitary pads. If the pain is not relieved by these simple measures the varices can be treated by injection. The veins are injected at several sites with small volumes (0.25 ml) of 3 per cent sodium tetradecyl sulfate (Sotradecol, STD, Trombovar), great care being taken to ensure that all sclerosant is placed in the lumen. Two sanitary pads are then applied and held in place with strong elastic pants. The veins cease to be tender after about 2 weeks and after several more weeks the thrombosed veins disappear.

If during pregnancy gross saphenofemoral reflux is present and the vulval veins communicate with it, then simple ligation under local anesthesia is safe and markedly reduces the vulval varicosities and edema. In general the policy is to avoid interventional treatment during pregnancy. If vulval and perivulval varices persist after pregnancy treatment is indicated when the patient so desires.

The perivulval varices may be a disfigurement without leg varices or pelvic symptoms. In this case they are easily eliminated by sclerotherapy as described previously. If associated with leg varices, particularly incompetence of the long saphenous vein, then surgery is the method of choice. After dealing with the long saphenous vein, the veins in the upper medial thigh can be removed by avulsion through small incisions, or better by the Müller techniques since the minute stab wounds do not require suture and leave no visible mark. When treated by surgery an on-table venogram will demonstrate the perineal connections, which can be identified and ligated to prevent bleeding. Any residual varices after surgery can be obliterated by sclerotherapy.

Varicose veins on the vulva and in the vagina with local vascular malformations or Klippel-Trenaunay lesions on the adjacent leg respond well to treatment by sclerotherapy.

Sometimes perivulval varices are associated with varices in the broad ligaments and symptoms of the pelvic congestion syndrome. When pelvic symptoms and varices are present, further investigations and treatment are required to prevent recurrence of leg varices and to eliminate the pelvic symptoms.

PELVIC CONGESTION SYNDROME

Many women experience pelvic pain in association with normal physiologic events such as ovulation, menstruation, coitus, and pregnancy. Other conditions giving rise to pelvic pain include infection, urinary tract disease, large bowel problems, orthopedic conditions, and genital lesions. Many generations of gynecologists have recognized a group of patients whose problem is chronic pelvic pain without evidence of inflammation or other obvious pathology; several causes have been postulated (3).

The pelvic congestion syndrome is a distinct clinical entity that is often overlooked (7). The varicosities may be confined to the perivulval area and buttocks or may involve the whole leg. Some patients have had repeated surgical treatment of leg veins without success because the proximal incompetence at the vulva was not recognized. Other patients present with pelvic pain but no gross external varices. Typically there is pelvic pain, of variable intensity, which is worse premenstrually and greatly increased by fatigue, standing, and especially coitus. Bladder irritability presenting as urgency rather than frequency is often present as a result of varicosities in the region of the trigone. When all investigations and specialist referrals have failed to find an explanation for the symptoms the general practitioner and the husband become less sympathetic and the patient's anxiety is increased. The final referral is then to the psychiatrist.

However, on examination varicosities are present on one or both sides of the vulva and these veins extend onto the medial aspect of the upper thigh behind the adductor tendon. Distally these veins may result in varicosities in the territory of the long saphenous system, yet the proximal long saphenous vein in the femoral triangle is normal. Often the varices spread across the posterior surface of the upper thigh and extend down to the popliteal fossa or lateral calf. They may communicate with the short saphenous vein through the Guacomini vein. Dilated veins may extend over the buttocks. These patients describe a sensation of perineal heaviness and dyspareunia. Retroversion of the uterus is frequently present.

Early Methods of Treatment and Development of Etiologic Theory

Although the pelvic congestion syndrome has been intermittently recognized for many years the treatment has been unsatisfactory because the etiology was not recognized. As different theories were postulated, so different groups of workers employed various methods with variable results.

The early gynecologic treatments concentrated on malposition of the uterus. Because it was thought that retroversion caused venous obstruction by kinking of the broad ligaments, a ventrosuspension operation was performed. Some gynecologists have also resorted to hysterectomy. Lately simpler solutions such as psychotherapy, ovarian suppression, and even oophorectomy have been used (8) without success. However, hysterectomy is probably effective in reducing the pelvic varices by mechanical interruption of the vessels.

It is now clear that some vulval varices and even recurrent leg varices arise from broad ligament varices, and when the typical history of the pelvic congestion syndrome exists it can be shown to be due to gross reflux in the ovarian veins. In these patients the ovarian veins must be visualized by selective ovarian venography. If grossly dilated, effective treatment is elimination of this reflux in addition to removal of the leg varices when present. In the treatment of leg varices the effective surgical treatment requires ligation of the superficial veins at their proximal source (i.e., where the perforating vein joins the deep system). If this is so, then ligation of the ovarian veins must be the correct treatment for the pelvic congestion syndrome.

Because Swedish workers could only demonstrate the left ovarian vein 20 years ago, they considered the pelvic congestion syndrome analogous to varicocele in the male and so only operated on the left side (9). The results reported were not highly successful and so this treatment was abandoned.

In South and Central America patients were frequently seen who have had multiple pregnancies, and in many of these the uterus is found to be enlarged and congested. Treatment in Brazil in this situation is by hysterectomy (10), which obviously reduces the vascularity of the broad ligaments and ovarian plexuses. When the uterus is not enlarged treatment is confined to the broad ligament and vulval varices. In Brazil the transperitoneal approach is used to either ligate the broad ligament varices or perform hysterectomy. A Mexican group (11) has used the retroperitoneal approach to ligate the incompetent pelvic veins and have combined this with sclerotherapy or local excision of the vulval veins.

For many years I have been studying this problem (7), as has Lechter in Columbia (12), and we independently came to the conclusion that retrograde flow in the ovarian veins was the primary problem and effective treatment must therefore eliminate this reflux. In a series of 50 patients Lechter and colleagues (13) have shown that multiple full-term pregnancies (four to 14; mean six) may cause enlargement of ovarian and pelvic veins, and reflux from these can explain vulval varices and the appearance of varices in the inner and posterior aspect of the upper thigh. Treatment by resection of the ovarian veins with ligation of the veins communicating to the uterine veins, plus vulval and leg varicectomy, gave excellent results. Lechter et al. were only able to catheterize the right ovarian veins in 13 of the 45 patients subjected to selective venography.

At operation they found dilated uteroovarian veins with no valve function, plexiform veins in the broad ligaments, and vulval varices. They used a retroperitoneal approach to expose and ligate the ovarian veins, bilaterally in 32 patients, right side only in 12, and left side only in six. During the period 1984–5 they only ligated the ovarian vein on the side involved, but then became convinced that both sides need to be treated because of the rich cross-communications in the pelvis.

I have also become convinced during the investigations and treatment of more than 500 women with vulval varices over a 20-year period that in selected cases the problem was due to incompetence of grossly dilated ovarian veins, and so, like Lechter, I now perform ovarian vein ligation (7).

Surgical Treatment: Ovarian Vein Ligation

When either or both of the ovarian veins have been shown to be grossly dilated and there are significant leg and vulval varices or bothersome symptoms of the pelvic congestion syndrome, an operation is offered to the patient. This operation involves a brief hospital stay and is relatively minor, with a rapid recovery because the peritoneal cavity is not entered. The ovarian veins are exposed through the retroperitoneal route and the left side is usually operated on first. The patient is placed in the supine position and a slight lateral table roll is helpful to give a better exposure of the retroperitoneal structures. A transverse incision is made in the crease line starting a thumb's breadth inside and above the anterior superior iliac spine and extending to the lateral border of the rectus sheath.

In thin patients a 3-inch long incision is sufficient, but for fatter patients a larger incision makes access easier. The muscles are split in a gridiron approach. Careful hemostasis ensures a clear field and avoids hematoma formation. The peritoneum is gently pushed forward until the psoas muscle is seen, as in the approach to lumbar sympathectomy. The ovarian vein is then seen as a longitudinal, wide, blue-colored vessel firmly embedded in the fascia and peritoneal fat. It may be surprisingly large and on the right side can be mistaken for the inferior vena cava. The vein is gently separated by sharp and blunt dissection, care being taken not to enter the peritoneal space.

The ureter must always be identified and will be found running posterior and medial to the ovarian vein. Large vessels may be present around the ureter, and sometimes these veins are in communication with the ovarian vein. The left ovarian vein is freed proximally up to the medial border of the lower pole of the kidney, where it is clamped and carefully divided between ligatures below the left renal vein. The ovarian vein is then reflected distally, dividing any communications. At the ovary the vein divides into at least two or three tributaries, and sometimes as many as six or seven, as it forms the ovarian plexus. These vessels are divided separately and a 3-inch length of vein is removed. Although the South Americans have recommended extending the dissection down into the broad ligament and pelvis, I consider this unnecessary. After ensuring that the wound is dry, it is closed in layers and with fine interrupted nylon to skin. Drainage is not used. A similar operation is then performed on the right side after rolling the table. Here care is taken because of the fragile union of the right ovarian vein and inferior vena cava. Having dealt with the incompetent ovarian veins, any varices present on the legs are then removed using the Müller technique and sometimes partial stripping.

The morning after surgery the abdominal wounds and any leg wounds are covered with short lengths of 1-inch micropore tape. Appropriate support stockings are applied to the legs after removing the bandages, and the patient is encouraged to walk every half hour and to sit out of bed. Urinary function is not disturbed, and the patient is discharged home on the second or third postoperative day. The sutures are removed a week later. The recovery is remarkably uneventful, and a patient who had a very severe pain with her periods noted how painless the period was during the postoperative week.

Recently a patient with severe symptoms making it difficult to stand during her third pregnancy found her life changed after ligation of the ovarian veins, and a fourth pregnancy was successful with no discomfort and no recurrence of the pelvic congestion syndrome.

Conclusion

It has been demonstrated that the pelvic congestion syndrome is due to incompetence of one or both of the ovarian veins, and this condition may also explain some recurrent leg vein problems. Ligation of the ovarian veins, which is a relatively simple and safe procedure, provides an effective cure for this disabling condition.

REFERENCES

1. Dixon JA, Mitchell WA: Venographic and surgical observations in vulval varicose veins. Surg Gynecol Obstet 1970;*131*:458–464.
2. Dodd H, Payling Wright H: Vulval varicose veins in pregnancy. Br Med J 1959;*1*:831–832.
3. Hobbs JT: The pelvic congestion syndrome. Practitioner 1976;*216*:529–540.
4. Katayama H, Kozuka T, Takashima T, Matsuura K, Yamaguchi K: Clinical survey on adverse reactions of iodinated contrast media—interim report. Nippon Igaku Hoshasen Gakkai Zasshi–Nippon Acta Radiologica 1988; *48*(2):214–216.
5. Palmer FJ: The RACR survey of intravenous contrast media reactions. Final report. Aust Radiol 1988;*32*:426–428.
6. Heinen G, Siegel D: Zur Frage des lokalen kontrast. Mittel Schadigung bei der Uterus Phlebography. Z Clin Gynak 1925;*87*:829.
7. Hobbs JT: The pelvic congestion syndrome. Br J Hosp Med 1990;*43*:200–206.

8. Beard RW, Reginalds PW, Pearce S: Pelvic pain in women. Br Med J 1986;*293*:1160–1162.
9. Edlundh KO: Pelvic varicosities in women. Acta Obstet Gynecol Scand 1964;*43*:399–407.
10. Figueiroa CLS: In 1st Congress of the Phlebology Society of Brasil, Recife, 23–26 November, 1988
11. Gomez ER, Villavicencio JL, Le Page P, Coffey J, Solander SM, Rich NM: The transperitoneal approach to the management of the pelvic varices, an anatomical clinical correlation [abstr]. American European Venous Symposium, Washington, 31 March–2 April.
12. Lechter A: Pelvic varices: Treatment. J Cardiovasc Surg 1985;*26*:111.
13. Lechter A, Alvarey A, Lopez G: Pelvic varices and gonadal veins. Phlebology 1987;*2*:181–188.

VI

SURGERY OF CHRONIC VENOUS INSUFFICIENCY

18

VALVE REPAIR AND SEGMENT TRANSPOSITION IN PRIMARY VALVULAR INSUFFICIENCY

Robert L. Kistner

The concept of direct surgical repair in carefully selected patients with incompetence of the deep veins in the lower extremity has evolved over the past two decades. The reason for performing surgical reconstruction in deep vein incompetence is to relieve the symptoms and improve the functional capacity of persons afflicted with the pain, swelling, and stasis changes of chronic venous insufficiency (CVI) states.

While nonsurgical management, consisting of elastic support, bed rest, and life-style change, can control the patient's symptoms, it does not correct the underlying problem and tends to impose restrictions on the individual's normal activities. Surgical repair, on the other hand, is designed to sufficiently correct the defect itself so the patient can return to full activity while remaining free of ulceration and pain.

To accomplish this goal, the surgical approach must be based upon thorough diagnosis of the abnormalities encountered in each clinical case. This diagnosis requires clinical, physiologic, and radiologic study of the extremity to plan the surgical approach that will produce maximal correction of the abnormalities in that leg.

RATIONALE OF SURGERY FOR PROXIMAL DEEP VEIN INCOMPETENCE

When valvular incompetence affects all the valves in the lower extremity veins, the erect patient has a column of blood extending from the heart level to the ankle in which to-and-fro motion of the blood occurs with the pumping action of the calf muscle. This leads to mechanical inefficiency for the venous return because some of the blood that is pumped by the calf during systole tends to reflux back down the leg during diastole. In this situation, restoring even a single competent valve along the course of the femoropopliteal vein cuts the incompetent column of blood from heart to ankle approximately in half and increases the mechanical efficiency of the calf pumping action by restoring one-way flow in the proximal vessels. However, restoring femoral vein valve function does not repair the incompetent perforator veins of the calf, nor does it repair the incompetent superficial veins in the lower leg. The management of these problems remains an important part of treatment and is best effected by conventional surgical measures for both the saphenous and the perforator veins when they are grossly abnormal.

Obstruction of the deep veins due to thrombophlebitis is often regarded as the major element in causing lower leg ulcers and stasis syndromes. This is incorrect. The major problem found in most patients with venous leg ulcers and stasis syndromes is loss of valve function rather than obstruction. As pointed out by Homans in 1916 (1) and Linton in 1952 (2), in most cases the obstructive phase of deep vein thrombophlebitis (DVT) is soon followed by recanalization of greater or lesser degree. The lingering problem that eventually leads to chronic stasis and ulcers is the loss of valvular function in the postthrombotic patient, just as it is in the patient with primary valvular incompetence.

The advent of careful diagnostic work-up of large groups of patients with chronic venous problems defines three distinct causes of valvular insufficiency. In addition to postthrombotic recanalization, primary valvular incompetence (PVI) and total aplasia of venous valves are identified. Aplasia is a rare but definite entity. PVI (3) is increasingly recognized as a frequent problem by those who perform descending venography in their CVI patients.

CONCEPT OF PRIMARY VALVULAR INCOMPETENCE

Primary valvular incompetence refers to a state in which the venous valves in the lower extremity are incompetent even though they are normally formed. They show no evidence of disease, such as thickening, scarring, or constriction. In PVI, the leading edge of the valve cusp has been found to be elongated, or stretched, and this elongated cusp causes incompetence because it prolapses when pressure is applied from above. The cause of the condition is not known. It may be due to stress or could reflect a basic weakness of the tissue itself. The process most resembles the stretched membrane of a hernia, in that the cusp is a stretched, normal membrane that responds to repair by surgical shortening. The prolapsing state is repaired by tightening up the leading edge of the valve, after which the valve is restored to normal function. In many of these patients, there is also thinning and stretching of the vein wall adjacent to the valve cusps, which responds to tightening of the outer wall of the vein at the level of the cusps.

PVI was first reported in a large group of patients by Bauer in 1948; he called it idiopathic incompetence (4). He found that nearly half of his patients with CVI had never had DVT, but did have severe venous reflux. Bauer was the first to perform descending venography in a large series of patients. Since he did not operate directly on the valves, his description of the condition was clinical and radiographic. Other sporadic reports of the condition appeared in the 1940s and 1950s (5,6).

The actual morphology of the stretched valve cusp was clarified by the successful surgical repair of incompetent valves in 1968 (7). At that time the existence of the stretched valve cusps was proven by direct observation, and the repair of these valves by shortening the cusps was accomplished. These findings have been corroborated by many surgeons, who have operated upon the stretched valve cusps and have repaired the incompetence state (7–10).

The recognition of PVI in a series of patients with severe venous insufficiency varies widely. There are multiple series in which PVI is present in 30 to 60 per cent of the cases (4,8,9,11) and there are other series in which PVI is rarely, if ever, found. Perhaps this difference is due to a variation in the technique of descending venography or to some mystery of patient selection.

In addition to those with pure PVI, many patients have proximal PVI in the superficial femoral vein, and distal postphlebitic valvular incompetence in the tibial and popliteal and even the distal superficial femoral veins. When valvular incompetence is limited to the thigh, the patient is usually asymptomatic and does not require surgical correction. When the distal veins also become incompetent, however, symptoms of CVI usually follow. This is true whether the distal incompetence is due to PVI or to postthrombotic recanalization. The occurrence of proximal PVI with distal postthrombotic incompetence is frequent enough to even suggest that proximal PVI may predispose to DVT in the lower leg. Further study of the natural history of these events is warranted.

The literature suggests that valvular incompetence limited to the tibial veins is likely to be well tolerated by the patient, but incompetence of the entire lower extremity deep venous system is poorly tolerated (12). While some patients have venous ulceration and stasis disease on the basis of deep venous incompetence limited to the calf, more frequently severe CVI patients have incompetence of the entire deep system.

DIAGNOSIS

The diagnosis of PVI requires descending venography to demonstrate the position and function of the individual valves. However, this is the last step in the work-up of the patient with chronic venous ulcers or stasis disease because it is the most complex.

An organized approach is needed to evaluate patients with advanced CVI. We classify the clinical state as mild, moderate, or severe. Particular attention is paid to finding out if the patient's normal life-style or occupation is limited by the venous disease, because these are the patients who may benefit from venous reconstruction. In the office, all patients are studied with Doppler, and valvular incompetence is mapped by using the Valsalva maneuver and local compressions throughout the extremity. A test of venous physiology, such as photoplethysmography, foot volumetry, or venous pressure, is an important step to separate true venous problems from other causes of leg symptoms.

The color flow duplex scan is now our choice as the best laboratory screening test for patency and competence of the deep venous system. It is accurate in identifying valvular incompetence in the separate veins of the extremity [e.g., the greater saphenous vein (GSV), superficial femoral vein (SFV), and profunda femoris vein (PFV)], and the degree of incompetence can be semiquantitated with this equipment. By using Valsalva and compression maneuvers, further localization of incompetent segments up and down the extremity can be observed.

Ascending venography confirms deep vein patency and defines anatomy, and, if done with ankle tourniquets and fluoroscopy, is the best test for defining incompetent perforator veins.

Descending venography (13) is performed with the patient semi-erect on a table adapted to fluoroscopy and capable of recording the study on videotape. The study must demonstrate the position of valves in the SFV, PFV, and GSV. Valve competence is defined as a valve that prevents reflux when the patient performs a forced Valsalva maneuver by blowing a pressure manometer over 30 mm Hg. When reflux occurs during Valsalva, its distal extent is traced by fluoroscopy and recorded on videotape.

After the patient is evaluated in this manner, the surgeon has a thorough knowledge of the anatomy and function in the venous system of the extremity. Patency and competence will have been checked in each segment of the venous tree, and the position and function of all proximal competent valves will be known. Based upon these findings the surgeon is able to devise a treatment program to address the specific problems of a given extremity. The treatment of venous incompetence should fit these specific problems. When a patient has severe saphenous incompetence, the GSV should be ligated. When there are large perforators with gross incompetence, they should be ligated. When the deep system is grossly incompetent, it should be repaired.

PLANNING THE SURGICAL REPAIR

Deep venous surgical reconstruction should be limited to the patient with a severe clinical syndrome who has a repairable problem and whose activity level has been seriously impaired by the disease. Patients who are inactive can be managed well nonsurgically. Valvuloplasty techniques are only applicable in patients who have PVI because the postphlebitic valve is scarred and shortened and cannot be repaired. The choice of reconstructive procedure for postphlebitic cases includes transposition of involved veins to adjacent veins that have competent proximal valves, or transplantation of veins that contain a competent functioning venous valve into the superficial femoral or popliteal vein.

SURGICAL TECHNIQUE OF VALVULOPLASTY

Three internal techniques (7,13,14) and two external techniques (15,16) are available to render an incompetent valve competent in PVI. In each of the internal techniques, the stretched leading edge of the valve cusp is shortened by suturing this edge to the vein wall. The differences in technique are based upon three different approaches to the commissure of the valve. In contrast, the external techniques reinforce the wall of the vein at the level of the valve cusp. Their mechanism of action is less well understood but probably involves deepening the valve cusp and reinforcing the weak vein wall.

Internal Techniques

The original technique for valve repair was first performed in 1968 and the first series of cases was reported in 1975 (17). In this method (7) the valve is exposed by a longitudinal incision directly through the commissure of the valve. The venotomy incision begins below the valve and is carried up directly between

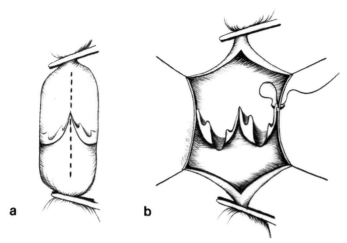

Figure 18–1. Internal valvuloplasty by Kistner method. *A*, Vertical incision through commissure. *B*, View of floppy valve after venotomy.

the cusps, through the commissure, and into the proximal vein. When the vein is opened the valve structure is clearly exposed and its morphology can be directly observed (Fig. 18–1). A precise anatomic repair can be done by placing interrupted sutures at the commissure. The sutures catch a segment of the stretched leading edge of the cusp and secure this edge to the side wall of the vein. The floppy elongated valve cusp is progressively shortened by a series of interrupted sutures at each commissure until the redundancy in the leading edge is corrected and the valve cusp lies straight across the face of the vein. The repair is anatomic and precise; 7-0 monofilament suture is used for the repair, which is done under loupe magnification.

The modification of this valvuloplasty by Raju (14) is done by a transverse venotomy made cephalad to the valve (Fig. 18–2), so the surgeon is looking down on the valve during repair. This is an easier venotomy but it may be more difficult to see the morphology of the valve. Time and care are needed to identify the leading edges of the valve cusp where the sutures will be placed. Stay sutures

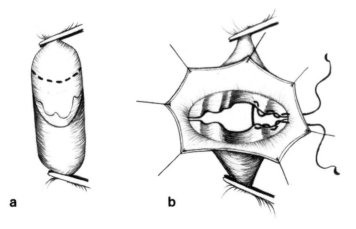

Figure 18–2. Internal valvuloplasty by Raju method. *A*, Horizontal incision above valve. *B*, View of valve from above and suture placement after venotomy.

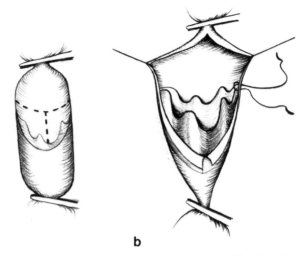

a   b

Figure 18–3.   Internal valvuloplasty by Sottiurai method. *A*, T-shaped incision above valve. *B*, View of valve during repair.

are used to stretch the vein open during repair. Repair is done with a fine suture placed in the edge of the two opposing valve cusps. The suture snakes along the valve edge and is brought out through the vein wall, where it is tied on the outside of the vein.

A third method, described by Sottiurai (10), combines elements of the first two procedures (Fig. 18–3). The venotomy is made transversely, cephalad to the valve, and is similar to the incision of Raju. Then a vertical incision is made down into the base of the cusp (Fig. 18–3). This affords a clear view of the valve cusps and the commissure on both sides. Repair is with interrupted sutures at the commissures placed under direct vision, in a manner similar to the interrupted sutures of the Kistner method.

The choice of operation is one of individual preference. Each repair is effective if done properly. The advantage of the internal approach is that it effects a precise repair of the prolapsing valve cusp, and its long-term record has been established in the literature as being 65 to 80 per cent successful over a 4-year follow-up (8,9,11,18). The disadvantages of the internal repair are that the operation is technically more demanding than the external approach and the opened vein makes anticoagulants important perioperatively.

External Techniques

The external approaches to valve repair were developed recently and their long-term effectiveness is yet to be established. Two external repairs are under trial, one by external suture and the other by an external cuff appliance.

The external suture technique has been used for 2 years. It consists of a series of interrupted 6-0 or 7-0 sutures placed along the decussating margin of the line of valve insertion on both sides of the vein (Figs. 18–4 and 18–5). The first suture is placed at the commissure and successive sutures are distal, each one progressing down the vein, coapting the margins of valve origin as they descend toward the base of the cusp. The suturing is done on both sides of the vein, beginning at the

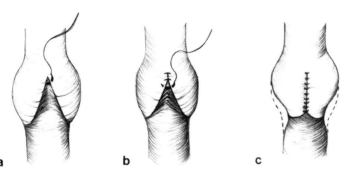

Figure 18–4.   External repair: view from outside vein. *A,* Suture engages one side of valve insertion. *B,* Third suture engaging both sides of valve insertion. *C,* Suture line completed, with mild narrowing of vein. From The Straub Foundation Proceedings, 1990;55:15.

commissure on each side. The end point is reached when the valve becomes competent; this is determined by releasing the proximal clamp and checking for valve competence. Usually five to seven sutures on each side of the vein are required to achieve competence; the lowest one to two sutures may produce a mild narrowing of the outside wall of the vein that approximates 20 to 30 per cent of the diameter of the vein. This technique results in a deeper, narrower valve pocket that prevents prolapse of the floppy cusp margin (Fig. 18–5). It also reinforces the vein wall by invaginating the often dilated weak vein wall that in some patients has developed between the decussating margins of the valve insertion.

The technique using an external cuff (Venocuff) was devised by Lane in Australia (16). It consists of a Silastic external cuff placed around the vein at the site of the valve. This cuff is tightened around the valve until the valve becomes competent. The technique was developed through extensive laboratory testing in an animal model and is now in clinical trial.

The advantages of external repairs are their simplicity and the fact that anticoagulants are unnecessary because the vein is not opened. Multiple valves can readily be done in a single operation, which may improve the results of deep vein reconstructive surgery.

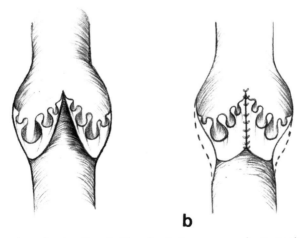

Figure 18–5.   External repair: view from inside vein. *A,* Appearance prior to repair showing divergence of valve margins. *B,* After repair, valve cusp is deeper and narrower. From The Straub Foundation Proceedings, 1990;55:15.

Results of Valvuloplasty for PVI

Direct reconstruction in PVI has been done long enough by a sufficient number of surgeons that we now know its 4-year results. Our report in 1982 (11) gave 4-year results (range, 1 to 13 years) in 32 cases. Raju reported results of his technique in 61 cases in 1988 (8), with follow-up longer than 2 yars. Eriksson reported a carefully worked-up series of 12 patients in 1986 who were followed for more than 3 years (9). In 1990, Sottiurai reported his 4-year results of 29 cases followed for 4.5 years (18).

In each of these series, careful preliminary work-up led to the operation and detailed objective follow-up included postoperative clinical and venographic testing. At 4 years (range, 2 to 13 years) of follow-up, these series all show 63 to 80 per cent good to excellent clinical results (Table 18–1). These patients have proven long-term competence of their repaired valves and have lived without recurrence of their ulcer or other stasis problems. In the 20 to 30 per cent of these patients in whom ulcers and symptoms have recurred, failure of the valve repair can usually be demonstrated. This correlation between clinical failure and recurrent valve leakage demonstrated by descending venography lends credence to the value of a competent proximal valve in these patients. Several of the patients in our series who have experienced recurrent postoperative valve leakage have had a second repair that has produced a good result.

In those patients who have good to excellent results we observe about 30 per cent who discard elastic support and still maintain an excellent result. We regard these patients as having been completely relieved of their venous insufficiency state.

All these investigations have observed a close relationship between the clinical results and competent valves found by postoperative venograms, but a rather poor correlation between the clinical state and postoperative physiologic tests, such as venous pressure and plethysmographic tests. This discrepancy is disappointing and must reflect continued abnormality in the deep veins in these patients. These patients are considered to be restored to a compensated state by the surgery, or to a state in which the residual abnormalities are compensated by the calf pump and by the complexity of the overall venous return system of the leg. Newer developments in the study of lower extremity hemodynamics may provide better means to estimate clinical improvement (19).

The causes of recurrence have been variable. Some were due to an inadequate original repair. In our series there was one recurrence that was due to a circumscribed hole in one valve cusp. When this hole was repaired, the patient achieved an excellent longer term result. Eriksson and Alzugren (9) reported the unexplained disappearance of the repaired valve in a few cases.

It is to be stressed that valve repair was used as just part of the treatment of complicated venous insufficiency for some of the patients in each of these

TABLE 18–1.   Valvuloplasty Results

	RAJU	SOTTIURAI	ERIKSSON	KISTNER
No. of valves repaired	61	29	12	32
Good results	63%	76%	67%	80%
Average follow-up (months)	24	56	36	72

series. All authors agree that the incompetent saphenous system requires treatment by ligation, with or without stripping of the GSV. Eriksson, Kistner, and Sottiurai selectively interrupted incompetent perforators in their patients, whereas Raju did not interrupt perforators. The role of perforators in these patients remains unclear.

The combination of saphenous and perforator surgery with valve repair has led to confusion and dispute as to whether the valve repair is truly responsible in many of the good results. In Eriksson's cases, the valve repair was only done after the patient had failed prior saphenous ligations and perforator interruptions. The same is true in some of the cases in both Sottiurai's and our series. In our series, we found some patients who required valve repair after saphenous and perforator surgery had failed; we also encountered the converse situation, in which saphenous or perforator surgery was necessary after valve repair did not completely control the insufficiency syndrome. Our present practice is to repair all systems that show severe incompetence in a given extremity. When the GSV has gross incompetence, it is ligated at the saphenofemoral junction. When perforators are both incompetent and grossly dilated, they are ligated. When perforators are incompetent but not grossly dilated, we use sclerotherapy. Valve repair is only used in patients with severe degrees of incompetence and advanced clinical syndromes.

TRANSPOSITION OF VENOUS SEGMENTS

The concept of transposing one venous segment that has no repairable proximal valve to an adjacent segment that has a normal proximal valve is called vein segment transposition (VST). This procedure was devised in 1977 to treat those patients who could not be managed by valve repair. This includes patients with postthrombotic destruction of the proximal SFV and PFV valves, and those with PVI in whom valve repair was not technically successful.

There are multiple technical possibilities for this procedure. Most frequently, an incompetent SFV is anastomosed to the PFV if it still has a good valve. Alternatively, the SFV could be transposed to the GSV when a good proximal valve is present in the GSV. In some cases, an incompetent PFV was transposed to the GSV when the SFV was occluded.

The transposition can be accomplished by end-to-end anastomosis, joining the distal incompetent vein segment to the competent proximal segment. It can also be done by placing the end of the incompetent distal segment into the side of the competent segment when there are both proximal and distal competent valves in the receiving segment (Fig. 18–6).

The experience with transposition surgery has been favorable in our series, with 70 per cent long-term good to excellent results at 2- to 4-year follow-up (11), but other series have had poor results (Table 18–2). In 1980, Queral et al. (20) reported excellent 1-year results with VST in cases in which perforator surgery was purposely not done; however, these patients showed clinical recurrence at an unacceptable rate 1 year later (21), indicating that VST does not replace perforator surgery. Raju (14) and Eriksson and Alzugren (9) found recurrence in their small series of three to four cases. Sottiurai found recurrence of valve reflux in 12 of 15 cases (18).

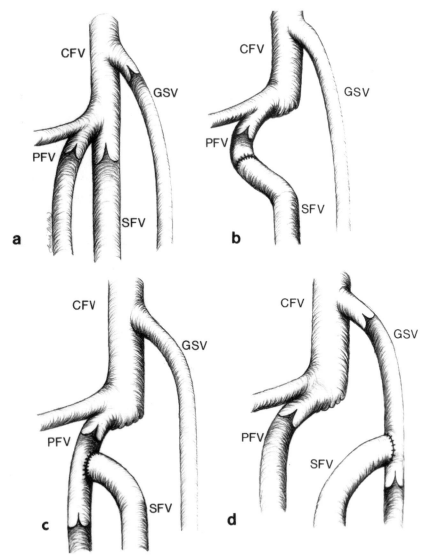

Figure 18–6. Transposition procedure. *A*, Normal anatomy. *B*, SFV-to-PFV transposition, end to end. *C*, SFV-to-PFV transposition, end to side. *D*, SFG-to-GSV transposition, end to side.

TABLE 18–2.   Transposition Results

	JOHNSON	SOTTIURAI	KISTNER
No. of operations	12	15	14
Good results	17%	20%	78%
Average follow-up (months)	24	66	36

The discrepancy in results with VST may reflect case selection and techniques of descending venography, or it may indicate that the receptor vein dilates with increased flow and renders the valve incompetent. It could be that a PFV valve that appears competent when the adjacent SFV has severe reflux actually is not competent when the refluxing SFV vein is no longer present and the PFV valve has to handle the whole load of the extremity.

The transposition procedure is a simple one and is often useful. However, it should not be generally used until it can be shown to function well in a sufficient number of patients. We continue to use it because our success rate with it remains high. For those who choose to try it, caution is choosing the patient is advised by careful selective preoperative venography and duplex scanning study, and by thorough testing of the valves at the time of surgery. As the Northwestern experience demonstrates (21), it is also necessary to perform appropriate ligations of incompetent saphenous and perforator veins.

GENERAL COMMENTS ON THE CONDUCT OF DEEP VEIN SURGERY

In the conduct of surgery on the deep veins several factors may be important. We always advocate the use of heparin during surgery for internal repairs, and think it may be advisable to continue its use in the first few postoperative days. Our practice in PVI cases is to use heparin during surgery and for the first 48 hr postoperatively, regulating the partial thromboplastin time to 1.5 times normal; this is followed by dextran for an additional 72 hr. In patients with prior DVT, we prefer heparin for 5 days and warfarin for 6 to 12 weeks because these patients are prone to develop recurrent DVT.

Surgery is done with wide exposure of the involved veins. Fine sutures and loupe magnification are important. The operating microscope may be an improvement but we have not used it.

With the advent of simpler techniques of valvuloplasty, such as external repair, the opportunity to repair multiple valves in a given extremity will be increased. One could look for improved results from repair of valves at different levels, such as SFV, PFV, popliteal, and tibial valves. Both the external suture technique and the Venocuff technique lend themselves to this idea.

Eriksson (22) has called attention to the incompetent PFV segment in patients with SFV-popliteal reflux. It is apparent that an incompetent PFV with large communication to the popliteal vein by way of PFV–popliteal collaterals will be an important cause of recurrent symptoms. We have identified such cases in our series and have successfully repaired them by eliminating the collaterals. This condition should be considered in the original surgical approach to the patient. Other solutions are to repair both the SFV and PFV valves, or to repair the distal popliteal or tibial valves.

CONCLUSIONS

Surgical repair of incompetent deep veins has now been done for over 20 years, and results from several important series have accumulated. Valvuloplasty by internal repair has shown consistent results in multiple series. Transposition surgery has a high failure rate in several series. New developments include external repair as a simplified method for PVI that will have wide appeal and permit repair of multiple valves in different segments, but results of the external repairs over time are not yet known. Primary valve incompetence has been established as a frequent problem that may stand alone as the cause of advanced venous insufficiency states or may coexist with postthrombotic valve destruction; it may even be an underlying predisposing agent of distal DVT in some patients. Deep valve repair is best usd in combination with ligation or sclerosis of grossly incompetent saphenous and perforator veins.

REFERENCES

1. Homans J: Operative treatment of varicose veins and ulcers. Surg Gynecol Obstet 1916;*22*:143–158.
2. Linton RR: Modern concepts in the treatment of the postphlebitic syndrome with ulceration of the lower extremity. Angiology 1952;*3*:431–439.
3. Kistner RL: Primary venous valve incompetence of the leg. Am J Surg 1980;*140*:218–224.
4. Bauer G: The etiology of leg ulcers and their treatment by resection of the popliteal vein. J Int Chir 1948;*8*:937–967.
5. Luke JC: The diagnosis of chronic enlargement of the leg with the description of a new syndrome. Surg Gynecol Obstet 1941;*73*:472–480.
6. Lockhart-Mummery HE, Smitham JH: Varicose ulcer: A study of the deep veins with special reference to retrograde venography. Br J Surg 1951;*38*:284–295.
7. Kistner RL: Transvenous repair of the incompetent femoral vein valve. *In* Bergan JJ, Yao JST, eds: Venous Problems. Chicago, Year Book Medical Publishers, 1978;493–509.
8. Raju S, Fredericks R: Valve reconstruction procedures for nonobstructive venous insufficiency: Rationale, techniques, and results in 107 procedures with 2-8 years follow-up. J Vasc Surg 1988;*7*:301–310.
9. Eriksson I, Alzugren B: Influence of the profunda femoris vein and venous hemodynamics of the limb. J Vasc Surg 1986;*4*:390–395.
10. Sottiurai VS: Technique in direct venous valvuloplasty. J Vasc Surg 1988;*8*:646–648.
11. Ferris EB, Kistner RL: Femoral vein reconstruction in the management of chronic venous insufficiency. Arch Surg 1982;*117*:1571–1579.
12. Burnand KG, O'Donnell TF, Thomas ML, et al: The relative importance of incompetent communicating veins in the production of varicose veins and venous ulcers. Surgery 1977;*82*:9–14.
13. Kistner RL, Fennui EB, Randhawa G, Kamida C: A method of performing descending venography. J Vasc Surg 1986;*4*:464–468.
14. Raju S: Valvuloplasty and valve transfer. Int Angiol 1985;*4*:419–424.
15. Kistner RL: Surgical technique external venous valve repair. The Straub Foundation Proceedings 1990;*55*:15–16.
16. Jessup G, Lane RJ: Repair of incompetent venous valves: A new technique. J Vasc Surg 1988;*8*:569–575.
17. Kistner RL: Surgical repair of the incompetent femoral valve. Arch Surg 1975;*110*:1336–1342.
18. Sottiurai VS: Comparison of the durability in valvuloplasty, vein transposition, and valve transplant. Presented at American Venous Forum, San Diego, California 2/23/90. J Cardiovasc Surg (submitted 1990).
19. Christopoulos D, Nicolaides AN, Szendro G: Venous reflux: Quantification and correlation with the clinical severity of chronic venous disease. Br J Surg 1988;*75*:352–356.
20. Queral LA, Whitehouse WM Jr, Flinn WR, et al: Surgical correction of chronic deep venous insufficiency by valvular transposition. Surgery 1980;*86*:688–695.
21. Johnson ND, Queral LA, Flinn WR, et al: Late objective assessment of venous valve surgery. Arch Surg 1981;*116*:1461–1466.
22. Eriksson I: Vein valve surgery for deep valvular incompetence. *In* Eklof B, Gjores JE, Theolesius O, Bergquist D, eds: Controversies in the Management of Venous Disorders. London, Butterworth Co, 1989.

19

POPLITEAL VEIN VALVE TRANSPLANTATION FOR DEEP VENOUS VALVULAR REFLUX: Rationale, Method, and Long-Term Clinical, Hemodynamic, and Anatomic Results

Thomas F. O'Donnell, Jr.

Although in the last several years interest in surgery for deep venous valvular incompetence has burgeoned, there are only a few series on this surgery available in the literature. Moreover, most fail to provide late anatomic and hemodynamic follow-up on the results of these procedures. To define the appropriate role of surgery for deep venous valvular incompetence several facts should be known:

1. The percentage of limbs with chronic venous insufficiency that have deep venous involvement.
2. The proportion of patients with valvular incompetence of the deep venous system rather than deep venous obstruction.
3. The anatomic level of valvular involvement.
4. The type, primary versus postthrombotic.
5. Appropriate indication for deep venous valvular reconstruction.
6. Immediate long-term clinical, hemodynamic, and anatomic results.

This chapter will explore these issues.

Table 19–1 summarizes the incidence of deep venous involvement in several series of patients evaluated for chronic venous insufficiency. From the outset it should be understood that bias enters into the selection of patients for the various series. Several of these reports are from tertiary university hospitals (2,4), where patients with both more complex and long-standing forms of chronic venous insufficiency may be referred, while other studies deal with only patients who were selected for surgery (5,6). The latter bias may yield a greater proportion of limbs with more advanced disease or alternatively select out only those limbs that were amenable to surgery. Finally, the clinical grade or stage of chronic venous in-

TABLE 19–1. Incidence of Deep Venous Disease[a]

SERIES	NUMBER OF LIMBS	CRITERIA FOR ENTRY	METHODS OF DIAGNOSIS[c]				SYSTEM INVOLVED (%)	
			Clin	Dop	AVP	Phleb	Superficial	Deep
Darke and Andress (1)	594	CVI	+	+		+	78	22
NEMCH (2)	346	CVI	+	+	+		35	65
Moore et al. (3)	174	PT	+	+			65	38
Raju and Fredericks (4)	147	PT	+		+	+	27[d]	73
St. Thomas' Hospital (5)	119	Surg	+		+	+	66	37
Schanzer and Peirce (6)	52	Surg	+		+	+	65	35

[a] Modified from O'Donnell TF: The surgical management of deep venous valvular incompetence. *In* Rutherford R. ed: Vascular Surgery, 3rd ed. Philadelphia. WB Saunders Company, 1989:1612.
[b] CVI, chronic venous insufficiency; PT, postthrombotic syndrome; Surg, candidate for surgery.
[c] Clin, clinical; Dop, bidirectional Doppler; AVP, ambulatory venous pressure; Phleb, ascending and/or descending phlebogram.
[d] Combined with superficial.

sufficiency biases results. Patients presenting with venous ulcer appear to have a higher proportion of deep venous involvement.

Darke and Andress's (1) series seems to be the least biased, because this study addressed consecutive patients presenting to a venous clinic. Of the nearly 500 patients who underwent both bidirectional Doppler examination and phlebography, over three quarters of the patients had superficial system involvement alone. By contrast, our series at New England Medical Center Hospital (NEMCH) (2) showed diametrically opposite results, with the incidence of deep venous involvement (65 per cent) three times greater than that reported by Darke and Andress. The relatively high proportion of deep venous involvement in our study was probably related to the increased number of limbs with stage III disease— 142 limbs (41 per cent of the series). Our results were similar to those of Raju and Fredericks (4), who assessed only patients with postthrombotic syndrome and found that approximately 73 per cent had deep venous involvement. Finally, two representative surgical series—those from St. Thomas' Hospital (5) and that of Schanzer and Peirce (6)—show a lower incidence of deep venous involvement. This finding probably represents a selection process of examining only those patients who were candidates for superficial venous surgery—ligation and stripping of the saphenous veins and/or subfascial ligation of incompetent perforating veins.

In summary, these data would suggest that as the clinical stage of the disease becomes more advanced, the probability of deep venous involvement is greater. For example, of our 142 limbs with stage III disease only 12 per cent had superficial venous involvement alone (2).

CAUSES OF DEEP VENOUS DISEASE

Table 19–2 summarizes the pathologic causes of deep venous insufficiency in several series. Several series, such as those of Darke and Andress (1), Pearce et al. (7), and Gooley and Sumner (9), detected no patients with obstruction as the cause of deep venous insufficiency. Raju and Fredericks (4), however, observed a 13 per cent incidence and we (2) noted a 5 per cent incidence of deep venous obstruction. These findings emphasize the fact that deep venous valvular incompetence with reflux is the commonest form of chronic deep venous disease.

LEVEL OF VALVULAR INCOMPETENCE

Several investigators have used either descending phlebography or bidirectional Doppler ultrasound assessment to define the anatomic location of deep venous valvular incompetence (Table 19–3). Most studies showed that distal valvular incompetence predominated. The popliteal vein segment was incompetent in over 80 per cent of limbs involved. In our recent study of 48 limbs with venous ulcer who underwent ascending and descending phlebography and venous hemodynamics, all limbs with significant reflux had reflux through the above-knee and below-knee popliteal segments (10). Shull and associates (11) demonstrated the important relationship between popliteal vein incompetence and the presence of venous ulcer in patients with previously documented deep venous thrombosis

TABLE 19–2. Types of Deep Venous Insufficiency[a]

SERIES	NUMBER OF LIMBS	CRITERIA FOR ENTRY[b]	METHODS OF DIAGNOSIS[c]				OBSTRUCTION (%)[d]
			Clin	Dop	AVP	Phleb	
Darke and Andress (1)	100	Ulcer	+	+		+	0
NEMCH (2)	346	CVI	+	+	+		5
Moore et al. (3)	113	PT	+	+	+		12
Raju and Fredericks (4)	100	PT	+		+	+	13
Schanzer and Peirce (6)	17	Surg	+		+	+	7
Pearce et al. (7)	48	PT	+		+		0
Borvins-Slot et al. (8)	194	PT	+	+			0
Gooley and Sumner (9)	74	PT	+	+	+		0

[a] From O'Donnell TF: The surgical management of deep venous valvular incompetence. *In* Rutherford R. ed: Vascular Surgery, 3rd ed. Philadelphia, WB Saunders Company. 1989:1613.
[b] *CVI, chronic venous insufficiency; PT,* postthrombotic syndrome; *Surg,* candidate for surgery.
[c] *Clin,* clinical; *Dop,* bidirectional Doppler; *AVP,* ambulatory venous pressure; *Phleb,* ascending and/or descending phlebogram.
[d] Remainder represents valvular incompetence.

TABLE 19–3. Location of Valvular Incompetence[a]

SERIES	NUMBER OF LIMBS	CRITERIA FOR ENTRY[a]	METHODS OF DIAGNOSIS[c]				VALVULAR INCOMPETENCE	
			Clin	Dop	AVP	Phleb	Proximal	Distal (Popliteal)
Darke and Andress (1)	100	Ulcer	+	+		+	19	88
NEMCH (2)	346	CVI	+	+	+		11	80
Moore et al. (3)	113	PT	+	+			22	78
Raju and Fredericks (4)	100	PT	+		+	+		
Schanzer and Peirce (6)	17	Surg	+		+	+		
Pearce et al. (7)	48	PT	+		+	+	47	14
Borvins-Slot et al. (8)	194	PT	+	+		+	14	86
Gooley and Sumner (9)	74	PT	+	+	+		54	46

[a] From O'Donnell TF: The surgical management of deep venous valvular incompetence. *In* Rutherford R. ed: Vascular Surgery. 3rd ed. Philadelphia. WB Saunders Company. 1989:1613.

[b] *CVI*, chronic venous insufficiency; *PT*, postthrombotic syndrome; *Surg*, candidate for surgery.

[c] *Clin*, clinical; *Dop*, bidirectional Doppler; *AVP*, ambulatory venous pressure; *Phleb*, ascending and/or descending phlebogram.

(DVT). Those patients with popliteal vein valvular incompetence had a high incidence of ulcers.

TYPE OF VALVULAR INCOMPETENCE

Most physicians assume that venous valvular incompetence is due to the destructive effects of a previous episode of deep venous thrombosis. In 1948 Bauer (12), however, reported that venous valvular incompetence could arise from a cause other than as a sequela to acute DVT. Kistner (13) has called attention to the entity of primary valvular incompetence (PVI). By means of high-quality descending phlebograms Kistner demonstrated that approximately 40 to 50 per cent of limbs with deep venous valvular reflux had PVI. Morphologically PVI presents with floppy, redundant, gossamer-like valves. The loss of fibroelastic tissue prevents normal coaptation of the valve cusps, while on phlebography none of the typical recanalization changes are observed in the area of the valves. In similar phlebographic studies Darke and Andress (1) corroborated this relative incidence of primary valvular incompetence. Partial valve leaflets may be visualized on ascending and descending phlebography. The importance of this finding is that it may alter the form of surgery performed.

We have recently observed the combination of characteristic postthrombotic changes distally at the popliteal vein level and below while the proximal (femoral) valves exhibit primary valvular incompetence. This mixed form of deep venous valvular incompetence might permit direct surgery on the femoral valve as the initial procedure and then, if deterioration occurs over time at this level, vein valve transplantation may be carried out at the popliteal level.

DEEP VENOUS REFLUX—PATHOPHYSIOLOGIC SEQUELAE

The basic hemodynamic abnormality in chronic venous insufficiency is transmission of the high pressure generated within the deep system during the systolic phase of the ambulatory cycle. Valvular incompetence with reflux increases deep venous pressure. Since venous pressure at the ankle level is directly related to the length of the uninterrupted column of blood cephalad to the point of measurement, the venous pressure may be quite high in the patient with popliteal vein valve incompetence. In the normal limb with competent deep venous valves the column of blood is divided into short segments, similar to locks in a canal. By contrast, in the patient with deep venous valvular reflux an uninterrupted column of blood may extend from the right atrium to the point of valvular incompetence in either the calf or distal popliteal vein (14). During the systolic phase of the calf muscle pump, venous pressure is high and reflux of blood is very rapid. The higher pressure generated within the deep system refluxes through the incompetent (communicating) veins to the superficial venous system. Microvascular changes then occur that lead to venous ulcer, as well described by Burnand et al. (15).

CLINICAL PRESENTATION

Patients with deep venous valvular reflux have a characteristic clinical picture. The pain experienced by a patient with deep venous valvular reflux is different than that experienced by a patient with deep venous obstruction. On standing the patient with reflux may observe the sudden development of leg heaviness. Our patients have described it as similar to "the sensation of water being poured into the leg and filling it up." After prolonged standing this complaint may be followed by a bursting type of heaviness in the calf that is quite incapacitating. This heaviness occurs independent of ambulation, in contrast to the situation in the patient with obstructive venous disease with venous claudication, who only experiences discomfort on ambulation. Edema is a common manifestation of deep venous reflux and is usually mild to moderate in degree, while predominating in the perimalleolar area. Cutaneous sequelae occur frequently in patients with long-standing deep venous reflux. Skin pigmentation secondary to brownish hemosiderin deposits is the initial sign. As the condition advances eczematous dermatitis develops and finally venous ulcer appears.

DIAGNOSTIC WORK-UP

We usually limit deep venous valvular reconstruction to patients with stage III disease, venous ulcer (14). Since presently this procedure may be considered experimental, it has not been applied to patients with limb swelling or early stage II disease. Certainly patients with advanced stage II disease with severe eczematous changes and intense pigmentary deposits may be candidates for reconstructive surgery. Our patients have severe ankle and calf swelling, advanced cutaneous pigmentary changes, and an active or recently healed ulcer.

Quantitative photoplethysmography by light reflection rheography is carried out as the initial screening study. Patients with deep venous involvement characteristically demonstrate venous refill times that are shortened to less than 10 sec. Compression of the superficial venous system by multiple tourniquets does not improve this shortened venous refill time. Following quantitative photoplethysmography patients next undergo bidirectional Doppler ultrasound assessment of valvular competency at the tibial, popliteal, and femoral vein levels. Proximal and distal compression as well as Valsalva maneuver help to determine valvular competence. Recent data from Strandness' group suggest that the Valsalva maneuver is the most important technique to determine valve competence (16).

Figure 19–1 shows the results of a typical sequence of studies in a patient with deep venous valvular reflux. The venous refill time is shortened to less than 5 sec, and Doppler auscultation of the popliteal vein reveals reflux. Spectral analysis at the time of duplex scanning supplements the bidirectional Doppler examination, and color duplex scanning may further simplify this examination. B-mode ultrasound examination provides anatomic information on the deep venous system. Valves in the superficial femoral, profunda femoris, popliteal, and tibial veins are examined for anatomic evidence of incompetence. Visualization of valve leaflets rather than a sclerotic valve site suggests primary valvular incompetence. Figure 19–2 demonstrates such a study.

We believe that all patients with advanced stage II and stage III disease who are candidates for surgery should undergo phlebographic studies (14). Ascending phlebography with multiple tourniquests to maximize visualization of the deep venous system is carried out first. In contrast to the phlebographic technique exployed for acute DVT, in evaluating chronic venous insufficiency the superficial

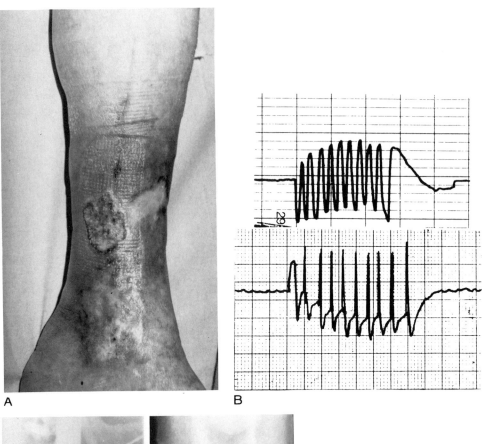

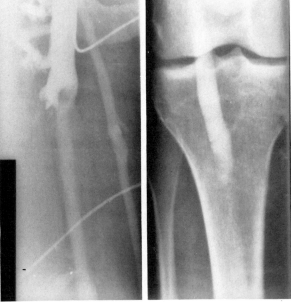

Figure 19–1. *A*, Clinical findings in a 42-year-old male with long-standing chronic stage III disease. *B*, Simultaneous venous pressure measurement and light reflection rheograph, which demonstrate shortened venous refill time and minimal change in light reflection and percentage decrease in venous pressure. *C*, Descending phlebogram that shows reflux to the infrapopliteal level secondary to incompetent valves.

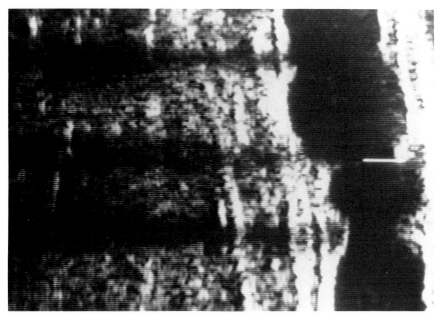

Figure 19–2. B-mode ultrasonogram of deep venous system demonstrating the presence of valve cusp structures but no valves.

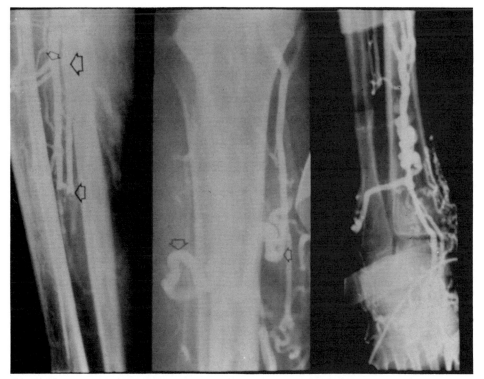

Figure 19–3. Ascending phlebograms from three various stages of chronic venous insufficiency. Progression of deep venous involvement from mild to severe is noted.

system is occluded by multiple tourniquets and the contrast material is infused by hand into the deep venous system, rather than by gravity (17). Visualization of the dye within the superficial venous system usually indicates paradoxical deep-to-superficial flow through incompetent perforating veins. The sites of these veins can be determined on fluoroscopy and then marked on the cut x-ray film. Typical signs of deep venous disease, such as recanalization, occlusion, or avalvular segments, are demonstrated (Fig. 19–3). Valve sites may be determined, which is of importance if direct valvular reconstruction is considered.

If no obstruction is noted in the deep system on ascending phlebography, then descending phlebography is performed next using the method of Kistner (18). The level to which the dye descends within the deep venous system determines the degree of valvular incompetence, so that patients with advanced venous disease typically have grade III or IV reflux (19).

In summary, a candidate for deep venous valvular reconstruction usually has stage III clinical disease, a venous refill time that is reduced to 10 sec or less by light reflection rheography, a patent deep venous system by ascending phlebography, and, finally, valvular incompetence to the below-knee popliteal or ankle level by descending phlebography.

SELECTION PROCESS

Despite the widespread enthusiasm noted in the available studies published in the literature, deep venous reconstructive surgery for valvular incompetence has played a limited role in the management of advanced chronic venous insufficiency. Table 19–4 compares the incidence of surgery for deep venous reflux as compiled from the contemporary literature. Kistner's incidence of deep venous reconstruction is approximately 25 per cent (20). In his assessment of nearly 800 limbs with deep venous valvular reflux, Raju (21) performed 89 procedures for an incidence of 14 per cent. This figure corresponds to our incidence of deep venous reconstructions performed in our institution for patients evaluated with stage III disease (14). It is apparent from this analysis that patients who undergo deep venous valvular reconstruction represent a highly selected group of patients (i.e., 75 per cent of patients with deep venous disease *do not* undergo reconstructive surgery). It is quite difficult to get hard data on the exact characteristics of those patients who do undergo deep venous reconstruction. In our small initial series of 10 patients who underwent popliteal vein valve transplantation the average duration of venous ulcer was 8 years (19).

TABLE 19–4.   Reported Incidence of Deep Venous Valvular Surgery

AUTHOR	APPROXIMATE POPULATION EVALUATED	TYPE OF SURGERY[a]			TOTAL	INCIDENCE (%)
		Valvulo	Transpo	Transpl		
Kistner (20)	>200	36	14	—	50	25
Raju (21)	774	71	18	—	89	14
Taheri et al. (22)				67	67	
NEMCH (14)	175	6	—	21	27	15.4

[a] *Valvulo,* valvuloplasty; *Transpo,* venous transposition; *Transpl,* vein valve transplant.

Most studies focus upon the efficacy of a particular type of nonsurgical or surgical therapy to heal the ulcer rather than to prevent recurrence. Browse (23) and Cranley (24) both have shown that over three quarters of ulcers can be healed with compression therapy and wound care. Prevention of ulcer recurrence, however, is too often neglected in the assessment of a treatment program's efficacy. It is the patient with repeated recurrent ulcer who is a candidate for deep venous reconstruction. Generally these patients would like to abandon the time-consuming and nonhygienic wound care that limits their active life-style. Thus, the efficacy of deep venous reconstruction should be judged on its ability to prevent recurrence, and not simply on its promotion of initial healing of the ulcer.

The second problem with the reported series on deep venous reconstruction is the lack of complete hemodynamic and anatomic follow-up. Some patients showed improvement in ambulatory venous pressure but not in venous refill time, whereas others demonstrated the converse. This lack of clear-cut hemodynamic benefit, despite clinical improvement, has remained a controversial point about the benefits of deep venous reconstructive surgery. Nicolaides pointed out that hemodynamic improvement may be present, but we may be measuring the wrong physiologic changes (25). Perhaps venous refill time and ambulatory venous pressures are too general a measurement. Nicolaides and his associates at St. Mary's Hospital in London have developed the air plethysmograph, which helps to dissect out the various components of venous physiology (25). In addition to ambulatory venous pressure, the degree of venous reflux and ejection fraction of the calf muscle pump are assessed by this technique. Such measurements should provide important documentation of the possible physiologic benefits of venous reconstructive surgery. Subsequently in this chapter we will report our results with this noninvasive assessment of venous function in patients undergoing popliteal vein valve transplant.

POPLITEAL VEIN VALVE TRANSPLANTATION

Approximately 8 years ago we initiated a clinical series of vein valve transplantation that differed from previous approaches to deep venous valvular reflux (26). This procedure employed the larger caliber axillary vein, which was transplanted to the above-knee popliteal vein. The rationale for this approach was twofold. The first advantage was to provide a better size match of the transplanted axillary vein segment to the host popliteal vein, which might prevent late dilation of the transplanted segment with subsequent valvular dysfunction. This latter situation had been encountered with transplantation to the superficial femoral vein segment. Although Taheri et al. (22) initially noted good clinical results with transplanting a brachial vein segment to the superficial femoral vein, they observed eventual dilation of the transplanted brachial vein segment. Valvular incompetence due to subsequent dilation of the transplanted segment as was observed with venous segment transposition is a theoretical disadvantage of employing the smaller caliber brachial vein. Despite using a larger diameter axillary vein segment, however, Raju and Fredericks (4) encountered progressive dilation and deterioration of valvular function when the femoral vein level was used. To avoid this problem the transplanted segment was encased in a Dacron graft.

The second advantage of popliteal vein valve transplant is to restore a functioning valve to the popliteal vein, where it can play a critical "gatekeeper" role above the calf muscle venous pump. The rationale for the gatekeeper role of the popliteal vein valve has been well demonstrated by previous investigators such as Schull et al. (11) and Moore et al. (3).

PRESENT LONG-TERM RESULTS WITH POPLITEAL VEIN VALVE TRANSPLANTATION

To assess the long-term benefits of deep venous valvular reconstruction by popliteal vein valve transplant we carried out clinical, hemodynamic, and phlebographic follow-up evaluation of 12 patients. It had been at least 3 years since surgery in all patients.

Preoperative Clinical Characteristics

The mean age of our patients was 49 years, and the left lower extremity was involved in nearly 90 per cent of the cases. Males outnumbered females in a 4:1 ratio. Venous ulcers were present for a mean length of time of 14 ± 4 years. The ulcer size on admission measured 3.5 ± 1.5 cm in diameter. Liposclerosis with severe induration was found in one third of patients. Fifty per cent of the patients had a previous history of DVT and two patients had a previously documented pulmonary embolus. Eighty per cent of the patients had prominent varicosities on admission. The majority of patients (80 per cent) had undergone a previous venous procedure, 60 per cent ligation and stripping, and 27 per cent subfascial ligation. Two patients had had their ulcer treated previously with split-thickness skin grafts.

Diagnostic Methods

Noninvasive Hemodynamic Evaluation

All patients underwent quantitative photoplethysmography by light reflection rheography, which is our standard initial screening study for patients with suspected chronic venous insufficiency. This method of assessing venous function has been described previously by us in detail (27).

Venous refill times were measured by light reflection rheography from completion of exercise to the point of a stable horizontal baseline. If the venous refill time was less than 25 sec, the test was repeated with a series of tourniquets to assess the contribution of the superficial venous system. Tourniquets were placed at above-knee, below-knee, and above-ankle levels and then were sequentially removed.

Complete normalization of venous refill time after tourniquet application was considered diagnostic of superficial venous insufficiency alone. If no improvement was observed with tourniquet compression of the superficial venous system, the limb was diagnosed as having deep venous insufficiency alone. Venous outflow obstruction was signified by slow or absent venous outflow during exercise. A shortened venous refill time that was unchanged after tourniquet compression,

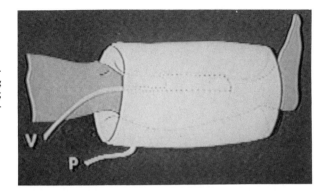

Figure 19–4. Air plethysmograph chamber (P) surrounds leg to assess limb volume changes; smaller inner sleeve (V) is for calibration.

with adequate venous filling demonstrated during exercise, was considered evidence of deep venous valvular incompetence.

Air plethysmography was carried out postoperatively in seven patients by the technique of Christopoulos and associates (25). This instrument (Fig. 19–4) is comprised of a 35-cm long air chamber of polyvinyl chloride that has a capacity of 5 liters. The chamber encases the entire leg from knee to ankle, and is connected to a pressure transducer and recorder. A smaller 1-liter bag is placed between the air chamber and the leg and used for calibration. The air plethysmograph is placed on the patient's leg in the supine position with the leg elevated to 45 degrees to empty the veins. The air chamber is then inflated to 6 torr and the leg kept in this elevated position for several minutes to achieve a stable baseline. The subject is then asked to stand with the weight on the opposite leg while holding onto a frame. An increase in the leg volume occurs as a result of venous filling. When a plateau is reached the veins are full. This measurement represents the functional venous volume (VV) (Fig. 19–5). Venous filling time 90 per cent (VFT 90) is defined as the time taken to reach 90 per cent of filling. The venous filling index (VFI) is derived from 90 per cent VV/VFT 90 and is expressed in milliliters per second.

The patient then is asked to do one toe stand with his weight on both legs and return to the initial position. The decrease in venous volume observed represents the ejected volume (EV), which is due to activation of the calf muscle

Figure 19–5. Typical volume changes with patient supine (*a*), with weight on nonexamined leg (*b*) and (*e*), following one toe stand (*c*), and following 10 toe stands (*d*). *VFT*, venous filling time; *VFT 90*, time to reach 90 per cent VFT; *VFI*, venous filling index, a measure of deep venous valvular reflux; *RVF*, residual volume fraction; *EF*, ejection fraction, a measure of venous pumping capacity; *EV*, ejected volume; *VV*, functional venous volume.

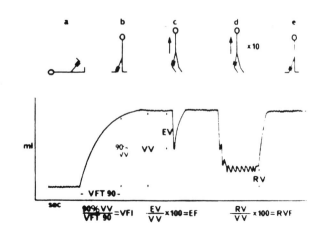

venous pump. After a new plateau is reached the patient performs 10 toe stands at a rate of 1/sec. A volume decrease to a new plateau is noted (Fig. 19–5). The residual volume (RV) is calculated from the original baseline value and the volume at the end of exercise. The ejection fraction (EF) with the first calf muscle contraction is derived from EF = EV/VV × 100 and the residual volume fraction from RV/VV × 100. Normalized units are employed to compare different clinical groups.

Phlebography

Ascending phlebography was performed by the method of Lea Thomas and McDonald (17), and descending phlebography was carried out by the technique of Kistner (18). The degree of reflux was classified by Kistner's criteria (18): grade I, reflux to upper thigh; grade II, reflux to knee; grade III, reflux to below knee; and grade IV, reflux to ankle.

Surgical Technique

The involved lower extremity and usually the contralateral upper extremity were prepped and draped, which allows for a two-team approach. The axillary vein was exposed through a longitudinal incision made parallel to the neurovascular bundle. The pressure and competence of axillary vein valves is determined by preoperative B-mode ultrasound imaging. Care was taken during the dissection of the axillary vein to avoid injury to the brachial plexus or other surrounding nerve structures. A segment of axillary vein was then tested for patency and valve function intraoperatively using a bidirectional Doppler probe. Usually, a segment of axillary vein measuring 6 to 8 cm and containing one valve was removed.

The popliteal vein was exposed through a standard above-knee approach commonly used in arterial reconstruction for femoral above-knee popliteal bypass, but the lower portion of this vein was the usual site of transplantation. The vein was dissected free from the concomitant arterial structures (Fig. 19–6). Usually, this dissection can be somewhat tedious if the vein has the characteristic post-thrombotic changes. After an approximately 8-cm segment of vein had been isolated it was encircled with vessel loops. Five thousand units of heparin were administered, and the vein was clamped with soft, rubber-shod, noncrushing vascular clamps. A 3- to 4-cm segment of vein was removed to receive the transplanted axillary vein valve-bearing segment.

The distal anastomosis of the interposition graft was usually done first with interrupted 7-0 monofilament suture. Once the four-quadrant interrupted sutures were placed, the transplanted vein segment was "parachuted" down into position (Fig. 19–6). The remaining sutures were then placed. In placing the sutures for both anastomoses, care must be taken to avoid entrapping the valvular mechanism. The proximal anastomosis was then performed in a similar manner. The vein segment was flushed before completion of the last portion of the proximal anastomosis. The operative site then underwent intraoperative evaluation (Fig. 19–7).

The patient was maintained on intravenous heparin perioperatively for 5 days and then converted to warfarin. To increase venous flow through the transplanted segment postoperatively, the patient was maintained on intermittent pneumatic

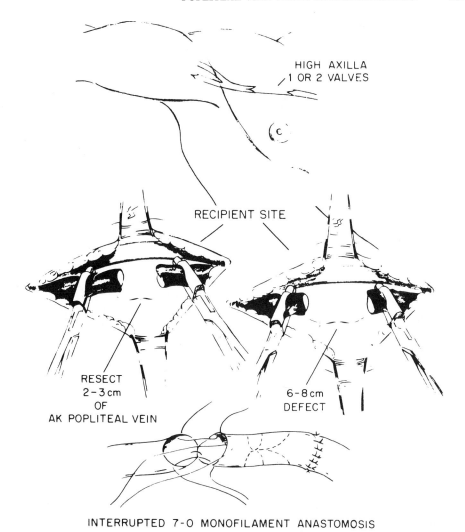

HIGH AXILLA
1 OR 2 VALVES

RECIPIENT SITE

RESECT
2-3 cm
OF
AK POPLITEAL VEIN

6-8 cm
DEFECT

INTERRUPTED 7-0 MONOFILAMENT ANASTOMOSIS

Figure 19–6. Popliteal vein valve transplantation following verification of the presence of a valve by B-mode ultrasound. The axillary vein is exposed and a valve-containing segment is harvested. The above-knee (*AK*) popliteal vein is dissected free and the valve-containing segment is placed as an interposition graft with interrupted 7-0 monofilament sutures.

compression (50 to 60 mm Hg) until fully ambulatory. The patient was usually up into a chair on the fourth or fifth day and ambulatory on day 6.

Preoperative Results

Noninvasive Hemodynamic Findings

The mean venous refill time was 7.1 ± 6 sec prior to popliteal vein valve transplant. Following surgery there was an insignificant rise to 10 sec.

Phlebography

Ascending phlebography showed incompetent perforating veins in 80 per cent of the patients. Descending phlebography revealed incompetent valves to the level of the midcalf (grade III reflux) in nine limbs and to the ankle level in three.

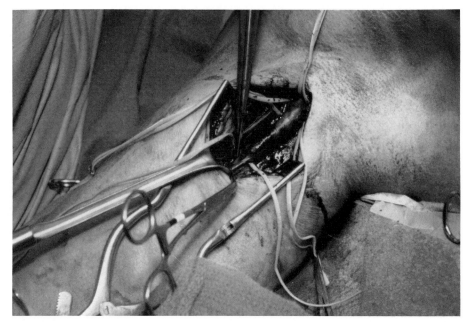

Figure 19–7. Perioperative photograph demonstrating valve competency. Column of blood is arrested by competent valve.

Postoperative Findings

Clinical Results

All ulcers healed following surgery. One ulcer recurred in the 12 limbs that underwent popliteal vein valve transplantation over a 44-month follow-up period. This ulcer reappeared 5 years after popliteal vein valve transplantation in a woman whose initial ascending phlebogram showed no incompetent perforating veins. Five years after surgery ascending and descending phlebography revealed patency and function of the transplanted valve segment, but multiple incompetent perforating veins were observed underlying the ulcer. The patient underwent a subfascial ligation with healing of the ulcer and presently, at 1 year following this last procedure, has a healed ulcer.

Phlebographic Results

All patients underwent ascending and descending phlebograms within 2 weeks following popliteal vein valve transplant. All transplanted segments were patent by ascending phlebography, but on descending phlebography one of the 12 showed minor valve leakage. Ascending and descending phlebograms were performed again on eight of the 12 patients at a mean of 4 years following popliteal vein valve transplant. All eight had patent transplanted popliteal vein segments. In one patient there was minor dilation of the transplanted segment. Descending phlebography demonstrated comptency of the transplanted valve segment in seven of the eight limbs examined. One patient, who had demonstrated partial incompetence on immediate postoperative phlebography, showed progression to frank incompetence several years after his procedure.

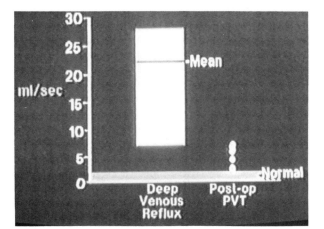

Figure 19–8. Assessment of venous filling index.

Late Hemodynamic Results—Quantitative Photoplethysmography

All patients had serial light reflection rheography studies at yearly intervals. Only one patient showed a significant improvement in venous refill time following popliteal vein valve transplant. The mean venous refill time was unchanged from preoperative or immediately postoperative values. No significant deterioration in venous refill time was observed in any patient.

Air Plethysmography

Seven patients had air plethysmographic studies performed at a mean of 39 months following popliteal vein valve transplant. All patients had concomitant ascending and descending phlebograms that proved both patency and function of the transplanted segment. Figure 19–8 demonstrates the results for assessment of the VFI, a measure of the degree of reflux, in these seven patients. These values are compared to normal control values (1.1 ml/sec) and to a mean value for patients with phlebographically demonstrated deep venous reflux (DVR) (22 ml/sec). The latter group was utilized rather than using the patients as their own controls because this test was not available to us to assess such patients 4 years ago. It is evident that the VFI (degree of reflux) is improved by popliteal vein valve transplant (4.4 ±1.7 ml/sec). Figure 19–9 compares the EF of patients

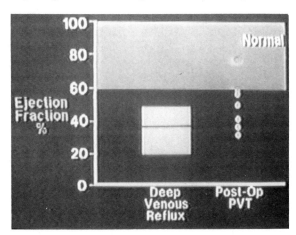

Figure 19–9. Ejection fraction of patients undergoing popliteal vein valve transplant, normal subjects, and patients with deep venous reflux.

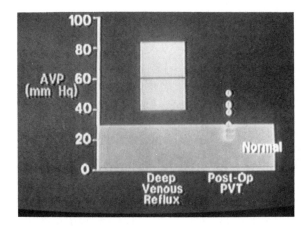

Figure 19–10. Ambulatory venous pressure as derived from residual volume fraction.

undergoing popliteal vein valve transplant (45 ±22 per cent) to normal (70 per cent) and DVR (38 per cent) groups. There was no clear trend toward improvement in the patients who had undergone popliteal vein valve transplant. A comparison of ambulatory venous pressure as derived from residual volume fraction is demonstrated in Figure 19–10. Like the VFI, ambulatory venous pressure in the popliteal vein valve transplant group (35 ±5 torr) appears to be improved toward normal (30 torr) from the values observed in the DVR group (72 torr). Thus, popliteal vein valve transplant appears to improve two components of venous hemodynamics, the VFI or degree of venous reflux, and the ambulatory venous pressure.

Discussion

Our results show long-term benefits to patients with chronic and recurrent venous ulcer following popliteal vein valve transplant, and late hemodynamic and anatomic studies demonstrate patency and morphologic function of the popliteal vein valve transplant. Although there was no alteration in venous refill time by photoplethysmography, hemodynamic assessment with air plethysmography revealed an improvement in both the VFI and residual venous volume as an indication of reduced venous reflux. As stated previously, our 12 patients represent a small percentage of those patients presenting with advanced chronic venous insufficiency. The long-standing nature of their venous ulcers is indicated by the long mean duration of recurrent ulcer (8 years) and the number of previous surgical procedures or failed conservative measures utilized to promote and maintain healing of the ulcer.

Popliteal vein valve transplant represents one of several techniques for correcting deep venous valvular reflux. In contrast to valvuloplasty, which directly repairs the valve, popliteal vein valve transplant is an indirect procedure that interposes a normal valve-containing segment from another vein into the area of venous reflex. The rationale for this technique is to provide an axillary vein segment that is of a comparable diameter to the recipient popliteal vein (14). This better size match may mitigate against either eventual dilation of the transplanted segment or flow-related intimal hyperplastic responses, both of which would adversely affect function of the transplanted valve segment. A second advantage of the popliteal position is to place a functioning valve above the calf muscle venous pump in a critical "gatekeeper" role. Several other investigators (3,11,12) have shown that function of the popliteal vein valve is very important in preventing venous ulcer.

HOW DO RESULTS OF POPLITEAL VEIN VALVE TRANSPLANT COMPARE TO THOSE OF OTHER PROCEDURES FOR DEEP VENOUS VALVULAR REFLUX

Table 19–5 summarizes the results of these various procedures and shows that there is a paucity of data available on long-term ulcer healing as well as late hemodynamic and anatomic results. Although not stated in the literature, Kistner's (13) late results with direct reconstruction of primary valvular incompetence by valvuloplasty reveal the best long-term patency and clinical relief. The disparity between Kistner and Sparkuhl's (20) results and those of the Northwestern group (29,30) with venous segment transfer may be related to two factors: 1) the site of transposition (the saphenous vein would appear to dilate more readily than the profunda femoris vein; the latter site is favored by Kistner); and 2) the lack of treatment of the incompetent perforating veins by the Northwestern group. In those few limbs that had subfascial ligation of incompetent perforating veins in the Northwestern series improvement in hemodynamics and the clinical state were maintained. Raju (4) noted deterioration in both the long-term ulcer healing rate and late ambulatory venous pressure measurements with superficial femoral vein valve transplantation. These findings helped shape our attitude toward developing a different procedure.

Our study revealed one patient who had recurrence of ulcer 5 years after her original popliteal vein valve transplantation, which had been unaccompanied by subfascial ligation of incompetent perforating veins. Her ulcer responded to a simple subfascial ligation after the patency and function of the transplanted segment were proven.

Despite the apparent excellent clinical results, the lodestone around the neck of deep venous valvular reconstruction is the lack of proven hemodynamic benefit. We (19) and others (4,13) have shown that the transplanted segments remain open while descending phlebography suggests function of the valve. Assessment with quantitative photoplethysmography and direct venous pressure measurements have yielded variable results. However, the data demonstrated in this chapter show clear-cut hemodynamic benefits to popliteal vein valve transplantation.

The technique of air plethysmography, which assesses venous dynamics in the whole leg, may overcome some of the previous problems encountered with segmental volume measuring devices. While venous reflux is assessed by descending phlebography or by duplex scanning, the VFI relates directly to the degree of venous reflux and is independent of the venous volume reservoir. As Christopoulos et al. (25) have shown, a normal VFI ranges from 0.6 to 1.7 ml/sec and is related to the rate of capillary venous filling. By contrast, patients with deep venous valvular incompetence have values that average 22 ml/sec as a result of reflux of blood in a paradoxical direction. Following deep venous valvular reconstruction our patients had a mean VFI of 4.4 $\pm$ 1.7 sec, not significantly different than the upper limits of normal values. Our measurements with air

TABLE 19–5. Comparison of Surgical Results[a]

AUTHOR	NUMBER OF LIMBS	PREOP ULCER (%)	ULCER HEALING (%)		PAIN RELIEF (%)		VRT[c] IMPROVED (%)		AVP[d] IMPROVED (%)		PATENT AND FUNCTIONING SEGMENT BY PHLEBOGRAPHY (%)	
			ST[b]	LT[b]	ST	LT	ST	LT	ST	LT	ST	LT
Primary valvuloplasty												
Ferris and Kistner (28)	32	?	83	—	—	—	64.1	—	86	—	88	—
Raju and Fredericks (4)	61	66	85	63	90	87	—	—	100	—	—	—
Venous transposition												
Ferris and Kistner (28)	14	?	80	—	64	—	—	—	92	—	100	57
Queral et al. (29)	12	33	100	—	75	—	92	—	50	—	75	—
Johnson et al. (30)	12	33	0	67	—	25	—	25	—	—	—	—
Femoral vein valve transplant												
Taheri et al. (22)	13	80	—	60	—	100	—	—	—	—	100	—
Taheri et al. (22)	43	40	—	94	—	75	—	—	89	89	90	90
Raju and Fredericks (4)	24	80	79	42	77	50	629	100	46	13	—	—

[a] From O'Donnell TF: The surgical management of deep venous valvular incompetence. *In* Rutherford R. ed: Vascular Surgery. 3rd ed. Philadelphia, WB Saunders Company. 1989:1617.
[b] *ST,* short term; *LT,* long term.
[c] *VRT,* venous reflux time.
[d] *AVP,* ambulatory venous pressure.

plethysmography showed a wide range of values for EF following popliteal vein valve transplant. In limbs with venous reflux there is not only an increased VV, but a decreased EF. No consistent improvement in EF was observed in our patients. This finding indicates that while reflux can be improved with popliteal vein valve transplant, little is done to the pumping capacity of the calf muscle venous pump.

Finally, the residual volume fraction has been shown by Christopoulos and associates (25) to be directly related to the ambulatory venous pressure at the end of a series of tip toe exercises. In patients with deep venous disease, venous emptying is altered so that the limb reaches a steady state in which blood ejected from the veins with each systolic contraction of the calf muscle pump is comparable to the amount of blood entering both from the capillaries and from venous reflux. Patients with deep venous valvular reflux, therefore, exhibit a greater fraction of reflux. Following popliteal vein valve transplant our data indicate a reduction in the residual volume fraction. Since residual volume fraction is an indirect measurement of ambulatory venous pressure, ambulatory venous pressure is also improved. Thus, popliteal vein valve transplantation appears to have its predominant hemodynamic effect in preventing reflux, as indicated by an improved VFI and a reduced residual volume fraction. The calf muscle pump function does not appear to be improved, as signified by the variable changes in ejection fraction.

PRESENT APPROACH TO PATIENTS WITH DEEP VENOUS REFLUX

In the patient with recurrent venous ulcer and deep venous reflux we search for PVI (Fig. 19–11). Ascending phlebography plays an important role in deter-

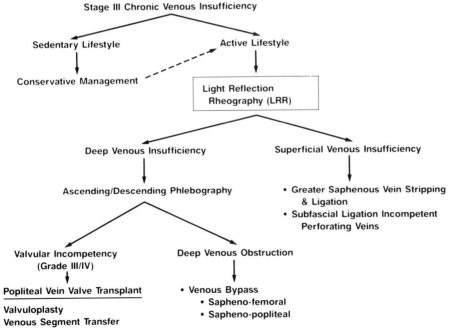

Figure 19–11. Overall treatment plan for patient and venous ulcer.

mining whether direct or indirect venous reconstruction is carried out. If the phlebogram and/or B-mode ultrasound image suggest the presence of valve leaflets at the common femoral or superficial vein level then this area is explored through an inguinal incision. Angioscopy is performed retrograde through the common femoral vein to determine whether valve leaflets and PVI are present. In the latter situation a valvuloplasty is performed by the method of Kistner (13). By contrast, if the valves are damaged, as suggested by phlebography or demonstrated directly by angioscopy, then a popliteal vein valve transplantation is carried out.

REFERENCES

1. Darke SF, Andress MR: The value of venography in the management of chronic venous disorders of the lower limbs. *In* Greenhalgh RM, ed: Diagnostic Techniques and Assessment Procedures in Vascular Surgery. London, Grune & Stratton, 1985.
2. McEnroe CS, O'Donnell TF, Mackey WC: Correlation of clinical findings with venous hemodynamics in 386 patients with chronic venous insufficiency. Am J Surg 1988;*156*:148–152.
3. Moore DJ, Himmel PD, Sumner DS: Distribution of venous valvular incompetence in patients with postphlebitic syndrome. J Vasc Surg 1986;*3*:49–57.
4. Raju S, Fredericks R: Valve reconstruction procedures for non-obstructive venous insufficiency: Rationale, techniques, and results in 107 procedures with 2-8 year follow-up. J Vasc Surg 1988; 7:301–810.
5. O'Donnell TF, Burnand KG, Browse NL: Is interruption of incompetent perforating veins really important to the management of chronic venous insufficiency? Surgery 1977;*82*:9–14.
6. Schanzer H, Peirce EC: A rational approach to surgery of the chronic venous stasis syndrome. Ann Surg 1982;*195*:25–29.
7. Pearce WH, Ricco JB, Queral LA, et al: Hemodynamic assessment of venous problems. Surgery 1983;*93*:715–721.
8. Borvins-Sol H, Vermeiden I, VanDam R: The detection of deep vein incompetence in 980 legs using Doppler in combination with spectral analysis. Second International Vascular Symposium, London, England, September, 1986.
9. Gooley NA, Sumner DS: Relationship of venous reflux to the site of venous valvular incompetence: Implications for venous reconstructive surgery. J Vasc Surg 1988;7:50–59.
10. O'Donnell TF, McEnroe CS, Mackey WC, et al: Long-term results with the management of venous ulcer. Arch Surg (in press).
11. Shull KC, Nicolaides AN, Fernandes JF, et al: Significance of popliteal reflux in relation to ambulatory venous pressure and ulceration. Arch Surg 1979;*114*:1304–1306.
12. Bauer G: The etiology of leg ulcers and their treatment by resection of the popliteal vein. J Int Chir 1948;*8*:937–967.
13. Kistner RL: Primary venous valve incompetence of the leg. Am J Surg 1980;*140*:218–224.
14. O'Donnell TF: The surgical management of deep venous valvular incompetence. *In* Rutherford R, ed: Vascular Surgery, 3rd ed. Philadelphia, WB Saunders Company, 1989;1612–1626.
15. Burnand KG, Whimster IW, Clemenson G, et al: The relationship between the number of capillaries in the skin of the venous ulcer bearing area of the lower leg and the fall in foot vein pressure during exercise. Br J Surg 1981;*68*:297–300.
16. van Bemmelen PS, Beach K, Bedford G, Strandness DE: The mechanism of venous valve closure. Arch Surg 1990;*125*:617–619.
17. Lea Thomas M, McDonald LM: Complications of phlebography of the leg. Br Med J 1978;*2*:307–315.
18. Kistner RL: Surgical repair of the incompetent femoral vein valve. Arch Surg 1975;*110*:1336–1342.
19. O'Donnell TF, Mackey WC, Shepard AD: Clinical, hemodynamic, and anatomic follow-up of direct venous reconstruction. Arch Surg 1987;*122*:474–477.
20. Kistner RL, Sparkuhl MD: Surgery in acute and chronic venous disease. Surgery 1979;*85*:31–43.
21. Raju S: Venous insufficiency of the lower limb and stasis ulceration. Changing concepts and management. Ann Surg 1983;*197*:688–697.
22. Taheri SA, Pendergast DR, Lazar E: Vein valve transplantation. Am J Surg 1985;*150*:201–202.
23. Browse NL: Venous ulceration: natural history and treatment. *In* Browse NL, Burnand KG, Lea Thomas M, eds: Diseases of the Vein. Pathology, Diagnosis and Treatment. London, Edward Arnold, 1988;411–419.

24. Cranley J: The management of venous disorders. *In* Rutherford R (ed): Vascular Surgery. Philadelphia, WB Saunders Company, 1989.

25. Christopoulos DG, Nicolaides AN, Szendro G, Irvine AT, et al: Air-plethysmography and the effect of elastic compression on venous hemodynamics of the leg. J Vasc Surg 1987;5:148–159.

26. O'Donnell TF, Shepard AD: Chronic venous insufficiency. *In* Jarrett F, Hirsch J, eds: Vascular Surgery of the Lower Extremity. St. Louis, CV Mosby, 1985.

27. Shepard AD, Mackey WC, O'Donnell TF, Heggerick PA: Light reflection rheography (LRR): A new non-invasive test of venous function. 1986;8:266–270.

28. Ferris EB, Kristner RL: Femoral vein reconstruction in the management of chronic venous insufficiency. Arch Surg 1982; *117*:1571–1579.

29. Queral LA, Whitehouse WM, Flinn WR, et al: Surgical correction of chronic deep venous insufficiency by valvular transposition. Surgery 1980;87:688–695.

30. Johnson HD, Queral LA, Flinn WR, et al: Late objective assessment of venous valve surgery. Arch Surg 1981;*116*:1461–1466.

20

EXPERIENCE WITH VENOUS RECONSTRUCTION IN PATIENTS WITH CHRONIC VENOUS INSUFFICIENCY

Seshadri Raju

Many fundamental aspects of venous reflux, including etiologic mechanisms and pathophysiology, are poorly understood. In this setting, valve reconstructive surgery should be considered experimental even though excellent to good empirical results have been obtained in selected patients with various procedures. Indeed, these encouraging results combined with dissatisfaction with traditional methods of treatment have provided a major impetus in recent years toward a better understanding of the pathophysiology of venous reflux.

HEMODYNAMIC BASIS OF STASIS ULCERATION

It is widely accepted as axiomatic that reflux stasis ulceration is the result of ambulatory venous hypertension. Yet in our experience roughly 25 per cent of patients with stasis ulceration have postexercise pressures of 50 mm Hg or less (Table 20–1). There are other examples of discordance in this perceived relationship between ambulatory venous pressure and stasis ulceration. For instance, it has been recognized that surgical procedures such as perforator ligation (1) or valve reconstruction (2) heal stasis ulceration even though postexercise pressures are improved only modestly or not at all. Large stasis ulcers often overlie a large ankle perforator vein. Ligation or sclerotherapy of a single such perforator may lead to the healing of the ulcer without affecting postexercise pressure (3,4).

Because it was clear that ambulatory venous pressure measurement did not accurately measure obvious clinical improvement, other parameters of reflux have been investigated. Valsalva-induced foot venous pressure elevation in the recumbent patient was found by us to be a superior index of reflux, especially with regard to surgical outcome (2). This simple test proved to be highly reproducible in reflux patients (5), with clear delineation between normal and refluxive limbs. Nevertheless, false-negatives occurred in stasis ulceration even with this technique (2), such that the negative predictive value was poor.

Since force = mass × acceleration, if reflux force is the basis of stasis

TABLE 20–1. **Ambulatory Venous Pressure Measurements in Stasis Ulcer Patients**[a]

PRESSURE AFTER EXERCISE (mm Hg)	NO. OF ULCER LIMBS	TOTAL LIMBS TESTED	INCIDENCE OF ULCERS (%)
<30	0	15	0
30–40	8	103	8
40–50	14	206	7
50–60	30	198	15
60–70	16	131	12
70–80	10	56	18
80–90	6	45	13
90–100	3	9	33
>100	0	0	0

[a] From Raju S, Fredericks R: Valve reconstruction procedures for nonobstructive venous insufficiency: rational, techniques and results in 107 procedures with two to eight year follow-up. J Vasc Surg 1988;3:301–310.

ulceration, both mass and acceleration should be considered. Obviously, reflux force or its components cannot be measured precisely in the clinical setting, but substitutes are available. Postexercise pressure can be used as an approximation for mass. Valsalva-induced foot venous pressure elevation may be used as a substitute for acceleration. A product of these two parameters can be used as an index for reflux force (RFI). A value of 150 was established as the upper limit for the RFI in normal volunteers. An increasing incidence of stasis ulceration can be demonstrated with increasing RFI (6). Virtually all patients with an RFI of over 1000 demonstrate stasis ulcers. More importantly, the negative predictive value for this measure appears to be excellent. The incidence of stasis ulceration among a group of reflux patients with RFIs of less than 150 was 2 per cent. In contrast, the negative predictive values of postexercise pressure measurement and Valsalva-induced foot venous pressure elevation individually are approximately 15 and 25 per cent, respectively.

It appears that patients who develop stasis ulceration despite a normal or below-normal postexercise pressure tend to have a high value for Valsalva-induced foot venous pressure elevation (6). The opposite situation apparently prevails in patients developing stasis ulceration despite a normal Valsalva-induced foot venous pressure elevation. High postexercise pressures are present in this circumstance. Thus, at least one of the two components of the RFI is always abnormal when stasis ulceration is present. The concept of the RFI can be better understood by the analogy that the force imparted and the damage suffered by a pedestrian when struck by a small automobile traveling at high speed can be identical to that produced by a heavier vehicle traveling at a much lower speed. The caliber and the competence of the perforator system have an obvious important role in allowing reflux forces within the deep venous system to be reflected at the superficial venous level.

ETIOLOGY OF STASIS ULCERATION

It has long been taught that the postphlebitic syndrome is the major etiologic mechanism for deep venous reflux. Primary cryptogenic reflux that is nonthrombotic in origin is generally believed to be rare even though the entity itself has been recognized since the early part of the century. It is well to remember that chronic venous insufficiency may be due to reflux, obstruction, or a combination of the two. While techniques to detect and measure reflux have been available, techniques for the diagnosis and quantification of chronic venous obstruction have been inadequate. It is clear that venography provides anatomic rather than physiologic information. Plethysmographic techniques suffer from lack of standardization and muscle movement artifacts. More importantly, these latter techniques have been typically employed in the resting limb. Obstructing veins may not become hemodynamically significant until the limb is exercised, because venous collaterals around a chronic venous obstruction may be entirely adequate in the resting limb. Resting foot venous pressure in the recumbent position was normal in 41 per cent of patients with radiographically proven venous obstruction (Fig. 20–1). When the arterial and venous flows were increased by inducing reactive hyperemia, significant elevation of foot venous pressure was demonstrated (7), exposing the inadequacy of collateralization under stress.

While several studies outlining the hemodynamic outcome of deep venous

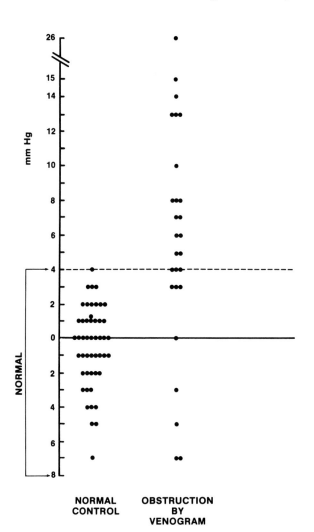

Figure 20–1. Supine arm/foot venous pressure differential in "normal" and venographically obstructed limbs. (From Raju S: A pressure-based technique for the detection of acute and chronic venous obstruction. Phlebology 1988;*3*:207–216.)

thrombosis have been reported, few have utilized hemodynamic measurements under circulatory stress. In one investigation in which this was accomplished (8), obstruction rather than reflux appeared to be the predominant injury in severely symptomatic limbs following deep venous thrombosis. Recent studies of deep venous thrombosis with duplex scanning have provided more detailed chronologic information than ever before, but this technique cannot replace precise hemodynamic measurements in these limbs. Thus the role of deep venous thrombosis as an etiologic factor in the generation of pure venous reflux remains an enigma. In an important prospective study (9), van Bemmelen and colleagues noted the occurrence of reflux in venous segments far removed from the site of venous thrombosis. This may be due to venous dilatation proximal to an obstructing thrombus or to some other mechanism not yet understood.

The relationship, if any, between postphlebitic reflux and cryptogenic reflux remains to be elucidated. It is clear, however, that cryptogenic reflux may lead to deep venous thrombosis from stasis. We have had occasion to perform venous valve reconstruction in several such patients who presented with calf vein thrombosis in association with reflux in the femoral and popliteal systems. Resolution of recurrent calf thrombosis was obtained with correction of valve reflux. A surprising number of patients presenting with deep venous thrombosis have venous reflux in the opposite extremity (8). These observations have prompted us to suggest that cryptogenic reflux may precipitate venous thrombosis, which in turn may lead to further reflux from valve destruction, thus completing a vicious cycle (Fig. 20–2).

Most symptomatic patients with venous reflux are found to have reflux at multiple levels (10). Isolated valve defects, such as at the popliteal level following a limited calf vein thrombus involving the popliteal valve, apparently generate relatively mild symptomatology (8). Furthermore, patients with multivalvular reflux benefit from reconstruction of only the superficial femoral or popliteal valve (2). It appears likely that there is not a single unique valve location in the venous system of the lower limb that is pivotal in preventing the malsequelae of venous reflux. Nicolaides and Yao (11) have shown that symptomatology was worse in a group of patients with venous obstruction in whom the popliteal valve was

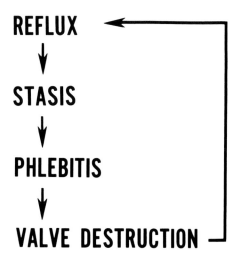

Figure 20–2. Primary reflux disease may predispose to thrombosis and valve destruction. This, in turn, may aggravate preexisting reflux. (From Raju S: Venous insufficiency of the lower limb and stasis ulceration–changing concepts and management. Ann Surg 1983;*197*:688–697.)

REFLUX

STASIS

PHLEBITIS

VALVE DESTRUCTION

incompetent. When the popliteal valve was competent, ulceration did not occur in this group of obstructed patients. Since the incompetence of the popliteal valve could have been a marker for the severity of venous obstruction in this group of patients, no definitive conclusions can be drawn with regard to the relative importance of popliteal reflux over other valvular sites. A thrombotic process must be extensive to involve valves at multiple levels. While complete resolution is certainly possible following such extensive thrombosis, the process of recanalization and resolution in all likelihood will be incomplete, leaving behind significant obstructive lesions in addition to valvular reflux.

DIAGNOSTIC PROFILE OF REFLUX VENOUS INSUFFICIENCY

It is generally impossible to differentiate chronic obstruction from reflux based on clinical grounds alone because both groups of patients present with a combination of pain, swelling, and/or ulceration. Laboratory and radiologic studies are required to make this differentiation. When patients with obstruction and combined obstruction/reflux are excluded, the remainder are found to have refluxive limbs predominantly of the cryptogenic variety (approximately 80 per cent). The other 20 per cent or so are postthrombotic, with characteristic stigmata such as collateral formation, vein wall thickening and recanalization, and obvious periphlebitis evident at the time of surgery. Patients with cryptogenic reflux often describe episodes of "phlebitis." Many had been hospitalized and given anticoagulants for episodes of leg swelling and tenderness. Positive venographic evidence is often lacking in such instances, and the current venogram is clean as a rule. It is difficult to ascertain whether these episodes represented periods of calf vein thrombosis of a limited nature or some other mechanism that temporarily exacerbated the symptomatology of venous reflux.

Descending venography performed at a 60 degree tilt, as described by Kistner et al. (12), is routinely performed in patients under consideration for surgical correction of reflux. Isolated saphenous venous reflux is extremely rare in this group of limbs, comprising less than 2 per cent in a large series analyzed from our institution (13). The great majority of patients have multiple-level reflux involving the femoral, popliteal, profunda, and saphenous veins in various combinations. Combined superficial and deep venous insufficiency involving the saphenous vein and one or more of the deep veins is found in approximately 16 per cent of patients. Even though the reflux may be confined to the thigh, patients are symptomatic when more than one venous system in the thigh (i.e., deep femoral, superficial femoral, or saphenous) is involved, suggesting that the quantity of reflux rather than the retrograde extension is more important in generation of symptoms (14). While perforator incompetence is fairly common in this group of patients, "pure" perforator insufficiency alone was a rare entity (2). Invariably, other deep system valve reflux was present on descending venography when perforator incompetence was identified in ascending venograms.

Photoplethysmography is widely used as a screening technique for venous insufficiency. Table 20–2 shows sensitivity and specificity data for this technique when a variety of other techniques are utilized as gold standards for comparison. While the level of sensitivity is acceptable, poor specificity is noted irrespective of the other technique used for comparison.

TABLE 20–2.   Sensitivity and Specificity Data for Photoplethysmography

TECHNIQUE USED FOR COMPARISON	n	SENSITIVITY (%)	SPECIFICITY (%)
Descending venography	208	74	37
Doppler ultrasound	814	85	62
Ambulatory venous pressure (<16-sec recovery time)	389	97	57
Valsalva-induced foot venous pressure elevation	315	96	48
Presence of stasis ulceration	87	90	—

INDICATIONS FOR VALVE RECONSTRUCTION PROCEDURES

Stasis ulceration and class III skin changes comprise the primary indications for valve reconstruction at the present time. Swelling frequently becomes worse temporarily following venous valve surgery. Long-term resolution of swelling, however, is quite good (2). When combined swelling and pain are present preoperatively, any residual swelling persisting after surgery is frequently painless and well tolerated by the patient. For these reasons, surgery may be offered to patients with leg swelling on a selective basis. Pain as a primary symptom presentation in the absence of skin changes or swelling offers difficult choices for the surgeon in patient selection. Because of the chronicity, many patients with severe reflux have lowered thresholds for pain and often present with personality changes. Some patients may malinger in an effort to establish a basis for disability. Since pain relief following surgery cannot be measured objectively, the utility of valve reconstruction and surgical outcome cannot be gauged adequately in this group of patients. Clinical judgment and severity of reflux as determined by objective laboratory and venographic criteria should be the guide to proper selection of patients for surgery.

VALVE RECONSTRUCTION

Surgical Approach

After a thorough work-up, the uppermost valve in the superficial femoral vein is approached through a groin incision. The presence of reflux through the valve should be established by a strip test at the time of surgery. A more complete description of the technique of internal valvuloplasty can be found elsewhere (2). The valve is approached through a transverse incision and plicated by two commissural sutures on either side. On gross inspection, the cryptogenic refluxive valve presents as a redundant structure with multiple folds and pleats at the free edges, much like the edge of lettuce. Approximately 20 per cent of the free edge of the valve at either commissure usually requires plication to achieve competence. This should be confirmed by a repeat strip test after closure of the transverse venotomy. Occasionally, the valve is found to be competent even before repair on a strip test following venoconstriction induced by surgical manipulation. In such cases, a formal internal valve repair is avoided and a Dacron jacket of 8 to 10 mm is fitted around the valve area to sustain it in the contracted position.

In approximately 20 per cent of cases, the valve cusp is found to be destroyed or deformed by a previous thrombotic process, preventing the possibility of a commissural repair. Axillary vein valve transfer is performed in such instances. To prepare for such an eventuality, one of the axillae is always prepared and kept ready at the time of surgery. It is our practice to ensheath the transferred axillary valve in an 8- to 10-mm Dacron sleeve to prevent late dilatation (2,15). An interesting feature of axillary vein transplantation is the high incidence of incompetent axillary valves (2,15). The significance of this finding in relationship to the possible global nature of valve reflux in these patients is intriguing.

More recently, we have resorted to an external valvuloplasty technique suggested by Kistner (personal communication). The technique is rapid and allows correction of multiple valve sites. With practice it has become possible routinely to correct reflux of the profunda, superficial femoral, and posterior tibial levels with this technique. Even though our experience is still very limited, a surprising number of patients have normalized their ambulatory venous pressures following this technique of multiple valve correction. This early observation would require verification with a larger experience and a much longer follow-up.

Complications and Postoperative Care

Heparin administered intraoperatively is not neutralized in these patients because they are particularly prone to develop deep venous thrombosis. A 7 per cent incidence has been noted in our series. More recently we have sustained continuous heparin infusion in the immediate postoperative period, and then gradually converted to low-dose warfarin (2.5 mg/day). Hematomas and seromas occur not infrequently and are managed aggressively by surgical evacuation and closed drainage. When thromboses occur, they usually involve the calf and spare the reconstructed valve. Deep venous thrombosis in the unoperated opposite extremity has also been observed.

Results

Initial experience with valve reconstruction has been gratifying (Table 20–3). With increasing experience and better selection of patients, the results should further improve.

TABLE 20–3.   Results of Valve Reconstruction Surgery (Follow-up 2 to 8 Years)

		POSTOPERATIVE IMPROVEMENT IN SYMPTOMS		
PROCEDURE	*n*	Pain	Swelling	Stasis Ulcer
Valvuloplasty	61	87%	83%	63%
Valvuloplasty/Dacron sleeve	10	60%	60%	50%
Axillary vein transfer	18	50%	39%	46%
Axillary vein transfer/ Dacron sleeve	6	50%	30%	33%
Dacron sleeve in situ	12	83%	91%	63%

Surgical Failures and Repeat Valve Surgery

When satisfactory resolution of symptoms is not obtained following valve reconstruction or when there is recurrence of symptoms after initial improvement, a thorough laboratory and radiologic investigation should be undertaken. In our experience, the recurrence rate of reflux through the operated valve following successful valvuloplasty is low. Higher failure rates are noted following axillary vein transplantation, thought to be due to late dilatation of the transferred valve.

When the primary valve repair is still intact, the basis for recurrent symptoms should be sought elsewhere. In some such cases, a deep venous thrombosis that has developed since surgery may be documented. In others, recurrent saphenous venous reflux and/or perforator incompetence may be identified. We have had good results in resolving recurrent symptoms by performing saphenous vein stripping and/or the Linton procedure as indicated in these instances. Occasionally there is recurrence of pain without an identifiable venographic basis or laboratory evidence of worsening reflux. Pain in these patients has a significant functional component and the patients may have been poorly selected initially. An occasional such patient has obtained satisfactory pain relief by implantation of a nerve stimulator or other neurosurgical procedure for pain relief.

VENOUS BYPASS FOR VENOUS OBSTRUCTION

A bypass procedure for obstruction should not be considered unless a pressure gradient is demonstrated at rest. A bypass procedure performed on the basis

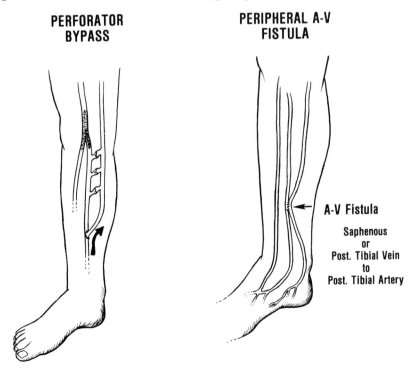

Figure 20–3. Surgical approaches for relief of distal venous obstruction (see text). *A-V*, arteriovenous; *Post.*, posterior.

of venographic appearance alone is unlikely to remain patent if a gradient is not present. A conduit adequate for the site of obstruction should be utilized.

The saphenous vein is generally too small to bypass a significant iliac vein obstruction. Residual symptoms are frequently present even when the saphenous vein bypass is demonstrated to be patent in such cases (16). We advocate the employment of a temporary arteriovenous fistula to dilate the saphenous vein conduit when used in this setting. Endothelial healing is usually complete by 6 weeks following venous surgery (17). For this reason, anticoagulation should be maintained for at least this period and probably much longer as prophylaxis against recurrent deep venous thrombosis. A temporary arteriovenous fistula, when utilized to increase flow and assist endothelial healing, should also be maintained for up to 6 weeks. Because there is a significant incidence of infection as well as distal venous hypertension in chronically maintained arteriovenous fistulas, most fistulas should be closed no later than 6 months after they are created.

Obstructive lesions of the popliteal vein and its tributaries more distally pose a difficult clinical problem. Direct saphenous vein–to–posterior tibial anastomosis (16) to bypass inefficient perforator collaterals (Fig. 20–3) has had a surprisingly good patency rate (four of six cases) with symptom resolution. In two cases, the perforator bypass thrombosed postoperatively but recanalized later to establish a useful outflow. We had employed peripheral arteriovenous fistulas (Fig. 20–3) in an effort to stimulate collateral formation in similar cases, but have abandoned this effort even though objective improvement was documented occasionally (16). Abandonment of this technique was stimulated by a high rate of spontaneous fistula closure (16) and the absence of symptomatic or objective improvement in the majority of patients so treated.

REFERENCES

1. Burnand KG, O'Donnell TF Jr, Lea TM, Browse NL: The relative importance of incompetent communicating veins in the production of varicose veins and venous ulcers. Surgery 1977; 82:9–14.
2. Raju S, Fredericks R: Valve reconstruction procedures for nonobstructive venous insufficiency: Rationale, techniques, and results in 107 procedures with two- to eight-year follow-up. J Vasc Surg 1988;7:301–310.
3. May R, Partsch H: Concluding remarks on the therapy of incompetent perforating veins. In May R, Parsch H, Staubesand J, eds: Perforating Veins. Baltimore: Urban & Schwarzenberg, 1981; 251.
4. Partsch H: Early functional results after the hook method in chronic venous incompetence. In May R, Parsch H, Staubesand J, eds: Perforating Veins. Baltimore: Urban & Schwarzenberg, 1981;234.
5. Raju S, Fredericks R: Evaluation of methods for detecting venous reflux: Perspectives in venous insufficiency. Arch Surg 1990 (in press).
6. Raju S, Fredericks R: Hemodynamic basis of stasis ulceration—an hypothesis. Arch Surg 1990 (in press).
7. Raju S: A pressure-based technique for the detection of acute and chronic venous obstruction. Phlebology 1988;3:207–216.
8. Raju S, Fredericks RK: Late hemodynamic sequelae of deep venous thrombosis. J Vasc Surg 1986;4:73–79.
9. van Bemmelen PS, Bedford G, Beach K, Strandness DE: Quantitative segmental evaluation of venous valvular reflux with duplex ultrasound scanning. J Vasc Surg 1989;10:425–431.
10. Raju S: Distribution of venous valvular incompetence in patients with the postphlebitic syndrome [letter]. J Vasc Surg 1986;4:536.
11. Nicolaides AN, Yao JST, eds: Investigation of Vascular Disorders. New York, Churchill Livingstone, 1981;493.

12. Kistner RL, Ferris EB, Randhawa G, Kamida O: A method of performing descending venography. J Vasc Surg 1986;*4*:464–468.
13. Morano JU, Raju S: Chronic venous insufficiency: Assessment with descending venography. Radiology 1990;*174*:441–444.
14. Raju S: Valve reconstruction procedures for chronic venous insufficiency. Semin Vasc Surg 1988; *1*:101–106.
15. Raju S: Venous insufficiency of the lower limb and stasis ulceration. Ann Surg 1983;*197*:688–697.
16. Raju S: New approaches to the diagnosis and treatment of venous obstruction. J Vasc Surg 1986; *4*:42–54.
17. Raju S, Perry JT: The response of venous valvular endothelium to autotransplantation and in vitro preservation. Surgery 1983;*94*:770–775.

21

RECONSTRUCTIVE VENOUS SURGERY

James S. T. Yao, William H. Pearce, and
Walter J. McCarthy

Unlike arterial reconstructive surgery, bypass for venous occlusion has yet to be established as a standard vascular surgical procedure. Difficulty associated with venous surgery includes the poor patency rate of venous bypass, especially when prosthetic material is used as a conduit. Selection of patients could be a problem. Quite often the extensive occlusive process and incompetent calf perforating veins preclude surgical correction in these patients. Even after correction of the occlusive process, venous valvular incompetency of major or perforating veins may remain a problem. After complete evaluation by contrast venography, only a small number of patients are candidates for venous reconstructive surgery. The present chapter reviews the experience of venous reconstructive surgery at Northwestern University Medical Center.

PATIENT SELECTION AND EVALUATION

In general, patients with recent thrombosis (within 1 year) should not be considered for bypass procedure. With time and intensive compression therapy, most swelling will respond to conservative management. Similarly, patients with venous ulcer must first undergo compression using a pressure-gradient elastic stocking together with attention to skin hygiene and avoidance of allergenic medication. Surgery is reserved for those patients who fail this plan of treatment. Prior to surgical correction, these patients must be subjected to venography and noninvasive studies.

Several noninvasive techniques are now available to evaluate venous dysfunction. The venous refilling time recorded by photoplethysmography is used primarily as a screening test. In most instances, the venous refilling time is shortened in patients with severe chronic venous insufficiency, with a value less than 10 sec. Venous refilling time indicates the presence of venous reflux. For venous obstruction, venous outflow test by impedance plethysmography is helpful.

Recent introduction of duplex scanning has extended noninvasive testing to include the selective determination of venous valve incompetency (1–13). The use of duplex scanning is vital to determine the results of venous valve surgery.

For preoperative evaluation, the use of duplex scanning is helpful to determine the suitability of the autogenous vein as a conduit. Evaluation of the jugular vein by venography is often difficult, but examination of its patency must be routine in all upper extremity venous reconstruction procedures. The availability of magnetic resonance imaging or duplex scanning has made the examination of patency of the jugular vein as an outflow pathway a simple procedure. The duplex scan is also helpful to determine graft patency, provided the technologist is familiar with the anatomic pathway of the bypass. The superficially placed venous bypass is ideal for duplex scanning. For objective determination of the results of venous reconstructive surgery, it is also desirable to determine ambulatory venous pressure before and after the procedure.

Once the patient is considered a surgical candidate, a complete evaluation of the veins by contrast venography is mandatory. For lower extremity venous obstruction, visualization of the inferior vena cava is necessary to complete the evaluation. Venography is helpful to determine the operability as well as the types of venous reconstruction.

VENOUS OCCLUSION OF UPPER EXTREMITIES

Venous reconstruction is often not needed in patients with occlusion of the subclavian vein, the innominate vein, or the superior vena cava. The rich collateral networks of the upper part of the body often provide enough decompression, and surgery is reserved for patients with severe obstruction. With more frequent use of an indwelling catheter for hyperalimentation or chemotherapy, total occlusion of the subclavian or innominate vein may cause disabling swelling. Another cause of upper extremity venous thrombosis is the presence of a permanent pacemaker wire. One of the interesting problems of upper extremity venous thrombosis is the development of subclavian vein thrombosis in patients who had a functioning arteriovenous fistula constructed for hemodialysis. The presence of a functioning arteriovenous fistula distal to an occluded subclavian or axillary vein invariably causes severe swelling, and a bypass procedure may be necessary. Although some authors have advocated ligation of the fistula (4), the use of a bypass graft helps to relieve the swelling and at the same time salvage the fistula for hemodialysis. Recently, several authors have reported success in preserving the arteriovenous fistula in these patients (5–7).

Marked swelling of the face or the extremity may be associated with superior vena cava occlusion due to invasive tumor compression. Typical symptoms include suffusion, dyspnea, cough, and, less commonly, pain, syncope, dysphagia, and hemoptysis. The most important physical findings are the increased collateral veins covering the anterior chest wall, distended neck veins, and edema of the face. In a recent review by the Mayo Clinic, the cause of superior vena cava occlusion is most commonly carcinoma of the lung, with suffusion as the most common presenting symptom (8).

Types of venous reconstruction depend on the anatomic site of the occlusion. In patients with occlusion of the subclavian or axillary vein, an autogenous vein or a polytetrafluoroethylene (PTFE) graft is used. We prefer to use the two-incision technique. The jugular vein is often used for decompression and the vein is exposed by placing an incision along the anterior border of the sternocleido-

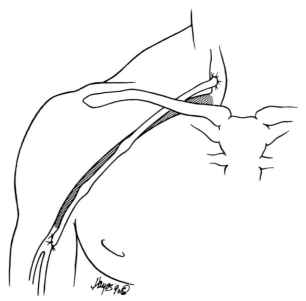

Figure 21–1. Autogenous saphenous vein bypass using the jugular vein for proximal anastomosis.

mastoid muscle. For distal anastomosis, the axillary vein is exposed in the upper arm (Fig. 21–1). Once the exposure of these two veins is complete, a tunnel is made subcutaneously underneath the clavicle. The long saphenous vein is then harvested from the thigh for vein grafting. After placing the vein graft through the tunnel, the anastomosis is constructed in an end-to-side manner.

As in all venovenous anstomoses, we prefer to excise a small portion of the host vein in an elliptical fashion and anastomose the vein graft in an end-to-side manner (Fig. 21–2). A similar maneuver is also used if a PTFE graft is used as the conduit. If the size of the saphenous vein is inadequate, the technique to

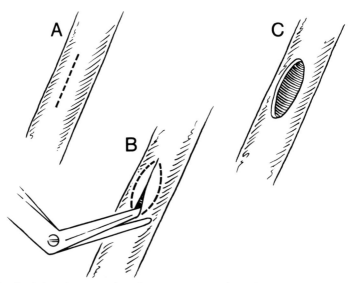

Figure 21–2. Technique in preparation of venous anastomosis. *A*, Venotomy. *B* and *C*, An elliptical incision is made in the recipient vein to avoid constriction.

construct a spiral vein graft suggested by Doty (9) may be used. This is done by wrapping the opened vein graft in a spiral manner over a small chest tube or rubber catheter of desired diameter. Polyethylene suture (6-0) is then used to suture the side of the vein in a continuous manner (Fig. 21–3). In the presence of a small saphenous vein, an alternate technique is to suture two opened saphenous veins into one graft using continuous sutures.

Surgical treatment of superior vena cava occlusion is needed in patients with persistent symptoms. Quite often the procedure is done for symptomatic relief in the presence of wide tumor spread. Because of obstruction involving the superior vena cava, we prefer to use the right atrium as the outflow decompression pathway. A jugular-to–right atrium graft is then constructed. The right atrium is approached through a median sternotomy and the jugular vein by the routine anterior approach (Fig. 21–4A). Choice of graft material depends on the projected longevity of the patient. A spiral vein graft should be used if the prognosis of the patient is favorable; otherwise a ring-reinforced PTFE graft is preferred. After the right atrium and the internal jugular vein are exposed, anastomosis is first performed in the jugular vein. The vein is then wrapped obliquely with the distal end sutured. An end-to-end anastomosis is then constructed between the graft and the jugular vein. After this is complete the other end of the graft is then anastomosed to the atrium (Fig. 21–4B).

VENOUS OCCLUSION OF THE LOWER EXTREMITIES

Chronic obstruction of the iliac or femoral veins may produce unrelenting swelling requiring surgical decompression. Procedures commonly used are the crossover vein graft of the saphenopopliteal bypass. The former was first described by Edurado C. Palma of Montevideo in 1958 (10) and subsequently popularized by Andrew Dale of Nashville, Tennessee (11,12). In recent years, European investigators have advocated the construction of a temporary arteriovenous fistula to maintain patency of these crossover grafts. For occlusion of the femoral vein, the more popular technique is the saphenopopliteal bypass (13). As devised by Palma and Warren independently, and as applied by Husni

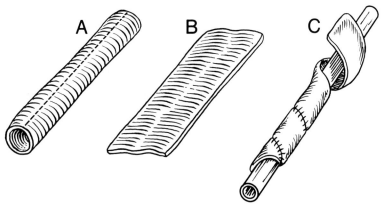

Figure 21–3. Technique in the reconstruction for spiral vein graft. *A*, Longitudinal opening of vein. *B*, Vein segment ready for wrapping. *C*, Construction of spinal graft.

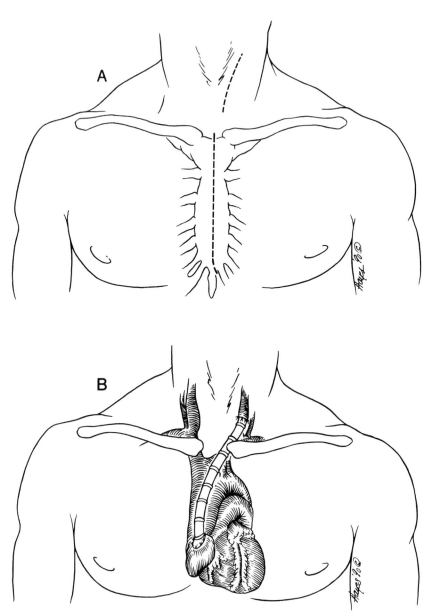

Figure 21–4. *A*, Simultaneous exposure of internal jugular vein and right atrium. The atrium is exposed through a median sternotomy. *B*, Internal jugular–to–right atrium bypass using ring-enforced PTFE graft.

(14) in this country and by Gruss (15) and May (16) in Europe, the saphenopopliteal bypass has great theoretical appeal. It employs Palma's principle of a single ven-ovenous anastomosis.

Femorofemoral Crossover Graft

The procedure is suitable for unilateral iliac vein occlusion with the presence of a rather normal contralateral venous system. On the side distal to the occlusion the patent common femoral vein is exposed by routine technique. On the donor side, the skin incision is extended to the distal thigh for exposure of the long saphenous vein (Fig. 21–5A). The femoral vein and the saphenofemoral junction are then carefully exposed. A subcutaneous tunnel is then made over the pubic bone, and the long saphenous vein is dissected free and transected after a desired length is achieved (Fig. 21–5B). Because of spasm, gentle manual dilation of the vein by connecting the distal end of the vein to a syringe filled with heparin-saline solution may be necessary. The graft is then tunneled over the pubic bone sub-cutaneously. Care must be taken to ensure no kinking of the saphenofemoral junction. The saphenous vein is then anastomosed to the femoral vein in an end-to-side manner (Fig. 21–5C). No attempt is made to construct a temporary fistula in these patients.

Saphenopopliteal Bypass

Candidates for this procedure must have a patent popliteal vein with a long saphenous vein free of disease and of adequate size. A medial skin incision is made in the lower part of the thigh along the course of the long saphenous vein (Fig. 21–6A). The saphenous vein is then exposed in a manner similar to that for femoropopliteal vein bypass. Following this the popliteal vein is exposed by plac-ing an incision medialy below the knee. The popliteal vein is then dissected free from the popliteal artery. A complete circumferential dissection is often not needed. For anastomosis, only an adequate portion of the anterior surface of the vein allowing the placement of a partial-occluding clamp is exposed. The popliteal vein is then palpated to ensure patency for bypass. Dissection of the long saphe-nous is continued following the course of the vein above the knee onto the calf wound. Once an adequate length is achieved, the vein is then dissected free from the bed and transected. Once again, the vein may need manual distention because of spasm during the dissection. The vein is then tunneled through the popliteal space between the heads of the gastrocnemius muscles. Placement of the saphe-nous vein through the anatomic channel prevents kinking and provides a better angle for distal anastomosis. After systemic heparinization, a partial-occluding clamp is then applied to the popliteal vein and a portion of the vein is excised. The saphenous vein is then anastomosed in an end-to-side manner (Fig. 21–6B).

POSTOPERATIVE CARE

Wound hematoma can cause graft occlusion as a result of compression; there-fore postoperative administration of heparin must be performed with great cau-tion. Other antithrombotic agents, such as dextran 40, may be used instead of

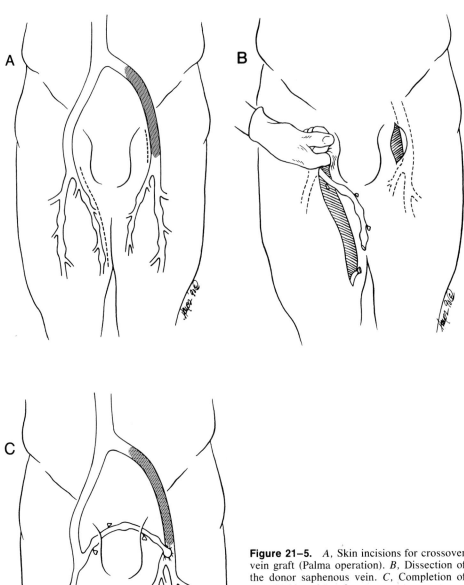

Figure 21–5. *A,* Skin incisions for crossover vein graft (Palma operation). *B,* Dissection of the donor saphenous vein. *C,* Completion of cross-pubic vein graft.

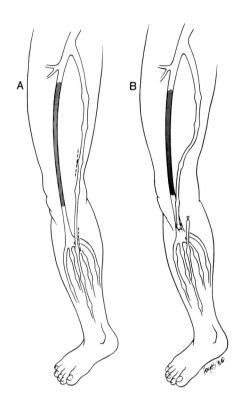

Figure 21–6. Preparation of saphenopopliteal vein graft. *A*, The saphenous vein is first dissected free below the knee and lower part of the midthigh. *B*, The saphenous vein is tunneled through the popliteal space for distal anastomosis onto the popliteal vein.

heparin. We have also found the use of mechanical compression as suggested by Hobson and his colleagues (17) to be helpful, and we believe it should be a part of routine postoperative care. The pump is used until the patient is fully ambulatory. Thereafter, the patient should be fitted for elastic support with a pressure-gradient (30 to 40 mm Hg) stocking. Many of these patients have a history of venous thrombosis; therefore long-term warfarin should be instituted during the immediate postoperative period. For evaluation of graft patency the availability of duplex scanning, especially the color-encoded imager, has been helpful. Venography is used when the results of duplex scanning are in doubt.

COMMENTS

Despite remarkable advances in arterial reconstructive surgery, venous bypass grafting has yet to be established as a standard modality in the treatment of chronic venous insufficiency. Other than occlusion, venous valve incompetency at either the femoral, the popliteal, or the level of the communicating veins further complicates the venous hemodynamics. Unless these two components are corrected, the result of bypass grafting is often disappointing. Fortunately, failure of these bypass grafts seldom causes limb loss, but many of these patients will revert to the original state with chronic swelling.

Most patients with upper extremity venous thrombosis seldom require a bypass procedure. Instead of a bypass graft using the long saphenous vein, others have advocated the use of cephalic vein crossover bypass (18) or the use of the internal jugular vein (19). In the latter, the distal end of the jugular vein is transected and ligated. The proximal end is then tunneled underneath the clavicle and anastomosed to the patent axillary vein. The causes of upper extremity venous thrombosis have changed dramatically in recent years, and catheter-induced thromboses are seen more frequently. In patients with renal failure, hemodialysis via an indwelling subclavian catheter is now a common procedure and late stenosis of the subclavian vein is not uncommon. If the patient subsequently requires an arteriovenous fistula, this may cause severe swelling of the entire arm because of outflow obstruction. Under this circumstance, the use of a vein graft often results in a dramatic decrease of swelling with salvage of the fistula. We have found that bypass grafting is a better technique than ligation of the fistula. Several authors have reported success using a bypass graft in these patients (5–7).

Perhaps the most challenging treatment is for superior vena cava occlusion. In addition to tumor compression, the placement of an indwelling catheter may result in the development of superior vena cava syndrome (20). For surgical decompression, an adequate conduit is prerequisite to success, and the technique suggested by Doty (9) should be followed if autogenous material is required. Otherwise, a ring-enforced PTFE graft appears to be an excellent substitute. Several investigators have reported good results in relief of symptoms in patients suffering from superior vena cava occlusion (see Chapter 36).

In highly selected cases, crossover femorofemoral or saphenopopliteal vein grafting may help to relieve obstructive symptoms. Although the construction of an arteriovenous fistula has been suggested by several investigators, reoperation to ligate the fistula is not always an easy undertaking, and several authors have suggested a simple technique to ligate the fistula (21,22). Even with an arteriovenous fistula to maintain graft patency, subsequent failure may occur immediately following ligation of the fistula. In Dale's report (12), he found a 75 per cent patency rate. Husni (23) reported a large group of autogenous bypasses, 71 without and 12 with arteriovenous fistula, in which patency of 72 to 78 per cent was achieved with follow-up to 3 years. Of these two reports, patients benefiting most from the procedure are those with extrinsic compression of the iliac vein by tumor. The best hemodynamic study of a large group of patients receiving femorofemoral crossover grafts has been accomplished by Halliday and his colleagues (24). In their study, they showed that a clinical assessment suggested that 89 per cent of femorofemoral grafts were patent when, in fact, objective proof was only obtained in 75 per cent of patients. Also, they have found the best clinical results are achieved in patients with venous claudication. When patients have progressed to ulceration, the patent graft may not be sufficient to heal the ulceration but will supplement ligation of perforators and removal of incompetent long and short saphenous veins. For saphenopopliteal bypass, a normal patent popliteal vein is needed. Because of the extensive involvement of thrombotic process in many patients, the popliteal vein is often not suitable for bypass. Therefore, cadidates for this procedure are rather limited. Also, the presence of a combined iliac vein thrombosis may further limit the validity of this procedure.

Techniques for venous bypass follow the guidelines of arterial surgery. Several technical points need to be emphasized. These include the construction of vein-to-vein anatomosis, control of the vein for anastomosis, and the construction of a spiral vein graft. For construction of an anastomosis, a venotomy with removal of an elliptical portion of the host vein is important to ensure adequate opening of the anastomosis. Unlike arterial surgery, the use of a partial-occluding clamp rather than individually isolating all branches minimizes unnecessary dissection. This is especially true for exposure of the popliteal vein for saphenopopliteal bypass. Surgeons must be familiar with the technique to construct a spiral vein graft. The latter is often needed for decompression of superior vena cava occlusion. Finally, great care in antithrombotic therapy is essential to the success of the operation. The use of a mechanical pump appears well suited as a routine adjunctive tool for postoperative care.

REFERENCES

1. Szendro G, Nicolaides AN, Zukowski AJ, et al: Duplex scanning in the assessment of deep venous incompetence. J Vasc Surg 1986;4:237–242.
2. van Bemmelen PS, Bedford G, Beach K, Strandness DE: Quantitative segmental evaluation of venous valvular reflux with duplex ultrasound scanning. J Vasc Surg 1989;10:425–438.
3. Gooley NA, Sumner DS: Relationship of venous reflux to the site. J Vasc Surg 1988;7:50–59.
4. Stone WJ, Wall MN, Powers TA: Massive upper extremity edema with arteriovenous fistula for hemodialysis. Nephron 1982;31:184–186.
5. Currier CB, Widder S, Ali A, et al: Surgical management of subclavian and axillary vein thrombosis in patients with a functioning arteriovenous fistula. Surgery 1986;100:25–28.
6. Campistol JM, Abad C, Torras A, Revert L: Salvage of upper arm access graft in the presence of symptomatic subclavian vein thrombosis. Nephron 1989;51:551–552.
7. Piotrowski JJ, Rutherford RB: Proximal vein thrombosis secondary to hemodialysis catheterization complicated by arteriovenous fistula. J Vasc Surg 1987;5:876–878.
8. Parish JM, Marschke RF, Dines DE, Lee RE: Etiologic considerations in superior vena cava syndrome. Mayo Clin Proc 1981;56:407–413.
9. Doty DB: Bypass of superior vena cava. Six years' experience with spiral vein graft for obstruction of superior vena cava due to benign and malignant disease. J Thorac Cardiovasc Surg 1982;83:326–337.
10. Palma EC, Riss F, Del Campo F, Tobler H: Tratamiento de los trastornos postflebiticos mediante anastomosis venosa safeno-femoral controlateral. Bull Soc Surg Uruguay 1958;29:135–145.
11. Dale WA: Chronic iliofemoral venous occlusion including seven cases of crossover vein grafting. Surgery 1966;59:117–132.
12. Dale WA: Peripheral venous reconstruction. In Dale WA, ed: Management of Vascular Surgical Problems. New York, McGraw-Hill Book Co, 1985;493–521.
13. Bergan JJ, Yao JST, Flinn WR, McCarthy WJ: Surgical treatment of venous obstruction and insufficiency. J Vasc Surg 1986;3:174–181.
14. Husni EA: Venous reconstruction in postphlebitic disease. Circulation 1971;43/44(suppl I):I-147–I-150.
15. Gruss JD: The saphenopopliteal bypass for chronic venous insufficiency (May-Husni operation). In Bergan JJ, Yao JST, eds: Surgery of the Veins. Orlando, FL, Grune & Stratton, Inc, 1985; 255–265.
16. May R: Der femoralisbypass beim postthrombotischen zustandsbild. Vasa 1972;1:267.
17. Hobson RW, Lee BC, Lynch TG, et al: Use of intermittent pneumatic compression of the calf in femoral venous reconstruction. Surg Gynecol Obstet 1984;159:285–286.
18. Hashmonai M, Schramek A, Farbstein J: Cephalic vein cross-over bypass for subclavian vein thrombosis: A case report. Surgery 1976;80:563–564.
19. Jacobson JH, Haimov M: Venous revascularization of the arm: Report of three cases. Surgery 1977;81:599–604.
20. Gore JM, Matsumoto AH, Layden JJ, et al: Superior vena cava syndrome. Its association with indwelling balloon-tipped pulmonary artery catheters. Arch Intern Med 1984;144:506–508.
21. Sanders RJ, Rosales C, Pearce WH: Creation and closure of temporary arteriovenous fistulas for venous reconstruction or thrombectomy: Description of technique. J Vasc Surg 1987;6:504–505.
22. Edwards WS: A-V fistula after venous reconstruction. A simplified method of producing and obliterating the shunt. Ann Surg 1982;196:669–671.
23. Husni EA: Reconstruction of veins: The need for objectivity. J Cardiovasc Surg 1983;24:525–528.
24. Halliday P, Harris J, May J: Femoro-femoral crossover grafts (Palma operation): A long-term follow-up study. In Bergan JJ, Yao JST, eds: Surgery of the Veins. Orlando, FL, Grune and Stratton, Inc, 1985;241–254.

22

VENOUS BYPASS FOR CHRONIC VENOUS INSUFFICIENCY

Joerg D. Gruss

There are two indications for direct venous bypass in chronic venous insufficiency. These are occlusion of the superficial femoral vein and occlusion of the common iliac vein. Variations of these conditions occur. For example, a total occlusion may be present in the superficial femoral vein and/or the popliteal vein with or without iliac vein occlusion. This may be present with or without extensive destruction of venous valves with consequent distal reflux. All of this may be a consequence of recanalized phlebothrombosis.

Because venous thrombosis is essentially a systemic disease, iliac venous occlusions and superficial femoral occlusions are actually commonly present coincidentally. Therefore, we have in the past carried out direct bypass operations, performing both the May-Husni and the Palma procedures simultaneously. However, in five patients in which this was done, occlusions occurred in three cases. Therefore, this operative approach has been abandoned (1–7).

As experience has developed, we now apply very strict indications to surgery involving venous bypass. This has limited the number of operations performed. Indications at present include severe postthrombotic syndrome with persistent tendency to swelling, leg ulceration, venous claudication, secondary varicose veins, and/or severe ankle pigmentation. In all cases consistent compression therapy, local therapy of venous ulcerations, and surgical interruption of incompetent perforating veins have been carried out before reconstructive surgery, bypass operations, or operations on the valvular apparatus.

The May-Husni operation and the Palma procedure have been quite satisfactory, but under no circumstances should they be carried out until 1 year has elapsed after the acute venous thrombosis episode. Early in our experience, we set a time limit of 6 months. Since that time, we have seen recanalization of the iliofemoral venous system under the direct influence of an arteriovenous fistula in a case of Palma procedure with a concomitant temporary arteriovenous fistula performed. The Palma transplant thrombosed, as soon as recanalization of the autologus vein occurred (Fig. 22–1).

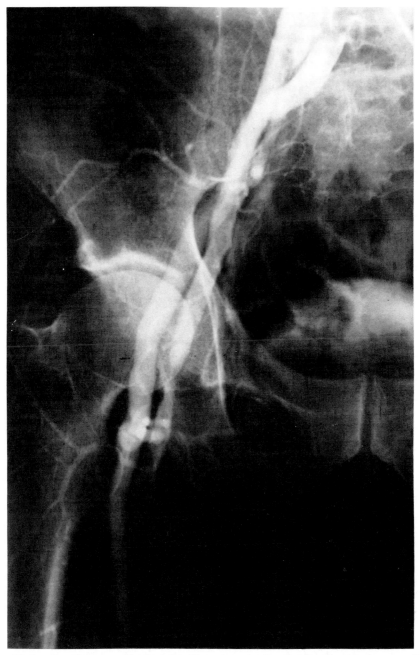

Figure 22–1. Complete recanalization of an iliac vein under the stimulus of an arteriovenous fistula in the right groin and occlusion of a Palma transplant.

SURGICAL REQUIREMENTS

Only patients with severe symptoms from chronic venous insufficiency are considered for direct venous reconstruction. In every case, operability is documented by ascending phlebography. Direct imaging of the iliofemoral veins is obtained. It has been estimated that an operable situation has been present in only approximately 2 per cent of patients with severe chronic venous insufficiency.

Patients with severely damaged leg and thigh veins and postthrombotic alterations in the iliofemoral venous system have not been considered for saphenopopliteal bypass. Likewise, patients with severe problems in the veins of the calf and thigh are no longer treated by us with a cross-pubic bypass (the Palma operation).

In addition to the anatomic situation of operability, there must be a functional indication for surgery. Good late results can only be obtained with strict selection of patients. We have found that measurement of venous pressure and venous occlusion plethysmographic volumetry has proved effective as methods of investigating pathologic venous function. Details of this follow.

It should be emphasized that the number of patients reported by us for surgical correction is small because of strict adherence to indications for surgery—that is, severely symptomatic chronic venous insufficiency; an isolated pathologic lesion in the femoral, popliteal, or iliac venous system; and supporting hemodynamic parameters. Therefore, 49 Palma operations in 47 patients and 14 May-Husni operations have been carried out between the years 1971 and 1989 (Table 22–1).

MAY-HUSNI OPERATION

Warren and Thayer (8) pointed out the possibility of reconstructing the postphlebitic damaged superficial femoral vein by transplantation of the ipsilateral greater saphenous vein to the subsartorial position in 1954. Subsequently, the suggestion was not taken up and was forgotten. This principle was later rediscovered independently and published by three authors, in 1970 by Husni (3), in 1972 by Frileux et al. (9), and in 1972 by May (10). In 1975, we modified that procedure by creating a temporary distal arteriovenous fistula at the level of the ankle (11,12).

TABLE 22–1. Reconstructive Vascular Interventions, July 1971 through December 1989

INTERVENTION	NO. OF PATIENTS
All types	12,379
Venous reconstructions	
May-Husni	14
Palma	49

Preoperative Evaluation

In studying the patients preoperatively and after phlebographic detection of the occlusion in the femoropopliteal venous system, a measurement of peripheral venous pressure is performed. Venipuncture at the dorsum of the foot is done and exercise with 10 toe stands is performed. The maximum fall of pressure for surgical candidates should not exceed one third of the resting pressure. For example, with a resting pressure of 90 mm Hg, the change in pressure may not be higher than 30 mm Hg. Absence of a fall in pressure, or even a rise in pressure, is thought to be better for prognosis (10,13).

Venous occlusion plethysmographic volumetry is carried out in both legs simultaneously. The strain-gauge plethysmograph is applied to the calf in the area of greatest circumference. After exercise with 10 toe stands, the decrease in volume on the affected side may be a maximum of one third of the fall in volume on the healthy side. The curves of venous pressure measurement and volumetry curves usually do correspond.

Surgical Procedure

The operation is carried out under general anesthesia with endotracheal intubation. The patient is positioned supine, the affected leg flexed at the hip and knee and slightly rotated outward. An incision 10 to 12 cm in length is placed on the proximal anteromedial leg. The greater saphenous vein is mobilized and manipulated with atraumatic technique using moistened rubber slings and not metal surgical instruments. Tributaries are closed and divided between metal clips.

Following mobilization of the saphenous vein, a fasciotomy is performed and the popliteal vein is mobilized using atraumatic techniques. If a double popliteal vein is encountered, the larger vein of the one with the fewest postthrombotic changes is chosen for anastomosis.

After a bolus of 5000 units of heparin, venous flow is interrupted digitally or with rubber slings. Either an end-to-side or end-to-end anastomosis is performed, depending upon the size match of the saphenous vein and the popliteal vein. In deeply situated popliteal veins, the end-to-end anastomosis obviates a hemodynamically unfavorable, steep anastomotic angle. It is necessary sometimes to transsect the pes anserinus in order to avoid angulation of the vein. When this is done, reanastomosis is unnecessary. When closing the fascia, a large gap is left so that the vein is not compressed in transit through the fascia.

Following the creation of the proximal anastomosis, the distal saphenous vein is mobilized at the ankle by means of an S-shaped incision. It is then anastomosed end to side to the posterior tibial artery. The back wall of the anastomosis is performed first under magnification, and then the anterior wall is closed. Magnification, although useful in creating the distal arteriovenous fistula, is not necessary for the saphenopopliteal anastomosis (11,13,14).

Nonabsorbable 6-0 monofilament polytetraflueoroethylene (PTFE) sutures have been used for the saphenopopliteal anastomosis and 8-0 sutures for the arteriovenous anastomosis. The arteriovenous anastomosis transmits arterial blood flow into the saphenous vein and from there through the perforating veins into the tibial venous trunks. This causes an increase in flow velocity in the tibial and peroneal veins and irrigates the saphenopopliteal anastomosis. It is believed that this increased flow velocity is essential to ensure patency of the anastomosis, especially when the calf muscle pump is at rest in the first few postoperative days.

After surgery, increasing doses of heparin are administered via constant intravenous perfusion. After 6 days postoperatively, there is a gradual changeover to oral anticoagulation. Mobilization of the patient is started on the fourth day after surgery. Patients with a peripheral arteriovenous fistula are not allowed to wear compression bandages or stockings because these may compromise the function of the fistula.

The arteriovenous anastomosis is allowed to function for 2 to 3 months. In the majority of cases, this can be closed by applying a tight elastic compression bandage. When local pressure is applied, the thrill and flow murmur of the fistula disappear after a few days. Surgical closure of the anastomosis has been necessary in only three of the nine cases performed to this date. Follow-up of the patient's course and prescription of compression therapy, as well as the estimation of functional results of treatment, are made at 6-month intervals postoperatively by measurement of ambulatory venous pressure and by plethysmography.

Results

Experience to date includes 14 May-Husni operations. Nine of these were performed with arteriovenous fistulas and five without. As indicated previously, the May-Husni operation has been combined with a Palma operation in five cases. Interestingly, in the two cases of continued patency of both bypasses, the transplants showed varicose dilation but venous pressure curves continued to show improvement in the postoperative state as compared to the preoperative estimates. Those patients have been followed since 1974 and 1979. In the patients with thrombosis, all three had occlusion of the saphenopopliteal bypass. None occluded the cross-pubic bypass of Palma.

In the patients with saphenopopliteal operations, all showed clearly improved venous pressure curves and volumetric curves immediately after operation or after the arteriovenous fistula had been closed. Follow-up examinations after 10 to 15 years show that the transplanted vein can develop varicose degeneration without decreasing its function (Table 22–2).

Of the 14 patients receiving May-Husni bypass, three developed postoperative thrombosis. In all three, the venous pressure curves deteriorated. These patients continue to suffer from severe chronic venous insufficiency and must be treated with strong compression bandaging.

Four patients with patent saphenopopliteal bypasses have exhibited worsening of the venous pressure and volumetric curves. These now correspond to preoperative curves. Seven patients with patent transplants show a lasting im-

TABLE 22–2. Long-Term Results of the May-Husni Operation in 14 Patients

	MAY-HUSNI PLUS PALMA	MAY-HUSNI ALONE
No. of patients	5	3
Graft thrombosis	3	
Worsening (varicose dilation)		4
Good function (varicose dilation in 4)	2	7

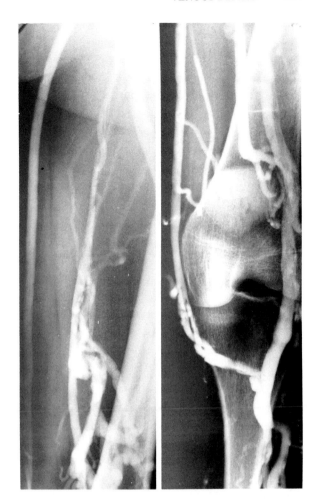

Figure 22–2. A functioning May-Husni operation after 7 years.

provement of function 10 to 15 years postoperatively. In two of these, the transplants are clearly varicose (Table 22–2).

It is appreciated that the number of patients is small and it is not possible at present to arrive at a reliable conclusion regarding the significance of the peripheral arteriovenous anastomosis with regard to success of the treatment (15) (Fig. 22–2).

PALMA OPERATION

Preoperative Evaluation

Before performing the Palma operation, pressure is measured in the common femoral vein bilaterally in the supine patient. In the horizontal position, venous pressure in the common femoral vein is between 4 and 6 mm Hg. Several authors (10,16) reported a somewhat higher pressure in the left femoral vein even under physiologic conditions. In unilateral occlusion of the iliofemoral veins, the resting pressure in the horizontal position of the patient is only slightly higher on the occluded side than the resting pressure on the contralateral side. In a well-collateralized iliofemoral vein occlusion, the venous pressure only rises slightly, even during exercise, by foot dorsiflexion. When this is encountered, the Palma operation is not indicated. Various authors (16,17) have suggested that the exercise performed in the horizontal position should consist of flexion and extension of the upper ankle joint. If the pressure rises in the femoral vein to at least double the resting pressure, and especially when the resting pressure itself is abnormally elevated, these findings are regarded as an indication for the Palma procedure. In brief, the exercise pressure must be at least 10 mm Hg when a resting pressure of 5 mm Hg is encountered (Figs. 22–3 and 22–4).

The curve obtained from the venous occlusion plethysmographic volumetry will correspond to the curve of venous pressure in patients with patent deep veins in the legs and thigh. This is because emptying of the venous sytem is impeded by a central obstruction to drainage. A rise of the femoral venous pressure to double or three times resting values corresponds to a fall in volume during exercise of, at the most, one third of the fall in volume in the normal, healthy side. Exercise in this instance is 10 toe stands.

Surgical Procedure

The Palma operation is carried out with the patient in the supine position under intubation anesthesia. The duration of the operation can be shortened by deploying a second surgical team. On the normal venous side, the termination of

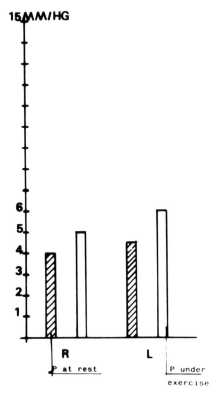

Figure 22–3.   No functional indication for a Palma operation.

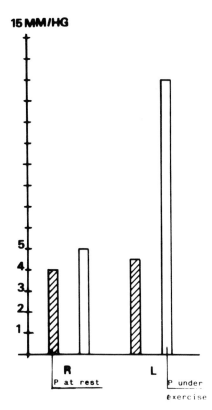

Figure 22–4. Good functional indication for a Palma operation, in which long-term success is expected.

the saphenous vein is exposed from a high inguinal incision. The vein is touched as little as possible with metal instruments and is manipulated only with moistened rubber slings. Venous branches or tributaries are closed with metal clips and divided.

In order to expose an adequate length of the greater saphenous vein on the normal side, two or three additional incisions are necessary. These are placed directly over the saphenous vein, and the vein itself is initially left in situ after mobilization. On the occluded side, the common femoral vein is exposed from a high inguinal incision. The vein is denuded as little as possible. This approach allows dissection of the femoral artery and its bifurcation, with placement of atraumatic rubber slings on the common femoral, the superficial femoral, and the deep femoral arteries. The greater saphenous vein, its tributaries, and any suprapubic collateral veins that may be present are carefully mobilized, avoiding damage to the structures. Any one of the tributary veins may be used as an arteriovenous fistula.

Before interruption of the venous circulation, the patient is systemically anticoagulated with 5000 units of heparin. The optimal sites for connection of the Palma transplant will be determined by inspection and palpation of the common femoral vein, the superficial femoral vein, and the proximal greater saphenous vein. At this time, it will be decided whether or not the anastomosis will be made end to end or end to side depending upon the caliber of the transplant vein itself.

When the saphenous vein on the normal side is too small in diameter or perhaps absent, consideration should be given to use of the ipsilateral greater saphenous vein as an inverse Palma transplant. Alternatively, a plastic prosthesis may be inserted.

Prior to performing the anastomosis on the affected side, blood flow is interrupted with rubber slings or hydragrip clamps. If an end-to-end anastomosis is chosen, the common femoral vein is severed obliquely. For an end-to-side anastomosis the vein is opened by a longitudinal, oblique incision. Suprapubic, bidigital tunneling is carried out and exact measurement of the length of the transplant is made with a marking thread. The saphenous vein to be used as a transplant is then severed transversely at the proper level. Torsion of this vein is carefully avoided, and the anterior wall of the vein may be marked with a suture. The vein is then tunneled without tension to the opposite side and anastomosed obliquely end to end or end to side to the common femoral vein. This anastomosis is carried out with continuous suture technique with a monofilament 6-0 PTFE suture (6,18,19).

In the inverse Palma operation, the greater saphenous vein on the occluded side is mobilized with the same careful, atraumatic technique described above. The vein is also tunneled suprapubically to the contralateral side after distal division. Since the vein of the occluded side is markedly dilated, many of the valves are already incompetent and elimination of these valves by valvotomy is practially always unnecessary.

In 1978, we began use of the spirally reinforced PTFE prosthesis using an 8 to 10-mm diameter graft (Fig. 22–5). Initially, the indication for this was an absent saphenous vein or an unsuitable saphenous vein bilaterally. The first PTFE Palma transplants were positioned subcutaneously suprapubically as in the original operation (Fig. 22–6). That first experience with the use of a PTFE prosthesis was favorable. During subsequent years, we have increasingly turned to preserving the greater saphenous vein for arterial or other reconstructions.

Apart from a few exceptions, we exclusively use PTFE prostheses for the

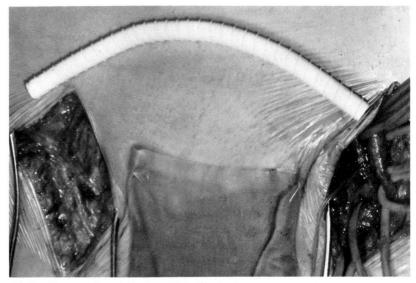

Figure 22–5. The use of a spiral-wrap PTFE prosthesis [Improflex (Impra Inc., Tempe, AZ)] as a Palma transplant ensures short- and long-term patency.

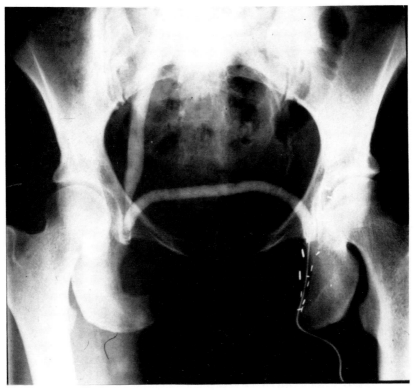

Figure 22–6. A PTFE prosthesis as Palma transplant in the original position placed subcutaneously.

Palma transplant today. Because of this, we have modified the surgical technique. The PTFE graft is connected on the occluded side end to end or end to side as in the classic Palma operation. However, the graft is led behind the inguinal ligament and behind the abdominal musculature to the contralateral side in a prevesical, suprapubic position. The connection on the recipient side is carried out obliquely end to side to the external iliac vein. We use a short, oblique incision in the lower abdomen as an approach to this structure. This modification ensures better protection of the transplant by abdominal musculature and produces the slightly S-shaped and hemodynamically more favorable transplant course (Fig. 22–7).

Because of the favorable PTFE experience, we have only carried out a single venous Palma operation in recent years. This was necessary in a young woman medical student who developed prosthesis infection after a successful PTFE Palma operation. The plastic prosthesis was removed and after conservative therapy had been applied for 6 months, an original, classic Palma operation was performed using the greater saphenous vein from the normal extremity. The severity of the postphlebitic venous stasis had entirely disabled the patient.

We always create a temporary arteriovenous fistula at the level of the groin when performing the original Palma operation and in doing the PTFE Palma transplant. In the early experience, we used the proximal part of the ipsilateral greater saphenous vein for this purpose. In order to protect this important vessel, the arteriovenous fistula now is created with a high branch of the greater saphenous

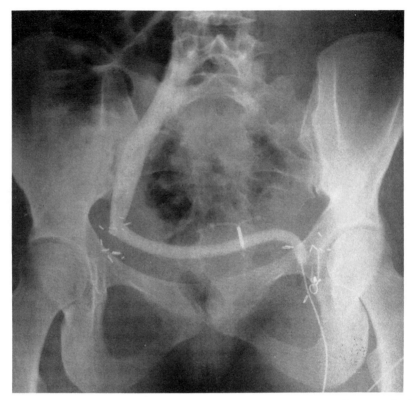

Figure 22–7.   A PTFE prosthesis as Palma transplant in the modified position, retrofascial.

vein, a branch of the deep femoral vein, or a suitable suprapubic collateral vein. The fistula is carried out end to side either to the common femoral artery or the superficial femoral artery. This is done with continuous 6-0 or 7-0 PTFE suture. The caliber of a suprapubic collateral vein that is too capacious may be reduced by enveloping it with a PTFE prosthesis segment.

Two points can be made with regard to surgical technique in creating the arteriovenous fistula. These ensure that later closure of the fistula will not entail any unnecessary difficulties. First, the fistula vein must be sufficiently long to be displaced into the subcutaneous tissue. Second, the fistula should be marked by a wire loop. This will later facilitate dissection and exposure of the fistula (7,12,14,20,21).

Finally, before conclusion of the operation, a fine plastic catheter is placed into a side branch of the greater saphenous vein or the superficial femoral vein in the immediate vicinity of the Palma anastomosis. The patient is anticoagulated intraoperatively and postoperatively with heparin via this catheter and, in addition, the catheter allows intraoperative and postoperative plebography (Fig. 22–8).

Results

Forty-nine Palma operations were carried out in 47 patients in the 18 years from July 1, 1971 to December 31, 1989. In one case, a PTFE prosthesis was

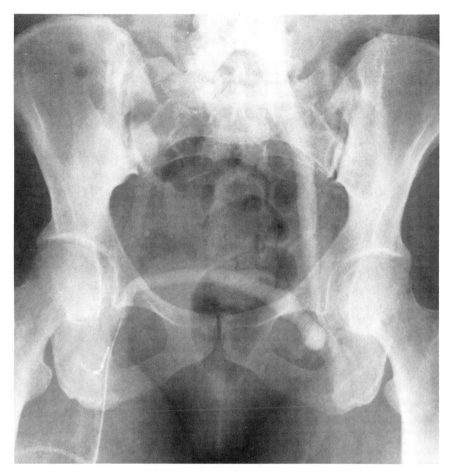

Figure 22–8. Phlebographic access to a venous Palma transplant via a thin intra-venous catheter placed in a venous side branch at surgery.

placed after occlusion of the venous Palma transplant. This graft has remained open over the long term. In another case a PTFE transplant was removed because of infection and was later replaced by a vein transplant, as indicated previously.

The mean age of patients operated upon has been 36 years at the time of the operation (range 16 to 68 years) (Table 22–3). Four patients were men and 43

TABLE 22–3. Characteristics of 47 Patients with 49 Palma Operations

Age (years)	
Mean	36
Range	16–68
Sex	
Male	4
Female	43
Occlusion	
Right	5
Left	44
Graft type	
Autologous	20
PTFE	29

TABLE 22–4.   Follow-up Results of 49 Palma Operations in 47 Patients

	TYPE OF GRAFT	
	Vein	PTFE
Patients operated	20	29
No. followed up	15	23
No. patient grafts	10	20
No. with recurrent postthrombotic syndrome	5	3

were women. The right iliofemoral segment was occluded in five cases, and the left in 44 cases. The autologous greater saphenous vein was used as a transplant 20 times and a spirally reinforced PTFE prosthesis was used 29 times. Fifteen of 20 venous Palma transplant patients were followed up (Table 22–4). Ten Palma transplants were still functioning at the time of follow-up examination. Of 29 PTFE operations, 23 were available for follow-up, and 20 of these were patent.

In the follow-up evaluation, measurement of venous pressure and venous occlusion plethysmographic volumetry were carried out routinely. However, ascending plebography was done only when indicated clinically. All patients with functioning venous or PTFE Palma transplants were free of subjective symptoms. They did not require elastic compression stockings or bandages and did not take venostatic medications. Five patients with venous transplants and three from the PTFE groups suffered from recurrent postthrombotic syndrome and had to wear long, class III elastic compression stockings continuously (Table 22–4).

A direct group comparison of venous and PTFE Palma operations is not possible. The patients were operated upon at different times with different indications. Most venous Palma operations were carried before 1978 and all PTFE Palma operations were performed after that date. In the first period of experience, venous pressures were not measured regularly. Until 1975, patients with severe postphlebitic syndrome were operated upon exclusively with phlebographic criteria.

Our results are comparable to those of Robert May, who reported on long-term patency of 16 grafts in a series of 22 total cases (16). After perfecting his surgical technique and emphasizing sparing of endothelium, he reported in 1980 on long-term patency of 13 venous transplants in 14 operations (Table 22–5).

Halliday performs the Palma transplant on the basis of clinical and phlebographic criteria without functional indications (22). In only four of 50 patients did he carry out an arteriovenous fistula. When this was done, he used the Krug modification. His reported cumulative 5-year patency rate was 75 per cent, with a standard deviation of 9 per cent (Table 22–6). The 10-year patency rate was 28 per cent with a standard deviation of 16 per cent. We continue to share May's view that the Krug modification, in which the venous Palma transplant is anas-

TABLE 22–5.   Long-Term Results in Two Series of Palma Operations by May

DATE OF REPORT	NO. OF OPERATIONS	NO. PATIENT
1971	22	16
1980	14	13

TABLE 22–6.   Long-Term Patency in 50 Palma Operations on 47 Patients
(Halliday)

	CUMULATIVE PATENCY	S.D.
5 years	75	9
10 years	28	16

tomosed side to side with the common femoral vein and the end of the saphenous vein is anastomosed to the side of the common femoral artery, results in an unfavorable hemodynamic situation. A high branch of the saphenous vein, when used for an arteriovenous fistula, is more favorable.

COMPLICATIONS

In the May-Husni operation, we observed that transplant thrombosis was followed by subsequent spontaneous recanalization only once. This was under the effect of a temporary distal arteriovenous fistula. Interestingly, in another case we had to carry out a laparotomy after a May-Husni operation because the patient had an intraabdominal hemorrhage from a ruptured ovarian cyst.

After the Palma operation, an extensive hematoma formed on the occluded side in two cases. This was controlled without operative intervention. As indicated above, infection occurred in a prosthetic graft after a Palma operation, and a successful correction was carried out with an autologous Palma transplant. In none of the patients with Palma operation have thromboembolic complications or early occlusions been observed.

SUMMARY AND CONCLUSIONS

Venous reconstructions should be carried out only with strict indications and confirmation of pathologic and physiologic parameters as indicated. It is to be expected that the number of patients who actually undergo such surgery will be exceedingly small. In our experience, only 63 venous reconstructions have been carried out during a time when 12,379 total vascular reconstructions were performed in our hospital.

The primary postoperative results after the May-Husni operation are favorable. However, long-term observation of these mostly young patients shows that the late results are unsatisfactory. After 10 to 15 years, only half (7 of 14) showed a satisfactory result. Even in those saphenopopliteal grafts that were still functioning well, a marked varicose degeneration was easily detected in two of the cases.

In contrast to the saphenopopliteal graft, the long-term results of the Palma operations are better. Varicose degeneration of the venous Palma transplant is not accompanied by loss of function. This is probably true because venous valves play a lesser role in the Palma procedure than they do in the saphenopopliteal procedure. The long-term results of the Palma operations with spirally reinforced PTFE prostheses are encouraging. After 10 years, 20 of 23 prostheses that have been followed proved to be patent. Six other grafts have been lost to follow-up. It appears to us to be justified to use the PTFE graft rather than the saphenous vein for primary Palma procedures, and it should be noted that this is a reversal of a previously held position.

REFERENCES

1. May R: Der Femoralisbypas beim postthrombotischen Zustandsbild. Vasa 1972;*1*:267.
2. May R: Venentransplantation beim postthrombotischen Zustandsbild. Actuelle Chir 1972;*7*:1.
3. Husni EA: In situ saphenopopliteal bypass graft for incompetence of the femoral and popliteal veins. Surg Gynecol Obstet 1970;*130*:297.
4. Husni EA: Clinical experience with femoralpopliteal venous reconstruction. *In* Bergan JJ, Yao JST, eds: Venous Problems. Chicago, Year Book Medical Publishers, 1978;485.
5. Palma CE, Esperon R: Tratamiento del sindrome postthrombo-flebitico mediante transplante de safena interna. Angiologie 1959;*11*:87.
6. Palma EC, Esperon R: Vein transplants and grafts in surgical treatment of the postphlebitic syndrome. J Cardiovasc Surg 1960;*1*:94–107.
7. Gruss JD, Vargas Montano H, Bartels D, Hanschke D, Fietze-Fischer B: Direct reconstructive venous surgery. Int Angio 1985;*4*:441.
8. Warren R, Thayer T: Transplantation of the saphenous vein for postphlebitic stasis. Surgery 1954;*35*:867.
9. Frileux C, Pillot-Bienayme P, Gillot C: Bypass of segmental obliterations of ilio-femoral venous axis by transposition of saphenous vein. J Cardiovasc Surg 1972;*13*:409.
10. May R: Chirurgie der Bein- und Beckenvenen. Stuttgart, Georg Thieme Verlag, 1974.
11. Gruss JD: Zur Modifikation des Femoralisbypass nach May. Vasa 1975;*4*:59.
12. Gruss JD, Bartels D, Tsafandakis E, et al: The AV fistula operation technique. *In* May R, Weber J, eds: Pelvic and Abdominal Veins. Amsterdam, Excerpta Medica, 1981;215.
13. Gruss JD: The saphenopopliteal bypass for chronic venous insufficiency (May-Husni operation). *In* Bergan JJ, Yao JST, eds: Surgery of the Veins. Orlando, FL, Grune & Stratton, Inc, 1985;255–265.
14. Gruss JD, Laubach K: Modifikation der Operationstechnik bei tiefer Becken- und Oberschenkelvenenthrombose. Thoraxchirurgie 1971;*19*:508.
15. May R: Spätergebnisse nach venösem Femoralisbypass. Vasa 1979;*8*:67.
16. May R, Weber J, eds: Pelvic and Abdominal Veins: Progress in Diagnostics and Therapy. International Congress Series 550. Amsterdam, Excerpta Medica, 1981.
17. Negus D, Cockett FB: Femoral vein pressures in postphlebitic iliac vein obstruction. Br J Surg 1967;*54*:522–525.
18. Dale WA: Reconstructive venous surgery. *In* Veith FJ, ed: Critical Problems in Vascular Surgery. New York, Appleton-Century-Crofts, 1982;199–213.
19. Dale WA: Crossover vein grafts for relief of iliofemoral venous block. Surgery 1965;*57*:608–612.
20. Kunlin J: Le rétablissement de la circulation veineuse par greffe en cas d'obliteration traumatique ou thrombophlébitique. Greffe de 18 cm entre la veine saphène interne et la veine iliaque externe. Thrombose après trois semaines de perméabilité. Présente par R. Leriche. Mem Acad Chir 1953;*79*:109.
21. Dumanian AV, Santschi DR, Park U, et al: Cross-over saphenous vein graft combined with a temporary femoral arteriovenous fistula. Vasc Surg 1968;*2*:116.
22. Halliday P, Harris J, May J: Femoro-femoral crossover grafts (Palma operation): A long term follow-up study. *In* Bergan JJ, Yao JST, eds: Surgery of the Veins. Orlando, FL, Grune & Stratton, Inc, 1985;241–254.

VII

THE SWOLLEN LEG

23

INVOLVEMENT OF THE LYMPHATIC SYSTEM IN CHRONIC VENOUS INSUFFICIENCY

Sharon L. Hammond, Edward R. Gomez,
James A. Coffey, Carl G. Lauer, Norman M. Rich,
and J. Leonel Villavicencio

The involvement of the lymphatic system in patients with chronic venous insufficiency (CVI) has received little attention, yet this involvement may have significant clinical and therapeutic implications. It is well recognized that both the lymphatic and venous systems share an early embryologic development. Sabin, in 1916, suggested that the lymphatics originated from the venous system and thereafter accompanied the veins in both the upper and lower extremities (1). Further support for this common origin was reported by Yoffey and Courtice, who described the lymph system as "off shoots" from the endothelium of veins (2).

In addition to a similar embryologic development, the lymphatics are known to course anatomically in close proximity to the venous trunks. The superficial lymphatic system originates from plexuses on the plantar surface of the foot, and continues through interdigital clefts to form collecting channels on the dorsum of the foot. These channels run along the pathway of the lesser and greater saphenous veins to drain into the superficial inguinal lymph nodes. The deep lymphatic vessels of the lower limb likewise accompany the deep vessels of the leg to the popliteal lymph nodes and then continue along the femoral vessels to reach the deep inguinal lymph nodes (3). This shared embryology and close anatomic relationship between the lymphatic and venous systems was recognized by early investigators, prompting them to speculate that the edema following venous thrombosis may have a lymphatic component.

HISTORICAL PERSPECTIVE

In designing an experimental model for iliofemoral thrombosis, Homans detected a significant component of lymphatic obstruction. He believed that this phenomenon occurred when the venous thrombosis was associated with an inflammatory process (4). Homans applied his experimental results to the clinical condition of phlegmasia alba dolens. It was his belief that this clinical condition could be altered by "releasing the lymph channels from the inflammatory pressure in which they are held, that is, in and about the sheath of the great vessels from the region of the common iliac vein down to the opening of the greater saphenous vein into the femoral and perhaps even lower in the thigh" (4).

Matas observed that elephantiasis could follow an episode of either venous or lymphatic obstruction (5), while Reichert further explored this concept through animal experimentation. Reichert demonstrated that division of the femoral vein could produce lymphatic edema through the interruption of small lymphatic vessels on the vein's surface (6).

Linton further acknowledged the lymphatic and venous system relationship in patients with the postphlebitic syndrome (7). He believed that the lymphatic obstruction was secondary to scarring and fibrosis that occurred in the perivascular tissue of the blood vessel, and he demonstrated lymphedema in 100 per cent of extremities with venous thrombosis (Fig. 23–1).

From this brief historical review, it is evident that the involvement of the lymphatic system and its contribution to the edema observed in patients with CVI has been strongly suspected by several investigators since the first publication of Homans. Many of us have been impressed by the large amounts of protein-rich fluid that virtually oozes from every pore of the limb of a patient with severe postphlebitic sequelae and wet eczema (Fig. 23–2). These clinical observations linking lymphatic disorders to venous pathology have been recently supported by the dramatic findings provided by new radiographic techniques and isotope exploration of the lymphatic system (8).

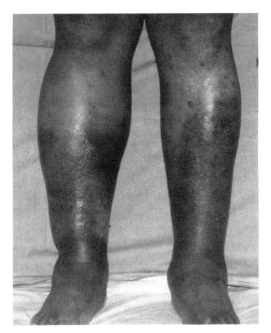

Figure 23–1. Pigmentation and edema in a patient with chronic venous insufficiency secondary to deep venous thrombosis occurring 7 years earlier. Swelling is more pronounced in the right leg.

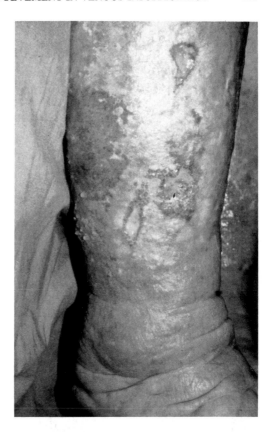

Figure 23–2. Severe postphlebitic sequelae in a patient who suffered a deep venous thrombosis 12 years earlier. Eczema, ulceration, and marked lymphatic oozing have produced incapacitating symptoms. Note the sweatlike lymph droplets on the posterior aspect of the leg.

EXPLORATION OF THE LYMPHATIC SYSTEM

Evaluation of the lymphatic system has progressed over the years from the era of injections of mercury in cadaver dissections to the modern techniques of radiographic visualization and nuclear scans. Initially, experimentation with vital dye injections was performed. Patent Blue dye, introduced by Hudack and McMaster and extensively used by Kinmonth, was subsequently used intradermally to facilitate localization of the lymphatics (9). As an 11 per cent solution it is readily diffusible into the tissues and selectively absorbed by the lymphatics. It is currently used as a valuable adjunct with radiographic lymphography to identify the location of the lymphatic vessels and facilitate their subsequent cannulation.

In 1956 Brunn and Engeset injected an oil-soluble contrast agent into the lymph nodes of a patient with lymphosarcoma, and demonstrated the lymph pathways (10). This method led to the use of water-soluble agents, which have the advantage of being able to be administered in larger volumes.

Kinmonth pioneered radiographic lymphography, which was the basis for the evaluation of the anatomy and structure of the lymphatic system (9). He introduced the classification of lymphedema based on the radiologic findings from lymphography. Kinmonth's classification of lymphedema into congenital or primary and acquired or secondary, as well as his lymphangiographic, morphologic, and anatomic organization of pathologic changes in patients with lymphedema, were cornerstones in the study of the lymphatic system. This classification served as the basis by which to compare other studies designed to explore the system. Kinmonth's lymphangiography can be compared to phlebography or arteriography in the vascular system. Its main deterrent is that its execution requires exquisite skill and great patience (Fig. 23–3).

The Kinmonth method for direct lymphography, which is still in current practice today, involves dissection of the lymphatic channel, cannulation, and subsequent injection of a contrast medium. Often the injections need to be performed under general anesthesia because of patient discomfort. Complications include not only discomfort, but allergic dye reactions and potential injury to the lymphatic system. The injury can occur either during the dissection of the lymphatic channel or from the injection of the contrast medium and subsequent inflammation of the lymphatic vessels, leading to lymphangitis. Although sharp anatomic detail can be obtained from this direct method of lymphatic visualization, it provides scarce information on the function of the lymphatic system.

Other methods that have been introduced to evaluate the lymphatic system include fluorescein microlymphography and indirect lymphography. In the former method, fluorescein dyes are injected intravenously as described by Bollinger et

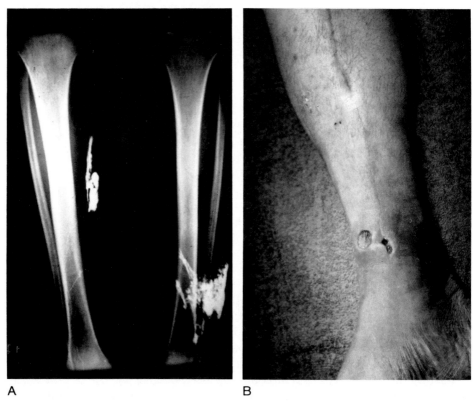

A   B

Figure 23–3.   *A*, Lymphangiogram obtained by direct cannulation of lymphatic channels on the foot. Observe the extensive contrast extravasation through areas of lymphatic disruption secondary to saphenous vein harvesting. *B*, This patient developed edema and areas of skin necrosis after saphenous vein harvesting for coronary artery bypass surgery.

al. (11). This method has been useful in differentiating swelling occurring in lymphedema from that due to CVI. Patients with CVI were found to have larger pericapillary areolas, known as "halos" (12). Indirect lymphography has employed a variety of reagents, including contrast media such as Iotasol (13). It can also be performed with the use of radionuclides. The latter method requires a specialized scintillation camera, but has the advantage in that it is performed in a noninvasive fashion.

Lymphoscintigraphy (LSC) as an imaging modality can simultaneously interpret morphologic and functional alterations occurring to the lymphatic system, by providing a visual image of the lymphatic flow patterns while assessing the lymphatic flow rate. As a diagnostic tool, isotopic scintigraphy was introduced by Sherman and Ter-Porgassian (14). Initially colloidal gold was the agent selected to visualize the lymph nodes. However, the radiation dose proved excessive and required the development of smaller particle sizes. Several colloids are currently in use. They include rhenium sulfide and antimony sulfide labeled with technetium. LSC has been used primarily in the lower extremity for the evaluation of swelling in patients with primary and secondary lymphedema, and in patients with venous disorders such as Klippel-Trenaunay syndrome, saphenous vein excision, transposition, and chronic venous insufficiency (8,15).

LYMPHOSCINTIGRAPHIC TECHNIQUE

LSC is performed at the Walter Reed Army Medical Center under a research protocol using technetium-99m–labeled antimony trisulfide colloid (Tc-Sb2S3) (Cadema Medical Products, Inc, Middletown, NY). The procedure requires the injection of the colloid subcutaneously into three interdigital web spaces of each foot. One millicurie (37 megabequerels) of Tc-Sb2S3 is mixed with 0.3 to 0.5 ml of normal saline for each foot injection. Prior to the injections the patient ambulates or performs stationary foot presses. Images are then obtained at 10-min intervals with the use of a gamma camera (General Electric Medical Systems Group, Milwaukee, WI) with a large field of view. Immediately after injection, three consecutive images over the pelvis are obtained at 10-min intervals anteriorly. Images are obtained with the patient supine. If inguinal nodes are not seen within 30 min, pelvic imaging is repeated at 1 hr; if there still is no visualization, pelvic imaging is repeated 2 and 4 hr after injection. If additional images are needed after 1 hr as a result of delayed visualization of the inguinal nodes, the patient then ambulates again before repeating the images. Assessment of LSC studies involves three components: 1) an interpretation of the drainage pattern, 2) the degree of visualization of the tracer in the groin nodes, and 3) the rate of flow. Figure 23–4 demonstrates a normal anatomic drainage, along with bilateral symmetric transit of the tracer to the inguinal nodes within 1 hr.

Abdominal LSC patterns include collateralization, lateral channels, dermal backflow, obstruction, lymphoceles, and reflux. The degree of visualization is considered normal when there is clear visualization of the tracer in the inguinal nodes. Abnormal visualization will show either an enhanced or a faint visualization of the isotope at the inguinal nodes. Flow is considered normal if there is activity of the tracer at the inguinal nodes within 30 min. Accelerated flow is described when visualization occurs on the initial 10-min image, and delayed flow is defined as the absence of inguinal node visualization at 60 min (Fig. 23–5).

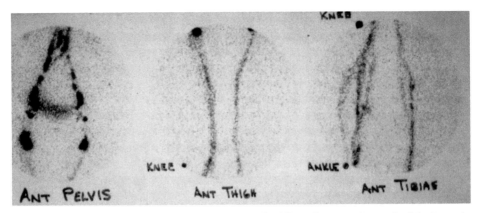

Figure 23–4. Normal lymphoscintigraphy demonstrating bilateral symmetric transit of the tracer to the inguinal nodes within 1 hr. The degree of tracer visualization is normal.

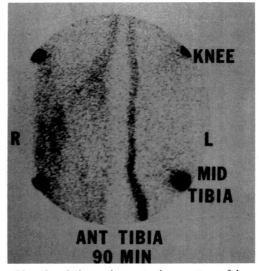

Figure 23–5. Abnormal lymphoscintigram demonstrating a pattern of dermal backflow in the right leg and delayed visualization at 90 min in a patient with lymphadema and lymphatic obstruction at the groin.

TABLE 23–1. Lymphoscintigraphic Flow Rates in Patients with Chronic Venous Insufficiency

AUTHOR	YEAR	PATIENTS	FLOW RATE
Battezatti and Domini (18)	1964	*a*	Accelerated
Stewart et al. (15)	1985	5	Accelerated
Weissleder and Weissleder (19)	1988	34	Delayed
Gloviczki et al. (17)	1989	4	Normal
		1	Accelerated
Collins et al. (8)	1989	10	Delayed

a Number of patients not specified.

The evaluation of LSC with the three components as described represents a semiquantitative analysis. Although quantitative studies have been described (16), interpretation of the data remains confusing. Using a semiquantitative method of interpretation, LSC has been shown to have a 92 per cent sensitivity and 100 per cent specificity in determining if the lymphatic system was normal or abnormal (17).

Several reports have been published on the use of LSC in the evaluation of the swollen extremity, but few investigators have included patients with CVI. In the studies that have evaluated swollen extremities in patients with CVI, the data have been conflicting. Some investigators have reported that there is an accelerated lymphatic flow in cases of CVI (15,18). Others have shown a normal flow rate, and still others have described a delayed transit time and obstructive lymphatic patterns (8,17,19). Table 23–1 summarizes the published series that have evaluated the swollen extremity by LSC and included patients with CVI.

WALTER REED ARMY MEDICAL CENTER EXPERIENCE

In an effort to expand on LSC studies previously published (8), a prospective study (20) was undertaken on 29 patients with CVI [nine females and 20 males, age range from 25 to 83 years (mean 63 years), with duration of disease from 1 to 50 years (mean 11 years)]. Nineteen patients had bilateral and 10 patients had unilateral CVI, providing a total of 48 extremities with CVI for evaluation. The 48 extremities were divided into two groups. Group A comprised 27 extremities with a documented history of deep venous thrombosis, and group B comprised 21 extremities with no history of deep venous thrombosis but with clinical examinations consistent with postphlebitic syndrome and noninvasive venous studies supporting the diagnosis for venous insufficiency (Table 23–2).

The degree of CVI was graded from 0 to 3 using the classification prepared by the Society for Vascular Surgery and the North American Chapter of the International Cardiovascular Society (21) (Table 23–3). Nineteen extremities were grade 3, with ulcer disease present; 17 extremities were grade 2, showing pig-

TABLE 23–2. Characteristics of 29 Patients with Chronic Venous Insufficiency

Sex	
Male	20
Female	9
Age (years)	
Mean	63
Range	25–83
Extremities	
Unilateral	10
Bilateral	19
Total	48
Etiology	
Postphlebitic (group A extremities)	27
Primary venous insufficiency[a] (group B extremities)	21
Duration of disease (years)	
Mean	11
Range	1–50

[a] Extremities having no history of thrombosis.

TABLE 23–3.   Classification of Chronic Venous Insufficiency[a]

CLASS	CURRENT SYMPTOMS
0	Asymptomatic
1	Mild (swelling)
2	Moderate (hyperpigmentation)
3	Severe (ulcerative changes)

[a] Adapted from Classification of the Subcommittee on Reporting Standards of Venous Disease (21).

TABLE 23–4.   Grade of Chronic Venous Insufficiency in 48 Lower Extremities

GRADE	NO. GROUP A EXTREMITIES	NO. GROUP B EXTREMITIES
0	2	2
1	6	2
2	12	5
3	8	11
Total	28	20

mentation; eight extremities were grade 1, with edema alone; and four extremities were grade 0, having normal clinical exams but abnormal noninvasive venous exams (Table 23–4). Twenty extremities had the presence or a history of cellulitis. No extremity had undergone previous operation. All patients underwent Doppler ultrasound, strain-gauge plethysmography, photoplethysmography, extremity circumference measurements at four levels, and LSC.

RESULTS

A total of 36 of 48 extremitites with CVI were found to have an abnormal LSC. This was statistically significant ($p < .01$). The abnormalities observed were both anatomic and functional in nature. Abnormal anatomic drainage patterns of obstruction identified by LSC included collateralization, lateral channels, dilated and prominent channels, dermal backflow, complete trunk obstruction, and crossover filling (Table 23–5).

TABLE 23–5.   Lymphoscintigraphic Patterns of Obstruction in Extremities with Chronic Venous Insufficiency

PATTERN	NO. EXTREMITIES
Collateralization	2
Lateral channels	1
Prominence	2
Dilation	2
Dermal backflow	2
Truncal interruption	1
Crossover filling	1
Total	11

TABLE 23–6. Patterns of Lymphoscintigraphic Visualization and Tracer Transit Time with Chronic Venous Insufficiency

	NO. EXTREMITIES
Visualization	
Enhanced	1
Decreased	7
Normal	40
Transit time	
Accelerated	2
Delayed	32
Normal	14

Functional changes revealed by LSC included abnormal visualization of the tracer at the groin nodes, as well as delay in the foot-to-groin transit of the radioactive tracer. The degree of visualization of the radioactive labeled tracer observed at the inguinal nodes, however, was altered in only eight extremities (seven extremities showed decreased visualization and one extremity demonstrated enhanced visualization). On the other hand, analysis of the transit time of the tracer revealed substantially different results. Thirty-two extremities showed delay in the transit time and only two extremities showed acceleration. Delayed transit of the lymphatic flow proved to be the most common abnormality revealed by LSC in patients with CVI (Table 23–6).

A correlation between the presence of an abnormal LSC and a history of thrombosis was also observed in this study. Eighty-three per cent of the patients in group A had an abnormal LSC versus 62 per cent of the patients in group B. Data also suggested that patients having the presence or a history of cellulitis had an increased chance for having an alteration of the lymphatic system (group A, 78 per cent; group B, 70 per cent).

DISCUSSION

The results of this prospective study (20) suggest that there is an important lymphatic involvement in patients with CVI, and are similar to those obtained by Weissleder and Weissleder in a study of 128 patients that included 34 patients with CVI (19). In that study, using LSC with technetium-99m–labeled albumin, all but seven extremities showed a delay in the transit of the tracer. Battezatti and Domini, on the other hand, described an acceleration of lymphatic flow in patients with postphlebitic edema, but did not elaborate on the number of patients studied or the nature of the venous disease (18). Similar results were reported by Stewart et al., who showed accelerated flow in 10 limbs with venous edema as well as an increased uptake at the inguinal nodes (15). However, they failed to describe the duration of venous disease in their patients. Since duration and type of venous disease were not specified in the latter two studies, analysis of these two studies and comparison of results with those obtained from Weissleder and Weissleder and our study is difficult.

Despite these controversial reports, it is clear from our analysis that patients with CVI have not only a certain degree of venous hypertension, but alterations that affect the lymphatic system as well. The accelerated flow that has been described on LSC probably represents an earlier stage in the process of venous thrombosis. This concept has been borne out in an experimental model for venous thrombosis. In their construction of an experimental design for acute venous hypertension in the canine, Leach and Browse were able to demonstrate an acceleration of lymphatic flow during the acute stages of venous thrombosis probably serves as a compensatory mechanism for clearance of the increased interstitial fluid, which is a consequence of the venous hypertension produced by the thrombotic process.

CVI produces a different lymphatic pattern, as suggested by Weissleder and Weissleder and our studies. Our patient population consisted of individuals with a long history of venous disease and a positive history for cellulitis and inflammation. Every new attack of cellulitis may produce increased destruction of cutaneous lymphatics and subsequent obstructive lymphatic patterns. It is therefore conceivable that after years of repeated episodes of inflammation and scarring, areas of narrowing and obstruction develop within the lymphatic vessels that produce alterations of the morphology and function of the lymphatic system.

The precise mechanism responsible for producing these lymphatic changes requires further clarification. Although the early investigators could only hypothesize that inflammation could lead to lymph stasis and lymphedema occurred after venous thrombosis, there are now data obtained through LSC to support this hypothesis. Results from LSC suggest that the lymphatic system is often impaired in patients with CVI. This impairment is reflected by the presence of anatomic changes, even though a delayed lymphatic flow rate is the most commonly observed anomaly. These changes may ultimately interfere with the clearance of interstitial fluid in extremities with chronic venous insufficiency and contribute to an increase in the clinical swelling observed. Further investigations are necessary to confirm this theory and substantiate the results observed with LSC.

The venous and lymphatic systems have both a similar embryologic origin and a close anatomic association. In venous pathology, this relationship becomes further magnified. Although few reports have described an alteration or involvement of the lymphatic system in patients with CVI, such a relationship does exist. Fluorescein studies have demonstrated a microlymphangiopathy, while LSC demonstrates anatomic as well as functional changes. A functional delay may represent subtle anatomic changes secondary to chronic inflammation and scarring over long periods of time, or may represent a true functional alteration.

These findings lend further support to the beneficial use of external elastic compression in CVI. More advanced cases of venous insufficiency with induration and ulceration may be best served with intermittent pneumatic compression, which has proven its usefulness in cases of severe lymphatic stasis.

REFERENCES

1. Sabin F: The origin and development of the lymphatic system. Johns Hopkins Hosp Rep 1916;*17*:347.
2. Moore KL: The cardiovascular system. *In* Moore KL, ed: The Developing Human, 2nd ed. Philadelphia, WB Saunders Company, 1977:248–285.
3. Woodburne RT: The superficial aspects of the limb. *In* Woodburne KL, ed: Essentials of Human Anatomy, 6th ed. New York, Oxford University Press, 1978;524–525.

4. Homans J: The operative treatment of phlegmasia alba dolens. N Engl J Med 1931;*204*:1025–1031.
5. Matas R: The surgical treatment of elephantiasis and elephantoid states, dependent upon chronic obstruction of the lymphatic and venous channel. Am J Trop Dis Prev Med 1913;*1*:60.
6. Reichert FL: The regeneration of lymphatics. Arch Surg 1926;*13*:871.
7. Linton RR: Post-thrombotic ulceration of the lower extremity: Its etiology and surgical treatment. Ann Surg 1953;*138*:582–591.
8. Collins PS, Villaviecencio JL, Abreu SH, et al: Abnormalities of lymphatic drainage in lower extremities: A lymphoscintigraphic study. J Vasc Surg 1989;9:145–152.
9. Kinmonth JB: Methods of lymphography. *In* Kinmonth JB, ed: The Lymphatics Surgery, Lymphography, and Disease of the Chyle and Lymph Systems, 2nd ed. London, Edward Arnold, 1902.
10. Brunn S, Engeset A: Lymphadenography. Acta Radiol 1956;*45*:389–395.
11. Bollinger A, Jager K, Siger F, Seglias J: Fluorescence microlymphography. Circulation 1981;*64*:1195–1200.
12. Saner H, Boss C, Mahler F: Demonstration of the pericapillary space after intravenous administration of sodium fluorescein. *In* Bollinger A, Partsch H, Wolfe JHN, eds: The Initial Lymphatic: New Methods and Findings; International Symposium Zurich, 1st ed. New York: Thiem-Stratton, 1985;94–97.
13. Wenzel-Hera BI, Partsch H, Urbanek A: Indirect lymphography with Iotasol. *In* Bollinger A, Partsch H, Wolfe JHN, eds: The Initial Lymphatics: New Methods and Findings; International Symposium Zurich, 1st ed. New York: Thieme-Stratton, 1985;94–97.
14. Sherman AI, Ter-Pogassian M: Lymph node concentration of radioactive colloidal gold following interstitial injection. Cancer 1953;6:1238–1240.
15. Stewert G, Gaunt JI, Croft DN, Browse NL: Isotope lymphography: A new method of investigating the role of the lymphatics in chronic limb edema. Br J Surg 1985;*72*:906–909.
16. Carena M, Campini R, Zelaschi G, et al: Quantitative lymphoscintigraphy. Eur J Nucl Med 1988;*14*:88–92.
17. Gloviczki P, Calcagno D, Schirger A, et al: Noninvasive evaluation of the swollen extremity: Experiences with 190 lymphoscintigraphic examinations. J Vasc Surg 1989;9:683–690.
18. Battezatti M, Domini I: The role of radioisotopes in the study of the physiopathology of the lymphatic system. J Cardiovasc Surg 1964;*56*:691–693.
19. Weissleder H, Weissleder R: Lymphedema: Evaluation of qualitative and quantitative lymphoscintigraphy in 238 patients. Radiology 1988;*167*:729–735.
20. Hammond SL, Gomez ER, Villavicencio JL: The post phlebitic syndrome and its impact on the lymphatic system: A lymphoscintigraphic analysis. Submitted for publication.
21. Porter JM, Clagett GP, Cranley J, et al: Reporting standards in venous disease. J Vasc Surg 1988;*8*:172–181.
22. Leach RD, Browse NL: Venous hypertension in dogs. J Vasc Surg 1985;*72*:275–278.

24

MICROSURGICAL TREATMENT FOR CHRONIC LYMPHEDEMA: An Unfulfilled Promise?

Peter Gloviczki

The natural history of chronic lymphedema is progressive swelling of the extremity, with induration and fibrosis of the subcutaneous tissue and hyperkeratosis and thickening of the skin. There is a decreased resistence to mycotic and bacterial infections, and frequent episodes of cellulitis and lymphangitis further destroy the lymphatic system. Without treatment, the disease causes significant cosmetic and functional problems in the limb, and the infectious complications may threaten the patient's life. Lymphangiosarcoma, a severe late complication of secondary lymphedema, is fortunately rare.

The mainstay of conservative treatment of chronic lymphedema has been the use of elastic compression with a bandage, gradual compression stocking, sleeve, or elastic garment. The use of intermittent pneumatic compression pumps has become popular, especially those with multiple cells for sequential compression. Prevention and immediate treatment of fungal, bacterial, or parasitic infection is necessary to prevent complications and further progression of the disease.

There have been few diseases, however, for which surgical treatment has been surrounded by more controversy than chronic lymphedema. The high number of different "excisional" and "physiologic" operations practiced around the world today is testimony to our frustration in dealing with this difficult problem. While the use of a debulking operation may be justified in advanced, disabling "elephantiasis," in patients with less severe disease such procedures can seldom be indicated.

The development of microsurgical techniques, with the ability to anastomose vessels less than 2 mm in diameter, promised new ways to treat obstructive lymphedema. Surgeons, enthusiastic from successful reconstructions for arterial occlusive disease, have suggested a similar strategy to treat the obstructed lymphatic system: bypass the obstruction with lymphovenous or with lymphatic grafting. Although experimental data were available as early as 1962 (1) and the first clinical applications of lymphovenous anastomoses were reported more than 30 years ago (2,3), microlymphatic surgery has been surrounded by doubt. Either the follow-up of the reported cases was short or objective documentation of the durability and late patency of the anastomoses was not convincing (2–14). In some reports the use of a concomitant resectional procedure made the evaluation of the microsurgical operation difficult (15,16). As one editor recently noted, it is uncertain whether these operations have been a promise unfulfilled or a promise that has been broken (17). In 1990, however, late results with lymphovenous anastomoses and lymphatic grafting performed in a large group of patients have been published by the two most productive microsurgical teams, headed by O'Brien in Australia (18) and Baumeister in Germany (19). Both papers documented long-term benefit following microsurgery.

To understand the rationale and technique of these microsurgical operations, a brief review of the anatomy of the lymphatic system of the extremities and the pathophysiology of the development of lymphedema is warranted.

ANATOMY OF THE LYMPHATIC SYSTEM

The lymphatic drainage of the lower extremity is divided into the superficial and the deep lymphatic systems (Fig. 24–1). The superficial system consists of a medial and a lateral group of lymph vessels (20). The medial bundle has five to 15 lymph vessels located in the anteromedial aspect of the extremity, which loosely follow the course of the greater saphenous vein. The lateral superficial lymphatic bundle consists of three to four lymph vessels that are located next to the lesser saphenous vein and either join a subfascial popliteal lymph node or join the medial superfical group above the knee. The deep lymphatic trunks follow the course of the anterior and posterior tibial and peroneal arteries and join a few subfascial popliteal lymph nodes. From here the deep femoral lymph vessels follow the course of the superficial femoral vein and enter into the inguinal nodes. There are three to 14 inguinal nodes, and although there is a superficial and a deep inguinal lymph node group, the difference between the two is not always obvious. The lymphatic drainage of the extremity is regional and there is no direct communication between the medial and lateral superficial lymphatic bundle distal to the knee. According to at least some authors (20), under normal conditions there is no significant communication present between the superficial and the deep lymphatic systems distal to the groin. Each of the main lymphatic groups collect lymph from their own region and not from others. Normally there are no significant direct communications between the main lymphatic vessels or nodes and the veins of the extremity.

Lymph drainage of the upper extremity follows a similar pattern (Fig. 24–2). Most of the lymph of the subcutaneous tissue is drained by the medial arm bundle, but there also is a superficial lateral group of lymph vessels and a deep system, which follows the course of the brachial artery and vein (21). Both the superficial and the deep systems enter the axillary lymph nodes. However, the lateral bundle, which may be an important collateral in case of axillary node dissection, carries most of the lymph to the supraclavicular nodes through the deltoideopectoral node group. Both the superficial and the deep lymph vessels can be used for lymphovenous or lympholymphatic anastomoses.

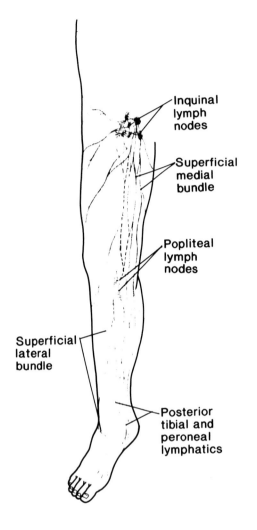

Figure 24–1. The lymphatic system of the lower extremity.

PATHOPHYSIOLOGY OF CHRONIC LYMPHEDEMA

Congenital or acquired insufficiency of the lymphatic transport results in lymph stasis and the accumulation of protein-rich interstitial fluid. However, chronic lymphedema develops only if the collateral lymphatic circulation becomes inadequate and the function of tissue macrophages, which aid in removal of macromolecules from the interstitial space, is exhausted. Other compensatory mechanisms, such as the function of spontaneous lymphovenous anastomoses, will also be insufficient.

Impairment of the lymphatic drainage results in significant changes in the lymphatic vessels and, even more importantly, in the subcutaneous tissue. Extensive proliferation of fibroblasts and sclerosis of the subcutaneous tissue have been observed, and the increased vascularity resembles changes seen in chronic inflammation (22–24). This raised questions about the effectiveness of microsurgical operations: Can restoration of the canalicular function of the lymph vessels

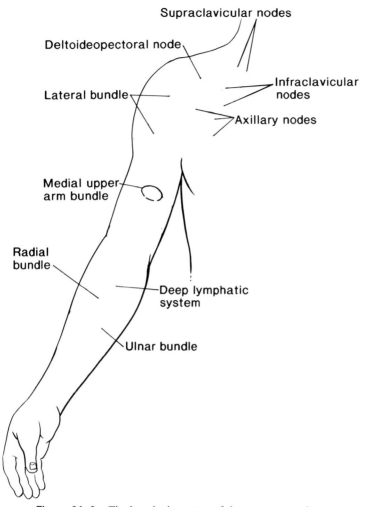

Figure 24–2. The lymphatic system of the upper extremity.

reverse the tissue changes that have already developed in chronic lymphedema (25)?

Secondary changes in the lymph vessels due to lymph stasis include fibrosis of the wall with loss of permeability and lymph concentration ability. The valves may also fibrose or become incompetent as a result of dilatation of the lymph vessels distal to the obstruction. The lymph vessel wall loses intrinsic contractility, and the muscle pump, which is an important element in lymphatic transport, will also be ineffective (22). Infection may result in obstructive lymphangitis with further destruction of the main and collateral lymphatic pathways. In the early phase of lymphedema there is an elevated intralymphatic pressure and normal lymphatic anatomy is preserved distal to the obstruction. Later, however, alteration in the interstitial tissue decreases interstitial and intralymphatic pressure (22). The quality of the lymphatic vessels suitable for anastomosis will also progressively deteriorate. The chances of successful microsurgical reconstruction in advanced chronic lymphedema are, therefore, truly diminished.

EXPERIMENTAL DATA

In experiments, objective evidence of patency of both microsurgical lymphovenous anastomoses and lymphatic grafting has been obtained. Performing lymphovenous anastomoses in dogs, Gilbert et al. (26) found a patency rate of 66 per cent between 6 and 12 weeks, a result similar to those obtained in our laboratory (27). In vivo cinelymphangiography gave us convincing evidence of patency up to 8 months after surgery. Scanning electron microscopy also confirmed patency (Fig. 24–3), and we observed complete endothelialization across the suture line by 4 weeks. Using an experimental model of severe obstructive lymphedema, however, Puckett et al. (28) failed to document patency of lymphovenous anastomoses at 3 weeks after the operation. His findings emphasize that the operation should be performed in the earlier stage of lymphedema, before significant tissue fibrosis and a complete loss of the valvular function of the lymphatics develop.

The technique of lymphatic grafting was developed by Baumeister (19,29,30). In experiments, he and his coworkers obtained 90 per cent patency of homologous

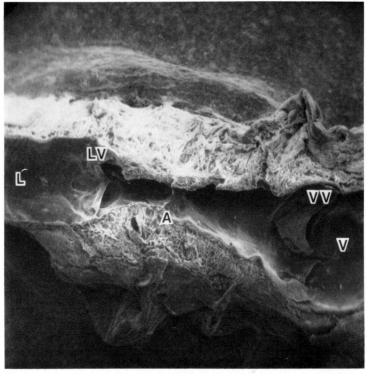

Figure 24–3. Scanning electron micrograph of a patent lymphovenous anastomosis 3 months after operation in a dog. *A*, anastomosis; *L*, lymph vessel; *LV*, lymphatic valve; *V*, vein; *VV*, venous valve. (Original magnification, ×10.) (From Gloviczki P, Hollier LH, Nora FE, Kaye MP: The natural history of microsurgical lymphovenous anastomoses: An experimental study. J Vasc Surg 1986;*4*:148–156.)

transplants of the abdominal thoracic duct in rats at 65 days after the procedure (31). Experimental lymphedema was successfully decreased with lymph vessel grafting in four dogs, confirming patency in all with contrast lymphangiography and lymphoscintigraphy (31).

CLINICAL APPLICATION

Nielubowicz was the first, in 1968, to report on successful lymph node–to–vein anastomoses in patients with lymphedema (2), and Yamada, in 1969, first performed lymph vessel–to–saphenous vein anastomoses in a 37-year-old patient with lower extremity secondary lymphedema (3). Microsurgical lymph vessel–to–vein anastomoses were subsequently reported by several authors (4–15), claiming success in patients with chronic secondary lymphedema of the upper or lower extremity. Encouraged by these favorable clinical reports and by our own experiments (22), our team at the Mayo Clinic has attempted microsurgical treatment in 26 patients with chronic lymphedema of the extremities. Results in the first 18 patients, 14 of whom had successful lymphovenous anastomosis operations, were reported previously (14). Since then, three additional patients have had lymphovenous anastomoses and five have had lymphatic grafting for unilateral lower extremity lymphedema.

PREOPERATIVE EVALUATION

In addition to obtaining a thorough history and performing a routine physical examination, blood tests, and chest roentgenogram, preoperative evaluation of patients with chronic leg swelling should include noninvasive venous studies and lymphoscintigraphy of the extremities. Patients with obstructive secondary lymphedema of the extremity may also have concomitant venous occlusion. We perform venous Doppler ultrasound evaluation and impedance plethysmography routinely, and duplex scanning of the deep veins selectively. Occlusion of the axillary-subclavian or iliofemoral vein results in venous hypertension and precludes the use of lymphovenous anastomosis. Computed tomography is performed routinely if the swelling began after puberty, or in any age group if malignancy is suspected. Patients with associated vascular malformation or suspected soft tissue tumor undergo nuclear magnetic resonance imaging.

Our current diagnostic test to prove that edema is of lymphatic origin is lymphoscintigraphy (32). We inject 400 to 500 μCi of technetium-99m–labeled antimony trisulfide colloid (Cadema Medical Products, Inc, Middletown, NY) in the second interdigital space of the hand or foot, with a small tuberculin syringe and a 24-gauge needle. The patients are asked to repeatedly squeeze a rubber ball or perform toe stands for a period of 3 min. Twelve-minute images are then obtained during a period of 1 hr. The gamma camera is positioned above the groin or the axilla. At 1 and 3 hr additional 5-min images are obtained of the trunk and affected extremity. Occasionally, delayed 6- or 24-hr images are obtained. In all normal patients, major regional (axillary or inguinal) lymph nodes were visualized at 1 hr. Although quantitative analysis of the data has been useful for some authors (33), we found semiquantitative evaluation of the lymphatic drainage and visual interpretation of the image pattern reliable to differentiate lymphedema from edemas of other origin (sensitivity: 92 per cent, specificity: 100 per cent) (30). Using lymphoscintigraphy alone we could not differentiate primary hypoplastic from secondary obstructive lymphedema, although there were certain image patterns that were characteristic of either the primary or the secondary type. Lymphoscintigraphy can be helpful in determining the site of the obstruction and it also can image major lymphatic vessels in the extremity that are suitable for microsurgery. The study, however, is primarily a functional and not an anatomic test. It determines the pattern of the lymphatic drainage of the area of the extremity where the labeled colloid is injected, but does not image all patent lymph vessels of the limb. During exploration using the operating microscope we could identify patent lymph channels even if they were not imaged by lymphoscintigraphy. In approximately 300 lymphoscintigraphic examinations, we observed no side effects and found this study to be safe and reliable.

The use of contrast lymphangiography has clearly been restricted in our practice. The procedure is painful, invasive, and difficult to repeat, and worsening of the lymphedema has been described by others (18) and also noted by us. We still use this test to confirm lymphangiectasia and reflux of the chyle to the pelvis or to the extremity if lymphoscintigraphy fails to give the definitive diagnosis (32). Occasionally, lymphangiography is still performed to exclude underlying malignancy or to localize a lymphatic fistula in the chest or abdomen.

PATIENT SELECTION

Good candidates for microsurgical reconstructions are patients with obstructive secondary lymphedema. On the upper extremity it is most frequently caused by axillary lymph node dissection, performed with mastectomy with or without irradiation. Inguinal lymphadenectomy in our series was the most frequent cause of lower extremity secondary lymphedema in patients who had cervical cancer or carcinoma of the prostate. Patients who had fewer episodes of cellulitis or who have lymphedema of short duration can expect a better surgical result (18).

PREOPERATIVE MANAGEMENT

Although most patients referred to us have had some form of compression treatment, we suggest they again undergo at least a 3-month trial of strict conservative management. The patients are fitted with a medium- or firm-compression elastic garment and are instructed to use an intermittent pneumatic compression pump at least twice daily. Proper skin care and the prevention of infections is emphasized.

We prefer to hospitalize patients with lower extremity edema 24 to 48 hr before operation to elevate the extremity and decrease the volume to facilitate dissection. Patients with upper extremity edema are hospitalized the morning of the operation. A first-generation cephalosporin is used perioperatively in every patient.

TECHNIQUE OF LYMPHOVENOUS ANASTOMOSIS

We have performed all of our operations under general anesthesia. In an attempt to visualize the lymph vessels, we inject 2 ml of Lymphazurine dye in the first interdigital space of the foot or hand and a similar dose about 10 to 15 cm distal to the incision site subcutaneously. The dye is massaged proximally manually with the help of an intermittent pneumatic compression pump. The sterile cuff is placed on the extremity distal to the incision. In many cases, however, because of the severe lymphatic stasis staining of the lymph vessels is not possible. For this reason, exploration and searching for the lymph channels under the operating microscope is performed. The most frequent site of anastomosis on the lower extremity is in the area just distal to the saphenofemoral junction. On the upper extremity the usual site of anastomosis is at the elbow or more proximally on the arm, in the medial bicipital fossa, subcutaneously or in the deep compartment. After the skin incision is made, lymph vessels, which usually measure 0.3 to 1.0 mm in diameter, are identified and marked by fine vessel loops. If epifascial dissection is completed, the search is continued subfascially. As many lymph vessels are dissected as possible. It is sometimes difficult to differentiate fibrosed lymph vessel from subcutaneous nerve or a fibrous cord. Under the microscope, however, the lumen of the transsected lymph vessel can be identified. Frequently clear or stained lymph dripping out of the lymph vessel is observed. The anastomosis is performed between the lymph vessels and a tributary of the saphenous vein using the operating microscope and standard microsurgical technique. We use 10-0 or 11-0 monofilament interrupted sutures and perform a tension-free anastomosis. Four to eight interrupted stitches are usually placed (Fig. 24–4). The wound is frequently irrigated with heparinized saline solution, but systemic heparinization is not done. Only the skin is closed, using interrupted vertical mattress nylon sutures. An Ace bandage, elevation and, on the lower extremity, an intermittent compression pump using low (40 to 50 mm Hg) pressures are used in the postoperative period to increase tissue pressure and facilitate flow through the anastomoses. The patient is fitted with an elastic garment or sleeve on the third postoperative day, before discharge.

TECHNIQUE OF LYMPHATIC GRAFTING

The technique of lymphatic grafting for both lower and upper extremity lymphedema was described in detail by Baumeister (19,30). Patients with secondary upper extremity lymphedema and those with secondary unilateral lower extremity lymphedema are candidates for this procedure. The lymphatic grafts are harvested from the normal leg. Two to four lymphatic vessels of the medial superficial lymphatic group of the donor extremity are dissected first under loupe magnification, using a single incision at the medial aspect of the thigh (Fig. 24–5). Two milliliters of Lymphazurine dye injected into the first interdigital space of the foot 15 min before the procedure facilitates dissection of the lymph vessels. In lower extremity lymphedema, lymph vessels are dissected under the microscope on the diseased side using a 5-cm long vertical skin incision just distal to the saphenofemoral junction. The lymphatic grafts are then divided on the normal side at the level of the knee and are tunneled subcutaneously to the contralateral groin

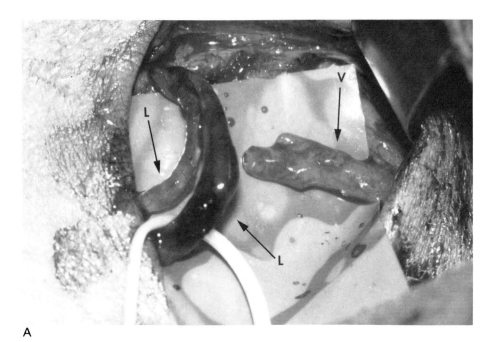

A

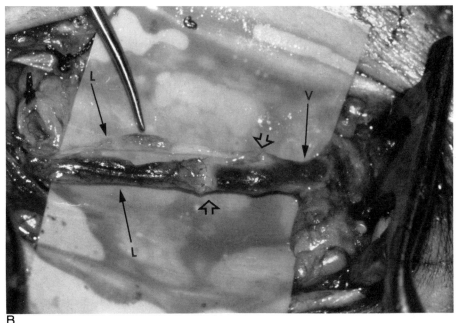

B

Figure 24–4. Microsurgical lymphovenous anastomosis performed at the right groin. *A*, Two dissected lymph vessels (*L*) and a tributary of the saphenous vein (*V*) with a side branch for anastomosis. *B*, Arrows indicate patent end-to-end lymphovenous anastomoses. [From Gloviczki P: Treatment of acquired lymphedema—medical and surgical. *In* Ernst CB, Stanley JC, eds: Current Therapy in Vascular Surgery—II. Toronto, B. C. Decker, Inc, 1990 (in press).]

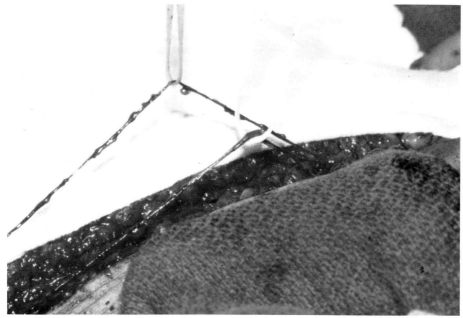

Figure 24–5. Two lymph vessels dissected on the medial aspect of the right thigh for suprapubic lymphatic grafting.

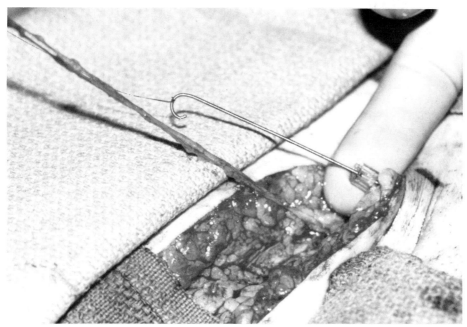

Figure 24–6. Tunneling of the two lymphatic grafts through a Silastic tube placed subcutaneously above the pubis. The lymphatic grafts are pulled through the drain with a 6-0 silk tied to a guide wire.

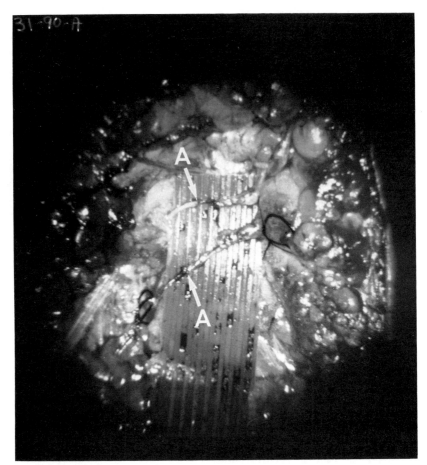

Figure 24–7. Anastomoses (*A*) between the lymphatic grafts and two superficial lymph vessels of the lymphedematous extremity.

through a Silastic tube (Fig. 24–6). Using the operating microscope and 11-0 mono-filament interrupted sutures, the lymphatic grafts are anastomosed end to end with four to six stitches to the lymph vessels of the edematous leg (Fig. 24–7). Closure and postoperative care is similar to that described for patients with lymphovenous anastomoses.

In patients with upper extremity lymphedema, the lymphatic grafts are completely removed from the thigh and are transplanted to the arm. The distal ends of the lymphatic grafts are anastomosed first end to end to lymph vessels of the medial arm bundle (Fig. 24–2), which were dissected at the medial aspect of the arm. The grafts are tunneled subcutaneously to the base of the neck, where end-to-end anastomoses are performed with descending lymph vessels of the neck, located just lateral to the internal jugular vein. On the left side, a direct anastomosis with the thoracic duct is avoided.

CLINICAL RESULTS

Results of the larger recent clinical series are tabulated in Table 24–1. In a group of 14 patients that we have operated on, we noted improvement in three

TABLE 24-1. Clinical Results of Microsurgical Lymphovenous Anastomoses

AUTHORS (REF.)	YEAR	NO. OF PATIENTS	EXTREMITY		FOLLOW-UP (MOS.)	RESULT EXCELLENT OR GOOD	METHODS OF ASSESSMENT		
			Upper	Lower			Volume	Lymphoscintigraphy	Lymphangiography
Krylov et al. (8)	1982	50	+		?	30%	+	—	—
Nieuborg (9)	1982	47	+		6–12	68%	+	—	—
Gong-Kang et al. (10)	1985	91		+	24[a]	79%	+	—	—
Zhu et al. (13)	1987	48		+(?)	6–52	33%	+	—	—
		185		+(?)	6–52	73%	+	—	—
Gloviczki et al. (14)	1988	6	+		36.6[a]	50% (3/6)	+	+	—
		8		+		25% (2/8)	+		
O'Brien et al. (18)	1990	46	+			54%	+	—	—
		30		+	51[a]	83%	+	—	—
		6[b]	+			33% (2/6)	+	—	—
		8[b]		+		50% (4/8)	+	—	—

[a] Mean.
[b] Lymphovenous anastomosis plus excisional procedure.

upper extremities and two lower extremities after an average follow-up of 46.2 months (14). There was no change in five extremities and in four the lymphedema progressed. Only one patient with primary lymphedema improved, but four of seven patients with secondary lymphedema showed improvement. In our patients objective evidence of the late patency of the anastomoses of this procedure could not be demonstrated.

The best documented long-term results with lymphovenous anastomoses were recently reported by O'Brien et al. (18). During the last 14 years they treated 134 patients with lymphovenous anastomoses, and 90 were available for long-term follow-up. Fifty-two of these patients had only lymphovenous anastomoses, and 38 had concomitant segmental resection performed. Seventy-three per cent of the patients from the lymphovenous anastomosis only group had subjective improvement with 42 per cent showing objective decrease in the volume of the extremity. The average reduction of the excess volume was 44 per cent. Of the second group of 38 patients who had lymphovenous anastomoses with an excisional procedure, 78 per cent had subjective improvement and 60 per cent had decreased volume of the extremity. Seventy-four per cent of all patients were able to discontinue conservative measures, with a mean follow-up of 4 years after operation.

Of the currently available tests, only contrast lymphangiography could document late patency of lymphovenous anastomosis. Lymphoscintigraphy provides only indirect evidence of patency, since the labeled colloid arriving in the vein is immediately removed by the venous circulation and cannot be imaged by a gamma camera. Because of the possibility of fibrosing lymphangitis and the inconvenience for the patients, none of the clinical series have used contrast lymphangiography for late follow-up. For this reason, objective documentation of late patency of lymphovenous anastomoses in patients at present is still not available.

Only one microsurgical team in Munich has well-documented long-term results with lymphatic grafting. Baumeister and Siuda recently reported on 55 patients who underwent lymph vessel transplantation for secondary lymphedema (19). Thirty-six of the 37 patients with upper extremity lymphedema had had previous mastectomy. Eighteen patients had unilateral lower extremity lymphedema. The mean interval between the onset of edema and the operation was 8 years, ranging from 12 months to 20 years. The effectiveness of the operations was evaluated by volume measurements. Patency of the lympholymphatic anastomosis could be confirmed by lymphoscintigraphy, because imaging of the patent lymphatic graft was possible by a gamma camera. To estimate improvement in lymphatic clearance, a lymphatic transport index was also calculated based on semiquantitative evaluation of lymphoscintigraphy.

Volume reduction was achieved in 80 per cent of patients, with follow-up over 3 years, and the lymphatic transport index, measured by semiquantitative evaluation of the lymphoscintigrams, showed a 30 per cent late improvement. Patency of several lymphatic grafts was documented by lymphoscintigraphy, although patency rate of the studied 30 grafts was not given by the authors. None of the patients developed lymphedema of the donor limb.

Our own experience with this operation is modest, and the early clinical results (Fig. 24–8) do not permit us to draw conclusion about the effectiveness of this procedure. Of the five patients that we operated on for unilateral lower extremity lymphedema, early lymphoscintigraphy showed improved transport and

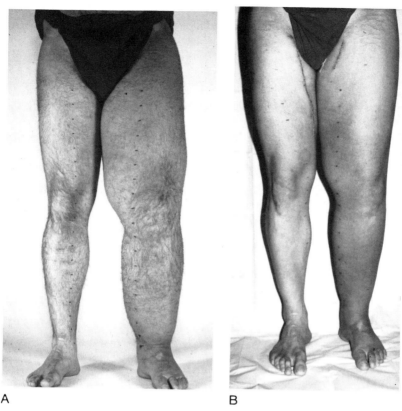

A   B

Figure 24–8. *A*, A 31-year-old male patient with secondary lymphedema of the left lower extremity. *B*, Postoperative picture of the same patient following suprapubic lymph vessel transplantation.

filling of contralateral inguinal nodes by the suprapubic graft in two patients (Fig. 24–9). Lymph is less coagulable than blood, and the pressure gradient across the lympholymphatic anastomosis is more favorable than across lymphovenous anastomosis. For these reasons, lymphatic grafting may have a somewhat better chance of late patency and function than lymphovenous anastomosis.

Figure 24–9. Lymphoscintigram 3 months after suprapubic lymphatic grafting for secondary lymphedema of the right lower extremity. Labeled colloid was injected into the right foot only. Arrow indicates suprapubic graft. Note intense filling of the left inguinal nodes. Preoperative lymphoscintigram in this patient showed no activity at the groins. [From Gloviczki P: Treatment of acquired lymphedema—medical and surgical. *In* Ernst CB, Stanley JC, eds: Current Therapy in Vascular Surgery—II. Toronto, B. C. Decker, Inc, 1990 (in press).]

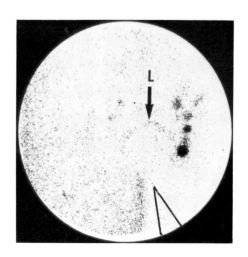

CONCLUSION

Lymphovenous anastomoses and lymphatic grafting are current microsurgical techniques to improve lymphatic drainage in chronic obstructive lymphedema. While with meticulous technique patent anastomoses can be performed between lymph vessels or between lymph vessel and vein, the long-term patency of these anastomoses in patients still needs to be objectively demonstrated. Fibrosis, loss of valvular function, and loss of intrinsic contractility of the lymph vessels, fibrosis of the subcutaneous tissue, decreased interstitial pressure, and loss of effective muscle pump are factors that, in the late stage of chronic lymphedema may render these operations ineffective. The most recent clinical data on lymphovenous anastomoses and lymphatic grafting confirm that patients with chronic lymphedema benefit from these procedures. The effectiveness of the operations, however, will have to be confirmed by other surgical teams and results have to be measured against currently practiced standard conservative treatment. It appears, however, that in the last decade of this century, microsurgical treatment for lymphedema has never been closer to fulfilling the promise that was made 30 years ago.

REFERENCES

1. Danese C, Bower R, Howard J: Experimental anastomoses of lymphatics. Arch Surg 1962;*84*:24–27.
2. Nielubowicz J, Olszewski W: Surgical lymphaticovenous shunts in patients with secondary lymphoedema. Br J Surg 1968;*55*:440–442.
3. Yamada Y: The studies on lymphatic venous anastomosis in lymphedema. Nagoya J Med Sci 1969;*32*:1–21.
4. Degni M: New technique of lymphatic-venous anastomosis (buried type) for the treatment of lymphedema. Vasa 1974;*3*:479–483.
5. Huang GK, Ru-Qi H, Zong-Zhao L, Yao-Liang S, Tie-De L, Gong-Ping P: Microlymphaticovenous anastomosis for treating lymphedema of the extremities and external genitalia. J Microsurg 1981;*3*:32–39.
6. Jamal S: Lymphovenous anastomosis in filarial lymphedema. Lymphology 1981;*14*:64–68.
7. Fox U, Montorsi M, Romagnoli G: Microsurgical treatment of lymphedemas of the limbs. Int Surg 1981;*66*:53–56.
8. Krylov V, Milanov N, Abalmasov K: Microlymphatic surgery of secondary lymphoedema of the upper limb. Ann Chir Gynaecol 1982;*71*:77–79.
9. Nieuborg, L: The Role of Lymphaticovenous Anastomoses in the Treatment of Postmastectomy Oedema. Alblasserdam, Holland: Offsetdrukkerij Kanters BV, 1982.
10. Gong-Kang H, Ru-Qi H, Zong-Zhao L, Yao-Liang S, Tie-De L, Gong-Ping P: Microlymphaticovenous anastomosis in the treatment of lower limb obstructive lymphedema: Analysis of 91 cases. Plast Reconstr Surg 1985;*76*:671–685.
11. Ingianni G, Holzmann T: Clinical experience with lympho-venous anastomosis for secondary lymphedema. Handchirurgie 1985;*17*:43–46.
12. Campisi C, Tosatti E, Casaccia M, et al: Microchirurgia dei linfatici. Minerva Chir 1986;*41*:469–481.
13. Zhu JK, Yu GZ, Liu JX, Pang SF, Lao ZG, Tang HY: Recent advances in microlymphatic surgery in China. Clin Orthop 1987;*215*:32–39.
14. Gloviczki P, Fisher J, Hollier LH, Pairolero PC, Schirger A, Wahner HW: Microsurgical lymphovenous anastomosis for treatment of lymphedema: A critical review. J Vasc Surg 1988;*7*:647–652.
15. O'Brien BM, Chait LA, Hurwitz PJ: Microlymphatic surgery. Orthop Clin North Am 1977;*8*:405–424.
16. O'Brien BMcC, Shafiroff BB: Microlymphaticovenous and resectional surgery in obstructive lymphedema. World J Surg 1979;*3*:3–15.
17. Baumeister RG, Siuda S, Bohmert H, Moser E: A microsurgical method for reconstruction of interrupted lymphatic pathways: Autologous lymph-vessel transplantation for treatment of lym-

phedemas. *In* Bergan JJ, Yao JST, ed: The Year Book of Vascular Surgery 1988. Chicago, Year Book Medical Publishers, 1988;241–242.

18. O'Brien BMcC, Mellow CG, Khazanchi RK, Dvir E, Kumar V, Pederson WC: Long-term results after microlymphatico-venous anastomoses for the treatment of obstructive lymphedema. Plast Reconstr Surg 1990;*85*:562–572.

19. Baumeister RG, Siuda S: Treatment of lymphedemas by microsurgical lymphatic grafting: What is proved? Plast Reconstr Surg 1990;*85*:64–76.

20. Pflug JJ, Calnan JS: The normal anatomy of the lymphatic system in the human leg. Br J Surg 1971;*58*:925–930.

21. Kubik S: The role of the lateral upper arm bundle and the lymphatic watersheds in the formation of collateral pathways in lymphedema. Acta Biol Acad Sci Hung 1980;*31*:191–200.

22. Olszewski W: Pathophysiological and clinical observations of obstructive lymphedema of the limbs. *In* Clodius L, ed: Lymphedema. Stuttgart, Thieme, 1977;79–102.

23. Casley-Smith JR, Gaffney RM: Excess plasma proteins as a cause of chronic inflammation and lymphoedema: Quantitative electron microscopy. J Pathol 1981;*133*:243–272.

24. Casley-Smith JR, Clodius L, Piller NB: Tissue changes in chronic experimental lymphoedema in dogs. Lymphology 1980;*13*:130–141.

25. Clodius L, Piller NB, Casley-Smith JR: The problems of lymphatic microsurgery for lymphedema. Lymphology 1981;*14*:69–76.

26. Gilbert A, O'Brien BMcC, Vorrath JW, Sykes PJ: Lymphaticovenous anastomosis by microvascular technique. Br J Plast Surg 1976;*29*:355–360.

27. Gloviczki P, Hollier LH, Nora FE, Kaye MP: The natural history of microsurgical lymphovenous anastomoses: An experimental study. J Vasc Surg 1986;*4*:148–156.

28. Puckett CL, Jacobs GR, Hurvitz JS, Silver D: Evaluation of lymphovenous anastomoses in obstructive lymphedema. Plast Reconstr Surg 1980;*66*:116–120.

29. Baumeister RG, Seifert J: Microsurgical lymph vessel transplantation for the treatment of lymphedema: Experimental and first clinical experiences. Lymphology 1981;*14*:90.

30. Baumeister RG, Siuda S, Bohmert H, Moser E: A microsurgical method for reconstruction of interrupted lymphatic pathways: Autologous lymph-vessel transplantation for treatment of lymphedemas. Scand J Plast Reconstr Surg 1986;*20*:141–146.

31. Baumeister RG, Seifert J, Wiebecke B: Homologous and autologous experimental lymph vessel transplantation: Initial experience. Int J Microsurg 1981;*3*:19–24.

32. Gloviczki P, Calcagno D, Schirger A, Pairolero PC, Cherry KJ, Hallet JW, Wahner HW: Noninvasive evaluation of the swollen extremity: Experiences with 190 lymphoscintigraphic examination. J Vasc Surg 1989;*9*:683–690.

33. Weissleder H, Weisleder R: Lymphedema: Evaluation of qualitative and quantitative lymphoscintigraphy in 238 patients. Radiology 1988;*167*:729–735.

25

VENOUS ANGIODYSPLASIA AND VENOUS MALFORMATIONS

William H. Pearce, James S. T. Yao,
B. Timothy Baxter, and Walter J. McCarthy

Venous malformations or angiodysplasia represent a portion of the spectrum of vascular malformations in which abnormalities of venous structures predominate. Unlike arteriovenous malformations, venous malformations are primary rather than secondary response to increased pressure and flow. Congenital venous malformations are common and range from discrete lesions to generalized ectasia and aplasia. For a full evaluation of these patients, a careful history and physical examination, along with the appropriate hemodynamic and radiographic investigations, are essential to define the extent of the lesion. On the basis of this information, it is possible to select the most appropriate mode of therapy. With localized superficial lesions, excision or sclerotherapy is effective. However, external support hose may be the only remedy for patients with diffuse ectasia and associated lymphatic involvement. This chapter will review the pathology, clinical evaluation, and treatment of venous angiodysplasia and malformations.

PATHOGENESIS AND CLASSIFICATION

Vascular malformations occur as a result of embryologic maldevelopment. The exact stage at which these events occur is unknown, and the nature of the malformation may not be readily apparent at birth. The development of the limb circulatory system is divided into three stages: 1) undifferentiated capillary network, 2) retiform plexus, and 3) formation of mature vessels (1,2). In the earliest phase, undifferentiated mesenchymal cell develop into cords with the development of angioblast. These early cells behave much like capillary cells, spontaneously forming tubelike structures when placed into tissue culture. Similarly, endothelial cells cultured from capillary hemangiomas continue to divide and express these characteristics (3). Later, in the retiform plexus stage, these structures coalesce, and with the flow of blood larger vessels develop with the retention of capillary beds. Alteration in the early hemodynamics of the embryo appears to play an important role in the development of venous malformations (4).

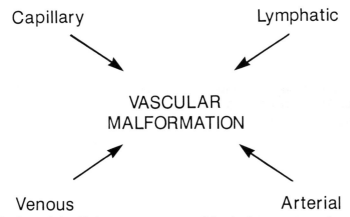

Figure 25–1.   Interrelationship between components of the circulatory system and vascular malformations.

Axial blood vessels nurture early limb development but eventually shrink, to be replaced by the major limb arteries. Residual axial arteries may remain patent in the lower extremity as a peristent sciatic artery. Similar abnormalities may develop in the venous system. Because the vascular bud is essential for limb growth, association skeletal anomalies may occur. Secondary skeletal changes also occur in response to increased flow (arteriovenous malformations) and venous stasis (Klippel-Trenaunay syndrome).

TABLE 25–1.   Characteristics of Vascular Birthmarks[a]

HEMANGIOMA	MALFORMATION
Clinical	
Usually nothing seen at birth; 30 per cent present as red macule	All present at birth; may not be evident
Rapid postnatal proliferation and slow involution	Commensurate growth; may expand as a result of trauma, sepsis, hormonal modulation
Female-to-male ratio 3:1	Female-to-male ratio 1:1
Cellular	
Plump endothelium, increased turnover	Flat endothelium, slow turnover
Increased mast cells	Normal mast cell count
Multilaminated basement membrane	Normal thin basement membrane
Capillary tubule formation in vitro	Poor endothelial growth in vitro
Hematologic	
Primary platelet trapping: thrombocytopenia (Kasabach-Merritt syndrome)	Primary stasis (venous); localized consumptive coagulopathy
Radiologic	
Angiographic findings: well circumscribed, intense lobular-parenchymal staining with equatorial vessels	Angiographic findings: diffuse, no parenchyma. Low flow: phleboliths, ectatic channels. High flow: enlarged, tortuous arteries with arteriovenous shunting
Skeletal	
Infrequent "mass effect" on adjacent bone; hypertrophy rare	Low flow: distortion, hypertrophy, or hypoplasia. High flow: destruction, distortion, or hypertrophy

[a] From Mulliken JB: Classification of vascular birthmarks. *In* Mulliken JB, Young AE, eds: Vascular Birthmarks: Hemangiomas and Malformations. Philadelphia, WB Saunders Company, 1988;35.

Maldevelopment of the vascular system may occur at any stage. As a result, a vascular malformation may contain some component of the arterial, venous, or lymphatic circulation (Fig. 25–1). Because of the wide variety of combinations of malformations, many eponyms and systems of classification have evolved. Since there is a basic biologic difference, vascular malformations may be divided into two broad categories, hemangiomas and vascular malformations (5,6). Strawberry, capillary, and capillary-cavernous lesions are considered hemangiomas, whereas port-wine stains, cavernous, venous, hemangiolymphangioma, and arteriovenous malformations are considered malformations. The features that distinguish these groups are listed in Table 25–1. Hemangiomas are usually not present at birth but grow rapidly in the newborn and infant. Vascular malformations, however, are commonly present at birth and grow with the child. Smaller lesions and lymphatic malformations are not readily apparent at birth but develop slowly and are recognized in older children.

MAJOR VENOUS ABNORMALITIES

Congenital venous malformations include agensis, duplication, ectasia, and avalvulosis. Although anomalies in pulmonary venous drainage may also occur, they will not be discussed in this chapter. Developmental abnormalities of the superior and inferior vena cava are uncommon (2 to 5 per cent) and represent arrest in the orderly maturation of the cardinal veins. Anomalies of the inferior vena cava (IVC) include persistent left-sided vena cava, duplication, and aplasia (0.2 to 0.5 per cent) (7,8). Duplication of the IVC represents the failure of the left sacrocardinal vein to lose its connection with the left subcardinal vein. Aplasia occurs when the right subcardinal vein fails to connect with the liver. Blood from the lower half of the body returns to the heart via the azygos system to the superior vena cava.

Congenital anomalies of the renal veins are more frequent. Multiple right renal veins occur in 15 per cent of cases, while abnormalities on the left are less frequent (9 per cent) (9–11). A circumferential aortic left renal vein occurs in 6 per cent and a retroaortic one in 3 per cent. The retroaortic left renal vein is associated with spontaneous aortorenal vein fistulas.

Abnormalities of the iliac vein are also common (20 per cent) and represent a form of dysplasia or compression of the left iliac vein by the right iliac artery. Venous compression of the left iliac vein or venous spurs in this location may predispose the patient to thrombosis (12,13). Congenital aplasia of the left iliac vein, however, will result in a massively dilated collateral (Fig. 25–2) that is often misinterpreted as an ectatic vessel. Congenital absence of the iliac vein and portions of the deep system of the leg are components of the Klippel-Trenaunay syndrome and Parkes-Weber syndrome (13).

Valvular Abnormalities

Congenital absence of venous valves occurs with varying clinical manifestations. Absence of venous valves in the iliac veins is common (50 per cent), with few clinical symptoms. When this absence occurs in combination with saphenofemoral incompetence, however, superficial varicose veins occur. Congenital

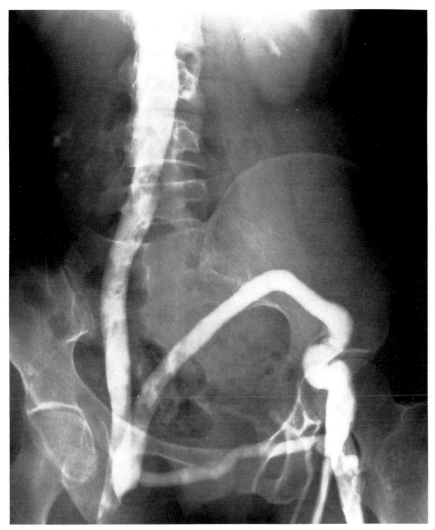

Figure 25–2.   Congenital left iliac vein aplasia with collateral drainage.

avalvulosis is exceedingly rare and is associated with venous ulcers, postural hypotension, and acrocyanosis (14,15). Whether valves become incompetent from a congenital floppy leaflet syndrome or are secondarily affected remains a controversy (16).

Venous Ectasia

Ectasia of the superficial and deep veins of the lower extremity occurs either as isolated discrete lesions or as diffuse involvement of the entire limb. Primary venous ectasia is either genuine diffuse phlebectasia or cutis marorata telangiectatica (a superficial skin lesion). Diffuse venous angiodysplasia is rare and may affect both the superficial and deep systems. Anatomically, these lesions are located in the subcutaneous, subfascial, or interosseous compartments. Intradermal lesions include port-wine stains and superficial varicosities. Subfascial lesions are

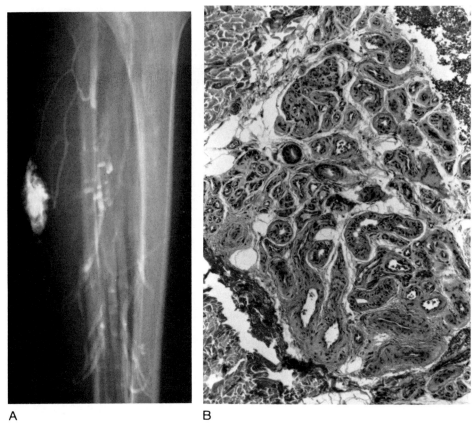

A   B

Figure 25–3. *A*, Venogram of a discrete venous malformation. *B*, Histology of mature venous channels.

manifested by hemarthrosis and muscle atrophy. Interosseous venous malformations (Gorham-Stout syndrome) are characterized by progressive bone destruction, pathologic fractures, limb shortening, and calcified phleboliths. These venous anomalies include localized venous dilations (Fig. 25–3) and extensive ectasia with reflux and venous aneurysms (Fig. 25–4). Secondary venous ectasia is found associated with deep vein hypoplasia (Klippel-Trenaunay syndrome), arteriovenous malformations (Parkes-Weber syndrome), valvular aplasia, or multiple spongy venous malformations.

Klippel-Trenaunay Syndrome

The Klippel-Trenaunay syndrome (KTS) is a mixed mesodermal abnormality that occurs sporadically without a familial tendency. This syndrome involves abnormalities of veins, capillaries, soft tissue, and skeletal elements (17–19). The disease is first recognized early after birth by the presence of a capillary nevus with limb hypertrophy and varicose veins. To avoid confusion with other syndromes, Schobinger has subclassified KTS into three types: type I—KTS without deep veins and without arteriovenous malformation; type II—KTS associated with arteriovenous malformations (Parkes-Weber syndrome); and type III—KTS

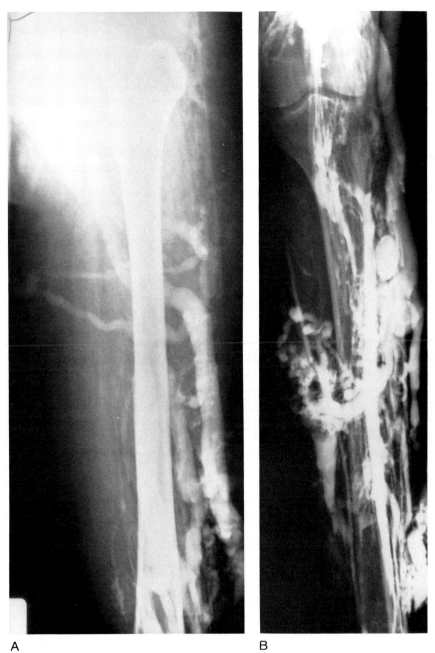

A   B

Figure 25–4. *A* and *B*, Venous ectasia with reflux, lateral vein, hypoplasia of deep veins, and venous aneurysm.

with anomalies of the deep veins and without arteriovenous malformations (20). The lower extremity is involed in 95 per cent of the patients and the upper extremity in 5 per cent. Limb hypertrophy occurs in 72 per cent, with both limb lengthening and calf enlargement. KTS is unilateral in 85 per cent, of cases and may involve both the upper and lower extremities in 15 per cent. Anomalies of the superficial veins of the leg are common (70 per cent), with the most common abnormality being a lateral vein that may extend from the lateral foot to the pelvis (Fig. 25–5). In addition, there may be extensive involvement of the deep system with both ectasia and hypoplasia (21). Twenty per cent of patients will have clinical evidence of pulmonary emboli, and 20 per cent will have rectal bleeding from pelvic varicosities (12).

Arterial and venous hemodynamics vary in KTS. A functioning arteriovenous malformation is not essential for limb hypertrophy. Venous outflow obstruction without change in blood flow may produce limb overgrowth (22). In addition,

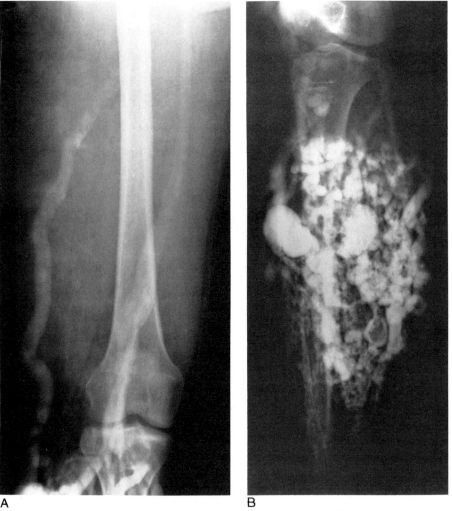

A   B

Figure 25–5. *A* and *B*, Lateral vein in association with venous ectasia. No arteriovenous malformation.

Ackroyd and colleagues found normal function of the calf muscle pump and rapid venous reflux in patients with KTS (23). In patients with a large cutaneous nevus, there is a slight increase in arterial flow without a detectable arteriovenous malformation. This increae is related to blood flow within the cutaneous nevus. In summary, KTS is a mixed malformation with combinations of venous, arterial, and soft tissue anomalies with variable alteration in limb hemodynamics.

Maffucci's Syndrome

Maffucci's syndrome is a rare disease in which both venous malformations and dyschondroplasia occur (13,24). The disease is present at birth in 25 per cent of cases, but the majority of patients develop symptoms in adolescence. Venous

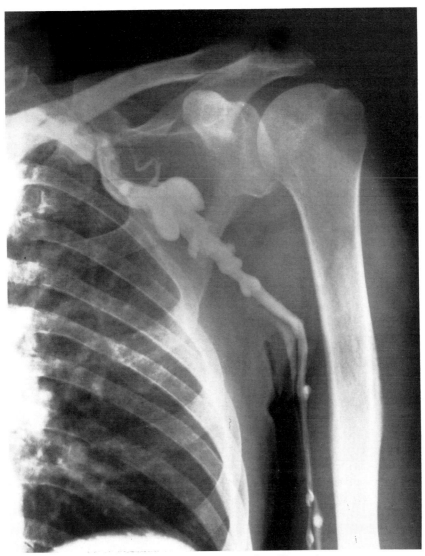

Figure 25–6. Venous aneurysm in axillary vein.

malformations include venous ectasia and cavernous lakes. The venous malformations often protrude from the limb and digits in grapelike clusters in association with deep venous anomalies. The malignant potential of the disease is 50 per cent, with chondrosarcoma, hemangiosarcoma, lymphangiosarcoma, and fibrosarcomas being the most common (25). Maffucci's syndrome occurs sporadically without a pattern of inheritance.

Venous Aneurysms

Secondary venous aneurysms occur frequently in patients with arteriovenous malformations in response to increased flow and turbulence. These "cirsoid" or "racemosem" aneurysms develop slowly and are a visible manifestation of an underlying arteriovenous malformation. Such secondary venous aneurysms also occur with chronic hemodialysis fistulas. Primary venous aneurysms, however, are uncommon, with only scattered case reports. Reported venous aneurysms include jugular, superior vena cava, portal, superior mesenteric, splenic, femoral, popliteal, saphenous, and axillary veins (Fig. 25–6). Although primary venous aneurysms rarely produce symptoms other than cosmetic ones, there is a single report of a popliteal aneurysm producing a pulmonary embolus (26).

CLINICAL EVALUATION

Because of the extensive overlap among the many types of congenital vascular malformations, it may be difficult to fully characterize the malformation on the basis of the history and physical examination. Frequently a cutaneous lesion (birthmark or varicosity) will be the only sign of the underlying lesion. In the evaluation of these patients, it is important to determine 1) the nature of the dominant lesion (venous, arterial, or lymphatic), 2) the anatomic extent, and 3) the local and systemic hemodynamic effects. Once the nature of the malformation has been clearly defined, it is then possible to determine therapy rationally. Both noninvasive testing and anatomic imaging are required to accomplish these goals.

The role of noninvasive testing is to define the hemodynamics of the vascular malformation. Noninvasive testing should be directed at answering a specific question. First, is there an increase in arterial blood flow and, if so, to what degree? Segmental limb pressure, pulse volume recording, and Doppler velocity waveforms are helpful but are not quantitative. Recently, we have used duplex scanning to determine velocity and to calculate flow. We then compare the blood flow in the symptomatic limb to that in the opposite extremity, because increased flow indicates the presence of arteriovenous shunting. In contrast, venous malformations do not have arteriovenous communications and, therefore, should not have a significant increase in arterial blood flow. Nevertheless, limb blood flow may be slightly increased with a large cutaneous nevus. Estimation of limb blood flow by duplex scanning is being currently used in the pre- and postintervention periods to evaluate the effectiveness of therapy.

The second question to be answered by noninvasive testing is: What is the nature of the hemodynamic abnormalities with a given malformation? Impedance plethysmography will determine venous outflow obstruction, and photoplethysmography will evaluate muscle pump function and venous reflux. Obtaining ambulatory venous pressure is rarely necessary. Duplex scanning may be valuable to evaluate the deep venous system for dysplasia and avalvulosis, unless there is diffuse ectasia. In this case, duplication and multiple dilated venous channels make interpretation impossible.

A variety of imaging techniques are needed to define the anatomic ramifications of the malformation. Both arteriography and venography are gold standards when intervention becomes necessary. Arteriography will visualize macroarteiovenous fistulas but will be normal with micro-, low-flow fistulas. In these cases, labeled microspheres (^{99m}Tc-labeled 250-μm human albumin microspheres) are injected intraarterially proximal to the arteriovenous fistula, and the degree of shunting is calculated. Less than 3 per cent of extremity blood flow is shunted in the normal limb (27). Because of the large blood volume with venous malformations, standard venography is generally inadequate and will require multiple injections. Closed-space venography is a superior technique in these patients because of its ability to delineate venous pathology with greater opacification and clearer detail (28,29).

Unfortunately, arteriography and venography are invasive and frequently underestimate the degree of soft tissue involvement. Magnetic resonance imaging (MRI) overcomes these problems because it does not require contrast and will differentiate soft tissue (i.e., muscle, fat, and blood vessels) (30). Furthermore, MRI generates transverse, frontal, and sagittal sections that are useful to orient the location of the malformation. In Maffucci's syndrome, MRI will help to distinguish hemangiomas from enchondromas and chondrosarcomas (31). Also, MRI is particularly suitable for infants and small children, in whom invasive procedures are often difficult to perform.

TREATMENT

The management of venous malformations is dependent upon the patient's syndrome and the anatomy of the malformation. Many venous malformations are only curiosities and do not require treatment. For example, aneurysms of the portal vein or congenital aplasia of the iliac vein do not require therapy. In other instances, the venous malformation is a potential hazard. Venous anomalies of the left renal vein and the IVC present special problems for aortic surgery (8). Knowledge of these abnormalities will prevent venous injury.

In patients with symptomatic venous malformations and angiodysplasia, therapeutic decisions require complete angiography and venography. Noninvasive evaluation is tailored to the patient's pathology. If the dominant lesion is superficial and localized, with a normal deep venous system, excision or stripping may be performed safely. Gorenstein et al. reported excellent cosmetic and functional results in 18 patients with superficial venous angiodysplasia. Four patients required multiple reexcisions (32). If the deep system is hypoplastic, however, excision of the superficial system may be harmful. A large lateral vein or cluster of veins may be the only venous drainage of the limb. Similarly, sclerotherapy of these anomalous veins may be equally disastrous. A variety of other surgical procedures are performed to control local symptoms, such as ligating a bleeding varicosity or ulcer débridement. Occasionally, epiphyseal stapling for leg length discrepancy is necessary in patients with KTS (5 per cent).

Elastic support remains the treatment of choice for complex venous malformation. Superficial venous reflux is common and is the predominant hemodynamic derangement in many patients with KTS. Swelling and limb discomfort may be relieved with external support. The support garment is fitted to the patient's needs and is usually a below-knee appliance. Elastic support is also important in mixed lesions with significant associated lymphedema.

SUMMARY

Venous malformations and angiodysplasia represent a diverse group of congenital abnormalities. The simplest method of categorization is to separate hemangiomas from vascular malformations. Within the group of vascular malformations, venous malformations are those lesions in which anomalies of mature venous structures predominate. In certain patients only the venous system will be involved, whereas in others there will be a mixture of arterial, venous, and lymphatic abnormalities. To understand venous malformations and to care for the patient, we must use both noninvasive and invasive techniques to define the nature of the dominant abnormality and its anatomic extent. In addition, the effects of the malformation upon the arterial and venous hemodynamics of the limb should be characterized.

REFERENCES

1. Sabin FR: Studies of the origin of blood vessels as seen in the living blastoderm. Contrib Embryol Carnegie Inst 1920;9:213.
2. Woollard HH: The development of the principal arterial system of the forelimb of the pig. Contrib Embryol Carnegie Inst 1922;14:139.
3. Mulliken JB, Zetter BR, Folkman J: In vitro characteristics of endothelium from hemangiomas and vascular malformations. Surgery 1982;92:348.
4. Woollard HH, Harpman JA: The relationship between the size of an artery and the capillary bed in the embryo. J Anat 1937;72:18.
5. Mulliken JB: Classification of vascular birthmarks. In Mulliken JB, Young AE: Vascular Birthmarks: Hemangiomas and Malformations. Philadelphia, WB Saunders Company, 1988;24–37.
6. Mulliken JB, Glowacki J: Hemangiomas and vascular malformations in infants and children: A classification based on endothelial characteristics. Plast Reconstr Surg 1982;69:412.
7. Chuang VP, Mena CE, Hoskins PA: Congenital anomalies of the inferior vena cava. Review of the embryogenesis and presentation of a simplified classification. Br J Radiol 1974;47:206–213.
8. Bartle EJ, Pearce WH, Sun JH, Rutherford RB: Infrarenal venous anomalies and aortic surgery: Avoiding vascular injury. J Vasc Surg 1987;6:590–593.
9. Mitty HA: Circumaortic renal collar: A potentially hazardous anomaly of the left renal vein. Am J Roentgenol Radium Ther Nucl Med 1975;125:307–310.
10. Davis CJ, Lundberg GD: Retroaortic left renal vein: A relatively frequent anomaly. Am J Clin Pathol 1968;50:700–703.
11. Beckmann CF, Abrams HL: Circumaortic venous ring: Incidence and significance. Am J Radiol 1979;132:561–565.
12. Browse NL, Burnand KG, Lea Thomas M: Congenital venous abnormalities. In Diseases of the Veins: Pathology, Diagnosis and Treatment. London, Edward Arnold, 1988;603–625.
13. Young AE: Venous and arterial malformations. In Mulliken JB, Young AE, eds: Vascular Birthmarks: Hemangiomas and Malformations. Philadelphia, WB Saunders Company, 1988;196–213.
14. Lodin A, Lindvall N, Gentele H: Congenital absence of venous valves as a cause of leg ulcers. Acta Chir Scand 1958;116:256.
15. Plate G, Brudin L, Eklof B, et al: Physiologic and therapeutic aspects in congenital vein valve aplasia of the lower limb. Ann Surg 1983;198:229.
16. Kistner RL: Surgical repair of the incompetent femoral vein valve. Arch Surg 1975;110:1336.

17. Baskerville PA, Ackroyd JS, Lea Thomas M, Browse NL: The Klippel-Trenaunay syndrome: Clinical, radiological and haemodynamic features and management. Br J Surg 1985;*72*:232–236.

18. Servelle M: Klippel and Trenaunay's syndrome: 768 operated cases. Ann Surg 1985;*201*:365–373.

19. Gloviczki P, Hollier LH, Telander RL, et al. Surgical implications of Klippel-Trenaunay syndrome. Ann Surg 1983;*197*:353–362.

20. Schobinger RC: Periphere Angiodysplasien. Bern: Hans Huber, 1977.

21. Phillips GN, Gordon DH, Martin EC, et al. The Klippel-Trenaunay syndrome: Clinical and radiologic aspects. Radiology 1978;*128*:429–434.

22. Lindenauer SM: The Klippel-Trenaunay syndrome: Varicosity, hypertrophy, and hemangioma with no arteriovenous fistulae. Ann Surg 1965;*162*:303.

23. Ackroyd JC, Baskerville PA, Young AE, Browse NL: The Pathophysiology of the Klippel-Trenaunay Syndrome. 5th International Workshop for Vascular Anomalies, Milan, 1984.

24. Lewis RJ, Ketcham AS: Maffucci's syndrome: Functional and neoplastic significance. J Bone Joint Surg [Am] 1973;*55*:1465.

25. Jaffe HL: Tumors and Tumorous Conditions of the Bones and Joints. Philadelphia, Lea & Febiger, 1958.

26. Jack CR Jr, Sharma R, Venuri RB: Popliteal venous aneurysm as a source of pulmonary emboli in a male: A case report. Angiology 1984;*35*:54–57.

27. Anderson BO, Rutherford RB, Jones DN, Pearce WH, Davis K: Congenital vascular malformations in the extremities of children: Newer approaches to diagnosis and management. Pediatrics, 1990 (in press).

28. Braun SD, Moore AV Jr, Mills SR, Ford K, Heaston DK, Miller GA, Dunnick NR: Closed-system venography in the evaluation of angiodysplastic lesions of the extremities. Am J Radiol 1983;*141*:1307–1310.

29. Boxt LM, Levin DC, Fellows KE. Direct puncture angiography in congenital venous malformations. Am J Radiol 1983;*140*:135–136.

30. Pearce WH, Rutherford RB, Whitehill TA, Davis K: Nuclear magnetic resonance imaging: Its diagnostic value in patients with congenital vascular malformations of the limbs. J Vasc Surg 1988;*8*:64–70.

31. Unger EC, Kessler HB, Howalyshyn MJ, Lackman RD, Morea GT: MR imaging of Maffucci syndrome: Case report. Am J Radiol 1988;*150*:351–353.

32. Gorenstein A, Katz S, Schiller M: Congenital angiodysplasia of the superficial venous system of the lower extremities in children. Ann Surg 1988;*207*:213–218.

26

ROLE OF ELASTIC SUPPORT IN TREATMENT OF THE CHRONICALLY SWOLLEN LIMB

George Johnson, Jr.

One of the most important therapeutic aids in the management of venous and lymphatic disease of the lower extremity has been elastic compression. This has been reported to decrease swelling (1) and increase femoral (2) vein flow velocity. Recently, using an air plethysmograph, Christopoulos et al. demonstrated a decrease in ambulatory venous pressure and an increase in venous refill time with therapeutic elastic stockings in patients with venous disease (3). Although physicians are becoming educated as to their requirements, indications, and use, patient education and compliance remains a problem. Industry has moved so rapidly over the past 50 years to supply easy-to-fit stockings with appropriate compression that it behooves the physician to continually reappraise his or her knowledge of what is available.

Several years ago some of the history and technology of the elastic stocking was presented (4). This review will briefly expand on this, update the current products available, and give some insight on future expectations.

CHARACTERISTICS OF ELASTIC STOCKINGS

There are several varieties of elastic stockings. The below-knee stocking is the most popular and satisifes the needs of most patients. However, there are certain patients that need various other types, such as the low-thigh, high-thigh, and leotard.

There are various types of stockings. The so-called "supphose" has some compression from the nylon knit and it is not graded. The "antiembolism" stocking is graded and has somewhat higher compression (18 mm Hg at the ankle) than the supphose. The low-compression graded stocking (20 to 30 mm Hg at the ankle) is a therapeutic stocking but in our experience has very few indications for its use. It might be more effective in preventing deep vein thrombosis than the current antiembolus stocking, although the expense would be greater. The most commonly used stocking is the 30 to 40 mm Hg compression at the ankle, below-knee elastic stocking. For people with lymphedema or massive swelling secondary to chronic venous insufficiency, a higher ankle pressure stocking is indicated.

With modern technology, industry claims to be able to produce a noncustom ("off-the-shelf" or "ready-to-wear") graded elastic stocking that fits a major portion of the population, yet delivers the prescribed compression at the ankle. The ankle circumference just above the medial malleolus ranges from 15 to 30 cm in the majority of the population. Elastic stocking companies' ankle circumference fitting sizes vary in number from three to six. Those with fewer sizes emphasize that less inventory is needed and, with modern technology, they are still able to appropriately fit most of the population. Thus their stockings deliver the same compression over a stretch of several centimeters circumference. These are usually low-modulus stockings made with high-elongation natural rubber or synthetic rubber.

How does the stocking industry use modern technology to achieve the claims made? The Germans and Swiss in the early part of this century became masters of the knitting process. Each had their own technique. Some of the technology and knowledge has moved to the United States. The machines are computer controlled to assure a standard product. Basically the knit construction, the elastomeric feed devices, and the yarn itself control the compression. Although most elastic stockings use nylon for the base knit, the elastomer yarn inlay varies significantly from company to company. Natural rubber (latex) was the original elastic yarn. Because of patient allergies and deterioration of rubber when exposed to certain chemicals, it is now usually wrapped with nylon or cotton.

Spandex is a generic name for a synthetic rubber made in the United States by the Dupont and Globe companies. It goes under trade names of Lycra (Dupont) and Glospan (Globe) and has various sizes or deniers. Unwrapped, it is a low-modulus material (same compression for a lot of stretch) and therefore has a relatively large fitting range. Some companies believe that wrapping the material alters the characteristics. Although initially developed to have all the characteristics of rubber, spandex is now being altered to give characteristics that will be more appropriate than rubber for elastic compression. It is nonreactive to the patient and it does not deteriorate when exposed to sunlight, soaps, or body secretions. Stockings with spandex use various sizes or deniers of the yarn and vary the amount of spandex relative to nylon, cotton, or silk yarn. There have been some suggestions that the durability of spandex is less than that of rubber, but this is probably not true for the better grades of spandex.

There continues to remain a small percentage of the population that cannot be fitted by noncustom stockings. For these, a custom-made stocking with a seam is still available. Historically, this was the first elastic stocking made. They were made on a flatbed knitting machine with the fabric having the same compression throughout. The graded compression was made by customizing the stocking to a specific measurement on the patient and then sewing it together.

This chapter will be devoted to the noncustom calf-length therapeutic elastic stocking with a 30 to 40 mm Hg compression at the ankle. It is recognized that there are many other stockings that are useful, such as the 40 to 50 and 50 to 60 mm Hg compression, thigh-length, and leotard stockings. Each one has a special application. The below-knee therapeutic stocking with 30 to 40 mm Hg compression usually benefits the patient, yet is sufficiently sheer that patients are relatively compliant in their use.

Tables 26–1 and 26–2 are based on information regarding therapeutic calf-length elastic stockings received from companies distributing them in the United States. This does not imply endorsement of any one stocking company. In my judgment, each characteristic has pros and cons. It behooves the physician to use the stocking that best fits the patient's needs. This is strongly influenced by availability and service.

Construction

The basic knit for all elastic stockings includes the knitted loop and the underlying inlay. Beyond this a description becomes too complicated for those without special technical knowledge to understand. Each company claims to have its own process, the details of which may be understood only by the plant technical developer (one of the most valuable personnel in the company). The manner in which the yarn is placed in the stocking is crucial. Some companies, by special knit techniques, line the stocking with silk or cotton so it will feel better on the skin of the patient.

Materials

Latex, spandex, nylon, cotton, or silk are the basic yarns used in knitting a stocking. Latex was the original elastic yarn. Unless a special knitting process is used, it is a high-modulus yarn, giving a lot of compression with little stretch. Stockings made from latex need to be covered or wrapped because of potential patient sensitivity and possible deterioration of the latex by sunlight, soaps, and body chemicals. For this reason it is covered or wrapped with cotton or nylon yarn. These stockings may be quite bulky.

Nylon, cotton, and silk are used in various stockings in different ways. Often nylon is used as the basic knitted loop in stocking. Nylon (Helenca) is used by some companies to wrap the latex. Other processes use cotton or silk to wrap, coat, or line spandex to make the stocking softer to the skin and easier to put on.

Sizes

The various sizes usually refer to ankle compression. Closed-toe stockings usually have two foot lengths; open toe stockings have only one. Usually the higher the modulus of the material used in the stockings, the less noncustom fitting range. Some companies rely on two length sizes to give proper fit; others increase the number of ankle circumference sizes. It would appear that the majority of the population can now be accurately fitted with noncustom fittings by most companies. The more sizes a company makes, the greater the inventory. The benefit, however, is that more patients can be readily fitted.

Color

The industry has the ability to dye the stocking to any color desired; however, this necessitates increasing the inventory of the stockings. The number of colors available is growing, although beige is still the standard and most acceptable color.

TABLE 26–1. Comparison of Some Therapeutic Elastic Stockings[a]

	BELL HORN		CAMP		JOBST[b]					MEDI STRUMPF[c]
	173	39/19	1600	1800	U	V	VZ	UC	FF	
Material										
Synthetic rubber	Y	Y	Y	Y	Y (L)[d]	Y	Y (L)	Y (L)	Y (L)	Y
Natural rubber										NO
Nylon	Y	Y	Y	Y	Y	Y	Y	Y	Y	Y
Wrapped	Y[e]	Y[e]	Y[e]			Y[f]	Y[f]	Y[f]	Y[f]	
Toe open (O)/closed (C)	O	O/C	O	O	C	O	O	O/C	O/C	O/C
Color[g]	Be	Be	Be	Be	Be/Bl	Be	Be	Be	Be/Bl	Be, G, off W, Bl
No. of circumference sizes										
Ankle	5	5	3	3	4	3	3	4	3	6
Calf	1	1	2	2	1	2	2	1	2	1
No. of lengths	1	1	2	2	1	2	1	1	1	2
No. of foot sizes	1	1	1	1	1	1	1	1	1	2[h]
Total no. of sizes	5	5	12	12	4	12	6	4	6	12[i]
Zipper							Y	Y		
Compression Guarantee (months)	6	6	none	none	varies with type					6
Suggested retail price ($)	40.00	25.00			40–45	66.50	79.00	83.50	57.50	varies with sheer

[a] All stockings are 30 to 40 mm Hg compression at the ankle, calf-length, off-the-shelf (noncustom) types. Style names or numbers are indicated below each manufacturer's name.
[b] U, Ultimate; V, Vairox; VZ, Vairox zipper; UC, UlcerCARE; FF, Fast-Fit.
[c] Additional sizes and sheer available.
[d] L, lycra.
[e] With nylon.
[f] With texturized nylon.
[g] Be, beige; Bl, black; G, gray; W, white.
[h] Closed toe only.
[i] Additional sizes and sheer available.

TABLE 26–2. Comparison of Some Therapeutic Elastic Stockings[a]

	JUZO[b]				SIGVARIS				VENOSAN	
	H	V	VS[c]	VA	902	802	500	202	2002	1002
Material										
Synthetic rubber	Y	Y	Y	Y	Y	Y		Y	Y	Y
Natural rubber							Y			
Nylon										
Wrapped	Y[d]	Y[d]	Y[d]	Y[d]	Y[e]	Y[e]	Y[e]	Y[f]	Y[f]	Y[d]
Toe open (O)/closed (C)	C	O/C	O/C	O	O	C	O	O	O	O/C
Color[g]	Bl, W[h]	Be	Be	Be	Be	Be/Bl	Be	Be	Be	Be
No. of circumference sizes										
Ankle	6	6	6	6	3	3	3	3	3	3
Calf	1	1	1	1	2	2	2	2	2	2
No. of lengths	2	2	2	2	2	2	2	2	2	2
No. of foot sizes	1	1	1	1	1	2	1	1	1	2[i]
Total no. of sizes	12	12	12	12	12	12	12	12	12	12[j]
Zipper										
Compression Guarantee (months)	12	12	12	12	4–6	4–6	4–6	4–6	6	6
Suggested retail price ($)					54.00	54.00	61.50	61.50		

[a] All stockings are 30 to 40 mm Hg compression at the ankle, calf-length, off-the-shelf, (noncustom) types. Style names or numbers are indicated below each manufacturer's name.
[b] H, Hostess; V, Varin Super; VS, Varin Soft; VA, Varilastic.
[c] Cotton inside option.
[d] With nylon.
[e] With Helenca.
[f] With coton.
[g] Be, beige; Bl, black; W, white.
[h] Plus eight other colors.
[i] Closed toe only.
[j] Twenty-four in closed toe.

Price

Suggested retail prices were made available by several companies; others declined to present this information (Tables 26–1 and 26–2). While these are price-oriented times, the price should not be the main consideration. Acceptability, durability, and reliability must be prime considerations.

NEW TECHNIQUES

It would seem that several rather great advances made in the therapeutic elastic stocking are about to be developed. The companies that produce synthetic rubber (Dupont and Globe) are rapidly improving the yarn. The durability and elasticity of the yarn per size is being rapidly improved. Knitting techniques are entering a new generation. Not only can different materials be placed in the stocking, but they can be placed in specific sites in the stocking, such as the lining. Double or two-layer stockings with different purposes and compression pressures are being evaluated with reported good results. Various techniques to facilitate putting the stocking on are being reported, some in the makeup of a stocking. Some facilitate putting the stocking on, such as the zipper or silk or nylon bootie sleeve for the foot, while others involve an accessory appliance. It is hoped that greater variety in colors will help increase patient compliance, although various colors have been tried before with little improvement in compliance. Perhaps users now are more conscious of their appearance. The increase of sizes available and the new knitting techniques and yarns should make the stocking more rapidly available to the consumer.

INDUSTRY STANDARDS

The stocking industry in the United States has been most cooperative with the physician. The industry has responded to our need for products. It has sought our advice in changing designs. It has sponsored education-oriented programs on numerous occasions. In spite of this, elastic stockings have no standards in this country.

Does the stocking deliver the compression advertised with the fit recommended? How long does the compression last? In Germany and Switzerland, the Hohenstein Institute evaluates stockings against certain set standards. The stockings are classified according to the ankle compression they deliver with the advertised fitting guide. Thus class I delivers 18.4 to 21.05 mm Hg compression at the ankle, class II 25.2 to 32.2, class III 36.5 to 46.6, and class IV greater than 59 mm Hg. The institute has a stamp of approval that assures the consumer that the stockings will deliver the compression advertised and will continue to deliver this for the period of time stated. If a stocking does not meet certain standards, insurance companies will not pay for it.

Although some stocking companies in this country guarantee that the advertised compression lasts for a certain period of time, this needs to be evaluated and confirmed by an unbiased testing institute for stockings sold in the United States, similar to the Hohenstein Institute. My judgment is that the stocking industry in the United States, as in Europe, would be extremely responsive if such an agency was developed. Although this could be monitored by the Food and Drug Administration, it is hoped that a completely unbiased organization, separate from a government agency sponsored by the stocking industry, could be set up as an independent entity to test and assure that elastic stockings meet certain standards.

SUMMARY

It is hoped that this brief review of available elastic stockings by a semi-informed prescriber will help the physician in giving the appropriate stocking to the consumer in this rapidly changing field. In spite of extraordinary detailed attempts to be fair and complete and to present the data in an accurate fashion, the fallibility of this technique and the author is recognized. Companies or products may have been overlooked. It is believed that the importance of presenting this type of information to the practicing physician outweighs any oversight or inaccuracy on the part of the reviewer.

Appreciation is expressed to all the companies reviewed in this manuscript. Without exception they were most cooperative and informative.

REFERENCES

1. Pierson S, Pierson D, Swallow R, Johnson G Jr: Efficacy of graded elastic compression in the lower leg. JAMA 1983;249:242–243.
2. Johnson G Jr, Kupper C, Farrar DJ, Swallow RT: Graded compression stockings. Custom vs noncustom. Arch Surg 1982;117:69–72.
3. Christopoulos DG, Nicolaides AN, Szendro G, et al: Air-plethysmography and the effect of elastic compression on venous hemodynamics of the leg. J Vasc Surg 1987;5:148–159.
4. Johnson GJ Jr: The role of elastic support in venous problems. In Bergan JJ, Yao JST, eds: Surgery of the Veins. Orlando, FL, Grune & Stratton, Inc, 1985;541–550.

VIII

MANAGEMENT OF CHRONIC VENOUS ULCERS

27

NONOPERATIVE TREATMENT OF VENOUS STASIS ULCER

John C. Mayberry, Gregory L. Moneta, Lloyd M. Taylor, Jr., and John M. Porter

The prevalence of lower extremity venous disease in our population is staggering. An estimated 27 per cent of the adult population have lower extremity venous abnormalities (1), an estimated 2 to 5 per cent have clinical manifestations of superficial or deep insufficiency (2), and 1.5 per cent have or have had venous stasis ulceration (2). Up to one third of patients with venous insufficiency or ulceration are limited in their ability to work outside the home (3). This clearly represents an important cause of time loss from work in the United States, considering both the remarkable chronicity of the problem and its frequent occurrence in patients in their peak working years. The slow healing and frequent recurrence of venous stasis ulcers are well known to medical practitioners. In spite of persistence and elaborate wound care protocols, both patient and physician frequently become frustrated with treatment failures. Many patients with lower extremity venous ulceration, especially those with recurrent disease, are eventually referred to a vascular surgeon. The competent vascular surgeon must be familiar with venous pathophysiology and possess a thorough understanding of the treatment options available to a discouraged patient in need of an acceptable and effective approach.

PATHOPHYSIOLOGY

Current theories on the pathogenesis of lower extremity venous stasis ulceration center on the damaging effects of ambulatory venous hypertension (4–6). In the normal human, competent valves in the calf muscle venous sinuses as well as the femoral, popliteal, and tibial veins maintain ankle ambulatory venous pressures below 30 torr (7) through the action of the calf muscle pump. In patients with deep venous valvular insufficiency the calf muscle pump is disabled and lower extremity venous pressure remains elevated with ambulation (8–10). The chronically elevated venous pressure is transmitted to the skin of the ankle region, causing dermal capillary proliferation (11), lymphatic destruction (12), and excessive colloid filtration (13), which result in regional edema, fibrin deposition, and a diffusion barrier to oxygen (14,15) (Fig. 27–1). Untreated, the skin of the

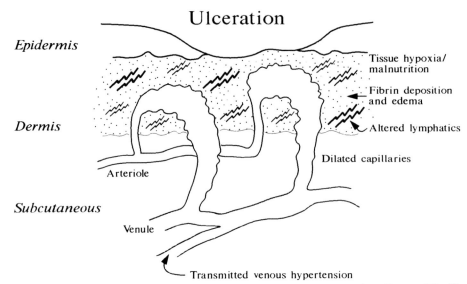

Ulceration

Epidermis

Tissue hypoxia/
malnutrition

Fibrin deposition
and edema

Dermis

Altered lymphatics

Dilated capillaries

Arteriole

Subcutaneous

Venule

Transmitted venous hypertension

Figure 27–1. The pathophysiology of venous stasis ulceration. (Adapted from Browse NL: The pathogenesis of venous ulceration: A hypothesis. J Vasc Surg 1988;7:470.)

lower extremity in patients with ambulatory venous hypertension demonstrates impaired wound healing and becomes prone to ulceration.

The etiology of lower extremity venous valvular insufficiency in most cases appears idiopathic. In our experience only 22 per cent of patients with venous ulceration have a well-documented history of lower extremity deep venous thrombosis (DVT) and thus may be accurately classified as having postthrombotic syndrome (16). Over three fourths of our patients with deep venous valvular incompetence and venous ulceration do not have a clear history of prior DVT. It is presently uncertain whether these patients develop valvular insufficiency as a consequence of a genetic defect or of the aging process, or as a sequela of prior episodes of subclinical DVT (17). The observation that evidence of residual venous changes compatible with prior DVT are frequently absent both phlebographically and by duplex scanning exam speaks against subclinical DVT (17). Interestingly, almost two thirds of venous ulcer patients exhibit edema and lipodermatosclerosis of the contralateral lower extremity with or without ulceration (16), indicating a striking bilaterality of the venous insufficiency process. We conclude that available evidence indicates that a significant majority of venous ulcer patients suffer from primary deep venous valvular incompetence unrelated to prior DVT.

Superficial venous insufficiency alone with a normal deep venous system can cause ulceration (4,18,19), although the frequency with which this occurs appears to differ greatly by geographic area. Cranley estimates that as many as 30 per cent of all venous ulcers result from isolated superficial venous insufficiency (20). In our experience and that of others, superficial venous insufficiency alone as the cause of venous ulceration is quite uncommon, accounting for less than 1 per cent of cases (17).

DIAGNOSIS

The optimal treatment of venous ankle ulceration is dependent upon the establishment of an accurate diagnosis. In our experience all patients with true venous ulceration will exhibit perimalleolar skin changes of lipodermatosclerosis (16) (Fig. 27–2). This is a histologic term referring to the pigmented, fibrous skin plaquing seen in malleolar and anterior tibial regions of afflicted individuals (21). Nearly all patients will have lower extremity edema (16). In patients who have been wearing an elastic stocking or wrapping their legs, edema may be minimal or absent, but all patients will have a history of recent lower extremity edema. The absence of typical venous skin changes or history of edema should cause one to doubt venous insufficiency as the cause of the ulceration. The differential diagnosis of lower extremity ulceration is remarkably long, although most of the listed causes are rare (Table 27–1) (21,22).

Confirmatory evidence of a venous etiology of lower extremity ulceration relies on established vascular lab examinations for the deep venous insufficiency. Deep venous valvular incompetence in the superficial femoral, popliteal, and tibial veins can be conveniently and accurately assessed by continuous-wave Doppler ultrasound or duplex scanning examination (21). Ankle venous refill time (VRT) can be measured noninvasively by photophlethysmography (PPG) (23). A VRT of less than 22 sec confirms venous insufficiency in our vascular lab. Careful attention to optimal PPG probe placement is essential. In our experience and that of others, the probe should be placed just above the medial malleolus (24). The gold standard test for venous insufficiency is invasively measured ambulatory venous pressure (AVP) (5). Invasive AVP, however, is only rarely required, usually in patients in whom the deep venous Doppler ultrasound or duplex scanning examination or the PPG-VRT are inconclusive. Venous ulceration is extremely unlikely in patients with an AVP less than 40 torr (25).

The measurement of both VRT and AVP (if done) should be repeated following the placement of a calf venous tourniquet that occludes the superficial

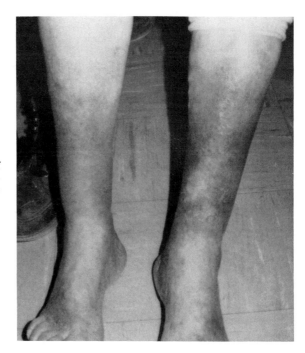

Figure 27–2. Perimalleolar skin of a patient with the typical lipodermatosclerotic changes of chronic venous insufficiency.

TABLE 27–1.   Differential Diagnosis of Nonvenous Leg Ulcer[a]

Traumatic	Dermatitic
Pressure ulcer	Allergic
Factitious	Bullous
Trench foot	Livido reticularis
Insect or animal bite	Atrophie blanche
Ischemic	Arteriovenous malformations
Infectious	Lymphedema
Bacterial	Arteriopathic
Tuberculous	Scleroderma
Tropical	Polyarteritis
Syphilitic	Rheumatoid
Iatrogenic	Pernio syndrome
Injection ulcer	Postpoliomyelitic
Warfarin induced (heterozygous protein	Systemic disease
C deficiency)	Heart failure
Cortisone abuse	Diabetes mellitus
Neoplastic/malignant	Blood cell dyscrasia
Orthopedic	Ulcerative colitis
Osteomyelitic	Malnutrition
Paget's disease	Other
Bony neoplasm	"Arterial" or "Martorell's" ulcer

[a] Adapted from Browse et al. (21) and Dodd and Cockett (22).

venous system. An unchanged VRT or AVP with the calf venous tourniquet excludes superficial venous insufficiency as a significant component. Improved venous hemodynamics following the calf venous tourniquet suggests combined superficial and deep venous insufficiency, whereas normalized measurements confirm isolated superficial venous insufficiency (4,22).

TREATMENT OPTIONS

Chronic deep venous insufficiency resulting in stasis ulceration of the lower extremity is not currently a curable disease. Effective palliation has focused on surgically eliminating and/or counteracting the effects of the transmission of the elevated venous pressure to the skin by external compression (Fig. 27–3). Potentially curative procedures such as venous valve reconstruction or transplantation continue to be investigated but have so far produced limited medium-term success (26,27).

Whatever the treatment modality, certain goals of therapy can be agreed upon (Table 27–2). Virtually all venous stasis ulcers can be healed with bed rest by prolonged elevation of the involved limb. However, the time required, frequency in excess of 1 month, is impractical and unnecessary for most patients. Alternative therapies have appropriately focused on allowing the patient to retain or quickly regain ambulatory status and to return to normal activity as soon as possible. Additionally, effective therapy must result in ulcer healing in a reasonable period of time. Healing that requires many months is generally unacceptable and ineffectual. Third, the issue of prevention of ulcer recurrence must be addressed. Most venous ulcers will recur quickly if the treatment program does not provide effective long-term preventive measures after initial ulcer healing. Finally, the

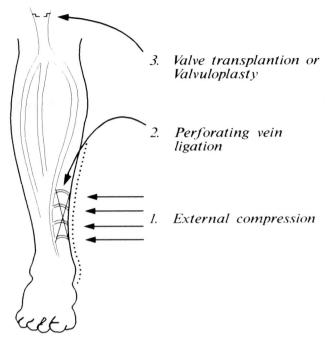

3. *Valve transplantion or Valvuloplasty*

2. *Perforating vein ligation*

1. *External compression*

Figure 27–3.   Treatment options for lower extremity venous stasis ulceration.

treatment obviously must be acceptable to the patient. Operative and nonoperative therapies alike clearly rely on patient compliance for optimal results.

OPERATIVE TREATMENT

Before describing the results of nonoperative treatment of venous stasis ulceration, a brief review of the theory and results of the most widely used surgical approaches to the healing of venous ulceration will be presented.

Varicose Vein Ligations and/or Stripping

In the rare patient with isolated superficial venous insufficiency resulting in significant ambulatory venous hypertension and ankle venous ulceration, surgical removal of the incompetent superficial varicose veins will be curative (4,18,19). Interestingly, we have not yet encountered such a patient in 20 years of vascular surgery practice, leading us to conclude that, at least in our region, isolated superficial venous incompetence is a rare or nonexistent cause of venous ulceration. The benefit of varicose vein extirpation in cases of combined superficial and deep venous insufficiency is at present unknown.

TABLE 27–2.   Goals of Treatment for Patients with Venous Stasis Ulceration

Return to ambulation quickly
Healing of the ulcer in a reasonable time frame
Prevention of recurrent ulceration
Patient tolerance/compliance

Subfascial Perforator Ligation

The perforating (or communicating) veins in patients with chronic deep venous insufficiency often become varicose and permit bidirectional blood flow between the superficial and deep venous systems through damaged or absent venous valves (28). It has been suggested (without confirmation) that obliteration of this communication prevents the transmission of chronically elevated ambulatory venous pressure to the skin and subcutaneous tissues. Extensive subfascial perforator ligations through longitudinal lower leg incisions became popular in the 1940s and 1950s (28,29). Initial enthusiasm was dampened, however, by frequent wound complications and ulcer recurrence. Series in the modern era have confirmed the above drawbacks (30–39). Wound complication rates vary from 2 to 44 per cent and recurrence rates from 6 to 55 per cent in long-term follow-up (Table 27–3). In addition, since in most of these series the routine use of postoperative elastic compression stockings is emphasized, the confounding role of compression therapy has never been differentially assessed. We suspect that much of the described success of perforator ligation may be more appropriately attributed to postoperative elastic compression stockings. Surgical obliteration of the perforating veins has therefore fallen short of its stated goals. This procedure has never been shown to prevent the transmission of the chronically elevated venous pressure to the skin and subcutaneous tissues.

Venous Valve Reconstruction or Transplantation

In recent years vascular surgeons have sought to directly address deep venous valvular incompetence with venous valve reconstruction or transplantation. Initial

TABLE 27–3.   **Representative Long-Term[a] Results following Subfascial Perforator Ligation for Venous Stasis Ulceration**

AUTHOR (REF.)	YEAR	NUMBER	HEALED (%)	WOUND COMPLICATIONS (%)	TOTAL RECURRENCE (%)	POSTOP STOCKINGS
Silver et al. (31)	1971	28	100	14	10	Yes
Thurston and Williams (32)	1973	89	100	12	13	Yes
Bowen (33)	1975	55	56	44	32	Yes
Burnand et al. (34)	1976	41	100	NR[b]	55[c]	NR
DePalma (35)	1979	53	100	2	6	Yes
Hyde et al. (36)	1981	109	100	15	24	Yes
Negus and Friedgood (37)	1983	77	100	22	13	Yes
Johnson et al. (38)	1985	37	100	14	41 (3 year)[d]	NR
					51 (5 year)[d]	NR
Cikrit et al. (39)	1988	27	100	26	22	Yes

[a] Mean of 3 years or greater.
[b] NR, not reported.
[c] Length of follow-up not given.
[d] Life-table recurrence.

reports demonstrated modest but variable early improvement in deep venous hemodynamic measurements but short-term deterioration (26,27). Clinical series are currently small and long-term follow-up is unavailable. Again the confounding effect of the use of postoperative elastic compression stockings has never been properly addressed. Venous valve reconstruction or transplantation surgery must for the present be regarded as an investigational procedure, certainly not recommended for general use. It is noteworthy in this regard that isolated proximal venous valve reconstruction or transplantation will not prevent the retrograde ejection of blood to the ankle and foot through incompetent tibial/soleal valves in the calf (40).

NONOPERATIVE TREATMENT

The cornerstone of effective nonoperative treatment of lower extremity venous stasis ulceration is limb compression therapy. The modalities commonly used include fitted, gradient elastic compression stockings, the Unna-style paste boot, the conventional Ace-type elastic bandage, and the recently marketed Circ-Aid Velcro-based appliance (41).

Although references to compression therapy date to the time of Hippocrates (21), satisfactory ulcer healing with elastic wraps was first clearly documented by Dickson-Wright in 1931 (42). In 1956 Anning reported on 100 venous ulcer patients treated with elastic wraps until healed, and then by compression stockings posthealing (43). He reported 100 per cent healing in an unspecified time and 59 per cent ulcer recurrence during 1 to 3 years' follow-up. Noncompliance with compression stockings posthealing was cited as the most common cause of recurrence. A similar study utilizing elastic wraps or plaster casts in an indigent patient setting revealed a 65 per cent healing rate but a 19 per cent 2-month recurrence rate (44). The use of Unna boots resulted in 30 per cent 3-month and 70 per cent 6-month healing (45,46).

Several adjunctive measures have been evaluated. Preliminary communications have suggested benefit from ulcer ultrasound therapy (45), intermittent pneumatic compression (47), superficial vein sclerotherapy (48), and oral pentoxyfylline (49). A recent publication reports benefit following the application of low-intensity laser energy to the ulcer (50). The long-term utility of these unconventional measures clearly has not been determined. Although some venous ulcer patients have been reported to be deficient in zinc, oral supplementation of this trace mineral has never been proven beneficial (51). Oral stanozolol, an anabolic steroid believed to stimulate blood fibrinolytic therapy, has been shown to be more effective than placebo in decreasing skin surface area involved with lipodermatosclerosis in patients wearing compression stockings (52). Its efficacy, if any, in venous ulcer patients is unknown.

Elastic Compression Stockings

The first elastic stocking was developed in the latter portion of the 19th century (53). The initial products, however, provided uniform or reverse-gradient compression from the ankle to the calf. Not until Conrad Jobst, an astute mechanical engineer suffering from venous ulceration himself, set to work on the

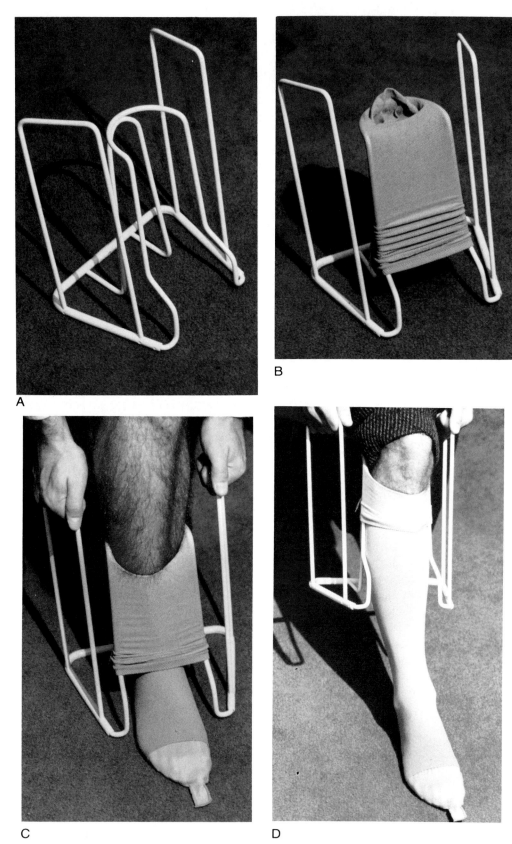

A

B

C

D

Figure 27–4. See legend on opposite page.

problem in the late 1940s did elastic compression stockings become available with a pressure gradient from the ankle up (54). The superiority of gradient compression over uniform compression has not been rigorously proven but has been suggested experimentally and is generally accepted (55). Currently gradient elastic compression stockings of varying lengths, strengths, and materials are readily available.

Gradient compression stockings, in spite of initial conflicting reports, probably do not affect deep venous hemodynamic measurements (56). Their beneficial effects appear to be related more to local compression. Stockings may favorably alter microvascular dynamics and regional Starling forces, leading to edema relief and secondarily to improvements in skin nutrition and oxygen delivery. Therefore elastic stockings do not "cure" ambulatory venous hypertension but appear to effectively counteract its deleterious effects on the skin.

Advantages and Disadvantages of Compression Appliances

Each compression appliance used for the treatment of venous ulcer has its own distinctive advantages and disadvantages. The advantage to using elastic wraps or the newer Circ-Aid device has been the relative ease of application. This may be particularly important in elderly, debilitated, or noncompliant patient groups. The Unna-type paste boot is also relatively easy to apply and has the additional benefit of needing replacement only after days. However, the drawback to any wrapped appliance has always been the inability to determine the amount of compression applied. Wrapped appliances usually lack a distal-to-proximal leg pressure gradient and may even result in a proximal tourniquet effect (57). In addition, Ace-type elastic wraps invariably lose their compressive effects after only 6 to 8 hr of normal activity (58). These drawbacks may in part explain the inferior published results of wrapped compressive devices. Compression stockings, on the other hand, reliably provide adequate pressure for up to 6 months with a proper distal-to-proximal gradient. Unusually configured legs can be accommodated by custom stocking manufacture (59).

A significant disadvantage of elastic compression stockings is the difficulty in application, which has frequently presented an insurmountable hurdle to the frail or elderly. Several developments in recent years have made a significant impact on this obstacle to treatment. The first is the advent of widespread home nursing care in the United States. Selected patients are visited at home on a daily basis by nurses and assisted with wound care and stocking placement. We have also recently begun using a stocking placement device called the Medi-Butler (Fig. 27–4). This sturdy metal appliance allows the stocking to be loaded for application by the patients themselves. By simply stepping into the loaded stocking and picking the device up the patient is able to apply the tight stocking without significant difficulty. In addition, the Jobst UlcerCARE system provides a gradient compression stocking with a zipper. Although we have not used this product, satisfactory preliminary results have been reported by others (60).

Figure 27–4. *A*, The Medi-Butler stocking placement device. *B*, The stocking loaded onto the device. *C* and *D*, The stocking being sequentially fitted onto the lower leg.

The Oregon Protocol

Over the past 20 years we have consistently maintained a nonoperative approach to the treatment of venous stasis ulceration, emphasizing the use of fitted, gradient elastic compression stockings (16). Our protocol has remained unchanged over this period (Table 27–4). All patients are treated with an initial period of bed rest with leg elevation either at home or in the hospital. Patients with large ulcerations, significant edema, cellulitis, or unsatisfactory home situations indicating a low likelihood of compliance with bed rest are recommended for hospital admission. The initial period of bed rest is variable, but a large majority of patients require only 5 to 7 days. Wound care consists of gauze dressing changes, daily soap and water ulcer cleansing, and intravenous or oral antibiotics if infection is present. Topical preparations, antiseptics, or antibiotic ointments are never applied directly to the ulcer.

Following resolution of edema and the initiation of healing, patients are fitted with elastic compression stockings and treated on an ambulatory basis. We begin with 30 to 40 torr below-knee gradient stockings. Only occasional patients require 40 to 50 torr stockings or above-knee stockings. Patients are instructed to wear their stockings at all times during the day and to remove them upon going to bed. Following daily ulcer cleansing, dry gauze is placed over the ulcer, followed by a below-knee noncompression nylon stocking over which the compression stocking may be placed without disrupting the dressing. Saline-soaked or moist dressings are not used since in our experience the resultant skin irritation frequently exacerbates the accompanying stasis dermatitis. Stasis dermatitis is effectively treated with topical corticoids. The patients must be cautioned, however, not to place any corticoid preparation directly on the ulcer. Patients with unusual ankle anatomy with depressions and crevices not effectively compressed by the stocking may have a sponge-rubber wedge placed locally under the stoking.

Periodic elevation of the ulcerated extremity is encouraged. All stockings must be replaced at least every 6 months or sooner if the fitting becomes loose. Patients are asked to purchase two pairs of stockings to allow for stocking laundering. Follow-up is obtained monthly until the ulcer heals and annually or semiannually thereafter. An ulcer photograph is obtained at each clinic visit. All patients are encouraged to continue wearing gradient elastic compression stockings indefinitely following healing.

Results

Following this protocol we achieved complete healing of the venous ulcer in 105 of 113, or 93 per cent, of our patients in a mean of 5.3 months (Fig. 27–5) (16). Ninety per cent, or 102 of 113, patients were consistently compliant with

---

TABLE 27–4. Oregon Protocol for Treatment of Venous Stasis Ulceration

1. Initial period of bed rest in hospital or at home.
2. Fitting with pressure-gradient elastic compression stocking when edema is adequately resolved.
3. Daily ulcer cleansing and dry gauze dressing changes.
4. Corticoid ointment to areas of stasis dermatitis surrounding ulcer, as needed.
5. Continued use of elastic compression stockings posthealing.

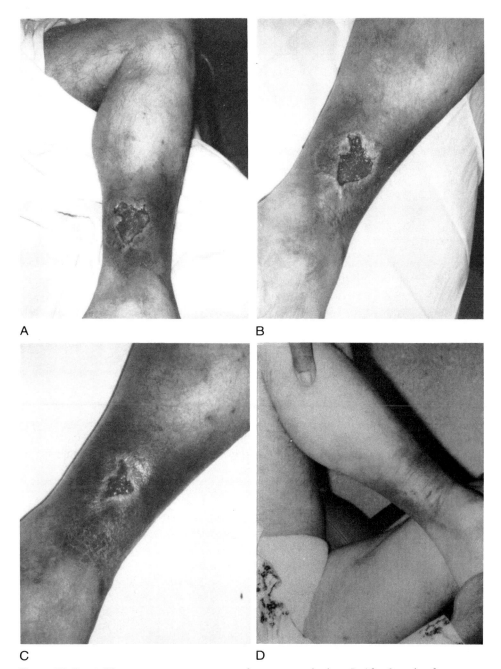

A   B

C   D

Figure 27–5. *A*, The pretreatment appearance of a venous stasis ulcer. *B*, After 2 weeks of treatment with our protocol. *C*, After 1 month of treatment. *D*, Complete healing at 2 months.

elastic stockings while their ulcer healed. Over two thirds of these patients were healed within 4 months. Following healing 73 patients were available for long-term follow-up. A total of 58 of 73 patients, or 79 per cent, were compliant with our recommendations for elastic compression stockings posthealing. To date, nine of 58, or 16 per cent, of these patients have experienced ulcer recurrence at a mean follow-up of 30 months. Recurrence rate calculated by the life-table method was 29 per cent at 5 years. In comparison all patients who were noncompliant with elastic compression stockings had an ulcer recurrence in the follow-up period. These nonoperative results are comparable to those obtained with venous surgery (Table 27–3) and are certainly superior to results in elastic wrap or Unna boot reports (43–46).

Unfortunately, virtually no ulcer recurrence data from other series have been calculated by the life-table method, despite the universal acceptance of the superiority of this method of presenting follow-up data. The striking apparent difference between our compliant patient overall recurrence rate of 16 per cent compared to our 5-year life-table recurrence rate of 29 per cent emphasizes the importance of the life-table method of data presentation.

Compliance

Many physicians are reluctant to utilize elastic compression stockings because of the perceived high incidence of patient noncompliance and dissatisfaction. However, as stated above, 90 per cent of our venous ulcer patients were consistently compliant with their prescribed stockings while healing. In posthealing follow-up, 79 per cent remained compliant. Our high compliance rate suggests that the above perceived drawbacks to stocking use have been overemphasized. Because we have a mixture of private and indigent patients and are not a center for the treatment of venous disease we believe our results are representative of the general population of venous ulcer patients. With appropriate persistence, practitioners in the community should expect to achieve similar or better compliance and healing results. It is our perception that patient compliance relates directly to the physician's expressed confidence in the method. We spend considerable time explaining to our patients the absolute importance of adherence to the elastic compression stocking regimen.

Peripheral Arterial Insufficiency

Approximately 10 per cent of our venous ulcer patients demonstrate significant peripheral arterial insufficiency [ankle-brachial systolic pressure ratio (ABI) 0.6 or less] concomitant with venous stasis ulceration. However, only two patients in 15 years have required concomitant lower extremity arterial revascularization. Both of these patients had an ABI of 0.5 or less. No patient with an ABI of 0.6 or greater required revascularization. All patients with an ABI of 0.6 ($n = 8$) were compliant with stockings and all healed their ulcerations in a mean of 4.2 months. This was not significantly different from the entire patient group (chi-square analysis).

Other Patient Characteristics

The following additional patient characteristics were analyzed statistically (logistic regression or chi-square analysis) and found to have no effect on initial ulcer healing or recurrence: ulcer size, previous venous ulcer, previous known DVT, diabetes, smoking, and PPG-VRT. The fact that a history of previous venous ulcer had no effect on healing or future recurrence brings up an interesting point.

Many authors have sought to define a recalcitrant ulcer patient group who would best respond to venous surgery (31,39). Twenty-seven per cent of our patients had a previous venous ulcer in the same leg. This group of patients, however, did not have a higher incidence of ulcer nonhealing or recurrence. The most important factor with regard to ulcer healing or the prevention of recurrence was compliance with elastic compression stockings. We are therefore currently unable to recognize a recalcitrant venous ulcer patient group except in relationship to stocking noncompliance. We are doubtful that persistent ulcers in noncompliant patients will be significantly improved by direct venous surgery.

CONCLUSION

Based on our results we believe a large majority of patients with venous ulceration can be effectively treated over the long term with elastic compression stockings. Using this regimen we have achieved overall ulcer healing of over 90 per cent, with a 29 per cent 5-year life-table recurrence rate. Undoubtedly a number of the delayed recurrences were due to partial noncompliance, because these patients promptly rehealed their ulcerations upon the renewed vigorous application of the same compressive therapy. We have not utilized vein stripping, perforator ligation, ulcer excision and skin grafting, sclerotherapy, or Unna paste boots to aid in ulcer healing in the past 20 years. In our experience, the problems of noncompliance and patient dissatisfaction with elastic compression stockings have been highly overemphasized. Adherence to a nonoperative protocol of venous ulcer treatment centering on the use of fitted, gradient elastic compression stockings provides both the physician and the patient an acceptable and effective method of venous ulcer treatment.

REFERENCES

1. Brand FN, Dannenberg AL, Abbott RD, Kannel WB: The epidemiology of varicose veins: The Framingham Study. Am J Prev Med 1988;4:96–101.
2. Madar G, Widmer LK, Zemp E, Maggs M: Varicose veins and chronic venous insufficiency—disorder or disease? A critical epidemiological review. Vasa 1986;15:126–134.
3. Prevalence of selected chronic conditions, United States 1979–81. Vital Health Stat [10] 155.
4. Burnand KG, O'Donnell TF, Thomas ML, Browse NL: The relative importance of incompetent communicating veins in the production of varicose veins and venous ulcers. Surgery 1977;82:9–14.
5. Porter JM, Rutherford RB, Clagett GP, et al: Reporting standards in venous disease. J Vasc Surg 1988;8:172–181.
6. Browse NL: The pathogenesis of venous ulceration: A hypothesis. J Vasc Surg 1988;7:468–472.
7. Pollack AA, Wood EH: Venous pressure in the saphenous vein at the ankle in man during exercise and changes in posture. J Appl Physiol 1949;1:649–662.
8. DeCamp PT, Schramel RJ, Ray CJ, et al: Ambulatory venous pressure determinations in post-phlebitic and related syndromes. Surgery 1950;29:365–380.
9. Sturup H, Hojensgard IC: Venous pressure in the deep veins of the lower extremity of patients with primary and post-thrombotic varicose veins. Acta Chir Scand 1950;99:518–525.
10. Bjordal RI: Pressure patterns in the saphenous system in patients with venous leg ulcers. Act Chir Scand 1971;137:495–501.
11. Burnand KG, Whimster I, Clemenson G, Thomas ML, Browse NL: The relationship between the number of capillaries in the skin of the ulcer-bearing area of the lower leg and the fall in foot vein pressure with exercise. Br J Surg 1981;68:297–300.
12. Butcher HR, Hoover AL: Abnormalities of human superficial cutaneous lymphatics associated with stasis ulcers, lymphedema, scars and cutaneous autografts. Ann Surg 1955;142:633–653.

13. Burnand G, Whimster I, Naidoo A, Browse NL: Pericapillary fibrin in the ulcer-bearing skin of the leg: The cause of lipodermatosclerosis and venous ulceration. Br Med J 1982;285:1071–1072.

14. Franzeck UK, Bollinger A, Huch R, Huch A: Transcutaneous oxygen tension, capillary morphology and density in patients with chronic venous incompetence (CVI). Circulation 1984; 70:806–811.

15. Moosa HH, Falanga V, Steed DL, et al: Oxygen diffusion in chronic venous ulceration. J Cardiovasc Surg 1987;28:464–467.

16. Mayberry JC, Moneta GL, Taylor LM, Porter JM: Fifteen year results of nonoperative therapy of chronic venous ulcer: The control series. Surgery 1990 (in press).

17. Raju S: Venous insufficiency of the lower limb and stasis ulceration: Changing concepts and management. Ann Surg 1983;197:688–697.

18. Sethia KK, Darke SG: Long saphenous incompetence as a cause of venous ulceration. Br J Surg 1984;71:754–755.

19. Hoare MC, Nicolaides AN, Miles CR, et al: The role of primary varicose veins in venous ulceration. Surgery 1982;92:450–453.

20. Cranley JJ: Nonoperative management of the postphlebitic syndrome and other forms of chronic deep venous insufficiency. In Rutherford RB, ed: Vascular Surgery, 3rd ed. Philadelphia, WB Saunders Company, 1989;1604.

21. Browse NL, Burnand KG, Thomas ML: Diseases of the Veins: Pathology, Diagnosis, and Treatment. London, Edward Arnold, 1988.

22. Dodd H, Cockett FB: The Pathology and Surgery of the Veins of the Lower Limb, 2nd ed. Edinburgh, Churchill Livingstone, 1976;297–314.

23. Abramowitz HB, Queral LA, Flinn WR, Nora PF, Peterson LK, Bergan JJ, Yao JST: The use of photoplethysmography in the assessment of venous insufficiency: A comparison to venous measurements. Surgery 1979;86:434.

24. Rosfors S: Venous photoplethysmography: Relationship between transducer position and regional distribution of venous insufficiency. J Vasc Surg 1990;11:436–440.

25. Shull KC, Nicolaides AN, Fernandes JF, et al: Significance of popliteal reflux in relation to ambulatory venous pressure and ulceration. Arch Surg 1979;114:1304–1306.

26. Bergan JJ, Yao JST, Flinn WR, McCarthy WJ: Surgical treatment of venous obstruction and insufficiency. J Vasc Surg 1986;3:174–181.

27. Raju S, Fredericks R: Valve reconstruction procedures for non-obstructive venous insufficiency: Rational, techniques, and results in 107 procedures with two- to eight-year follow-up. J Vasc Surg 1988;7:301–310.

28. Linton RR: The post-thrombotic ulceration of the lower extremity: Its etiology and surgical treatment. Ann Surg 1953;138:415–432.

29. Cockett FB: The pathology and treatment of venous ulcers of the leg. Br J Surg 1955;43:260–278.

30. Cranley JJ, Krause RJ, Strasser ES: Chronic venous insufficiency of the lower extremity. Surgery 1961;49:48–58.

31. Silver D, Gleysteen JJ, Rhodes GR, et al: Surgical treatment of the refractory postphlebitic ulcer. Arch Surg 1971;103:554–560.

32. Thurston OG, Williams HTG: Chronic venous insufficiency of the lower extremity: Pathogenesis and surgical treatment. Arch Surg 1973;106:537–539.

33. Bowen FH: Subfascial ligation (Linton operation) of the perforating leg veins to treat post-thrombophlebitic syndrome. Am Surg 1975;41:148–151.

34. Burnand KG, O'Donnell TF, Thomas ML, Browse NL: Relation between postphlebitic changes in the deep veins and results of surgical treatment of venous ulcers. Lancet 1976;1:936–938.

35. DePalma RG: Surgical therapy for venous stasis: Results of a modified Linton operation. Am J Surg 1979;137:810–813.

36. Hyde GL, Litton TC, Hull DA: Long term results of subfascial vein ligation for venous stasis disease. Surg Gynecol Obstet 1981;153:683–686.

37. Negus D, Friedgood A: The effective management of venous ulceration. Br J Surg 1983;70:623–627.

38. Johnson WC, O'Hara ET, Corey C, et al: Venous stasis ulceration: Effectiveness of subfascial ligation. Arch Surg 1985;120:797–800.

39. Cikrit DF, Nichols WK, Silver D: Surgical management of refractory venous stasis ulceration. J Vasc Surg 1988;7:473–478.

40. Sumner DS: Site of valve incompetence in chronic venous insufficiency: A possible reason that valve reconstruction may not work. In Veith FJ, ed: Current Critical Problems in Vascular Surgery. St. Louis, Quality Medical Publishing, 1989;133–138.

41. Villavicencio JL, Rich NM, Salander JM, et al: Leg ulcers of venous origin. In Cameron JL, ed: Current Surgical Therapy. Toronto, BC Decker Inc, 1989;610–18.

42. Dickson-Wright A: The treatment of indolent ulcer of the leg. Lancet 1983;1:457–460.

43. Anning ST: Leg ulcers—the results of treatment. Angiology 1956;7:505–516.
44. Kitahama A, Elliott LF, Kerstein MD, Menendez CV: Leg ulcer: Conservative management or surgical treatment? JAMA 1982;247:197–199.
45. Callam MJ, Harper DR, Dale JJ, Ruckley CV, Prescott RJ: A controlled trial of weekly ultrasound therapy in chronic leg ulceration. Lancet 1987;2:204–205.
46. Kikta MJ, Schuler JJ, Meyer JP, et al: A prospective, randomized trial of Unna's boots versus hydroactive dressing in the treatment of venous stasis ulcers. J Vasc Surg 1988;7:478–483.
47. Pekanmaki K, Kolari PJ, Kiistala U: Intermittent pneumatic compression treatment for post-thrombotic leg ulcers. Clin Exp Dermatol 1987;12:350–353.
48. Queral LA, Criado FJ, Lilly MP, Rudolphi D: The role of sclerotherapy as an adjunct to Unna's boot for treating venous ulcers: A prospective study. J Vasc Surg 1990;11:572–575.
49. Colgan MP, Dormandy J, Jones P, Schraibman I, Shanik D, Young R: The efficacy of Trental in the treatment of venous ulceration. Br Med J 1990 (in press).
50. Sugrue ME, Carolan J, Leen EJ, Feeley TM, Moore DJ, Shanik GD: The use of infrared laser therapy in the treatment of venous ulceration. Ann Vasc Surg 1990;4:179–181.
51. Myers MB, Cherry G: Zinc and the healing of chronic leg ulcers. Am J Surg 1970;120:77–81.
52. Burnand K, Clemenson G, Morland M, Jarrett PEM, Browse NL: Venous lipodermatosclerosis: Treatment by fibrionlytic enhancement and elastic compression. Br Med J 1980;280:7–11.
53. Johnson G Jr: The role of elastic support in venous problems. In Bergan JJ, Yao JST, eds: Surgery of the Veins. Orlando, FL, Grune & Stratton, 1985;541–550.
54. Bergan JJ: Conrad Jobst and the development of pressure gradient therapy for venous disease. In Bergan JJ, Yao JST, eds: Surgery of the Veins. Orlando, FL, Grune & Stratton, 1985;529–540.
55. Lewis CE, Antoine J, Mueller C, et al: Elastic compression in the prevention of venous stasis: A critical reevaluation. Am J Surg 1976;132:739–743.
56. Mayberry JC, Moneta GL, De Frang RD, Porter JM: The influence of elastic compression stockings on deep venous hemodynamics. J Vasc Surg 1991 (in press).
57. Lawrence D, Kakkar VV: Graduated, static, external compression of the lower limb: A physiological assessment. Br J Surg 1980;67:119.
58. Raj TB, Goddard M, Makin GS: How long do compression bandages maintain their pressure during ambulatory treatment of varicose veins? Br J Surg 1980;67:122–124.
59. Horner J, Lowth LC, Nicolaides AN: A pressure profile for elastic stockings. Br Med J 1980;280:818.
60. Young JR, Terwoord BA: Jobst^R UlcerCARE: A Systematic Approach for Management of Venous Leg Ulcers. Cleveland, OH, Cleveland Clinic Foundation and Jobst Institute, 1989.

28

SURGICAL TREATMENT OF CHRONIC VENOUS ULCERATION

Ralph G. DePalma

Linton (1) in 1938 taught that it was important to interrupt incompetent communicating and perforating veins to control the skin changes of venous stasis. Subsequent operations to alleviate dermatitis, induration, and stasis ulceration due to venous insufficiency have included techniques for subfascial (2) and extrafascial (2,3) ligation (3) of perforating veins along with skin grafting of ulcers.

In 1975, the author (4) described a modified operation using Linton's principles to interrupt perforating and communicating veins to minimize transmission of venous hypertension to the skin and subcutaneous tissues. This procedure had as its goal complete interruption of incompetent perforating and communicating veins and grafting of skin ulcers in one operation. It differed from the traditional approach in that rather than creating a longitudinal skin flap, regarded as hazardous for healing, a series of bipedicled flaps in the natural skin lines were fashioned. These provided access to offending veins in the lower part of the leg. In 1979, a follow-up report (5) detailed experience in 68 extremities among 53 patients followed up to 12 years. Four recurrences were described during that period; two related to failures to continue to wear support stockings, and in two others lateral recurrences related to later development of the short saphenous and lateral perforator incompetence. At that time, the indications for surgery were broadened to include more elderly patients and selected patients with corrected arterial insufficiency exhibiting continued venous ulceration. The flap incision in the skin lines afforded safer immediate postoperative healing and durable long-term results.

This chapter describes further evolution of techniques to interrupt communicating and perforating veins to control venous ulceration. Extrafascial and subfascial interruption has been practiced using the previously described skin line incisions. However, since 1985 a further modification used a shearing phlebotome described by Edwards (6) and others (7) to divide the perforating veins of the posteromedial arcade.

PATIENT SELECTION

Patients were referred for operation after failure of conservative treatment, including Unna paste boots, bed rest and elevation, support stockings, and various other types of therapy. In the period of May 1980 through January 1990, 40 extremities in 32 patients were operated on using both earlier techniques and adding, where appropriate, the sharing operation after 1985. The patients ranged in age from 27 through 64 years. Twenty-two were women. Twenty-two patients had deep venous disease, 14 of these thrombotic. Thirty-two operations were done for medial ulceration, seven for lateral ulceration, and one for both medial and lateral incompetence and ulceration. All patients were examined for adequacy of the arterial circulation and, within this series, there were no instances of arterial compromise.

Superficial venous incompetency was first evaluated by physical examination with the patient standing and the examiner palpating the long and short saphenous systems. Sequential tourniquets were then used to evaluate levels of venous incompetence and major leak points. Since 1985 the examination has been supplemented using a Doppler ultrasound probe to define leakage points at the saphenofemoral junction as well as in the popliteal fossa and in the leg for key posterior arcade perforators. Since 1987, all surgical candidates have undergone imaging using a QUAD 1 Quantum Angiodynograph ultrasound system to examine the deep venous veins to define deep thrombosis or valvular insufficiency. To supplement these examinations, especially to plan ligations at the infracrural region posteromedially, intraoperative varicography was used eight times. Preoperative venography delineated vena cava occlusion in one patient and further documented the status of the deep veins in five additional patients.

PREOPERATIVE CARE

With information about major leak areas, operations were planned. These procedures aimed to remove incompetent superficial systems and to interrupt incompetent perforators relating to areas of venous ulceration. There were 11 hospital admissions for intensive treatment of infected ulcerations for 2 to 3 days prior to operation. As described previously (4), strict bed rest was enforced, with the extremity elevated prior to surgery, treatment of ulcers with wet-to-dry dressings, and systemic antibiotics. This made possible a comprehensive operation done in one stage. Puritic dermatitis was treated with triamcinolone cream (0.025 per cent). Systemic steroids were required to control itching in two instances of severe dermatophytid reactions. Whenever possible, patients are now treated on ambulatory basis to avoid the time constraints of hospitalization; within the last 4 years, all but two patients were admitted to the hospital on the day of surgery.

OPERATIVE TECHNIQUE

In 24 operations done after 1985, the previous operative technique was altered for the medial perforator approach by using a shearing phlebotome (Fig. 28–1).

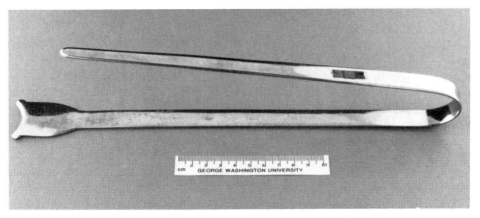

Figure 28–1.   Configuration of Edwards (6) shearing phlebotome.

Operations for lateral incompetence were done as previously described (3,5) without the use of the phlebotome. Either general or regional anesthesia was used.

For medial ulceration, particular attention was directed toward division of the posterior arcade perforators (Fig. 28–2). When the long or short saphenous veins were incompetent, these were stripped as related to the ulcerated area. At times it was difficult to decide on the contribution to venous hypertension of the

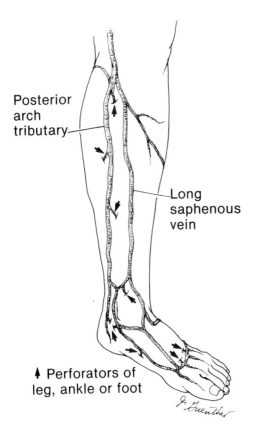

Figure 28–2.   Long saphenous vein and posterior arch tributary with arrangement of commonly observed perforating veins. Note perforating veins of foot and relative size of the posterior arch tributary as compared to long saphenous.

Posterior arch tributary

Long saphenous vein

↟ Perforators of leg, ankle or foot

long saphenous, short saphenous, or a highly located perforator at the posteromedial aspect of the calf. In these instances, intraoperative varicography was
performed (Fig. 28–3). With these findings, the short saphenous vein was divided
and the long saphenous vein stripped as well as ligating large perforators through
appropriate parallel incisions. Whenever the long saphenous vein was incompetent in the thigh, it was always stripped. If it was incompetent in the leg, it was

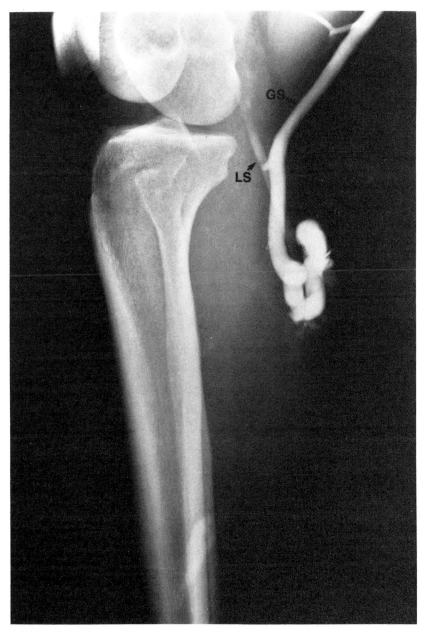

Figure 28–3.   Varicosity related to perforating vein with incompetent greater saphenous (*GS*) vein
and contribution from lesser saphenous (*LS*) vein located in upper medial calf.

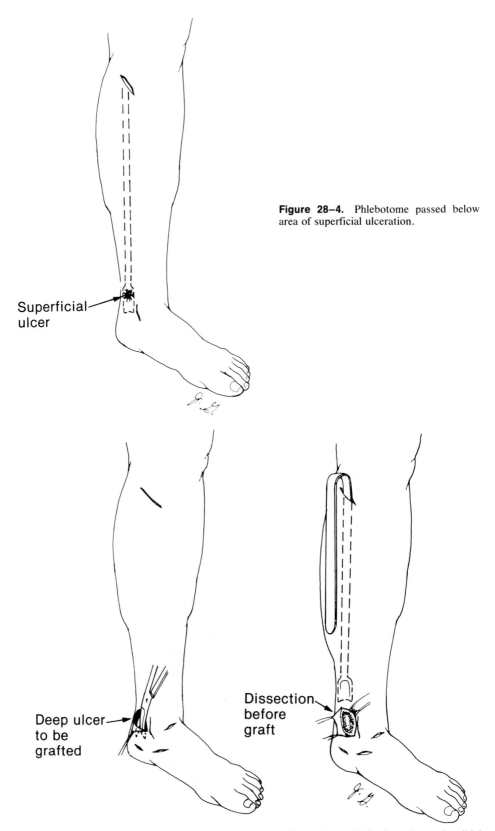

Figure 28–4. Phlebotome passed below area of superficial ulceration.

Superficial ulcer

Deep ulcer to be grafted

Dissection before graft

Figure 28–5. Phlebotome passed after formal excision of deep ulcer with ligation of posterior tibial tributaries.

400

removed from ankle to knee. Stripping, combined with varicography in some cases, is considered important for control of medial infracrural incompetence. One ulcer recurrence clearly related to failure to obliterate the troublesome complex (Fig. 28–3).

When the skin exhibited minimal liposclerosis or effacement between the skin and the fascia, the shearing phlebotome was passed in a subcutaneous plane below the malleolar level (Fig. 28–4) posteriorly. However, with liposclerosis and marked effacement with the formation of a "bottle leg," excision of the ulcer was carried out to expose the posterior tibial vein; in this case the shearing phlebotome was passed along the axis of the posterior arcade subfascially to an area just above the malleolus (Fig. 28–5). Before stripping or shearing, the operating table was placed in a 15 degrees head-down position. The legs were then kept elevated above the atrial level at all times in the immediate postoperative period.

Figure 28–6 shows the axis of passage of the phlebotome, with the stippled area illustrating some of the flap elevation. In many cases counterincisions were used. For deep ulceration excision, ligation of posterior tibial vein branches was carried out under direct vision using 3-0 chromic catgut. Skin grafts of 0.014 to 0.016 inch were applied after perforator division, suturing the graft with 5-0 silk. For superficial ulceration and minimal induration, excision was not often required with the shearing procedure. In these cases pressure dressings were applied immediately after shearing the perforators. Large high-pressure veins were ligated through the usual parallel incision as needed.

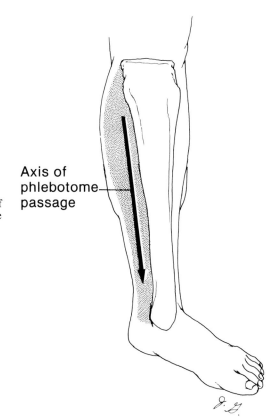

Figure 28–6. Proper axis for passage of phlebotome. Care is taken not to impinge upon the tibial area.

Axis of phlebotome passage

POSTOPERATIVE CARE

In cases requiring skin grafts, the patient remained at strict bed rest in a posterior splint for immobilization for at least 7 days. All patients receive broad-spectrum antibiotics postoperatively for 7 to 10 days. Intermittent sequential compression was applied to the contralateral leg; this was begun intraoperatively. Beginning 24 to 36 hr postoperatively, patients received from 4000 to 6000 units of heparin subcutaneously ever 12 hr when bed rest was required. When skin grafts were not required, patients were kept in bed with the legs elevated for 3 to 4 days, then ambulation with pressure dressings was begun.

All patients were fitted with pressure-gradient support stockings with pressures ranging from 30 to 50 mm Hg at the ankle before or shortly after leaving the hospital. The supports were fitted immediately after removal of dressings when swelling was minimal. Patients were instructed to don these stockings daily upon arising and to wear them until retiring. Triamcinolone cream (0.025 per cent) was applied nightly to areas of hyperpigmented skin. Patients with pruritis were urged to minimize the use of soap and water on affected areas.

RESULTS

There was no operative mortality; pulmonary emboli did not occur. Using the skin line incisions, there was primary healing in all except one patient, in whom healing at the ankle was delayed for a period of 21 days. Figures 28–7 and 28–8 illustrate the typical appearance of incisions in two patients 10 days and 8 weeks, respectively, after operation. Note that the effect of the shearing operation has reduced but not eliminated incisions for high-pressure veins. In 12 extremities in which skin grafts were applied, hospitalization postoperatively ranged from 7 to 18 days. The instances comprising the two longest periods of hospitalization occurred in a man with vena caval occlusion (see later in this section). There was one minor complication early in the experience with the phlebotome. This operation was required to correct recurrent ulceration following a Linton-type procedure performed elsewhere. In a small leg in a 55-year-old woman, the phlebotome was directed anteriorly, causing a linear 7 cm × 3 mm superficial slough that healed after 25 days of outpatient treatment. The skin graft took primarily. There was also transient saphenous neuropathy in this case, which was not later troublesome. Since adopting a policy of passing the phlebotome only once in the same axis and keeping it posterior to the medial border of the tibia, this complication has not been seen again.

Of the 32 patients operated on since 1980, one has died of lung cancer and two have been lost to follow-up. The others have been reevaluated in the George Washington clinic or by the author's staff in Reno, Nevada. There were four recurrences. The most troublesome occurred in a man operated on 15 years after vena caval ligation. This 57-year-old clerk was initially treated in 1983 with bilateral staged modified Linton procedures with skin grafting. He remained in the hospital 15 and 18 days for the two surgeries. His stasis changes recurred twice in the interval between 1983 and 1986. He required hospitalization for diffuse cellulitis and lymphangitis but not for breakdown of the skin-grafted areas. Each recurrent episode related to his noncompliance with support stockings. Since 1986

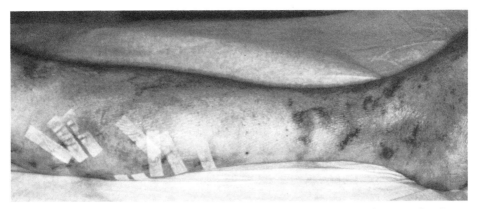

Figure 28–7. Male patient, age 60, 10 days after modified Linton and shearing operation for superficial ulceration. Note additional incisions for ligation of large perforators as needed.

he has been compliant with support stockings. He has been offered caval bypass, which he has refused. Currently his skin has remained healed and he continues to be employed.

The second patient with ulcer recurrence was a 35-year-old morbidly obese postal employee who was operated on in 1984, receiving a skin graft for malleolar ulceration and a modified Linton operation with saphenous stripping from ankle to knee. She stopped wearing support stockings in the fall of 1988. Ulceration occurred in the upper third of the leg at an incision site where a residual problematic perforator appeared in the infracrural area. She was treated by the application of Unna paste boots and reintroduction of support.

The third recurrence occurred in a 62-year-old rancher, operated upon in 1982 in Reno, Nevada, with recurrent medial ulceration beginning about 24 months postoperatively. This patient was last seen in September, 1982; the ulcer is now said to measure 12 × 6 cm and he is reported to be wearing supports.

The fourth recurrence, a minor one, involved the lateral aspect of a severely

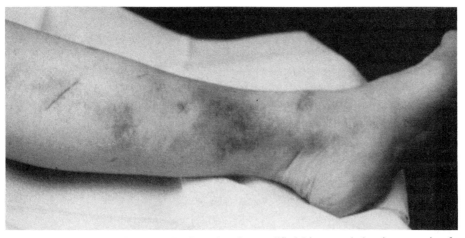

Figure 28–8. Female patient, age 50, 8 weeks after modified Linton and shearing operation for supramalleolar ulceration. Note healing without graft and location of ancillary incisions in skin lines.

involved "bottle"-deformed leg. This lateral recurrence followed an extensive medial ligation in a 58-year-old female grocery clerk who remained healed for 8 years. Because of her deformity, she required extensive padding under elastic wraps rather than supports. A new ulceration appeared laterally long after correction of the woody, calcified medial ulcer. A pattern of lateral recurrence has been noted before (5), suggesting transmission of venous hypertension through the lateral perforators after medial correction.

COMMENTS

Our experience has applied to patients with stasis ulceration of undoubtedly varying etiologies. While changes at the capillary level contributing to skin stasis changes are poorly defined, venous hypertension appears to be a common denominator. No evaluation of muscle pump function has been made. However, all these patients were ambulatory; all exhibited good range of motion at the ankle and most had supple calf muscles. Irrespective of the underlying etiology of venous hypertension, interruption or disconnection of the high venous pressure circuit from the skin and subcutis appeared to promote ulcer healing. This state is maintained by elastic support. While support will always be required, lighter and more comfortable weights can often be prescribed after operation.

The patients are relieved of time-consuming and expensive clinic care following surgery. The individual must recognize the requirement for indefinite use of graded support hose and must continue to care for affected skin properly. Triamcinolone (0.025 per cent) applied to areas of hyperpigmentation is effective in the long term. It should be applied sparingly on retiring. Its use during the day will destroy the integrity of elastic supports. Both excessive bathing and exposure to sunlight are also to be avoided.

In summary, risks of operation are minimal and, with the technique described, satisfactory healing of ulceration can be achieved in most cases. It is important that the operation be designed to deal as completely as possible with transmission of venous hypertension to affected skin as well as providing new skin coverage for areas of extreme stasis change.

REFERENCES

1. Linton RR: The communicating veins of the lower leg and the operative technique for their ligation. Ann Surg 1938;*107*:582.
2. Linton RR: The post thrombotic ulceration of the lower extremity: Its etiology and surgical treatment. Ann Surg 1953;*138*:415.
3. Dodd H, Cockett FB: The Pathology and Surgery of Veins of the Lower Limb. Edinburgh, E. S. Livingston Ltd, 1956;424–447.
4. DePalma RG: Surgical therapy for venous stasis surgery. Surgery 1975;*76*:910.
5. DePalma RG: Surgical therapy for venous stasis: Results of a modified Linton operation. Am J Surg 1979;*137*:810.
6. Edwards JM: Shearing operation for incompetent perforating veins. Br J Surg 1976;*63*:885.
7. Simpson CJ, Smellie GD: The phlebotome in the management of incompetent perforating veins and venous ulceration. J Cardiovasc Surg 1987;*28*:279.

IX

UPPER EXTREMITY VENOUS PROBLEMS

29

CHANGING CONCEPTS AND PRESENT-DAY ETIOLOGY OF UPPER EXTREMITY VENOUS THROMBOSIS

Walter J. McCarthy, Robert L. Vogelzang, and John J. Bergan

An obscure disease until recently, thrombosis of the axillary and subclavian veins is made interesting by diverse etiology and an enduring controversy over its proper treatment. Paget reported spontaneous thrombosis involving veins of the upper extremity in 1875, and classified this condition as "gouty phlebitis" (1). In his work he reviewed cases reported in 1862 by Mackenzie and in 1869 by Humphry, which were similar. The first detailed clinical description is attributed to von Schroetter in 1884, and thus the general condition of primary axillary or subclavian thrombosis is sometimes referred to as the Paget-Schroetter syndrome (2).

Venous thrombosis of the axillary and subclavian vein can be divided into primary and secondary types. Primary thrombosis is usually attributed to external venous trauma by a restrictive thoracic inlet. The often-used term "effort thrombosis" describes the temporal relation to athletic or occupational exertions of the upper extremity. Early reports, previous to 1950, were almost completely composed of such cases of primary or effort thrombosis. This is in contrast to current observations of subclavian vein thrombosis following iatrogenic trauma. Thus, secondary subclavian thrombosis has become almost commonplace in modern medical centers, related to cardiac pacemakers, venous hemodialysis, and all other types of central venous cannulation or manipulation.

PRESENTATION OF THROMBOSIS

Primary or effort thrombosis presents in a characteristic way. A young Michael DeBakey, writing in 1942 (3), described the presentation: "thrombosis occurs most commonly in the male and in the right arm, and when the left side is involved, it is usually in left-handed patients or those having exerted an unusual strain on this arm. Whereas rarely it may develop spontaneously like a bolt out of the blue and without rhyme or reason, the patient finding his arm stiff and swollen on awakening, usually the condition is observed in young, robust, muscular individuals and following some type of sudden or unusual effort or strain. It would seem that these forms of preceding muscular exertions vary considerably from sudden severe, violent efforts to simple banal acts." The commonly reported right arm–to–left arm ratio is about 2:1.

Rudolph Matas summarized the worldwide experience in 1934 and listed causal strains of the arm, including "checking and restraining a wild horse, fall from a horse on the abducted arm, a woman stricken after beating wash clothes with a heavy stick, and vigorous stirring of a Christmas pudding" (4). He also reported such curious causes as "vicious swinging with a golf club, an unusual twist in pitching a baseball, exertion at tennis, and cracking a long whip over a wagon team." Nearly every author adds an unusual extremity strain. Several of interest from the Northwestern University experience include one patient injured while placing a hard top to winterize a convertible sports car and two stockbrokers stricken while frantically waving their arms on the Mercantile Exchange floor.

This condition of effort thrombosis afflicts men much more commonly than women, with a ratio of about 4:1. Occurrence is usually in the second or third decade of life, peaking at about age 28.

E. S. R. Hughes' review of the first 320 reported cases in 1949 lends some accurate description of the signs and symptoms that is highly applicable today (5). "Swelling is the usual initial complaint involving the whole arm from fingers to the shoulder and frequently the lower neck or breast is involved. The swollen arm, while firm, rarely pits with finger pressure. The skin of the afflicted extremity is slightly cyanotic but may be mottled, and this coloration is more obvious in the hand and lower part of the forearm. Superficial veins are more prominent than usual as they act to form collateral circulation. . . . A firm, tender cord may or may not be palpable in the axilla" (6).

Also in 1949, Kleinsasser quantitated the above observations by Hughes with a review of 66 cases (7). At the time of hospital admission, swelling was present in 84.7 per cent, pain in 50.0 per cent, cyanosis 37.5 per cent, and prominent collateral veins in 26.4 per cent of all patients. On occasion, numbness, aching, stiffness, heaviness, and tightness were reported. Progression to gangrene with phlegmasia cerulia dolens has been reported but is extraordinarily rare.

ETIOLOGY OF PRIMARY OR EFFORT THROMBOSIS

Effort or primary thrombosis is actually due to chronic compression of the subclavian or axillary vein in the thoracic inlet (6). Vigorous debate over the course of a century attributes this compression to various structures, including the head of the humerus acting through the subscapularis muscle, the tendon of the pectoralis minor muscle, the subclavius muscle, or the costocoracoid ligament. Even the phrenic or accessory phrenic nerves have been implicated (8). In fact, it appears that the subclavian vein is usually compromised as it passes over the first rib, in front of the anterior scalene muscle, and behind the medial aspect of the clavicle (9). Motion of the upper extremity causes a scissoring action against the vein in some individuals.

Evidence for chronic compression of the subclavian vein preceding acute thrombosis is circumstantial but strong. A distinct group of patients exist who

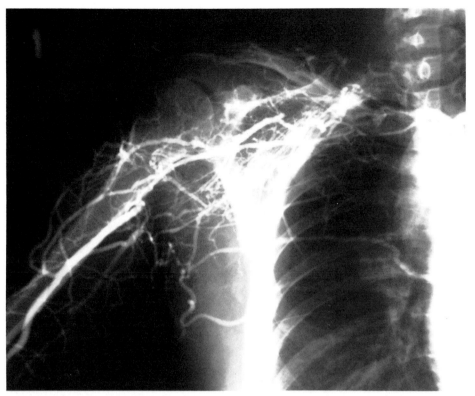

Figure 29–1.   A 47-year-old woman studied after acute thrombosis related to athletic exertion. Notice the numerous very tiny collaterals.

have symptomatic swelling of their upper extremity along with coexisting elevated venous pressures and intermittent vein compression seen on dynamic venography (10,11). Another observation is that patients with known subclavian thrombosis may, when studied venographically, have an opposite extremity afflicted with severe compression of the vein, but without thrombosis (12). In addition, surgical description of subclavian vein exploration after thrombotic lysis often includes a description of perivenous fibrosis (9). It seems logical to conclude that the subclavian vein is damaged by stretching and compression over time and eventually some major or minor event precipitates actual thrombosis (Fig. 29–1).

ETIOLOGY OF SECONDARY THROMBOSIS

Secondary axillary or subclavian vein thrombosis should be defined to include all causes other than compression and damage of the vein within the shoulder itself. Thus, injury by various types of hyperalimentation, dialysis, and chemotherapy catheters would be included. In addition, thrombosis precipitated by local tumor, local radiation, hypertonic or sclerotic solutions, and hypercoagulability would also be included.

A recent retrospective review of this condition at Northwestern Memorial Hospital identified 67 patients whose thrombosis was objectively confirmed by either venography or duplex scanning. Only seven patients from this entire group would be categorized as having primary effort thrombosis in the usual sense. Most of the others were patients with terminal cancer. Six had renal failure requiring subclavian venous dialysis catheters, 12 had miscellaneous other central lines placed, and 40 had widespread carcinoma. Most of the cancer patients had at one time undergone subclavian catheter placement, and some were on chronic chemotherapy with indwelling catheters.

Specific causes of secondary subclavian and axillary venous thrombosis have been studied prospectively, and their review is of interest. Not only does the condition appear to be extraordinarily common following certain types of central venous manipulation, but the long-term sequelae are nearly universally benign. Categories of secondary venous thrombosis will be reviewed along with their treatment not only as a guide to presentation and therapy but also to suggest lessons related to primary effort thrombosis.

Venous Thrombosis with Long-Term Transvenous Cardiac Pacing

With the availability of implantable, long-term cardiac pacemakers placed through a transvenous route, some venous thrombosis seems inevitable (13). Rarely, however, are patients symptomatic (14). Williams et al. reviewed 212 consecutive pacemakers placed between 1970 and 1977 at a single institution and found only five with symptomatic thrombosis of the subclavian vein (15). All five were treated with heparin anticoagulation followed by short-term warfarin therapy. In each case, elevation of the arm and anticoagulation resulted in prompt resolution of the symptoms, and none of the patients required pacemaker wire removal. Crook et al. investigated 125 patients paced through cephalic vein access and identified only three symptomatic subclavian thromboses (16). Other investigators have reported a low incidence of symptoms following subclavian thrombosis, but it remained for Stoney et al. to study this complication venographically (17). They evaluated 32 patients presenting for elective pacer replacement by performing upper extremity venograms. All electrodes had been functioning for 2 years or more except one studied at 18 months. The results are remarkable in that only seven patients (21 per cent) had normal venograms. Less than 50 per cent luminal stenosis was seen in 15 per cent, severe luminal stenosis of 50 to 90 per cent was present in 15 patients (44 per cent), and seven patients (21 per cent) had total venous obstruction. It was noted that symptoms were extraordinarily rare in this group, and only one patient actually presented with arm edema. The authors summarized their experience by stating that, although venous thrombosis is frequent after placement of permanent pacemakers, this complication almost never creates a clinical problem.

Indwelling Subclavian Hemodialysis Catheters

Temporary use of indwelling subclavian vein hemodialysis catheters has become common since their introduction in 1977. These useful devices can be readily placed at the bedside and offer immediate access for dialysis while more permanent fistulas or shunts are constructed surgically and allowed to mature. Evidence that these catheters may cause subclavian vein damage with thrombosis is not surprising, although the exact incidence of this occurrence is unknown. Reports on this topic have been limited to small series with anecdotal observations (18).

El-Nachef et al. believe that larger diameter catheters are more likely to cause subclavian thrombosis (19), but a comment from Bennett and Stewart reported similar problems using smaller single-lumen dialysis catheters (20). A recurrent observation is that the subclavian vein is unlikely to recanalize in patients after the dialysis catheter has been removed. Similar to the observations regarding patients with pacemaker venous thrombosis, patients rarely have significant complications from the subclavian vein thrombosis alone. It appears that many or most patients are in fact asymptomatic but may become suddenly compromised if an arteriovenous fistula is established in the affected arm.

McCauley et al. reported on the onset of severe arm edema following arteriovenous fistula surgery below a previously thrombosed subclavian vein (18). They suggested the consideration of radionuclide venograms or conventional venograms prior to constructing an arteriovenous fistula for patients who have had previous chronic subclavian catheters. On the basis of a similar experience at Northwestern Memorial Hospital, we would suggest the consideration of duplex scanning in such patients to establish that subclavian vein continuity exists before arteriovenous fistula surgery is performed.

The management of individuals with a functioning arm fistula and massive edema can be challenging. Currier and colleagues reported on six such patients, all with thrombosed subclavian veins, who had 6-mm polytetrafluoroethylene grafts placed from the axillary vein to the internal jugular vein for outflow continuity (21). Half of their patients maintained patent venous bypasses 1 to 3 years after operation, while the other three had graft thrombosis and required fistula ligation to control arm swelling. Our experience at Northwestern University and that of others (22) includes subclavian vein reconstruction using saphenous vein spiral grafting for axillary-to–central venous bypass.

The best advice related to this problem, perhaps, is to appreciate potential subclavian vein thrombosis related to dialysis catheters and to diagnose the condition before an arm arteriovenous fistula is placed. In addition, prolonged reliance on indwelling subclavian dialysis catheters might be avoided whenever possible.

Subclavian Hyperalimentation Catheters

Occurrence of venous thrombosis related to central venous catheter placement is very common (23) (Fig. 29–2). A prospective study using venography conducted by Jeejeebhoy et al. demonstrated a 90 per cent incidence of catheter-related thrombus (24). Usually this was a small amount attached to the catheter, but 13 per cent of the patients had some actual mural venous thrombus and 7 per cent had complete subclavian occlusion. Horattas et al. reviewed 33 of their cases of upper extremity deep venous thrombosis (25). One significant conclusion was that no obvious thrombosis was identified as being due to commonly used 16-gauge single-lumen catheters. Rather, this problem seemed more likely with multilumen or other large-bore catheters, shunts, or constant infusion delivery systems (Fig. 29–3). The authors also summarized recent articles on this topic, identifying nine prospective studies from which 152 cases of thrombus were identified in 539 patients undergoing subclavian venous catheterization. This 28 per cent

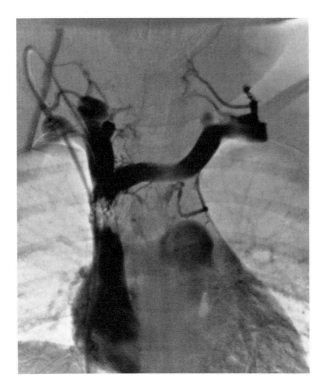

Figure 29–2. Thrombus has formed in the superior vena cava in relation to an internal jugular central catheter. This is interesting because there is no other thrombus present in the system.

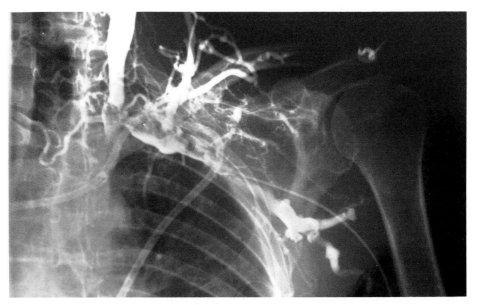

Figure 29–3. A left subclavian vein triple-lumen catheter is seen surrounded by thrombus. This material extends into the internal jugular vein.

incidence is quite striking. In their series, Harattas et al. identified a 12 per cent incidence of upper extremity–related pulmonary embolization. Therapy for subclavian vein thrombosis is usually simple, and patients almost always do well after removal of the predisposing catheter and anticoagulation with heparin followed by warfarin therapy. Reduction of the venous thrombosis by adding heparin to hyperalimentation fluid is suggested by some but remains controversial, because additional bleeding complications and heparin-induced thrombocytopenia are a risk (26).

Radiation Therapy for Carcinoma

Arterial occlusion is well known following radiation therapy and often involves the carotid, subclavian, or iliac vessels (27). It thus seems analogous that major venous thrombosis might also result from this treatment. Wilson and coauthors reported on two patients treated with external beam radiation and tamoxifen who presented with ipsilateral arm swelling (28). These women were examined 4 and 3 years after their initial radiation therapy, and both were free of tumor when examined. Venography demonstrated subclavian vein thrombosis in both cases, and both patients responded well to anticoagulation therapy. The authors speculated that radiation-induced fibrosis was a major etiology in both cases. In reviewing 235 patients with combined chemotherapy and mantle radiotherapy for lymphoma, Schreiber and Kapp identified four who developed subclavian vein thrombosis in the posttreatment period (29). These cases were thought to be unique because all lymphoma had presented with mediastinal disease, and there was clear x-ray evidence of fibrosis surrounding the axillary and subclavian vein without any active malignant disease present. Of interest is that three of the four patients had venous thrombosis in the same arm in which they had received the majority of their chemotherapy. Thus the influence of the chemotherapy infusions could be significant.

Patients with Malignant Disease

An association with malignant disease is well known with axillary and subclavian venous thrombosis (30), and most patients in the series gathered at Northwestern University had that association (Fig. 29–4). Schreiber and Kapp reviewed the entire relevant literature, excluding patients with malignancy in whom an infusion catheter was used in the subclavian vein (29). Thus, about 50 reported cases were available, and almost all patients had evidence of direct compression about the subclavian vein by tumor or a so-called migratory thrombophlebitis when they were diagnosed. Again, selecting cases seemingly unrelated to central venous cannulation, Hung reviewed six axillary-subclavian venous thromboses related to malignancy (27). In half, the thrombosis seemed to be caused by compression of adjacent tumor, and the rest more likely were related to a hypercoagulable state associated with the coexisting malignancy. In each case anticoagulation was administered, and four patients had complete recovery from their symptoms. One patient had some moderate swelling, and a single patient continued to have pain and swelling of the affected arm until he expired of a cause related to his malignancy.

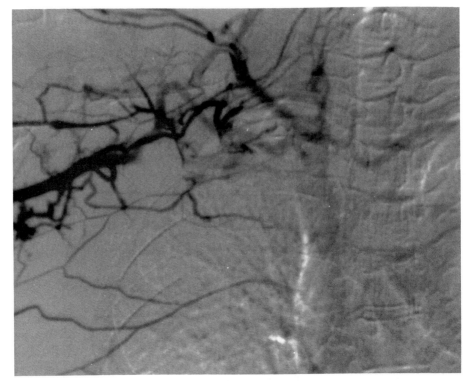

Figure 29–4.   A patient with end-stage ovarian cancer was studied after acute thrombosis of the right axillary subclavian vein.

Malignancy seems to be a common coexisting factor with axillary subclavian vein thrombosis, but it is usually further complicated by subclavian venous puncture or chemotherapy infusion (31) (Fig. 29–5). It seems that patients usually do well if heparin followed by warfarin anticoagulation can be maintained.

Miscellaneous Causes of Thrombosis

Infectious etiology of this condition must be rare but is discussed by Surkin et al. in a case of severe otitis media (32). Apparently, this precipitated thrombosis of the internal jugular vein, which later went on to subclavian vein thrombosis. A review of eight patients treated in Sri Lanka identifies filariasis as the etiology of subclavian thrombosis (33). The authors noted the endemicity of filariasis in Sri Lanka and the greatly enlarged lymph nodes and funiculitis in some of their patients. It is known that superficial thrombophlebitis is not an uncommon manifestation of filariasis.

While it seems logical that hypercoagulable states should predispose to upper extremity venous thrombosis, that premise has been hard to prove. Several case reports outline this problem in women taking estrogen-containing birth control pills (34,35). However, the etiologic connection seems unproven. Detailed hematologic parameters are reported by Sundqvist et al. in 60 consecutive patients with venographically verified deep venous thrombosis of the arm seen in Malmo,

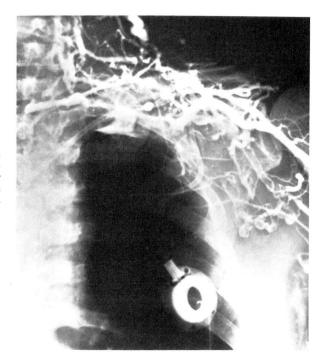

Figure 29–5. Thrombus within the subclavian vein is seen surrounding a Portacath placed for chemotherapy infusion. Notice the significant collateral circulation present.

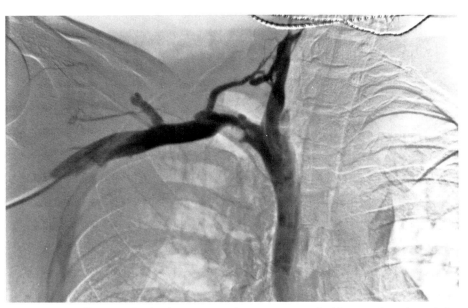

Figure 29–6. Effort thrombosis of a young man's arm was treated with systemic anticoagulation. Three weeks following anticoagulation for effort thrombosis, reevaluation demonstrates stenosis of the right subclavian vein.

Sweden (36). No factors, including antithrombin III, seemed abnormal compared to controls except a 49 per cent incidence of decreased fibrinolytic activity. The authors believe this was significant and may contribute to the mechanism of pathogenesis.

PROGNOSIS AND THERAPY

The reported prognosis following axillary-subclavian vein thrombosis differs between primary or effort types and those due to secondary causes (37). This is largely difficult to understand, but the observation seems borne out by most reports (38). Therefore, appropriate therapy may be different in these two groups.

Because of postthrombosis pain and edema, patients with effort-induced thrombosis may require generally more aggressive and sometimes surgical therapy when compared to the secondary group (38–41). This approach is supported by DeWeese and Machleder, whose reports are detailed elsewhere in this volume (Chapters 30 and 31, respectively), and by others (42,43). Kunkel and Machleder reported on 25 consecutive patients treated with thrombolytic agents and, in 17 patients, first rib resection to alleviate venous compression (44). This is logical, because the predisposing compression still remains following clot lysis (Figs. 29–6 and 29–7). Functional postoperative results are excellent; however, no control group using simple anticoagulation techniques is compared side by side. Although unproven, this more aggressive treatment, particularly using urokinase, may be appropriate for true effort-induced venous thrombosis.

Venous thrombosis related to secondary occlusion, usually complicating subclavian vein manipulation with various catheters, is usually an asymptomatic or barely symptomatic circumstance (45). Standard anticoagulation therapy using initially heparin, then warfarin, seems most appropriate. Thrombolytic therapy has some disadvantages and no proven benefit in uncomplicated cases (46,47) (Fig. 29–8). In general, if the predisposing subclavian catheter can be removed, this seems most appropriate. However, experience with chronic cardiac pacemaking wires demonstrates that the catheter may be left in place without deleterious result. The goal of anticoagulation is to reduce extended thrombosis and avoid the possibility of pulmonary embolus, which has been recorded in up to 12 per cent of some series of upper extremity venous thrombosis (48). A subset of patients have strong contraindications for anticoagulation therapy, and their treatment is controversial. There is no device comparable to the Greenfield vena caval filter that is applicable to the upper extremity. Thus, patients with known axillary-subclavian venous thrombosis at Northwestern Memorial Hospital and solid contraindication to anticoagulation have simply been treated with elevation and compressive dressings. This therapy has been largely successful, but the risk of a fatal pulmonary embolus, while minute, does exist.

The use of thrombolytic therapy, operative thrombectomy, or rib resection in secondary venous thrombosis seems largely unnecessary. At this time, it should be restricted to those with severe arm edema refractory to standard anticoagulation.

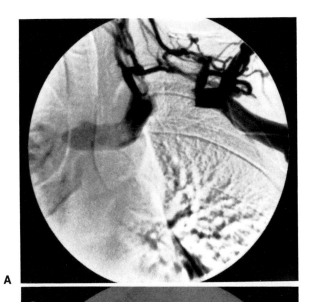

Figure 29–7. *A*, Acute effort thrombosis of the left subclavian vein treated with urokinase infusion. *B*, Urokinase was followed by balloon dilatation angioplasty of the subclavian vein. *C*, Immediately following balloon angioplasty there was wide patency in a neutral position, but with the upper extremity positioned in hyperabduction a tight stenosis of the subclavian vein is seen.

post balloon and 4 hrs UK

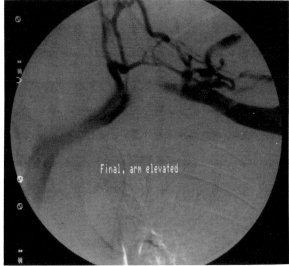

Final, arm elevated

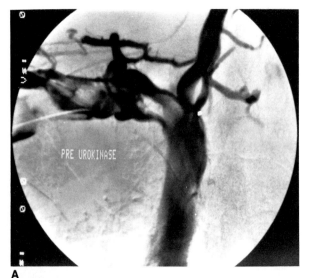

A

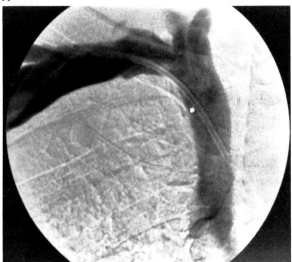

B

Figure 29–8. *A*, This patient presented with thrombosis surrounding a central line placed to treat end-stage lung cancer. Urokinase was used for 6 hr to lyse this thrombus. *B*, Six hours after treatment, the patient was admitted to the angiography suite and became acutely short of breath, but was found to have a remarkably normal-appearing subclavian vein. *C*, A ventilation-perfusion scan demonstrates multiple perfusion defects consistent with and confirming clinical suspicion of significant pulmonary embolism.

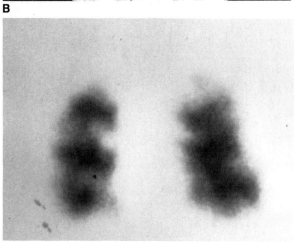

C

REFERENCES

1. Paget J: Clinical Lectures and Essays. London, Longmans, Green and Co, 1875.
2. Sampson JJ: An apparent causal mechanism of primary thrombosis of the axillary and subclavian veins. Am Heart J 1942;*21*:313–327.
3. DeBakey M, Ochsner A, Smith MC: Primary thrombosis of the axillary vein. New Orleans Med Surg J 1942;*95*:62–70.
4. Matas R: On the so-called primary thrombosis of the axillary vein caused by strain. Am J Surg 1934;*24*:642–666.
5. Hughes ESR: Venous obstruction in the upper extremity (Paget-Schroetter's syndrome). Int Abstr Surg 1949;*88*:89–127.
6. Hughes ESR: Venous obstruction in the upper extremity. Br J Surg 1948;*36*:155–163.
7. Kleinsasser LJ: "Effort" thrombosis of the axillary and subclavian veins. Arch Surg 1949;*59*:258–274.
8. Jackson NJ, Nanson EM: Intermittent subclavian vein obstruction. Br J Surg 1961;*49*:303–306.
9. DeWeese JA, Adams JT, Gaiser DL: Subclavian venous thrombectomy. Circulation, 1970;*41–42*(suppl II):II-158–II-164.
10. Adams JT, DeWeese JA, Mahoney EB, Rob CG: Intermittent subclavian vein obstruction without thrombosis. Surgery 1968;*63*:147–165.
11. Bass DH, Stein D: Intermittent obstruction of the subclavian vein: A case report. South African J Surg 1985;*23*:35–36.
12. Daskalakis E, Bouhoutsos J: Subclavian and axillary vein compression of musculoskeletal origin. Br J Surg 1980;*67*:573–576.
13. Rubio PA, Coan JD, Farrell EM, Berkman NL: Subclavian thrombosis secondary to transvenous pacing wire. South Med J 1980;*73*:1547.
14. Bradof J, Sands MJ Jr, Lakin PC: Symptomatic venous thrombosis of the upper extremity complicating permanent transvenous pacing: Reversal with streptokinase infusion. Am Heart J 1982;*104*:1112–1113.
15. Williams EH, Tyers GFO, Shaffer CW: Symptomatic deep venous thrombosis of the arm associated with permanent transvenous pacing electrodes. Chest 1978;*73*:613–615.
16. Crook BRM, Gishen P, Robinson CR, Oram S: Occlusion of the subclavian vein associated with cephalic vein pacemaker electrodes. Br J Surg 1977;*64*:329–331.
17. Stoney WS, Addlestone RB, Alford WC, Burrus GR, Frist RA, Thomas CS Jr: The incidence of venous thrombosis following long-term transvenous pacing. Ann Thorac Surg 1976;*22*:166–170.
18. McCauley J, Waszkiewicz M, Kovalak JA, Sorkin MI: Bilateral occlusion of the subclavian veins due to chronic indwelling subclavian catheters. Milit Med 1987;*152*(11):571–573.
19. El-Nachef WM, Rashad F, Ricanati ES: Occlusion of the subclavian vein: A complication of indwelling subclavian venous catheters for hemodialysis. Clin Nephrol 1985;*24*:42–46.
20. Bennett WM, Sterwart WK: Subclavian vein thrombosis with single-lumen venous catheters for hemodialysis [Letter]. Clin Nephrol 1986;*25*:54.
21. Currier CB Jr, Widder S, Ali A, Kuusisto E, Sidawy A: Surgical management of subclavian and axillary vein thrombosis in patients with a functioning arteriovenous fistula. Surgery 1986;*100*:25–28.
22. Jain KM, Smejkal R: Use of spiral vein graft to bypass occluded subclavian vein. Case Report. J Cardiovasc Surg 1988;*29*:572–573.
23. Rubenstein M, Creger WP: Successful streptokinase therapy for catheter-induced subclavian vein thrombosis. Arch Intern Med 1980;*140*:1370–1371.
24. Jeejeebhoy KN, Langer B, Tsallas GT, Chu RC, Kuksis A, Anderson GH: Total parenteral nutrition at home: Studies in patients surviving four months to five years. Gastroenterology 1976;*71*:943–953.
25. Horattas MC, Wright DJ, Fenton AH, Evans DM, Oddi MA, Kamienski RW, Shields EF: Changing concepts of deep venous thrombosis of the upper extremity—report of a series and review of the literature. Surgery 1988;*104*:561–567.
26. Smith VC, Hallett JW Jr: Subclavian vein thrombosis during prolonged catheterization for parenteral nutrition: Early management and long-term follow-up. South Med J 1983;*76*:603–606.
27. Hung SSJ: Deep vein thrombosis of the arm associated with malignancy. Cancer 1989;*64*:531–535.
28. Wilson CB, Lambert HE, Scott RD: Subclavian and axillary vein thrombosis following radiotherapy for carcinoma of the breast. Clin Radiol 1987;*38*:95–96.
29. Schreiber DP, Kapp DS: Axillary-subclavian vein thrombosis following combination chemotherapy and radiation therapy in lymphoma. Brief Communication. Int J Radiat Oncol Biol Phys 1986;*12*:391–395.
30. Mason BA: Axillary-subclavian vein occlusion in patients with lung neoplasms. Cancer 1981;*48*:1886–1889.

31. Lokich JJ, Becker B: Subclavian vein thrombosis in patients treated with infusion chemotherapy for advanced malignancy. Cancer 1983;*52*:1586–1589.

32. Surkin MI, Kessler SM, Green RP, Lucente FE: Subclavian vein thrombosis secondary to chronic otitis media. A Case Report. Ann Otol Rhinol Laryngol 1983;*92*:45–48.

33. Nagaratnam N, Fernando DJS, Deen MFO, Kulasegaram V, Ismail MM: Benign obstruction of subclavian and axillary veins possibly due to filariasis. Br J Surg 1976;*63*:379–380.

34. Beal JM, Ed: Subclavian vein thrombosis. Surgical Grand Rounds. Illinois Med J 1975;*5*:444–446.

35. Stricker SJ, Sowers DK, Sowers JR, Sirridge MS: "Effort thrombosis" of the subclavian vein associated with oral contraceptives. Case Report. Ann Emerg Med 1981;*10*:596–599.

36. Sundqvist SB, Hedner U, Kullenberg HKE, Bergentz SE: Deep venous thrombosis of the arm: A study of coagulation and fibrinolysis. Br Med J 1981;*283*:265–267.

37. Lindblad B, Tengborn L, Bergqvist D: Deep vein thrombosis of the axillary-subclavian veins: Epidemiologic data, effects of different types of treatment and late sequele. Eur J Vasc Surg 1988;*2*:161–165.

38. Donayre CE, White GH, Mehringer SM, Wilson SE: Pathogenesis determines late morbidity of axillosubclavian vein thrombosis. Am J Surg 1986;*152*:179–184.

39. Human L: An unusual case of effort thrombosis of the subclavian vein successfully treated by resection and saphenous vein grafting. Vasc Surg 1990;*Jan-Feb*:60–64.

40. Hansen B, Feins RS, Detmer DE: Simple extra-anatomic jugular vein bypass for subclavian vein thrombosis. J Vasc Surg 1985;*2*:921–923.

41. Aziz S, Straehley CJ, Whelan TJ Jr: Effort-related axillosubclavian vein thrombosis: A new theory of pathogenesis and a plea for direct surgical intervention. Am J Surg 1986;*152*:57–61.

42. Rauwerda JA, Bakker FC, van den Broek TAA, Dwars BJ: Spontaneous subclavian vein thrombosis: A successful combined approach of local thrombolytic therapy followed by first-rib resection. Surgery 1988;*103*:477–480.

43. Swenson WM, Rennich D, Capp KA, James EC: Axillary vein thrombosis due to thoracic outlet syndrome. AORN J 1987;*46*:878–886.

44. Kunkel JM, Machleder HI: Treatment of Paget-Schroetter syndrome. Arch Surg 1989;*124*:1153–1158.

45. Demeter SL, Pritchard JS, Piedad OH, Cordasco EM, Taherj S: Upper extremity thrombosis: Etiology and prognosis. Angiology 1982;*11*:743–755.

46. Jones JC, Balkcom IL, Worman RK: Pulmonary embolus after treatment for subclavian-axillary vein thrombosis. Postgrad Med 1987;*82*:244–249.

47. Ameli FM, Minas T, Weiss M, Provan JL: Consequences of "conservative" conventional management of axillary vein thrombosis. Can J Surg 1987;*30*:167–169.

48. Sassu GP, Chisholm CD, Howell JM, Huang E: A rare etiology for pulmonary embolism: Basilic vein thrombosis. J Emerg Med 1990;*8*:45–49.

30

RESULTS OF SURGICAL TREATMENT OF AXILLARY-SUBCLAVIAN VENOUS THROMBOSIS

James A. DeWeese

Thrombosis of the axillary-subclavian veins is rare. It may occur as a result of external compression or as a result of introduction of foreign objects or chemicals into the veins. Obstruction of the veins produces distention of the veins, swelling, reddish-blue discoloration of the skin, and pain. The classical management of the problem has consisted of elevation of the arms and anticoagulation. Early reports of the use of thrombolytic therapy for acute thrombosis have been encouraging. However, following anticoagulation or thrombolytic therapy, persistent or intermittent symptoms may result from continued obstruction of the major veins or positional compression of collateral veins. Surgical treatment in the form of thrombectomy for acute thrombosis, bypasses of obstructed veins, or decompression of the thoracic outlet for prevention of thrombosis or relief of postthrombotic symptoms is also possible. Favorable results have been reported and further evaluations appear warranted.

ANATOMIC CONSIDERATIONS

The superficial veins of the ulnar aspect of the lower arm drain through the median antebrachial and median antecubital veins into the basilic vein, which joins the brachial vein to become the axillary vein. There is also drainage on the radial side of the arm into the cephalic vein, which joins the axillary vein in the deltipectoral groove just lateral to the clavicle. The axillary vein becomes the subclavian vein at the outer border of the first rib and joins the internal jugular vein at the base of the neck to become the innominate vein, which joins the opposite innominate vein to become the superior vena cava.

The subclavian vein passes anterior to the first rib and posterior to the clavicle to enter the costoclavicular space. This space is bounded anteriorly by the clavicle and the underlying subclavius muscle and clavipectoral fascia. Its posterior limits are the anterior scalene muscle and first rib. It is important to remember that the vein lies anterior to the anterior scalene muscle, whereas the subclavian artery and cords of the brachial plexus lie posterior to it.

The costoclavicular space may be narrowed in two positions. The first position is the military position, in which the patient sits with his shoulders back and downward. The clavicle and first rib are approximated much like the blade of a scissors. The second position that narrows the costoclavicular space consists of hyperabduction and external rotation of the arm. With hyperabduction alone and forward extension of the arm the costoclavicular space may be widened, but with hyperabduction of the arm to beyond 90 degrees and external rotation of the bent lower arm the clavicle rotates backward and downward toward the first rib. The site of compression has been variously described as occurring between the clavicle and first rib, the clavicle and anterior scalene muscle, the subclavius muscle and first rib, or the costocoracoid ligament and first rib (1–3).

PATHOGENESIS

There are two distinct types of venous thrombosis of the upper extremity. The first is related to an external compression or trauma to the vein. The second type follows the introduction of foreign materials into the veins.

Primary Thrombosis

Sir James Paget is credited with first describing an upper extremity venous thrombosis in 1875, which he described as "a gouty phlebitis" (4). Von Schroetter in 1884 reported a similar case in a healthy man who was painting at the time the thrombosis occurred. Hughes in 1949, in his excellent review of 320 reported cases of upper extremity venous thrombosis, termed the condition "Paget-Schroetter's syndrome" (5). However, it was also termed "primary thrombosis" by Matas (6), "spontaneous thrombosis" by French (7), "traumatic thrombosis" by Roelsen (8), and "effort thrombosis" by Kleinsasser (9) and others (10,11). Hughes reported that the cause of the thrombosis was effort, anatomic, or trauma in 188 of 320 patients and spontaneous, or in other words unknown, in 110. Only 18 could be attributed to heart failure, infection, polycythemia, or a hypercoagulable state (5). No cases of thrombosis secondary to intravenous foreign material were described (5,12). The activities preceding acute thrombosis of the arm veins included throwing a football or baseball, playing handball or tennis, swimming, chopping wood, painting ceilings, pulling a propellor, rowing a boat, washing walls, starting an outboard, lifting weights, carrying a heavy suitcase, wearing a figure-of-8 splint, falling asleep with the arm over the back of a chair, and hanging with the arm hooked over a ladder rung (5,9–11).

It would appear that the most usual causes of thrombosis are related to external trauma or compression of the veins, as may occur with sudden or repetitive movements or unusual positioning of the arm.

Iatrogenic Thrombosis

In 1967 Coon and Willis reported that six of 60 cases of axillary and subclavian vein thrombosis were related to catheterization of arm veins (13). In 1986 Donayre et al. reported 10 of 41 thromboses to be catheter induced (14). Horattas et al., in 1988, attributed 13 of 33 arm thromboses to catheters (12).

Intimal injury with localized and possibly secondary ascending thrombosis of the arm veins is a recognized complication of the intravenous injection of many chemicals, including hypertonic solutions, potassium chloride, and even antibiotics. The central venous placement of catheters for short-term monitoring or long-term parenteral nutrition or chemotherapy may also present problems. Brismar et al. performed phlebograms on 53 patients before and after prolonged parenteral nutrition. Sleeve thrombi were identified on removal of the catheter in 42 per cent of the patients. The thrombi were occlusive in 8 per cent of the arms (15). Fabri et al. indicated that thrombi have been identified in 7 to 71 per cent of subclavian veins during total parenteral nutrition with polyvinyl catheters. Using radionuclide phlebograms they showed a significant reduction in the incidence of thrombi by adding heparin to the parenteral solution (16). Stoney et al. reviewed reports of subclavian and innominate venous thrombosis documented by phlebograms in patients with permanent pacemakers. Venous thrombosis was documented in 31 percent (63/203) of the patients (17).

SIGNS AND SYMPTOMS

Signs and symptoms of primary or effort thrombosis usually occur within 72 hr of the inciting event and consist of aching pain, heaviness, swelling of the whole arm, bluish-red discoloration, and venous distention. The cord of the thrombosed basilic or axillary vein may be left. Some patients may have had intermittent, less severe symptoms lasting during effort but not persisting (18). Phlegmasia cerulea dolens and venous gangrene may rarely be seen (10). Although it was originally believed that pulmonary embolism was not a threat, Horattas et al. reviewed 218 reported cases of thrombosis and found a 12 per cent incidence of nonfatal pulmonary emboli and a 3 per cent incidence of fatal pulmonary emboli (12).

Iatrogenic venous thrombosis, on the other hand, infrequently causes significant occlusion or symptoms. Torosian et al. reviewed the reported cases of subclavian venous thrombosis following prolonged central venous catheterization studied by phlebographic or radionuclide scans (19). Although thrombi have been identified in 20 to 70 per cent of the patients, only 3 to 5 per cent have been symptomatic. Stoney et al. reviewed 203 reported patients with permanent pacemaker electrodes who have venous thrombosis by phlebogram. Total occlusion was present in 15 per cent but only 5 per cent had arm edema (17).

DIAGNOSIS

Venous pressures are elevated acutely following thrombotic occlusion of the vein (11). Doppler ultrasound studies and color Doppler sonographic imaging may be useful, but visualization of the subclavian vein may be hampered by the clavicle (20–22). Phlebography provides the most definitive method for the diagnosis and evaluation of venous forms of treatment. It is important that the injection be made into the medial antecubital vein and not the cephalic vein for best visualization of the basilic and axillary veins (23,24).

TREATMENT

Nonoperative Treatment

The accepted nonoperative management of axillary-subclavian vein thrombosis for many years has been elevation and anticoagulation. Early and late morbidity was decreased in patients treated with anticoagulants in comparative studies of small groups of patients (11,13,25). Even with anticoagulation complete recovery is uncommon in patients with primary or effort thrombosis. Residual symptoms have been reported in 40 to 85 per cent of patients (11,26,27). Phlebograms of symptomatic patients frequently demonstrate large first rib collaterals between the axillary vein and the internal jugular vein in the neutral position of the arm that are obstructed during elevation of the arm or in the military position, either of which causes narrowing of the costoclavicular space (10,11,21,28). Similar problems have not been reported following iatrogenic thrombosis. Significant residual symptoms occurred in only two of 23 patients with iatrogenic thrombosis, as opposed to eight of 17 patients with thrombosis secondary to external compression reported by Donayre et al. (14).

Thrombolytic therapy is being used with increasing frequency for the initial treatment of axillary-subclavian thrombosis. When streptokinase is used it is used intravenously with a loading dose of 250,000 units followed by 10,000 units/hr continuously for 2 to 3 days; this has been successful in most reported cases (29,30). Streptokinase has also been infused into the thrombus itself, with mixed results (31–34). The best results were obtained when longer periods of 5 to 8 days of infusion were used (32). Others have reported better results with urokinase administered at doses of 1000 units/kg/hr or 1000 units/min directly into the thrombus (33,34). Good results are also seen in the treatment of some but not all patients with iatrogenic thrombosis (31,33). Recurrences are common following initially successful lysis (35).

Surgical Treatment

There has been increasing agreement that effort and even "spontaneous" axillary-subclavian venous thrombosis occurs as a result of repeated external compression of the subclavian veins by structures lining the costoclavicular space. The compression of the subclavian vein and resulting venous hypertension may occur intermittently prior to thrombosis. In addition, positional compression of the collateral veins around the obstructed subclavian vein may cause intermittent venous hypertension. This has resulted in numerous reports of operations performed that remove portions of the structures that line this space, including the first rib, clavicle, subclavius muscle, and anterior scalene muscle. These operations have been performed to prevent thrombosis, to prevent rethrombosis following thrombectomy or thrombolytic therapy, or to prevent recurrent symptoms following venous thrombosis. Congenital or postthrombotic stenosis has been treated by balloon angioplasty or excision of intraluminal residuals of the thrombus and patch grafting. Obstructed veins have been replaced or bypassed.

Operations for Intermittent Venous Obstruction

There are patients who will develop symptoms of subclavian vein obstruction—increases of brachial venous pressures and phlebographic evidence of occlusion of the vein—only when the arm is abducted and externally rotated or pulled backward and downward, as in the military position (3,18). Anterior scalenotomy and/or resection of the subclavius muscle has not routinely relieved the venous compression (3,18,36,37). First rib resection has more successfully relieved the symptoms (18,28,38–40). Resection of the medial half of the clavicle has also been successful (18).

Operation for Acute Thrombosis

DeWeese et al., in 1979, were able to find 22 reported instances of thrombectomy for acute axillary-subclavian venous thrombosis (41), including that first described by Bazy in 1926 (42). Of those reported in which details were available, almost all followed stressful use of the arm. The approach to the thrombosed segments of the veins is not clearly described, but at least four operations, including those reported by Dale (43) and Drapanas and Curran (44) and later Inahara (45), were performed through the axillary vein, with removal of thrombus from the subclavian vein with a Fogerty catheter or suction catheter (41). Cure or improvement was described in almost all cases. Four of five postoperative phlebograms were described as showing patency without collaterals (41).

We also described our experiences with an additional six thrombectomies (21,41). All were approached through a supraclavicular incision. Only three of the patients described stressful use of the arm. Two patients were "painting ceilings" and one patient was "twisting a large dowel" prior to onset of symptoms. Nonetheless, perivenous adhesions and thickening and narrowing of subclavian veins near their junction with the internal jugular veins, consistent with trauma, were seen in all six explorations. The first and second operations were performed without resection of the clavicle. The second patient was found to have an old organized thrombus lining the wall of the vein, with an intraluminal red thrombus. The preoperative phlebogram had demonstrated a large supraclavicular collateral vein around the area of occlusion. Postoperatively the patient continued to be symptomatic. He was found to have elevated venous pressures and a phlebographic demonstration of occlusion of the large collateral vein with abduction of his arm or when in the military position (Fig. 30–1). The remaining four thrombectomies were therefore performed following extraperiosteal resection of the medial one half of the clavicle (Fig. 30–2). This was done to provide easier exposure of the proximal subclavian vein and to prevent recurrent symptoms should the vein rethrombose. The second patient who required late claviculectomy has remained asymptomatic. He was demonstrated to have patency of the axillary vein and visualization of the "first rib collateral vein" by color Doppler studies in both the relaxed and stress positioning of his arm 27 years following his operation (21). Three of the five successful thrombectomies were demonstrated to be patent by phlebography 14 months, 6 months, and 3 months postoperatively (Fig. 30–3). These patients had no recurrence of thrombosis and had only minor complaints of periodic aching of the shoulder with excessive use of the arm. At follow-up 14, 22, and 24 years following operation, color Doppler studies on the three patients demonstrated patent axillary and subclavian veins without collaterals (21).

The remaining two of the five successful thrombectomies were found to have normal venous pressures equal to those in the opposite arm 12 and 16 months postoperatively and remained asymptomatic when last seen 48 and 52 months

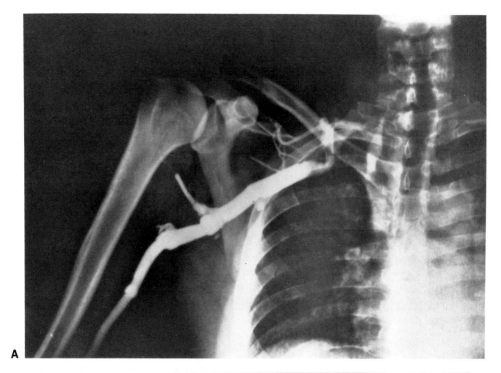

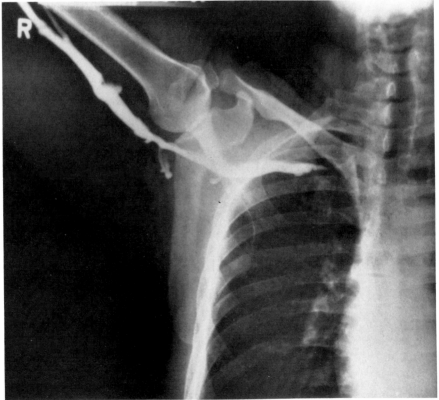

Figure 30–1. See legend on opposite page.

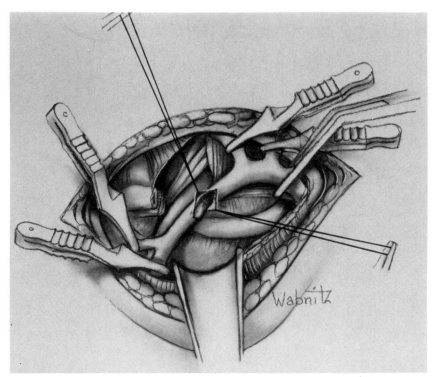

Figure 30–2. Surgical technique for venous thrombectomy. An incision is made over the medial half of the clavicle and it is resected. The jugular, axillary, and innominate veins are controlled. A longitudinal venotomy is made over the most proximal extent of the palpable thrombus. Thrombi are removed with instruments or a Fogarty thrombectomy balloon catheter. The venotomy is then closed with fine sutures. (From DeWeese JA: Management of subclavian venous obstruction. *In* Bergan JJ, Yao JST, eds: Current Problems in Surgery. Orlando, FL, Grune & Stratton, 1985;365–382.)

following operation (41). Aziz et al. had a similar good experience with medial claviculectomy and thrombectomy for acute thrombosis of 1 and 7 days' duration. These two patients were asymptomatic 6 years and 20 years following operation (46). Campbell et al. also performed claviculectomy and thrombectomy with a vein patency in one patient with acute thrombosis secondary to a catheter, but, as they stated, "the patient probably also would have done well without operation" (20). Roos, in 1971, reported "encouraging results" using a transaxillary approach accompanied by a resection of the first rib in two patients who had thrombectomy of the subclavian vein. He also emphasized the importance of decompression of the costoclavicular space by either first rib resection or claviculectomy for prevention of recurrence (40). Urschel and Razzuk also considered thrombectomy with transaxillary first rib resection to be a useful procedure in four patients (38). It must be concluded that thrombectomy within the first 7 days

←——

Figure 30–1. Phlebograms of patient with intermittent postthrombotic venous obstruction of the upper extremity. *A*, Phlebogram with the arm at the side and with a venous pressure of 21 cm saline. Large first rib bypass collaterals circumvent the obstructed subclavian vein. *B*, Phlebogram with the arm abducted and a venous pressure of 75 cm saline. The large collateral vein is occluded in the costoclavicular space. (From Adams JT, McEvoy RK, DeWeese JA: Primary deep venous thrombosis of upper extremity. Arch Surg 1965;*91*:39. Copyright 1965, American Medical Association.)

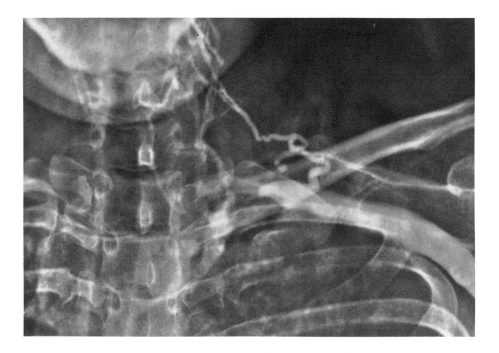

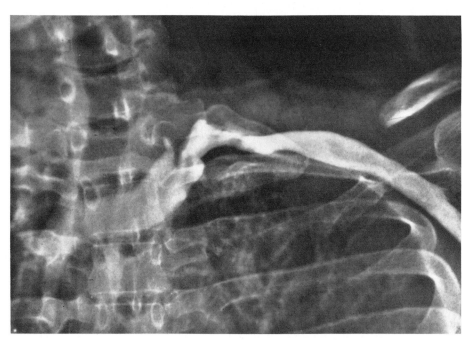

Figure 30–3.   Phlebograms before and after subclavian venous thrombectomy. *A*, Preoperative phlebogram shows a localized thrombosis of the left subclavian vein with small first rib collaterals. *B*, A phlebogram taken 6 months after thrombectomy and excision of the medial half of the left clavicle showing a patent vein without collaterals. (From DeWeese JA, Adams JT, Gaiser DL: Subclavian venous thrombectomy. Circulation 1970;*41-42*(suppl II):II-159, by permission of the American Heart Association, Inc.)

of onset of primary thrombosis can provide rapid relief of symptoms and long-term patency and should still be considered in young otherwise healthy individuals.

Operations for Postthrombotic Symptoms

Symptoms of recurrent swelling and pain are common following acute axillary-subclavian thrombosis. This may be 1) secondary to residual stenotic lesions, 2) continued intermittent compression of recanalized veins to the costoclavicular space, or 3) occlusions with large collaterals that may be intermittently compressed in the costoclavicular space (Fig. 30–1). Operations described for treatment include local removal of postthrombotic lesions with patch grafting of the vein, balloon angioplasty, removal of the first rib or clavicle, and various types of venous reconstructions.

THROMBOENDOPHLEBECTOMY AND PATCH GRAFTING.   Aziz et al. reported exploration of occluded subclavian veins in two patients 23 days and 90 days following acute thrombosis. They removed organized thrombus and/or fibrous intimal stenosis, which they called "endovenectomy," and then applied a venous patch graft (46). The medial half of the clavicle was also excised. Postoperative phlebograms demonstrated patent veins, and the patients were asymptomatic 6 months later. Green reported a similar experience in one patient with patency demonstrated by color Doppler 18 months postoperatively (personal communication). Mehigan reported similar cases successfully managed with "removal of internal webs" from the subclavian vein after transaxiallary first rib resection (47). Beaujain had a similar good experience with late treatment of two patients with residual stenotic lesions, but resected the first rib through an anterior trap door approach (personal communication, 1977). Campbell et al. reported on three patients with localized obstruction who had intraluminal resection of postthrombotic material and patch grafting following claviculectomy. None remained patent but only one patient had significant symptoms (20).

BALLOON ANGIOPLASTY.   Balloon angioplasty has also been used for treatment of the stenotic lesions seen after effort or iatrogenic thrombosis. It has not been as successful when used early after thrombosis as it has been in later cases (33,34).

FIRST RIB RESECTION.   Strange-Vognsen et al. performed phlebograms in the neutral supine position with the arm at the side and also with the arm abducted 90 degrees and rotated outward at the shoulder in 21 patients following successful lytic therapy (35). Phlebographic signs of venous compression in the costoclavicular space were identified in the normal and or exaggerated position in 12 patients. Two of these 12 patients suffered rethrombosis within a short period of time before first rib resection could be performed. None of the 10 other patients who had first rib resection suffered rethrombosis during a 1- to 6-year follow-up period (35). Rauwerda et al. reported on five patients who had successful thrombolysis of the subclavian vein and underwent first rib resection 3 to 12 weeks later. The patients remained asymptomatic without rethrombosis 6 to 37 months later (32). Druy et al. performed first rib resection on two patients following successful thrombolytic therapy. One remained asymptomatic 2 years later but the other patient suffered recurrence while playing tennis 4 months following operation (33). Landercasper et al. also performed first rib resection following successful thrombolytic therapy in two patients who remained asymptomatic 17 and

30 months later (30). Taylor et al. reported two similar successful cases (29). There are patients who are treated only with anticoagulants who also will recanalize their axillosubclavian veins, but continue to have intermittent symptomatic compression of the vein, who may also be relieved by first rib resection (34).

In addition to preventing positional compression and trauma to the subclavian vein, first rib resection also prevents compression of the large first rib collateral vein around subclavian veins that remain occluded following thrombosis (24). Patients may be selected for operation by performing venous pressure studies and phlebograms with the arms in neutral position and in an exaggerated military position (10). Glass described four patients who had "stress" thrombosis of the axillary-subclavian vein with large collateral veins whose symptoms were relieved by first rib resection (28). Roos (40), Urschel and Razzuk (38) and Kunkel and Machleder (34) also reported success with relief of postthrombotic symptoms that can be attributed to the prevention of compression of the subclavian vein by the removal of the first rib. It must be understood that much of the long-term success of the thrombectomies performed by Roos, Urschel, and others may be the result of the decompression of the costoclavicular space by resection of the first rib. The same can be said for the success of Mehigan (47) and Aziz et al. (46) in treating postthrombotic subclavian vein stenosis with venoplasty and first rib resection.

CLAVICULECTOMY.   Removal of the medial half or two thirds of the clavicle may also prevent compression of the subclavian vein or postthrombotic collaterals but has not been as popular as first rib resection. It is presumed that resection of the clavicle causes cosmetic deformity and disability, which has not been true in our experience. Medial claviculectomy successfully relieved the symptoms of two patients with intermittent subclavian vein obstruction, as reported by Adams et al. (18). Kunkel and Machleder reported on a patient who remained symptomatic following a first rib resection for postthrombotic discomfort who was relieved by a medial clavicular resection (34). A medial claviculectomy was performed by ourselves on a patient with a large postthrombotic first rib collateral vein, with immediate relief of symptoms; this patient is still asymptomatic 27 years later (10,21). The long-term successes of Aziz et al. (46), Campbell et al. (20), and ourselves (21) in performing venous thrombectomy acutely and of Aziz et al. (46), Mehigan (47), and Green (personal communication) in performing venoplasty may well attest to the ability of claviculectomy to adequately decompress the costoclavicular space and either prevent rethrombosis or relieve any compression of collateral veins should rethrombosis occur.

VENOUS RECONSTRUCTION.   If the axillary-subclavian veins remain obstructed following acute thrombosis, venous hypertension and swelling may persist unless adequate collaterals develop. In such patients a successful replacement or bypass of the obstructed vein should be of benefit. There are a few reports of such procedures. Witte and Smith bypassed an obstructed subclavian vein by dividing the ipsilateral internal jugular vein high in the neck and anastomosing it end to end to the distal subclavian vein (48) (Fig. 30–4). The venous pressure fell from 35 to 10 cm H_2O, and patency of the bypass was confirmed by phlebography 9 months later. The medial half of the clavicle was also removed. Jacobson and Haimov performed a similar operation but did not resect the clavicle and tunneled the jugular vein beneath the clavicle to perform an end-to-side anastomosis to the axillary vein (49). Patency was established by phlebography 6 months following

Figure   30–4. Diagrammatic representation of axillojugular venous bypass. The internal jugular vein has been mobilized, ligated high in the neck, and divided. It is then anastomosed to the patent axillary or subclavian vein distal to the venous obstruction. A claviculectomy may also be performed. (From DeWeese JA: Management of subclavian venous obstruction. *In* Bergan JJ, Yao JST, eds: Current Problems in Surgery. Orlando, FL, Grune & Stratten, 1985;365–382.)

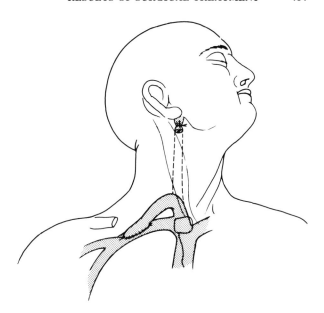

operation. Blebea et al. performed three jugulosubclavian bypasses following resection of the medial clavicle, with patency demonstrated by phlebography and color Doppler studies 8, 1.2, and 11.5 months later (21). Jacobson and Haimov also bypassed a postthrombotic occluded axillosubclavian vein by dividing the ipsilateral internal jugular vein high in the neck and anastomosing it to the cephalic vein (49). An arteriovenous fistula was constructed between the cephalic vein and the radial artery at the wrist level that was closed 3 weeks after the operation. A phlebogram performed 6 months later showed patency of the reconstruction.

Inahara used an autogenous saphenous vein to bypass an obstructed subclavian vein with end-to-side anastomosis to the axillary and internal jugular vein following resection of the medial clavicle. A phlebogram established patency 4 months after operation (45). Rabinowitz and Goldfarb performed a similar procedure but used a radial artery–to–cephalic vein fistula for 3 weeks after operation. Although not mentioned in their paper, the postoperative phlebogram demonstrating patency of a small vein graft also suggests that the clavicle had been removed (50). Hashmonai et al. performed a crossover bypass of an obstructed axillosubclavian vein by mobilizing the contralateral cephalic vein and tunneling it to the ipsilateral shoulder vein, performing an end-to-side anastomosis between the cephalic veins (51). An arteriovenous fistula was used for 6 weeks, and later phlebograms confirmed venous patency.

Bypass operations have been effective in providing additional collateral flow and have remained patent. However since most patients have also had claviculectomy as well as bypass, one must question if they would have had equal improvement with claviculectomy alone.

REFERENCES

1. Falconer MA, Weddell GL: Costoclavicular compression of subclavian artery and vein. Lancet 1943;2:539.
2. Horwitz O, Zinsser HF Jr: Subclavian vein obstruction. Report of a case studied by venography and relieved by surgery. JAMA 1953;151:997–999.

432   DeWeese

3. McCleery RS, Kesterson JE, Kirtley JA, Love RB: Subclavius and anterior scalene muscle compression as a cause of intermittent obstruction of subclavian vein by the first rib and clavicle, with special reference to the prominence of chest veins as a sign of collateral circulation. Am Heart J 1940;*19*:292.
4. Paget J: Clinical Lectures and Essays. London, Longmans, Green & Co, 1875.
5. Hughes ESR: Venous obstruction in the upper extremity (Paget-Schroetter's syndrome): A review of 320 cases. Int Abstr Surg 1949;*88*:89–123.
6. Matas R: So-called primary thrombosis of axillary vein caused by strain: Report of case, diagnosis, pathology, and treatment. Am J Surg 1934;*24*:642–666.
7. French GE: Spontaneous thrombosis of axillary vein. Br Med J 1944;*2*:271.
8. Roelsen E: So-called traumatic thrombosis of axillary and subclavian veins. Acta Med Scand 1939;*98*:589–622.
9. Kleinsasser LJ: "Effort" thrombosis of the axillary and subclavian veins. Arch Surg 1974;*59*:258–274.
10. Adams JT, McEvoy RK, DeWeese JA: Primary deep venous thrombosis of upper extremity. Arch Surg 1965;*91*:29–42.
11. Adams JT, DeWeese JA: "Effort" thrombosis of the axillary and subclavian veins. J Trauma 1971;*11*:923–929.
12. Horattas MC, Wright DJ, Fenton AH, Evans DM, Oddi MA, Kamienski RW, Shields EF: Changing concepts of deep venous thrombosis of the upper extremity—report of a series and review of the literature. Surgery 1988;*104*:561–568.
13. Coon WW, Willis PW III: Thrombosis of axillary and subclavian veins. Arch Surg 1967;*94*:657–663.
14. Donayre CE, White GH, Mehringer SM, Wilson SE: Pathogenesis determines late morbidity of axillosubclavian vein thrombosis. Am J Surg 1986;*152*:179–184.
15. Brismar B, Hardstedt C, Jacobson S: Diagnosis of thrombosis by catheter phlebography after prolonged central venous catheterization. Ann Surg 1981;*194*:779–783.
16. Fabri PJ, Mirtallo JM, Ruberg RL, Kudsk KA, Denning DA, Ellison EC, Schaffer P: Incidence and prevention of thrombosis of the subclavian vein during total parenteral nutrition. Surg Gynecol Obstet 1982;*155*:238–240.
17. Stoney WS, Addlestone RB, Alford WC Jr, Burrus GR, Frist RA, Thomas CS Jr: The incidence of venous thrombosis following long-term transvenous pacing. Ann Thorac Surg 1976;*22*:166–170.
18. Adams JT, DeWeese JA, Mahoney EB, Rob CG: Intermittent subclavian vein obstruction. Surgery 1968;*63*:147–165.
19. Torosian MH, Meranze S, McLean G, Mullen JL: Central venous access with occlusive superior central venous thrombosis. Ann Surg 1986;*203*:30–33.
20. Campbell CB, Chandler JG, Tegtmeyer CJ, Bernstein EF: Axillary, subclavian, and brachiocephalic vein obstruction. Surgery 1977;*82*:816–826.
21. Blebea J, DeWeese JA, Ouriel K, Ricotta JJ, Green RM: Long-term results of surgical therapy for axillary subclavian vein thrombosis. (in press)
22. Knudson GJ, Wiedmeyer DA, Erickson SJ, et al: Color Doppler sonographic imaging in the assessment of upper extremity deep venous thrombosis. AJR 1990;*154*:399–403.
23. DeWeese JA, Rogoff SM: Phlebography. *In* Schobinger RA, Ruzick FF Jr, eds: Vascular Roentgenology. New York, MacMillan, 1964;482–485.
24. DeWeese JA: Phlebography. *In* Dudley H, Carter D, Russell RCG, eds: Vascular Surgery. London, Butterworth & Co, Ltd, 1985;263–270.
25. Gloviczki P, Kasmier FJ, Hollier LH: Axillary-subclavian venous occlusion: The morbidity of a nonlethal disease. J Vasc Surg 1986;*4*:333–337.
26. Crowell LL: Effort thrombosis of the subclavian and axillary veins: Review of the literature and case report with two year follow-up and venography. Ann Intern Med 1960;*52*:1337–1343.
27. Tilney NL, Griffiths HJG, Edwards EA: Natural history of major venous thrombosis of the upper extremity. Arch Surg 1970;*101*:792–796.
28. Glass BA: The relationship of axillary venous thrombosis to the thoracic outlet compression syndrome. Ann Thorac Surg 1975;*19*:613.
29. Taylor LM Jr, McAllister WR, Dennis DL, Porter JM: Thrombolytic therapy followed by first rib resection for spontaneous ("effort") subclavian vein thrombosis. Am J Surg 1985;*149*:644–647.
30. Landercasper J, Gall W, Fischer M, Boyd WC, Dahlberg PJ, Kisken WA, Boland T: Thrombolytic therapy of axillary-subclavian venous thrombosis. Arch Surg 1987;*122*:1072–1075.
31. Steed DL, Teodori MF, Peitzman AB, McAuley CE, Kapoor WN, Webster MW: Streptokinase in the treatment of subclavian vein thrombosis. J Vasc Surg 1986;*4*:28–32.
32. Rauwerda JA, Bakker FC, van den Broek TAA, Dwars BJ: Spontaneous subclavian vein thrombosis: a successful combined approach of local thrombolytic therapy followed by first-rib resection. Surgery 1988;*103*:477–480.

33. Druy EM, Trout HH III, Giordano JM, Hix WR: Lytic therapy in the treatment of axillary and subclavian vein thrombosis. J Vasc Surg 1985;*2*:821–827.
34. Kunkel JM, Machleder HI: Treatment of Paget-Schroetter syndrome. Arch Surg 1989;*125*:1153–1158.
35. Strange-Vognsen HH, Hauch O, Andersen J, Struckmann J: Resection of the first rib following deep arm vein thrombolysis in patients with thoracic outlet syndrome. J Cardiovasc Surg 1989;*30*:430–433.
36. McCleery RS, Kesterson JE, Kirtley JA, et al: Subclavius and anterior scalene muscle compression as a cause of intermittent obstruction of the subclavian vein. Ann Surg 1951;*133*:588–602.
37. McLaughlin CW Jr, Popma AM: Intermittent obstruction of the subclavian vein. JAMA 1939;*113*:1960.
38. Urschel HC Jr, Razzuk MA: Letter. N Engl J Med 1972;*287*:567.
39. Schubart PJ, Haeberlin JR, Porter JM: Intermittent subclavian venous obstruction: Utility of venous pressure gradients. Surgery 1986;*99*:365–368.
40. Roos DB: Experience with first rib resection for thoracic outlet syndrome. Ann Surg 1971;*173*:429–442.
41. DeWeese JA, Adams JT, Gaiser DL: Subclavian venous thrombectomy. Circulation 1970;*41-42*(suppl II):II-158–II-164.
42. Bazy L: Thrombose de la veine axillaire droit: Bull Soc Chir Paris, 1926;*52*:529.
43. Dale WA: Discussion. *In* DeWeese JA, Adams JT, Gaiser DL: Subclavian venous thrombectomy. Circulation 1970;*41-42*(suppl II):II-158–II-163.
44. Drapanas T, Curran WL: Thrombectomy in the treatment of "effort" thrombosis of the axillary and subclavian veins. J Trauma 1966;*6*:107–119.
45. Inahara T: Surgical treatment of "effort" thrombosis of the axillary and subclavian veins. Am Surg 1968;*34*:470–483.
46. Aziz S, Straehley CJ, Whelan TJ: Effort-related axillosubclavian vein thrombosis. Am J Surg 1986;*152*:57–61.
47. Mehigan JT: Discussion. Aziz S, Straehley CJ, Whelan TJ: Effort-related axillosubclavian vein thrombosis. Am J Surg 1986;*152*:60.
48. Witte CL, Smith CA: Single anastomosis vein bypass for subclavian vein obstruction. Arch Surg 1966;*93*:664–666.
49. Jacobson JSH, Haimov M: Venous revascularization of the arm: Report of three cases. Surgery 1977;*81*:599–604.
50. Rabinowitz R, Goldfarb D: Surgical treatment of axillosubclavian venous thrombosis: A Case Report. Surgery 1971;*70*:703–706.
51. Hashmonai M, Schramek A, Farbstein J: Cephalic vein cross-over bypass for subclavian vein thrombosis: A Case Report. Surgery 1976;*80*:563–564.

31

THROMBOLYTIC THERAPY AND THORACIC OUTLET DECOMPRESSION IN SUBCLAVIAN-AXILLARY VENOUS THROMBOSIS

Herbert I. Machleder

In 1949, Hughes analyzed 320 cases of spontaneous upper extremity venous thrombosis collected from the medical literature and recognized the first two descriptions by naming the entity the "Paget-Schroetter syndrome" (1). Over the course of subsequent investigations it has become evident that, in contrast to the apparent spontaneous nature of the event, there is an underlying chronic venous compressive anomaly at the thoracic outlet (2).

Despite increasing recognition of this syndrome and innovative approaches to management, there have been areas of disagreement with regard to optimal therapy (3–5). The 167 reports in Hughes' literature review averaged two patients per paper, with no series containing more than 10 patients. This paucity of concentrated experience, particularly in view of major improvements in pharmacologic, interventional radiologic, and surgical techniques, inhibited the development of a comprehensive and effective therapeutic approach.

In 1985 a clinical management strategy based on contemporary concepts of pathophysiology and a multidisciplinary approach to therapy was initiated at the UCLA Medical Center. Flexibility was incorporated in the clinical algorithm, to accommodate the stage of illness at which the patient was referred as well as the effects of antecedent treatment (Fig. 31–1). The results of this therapeutic approach were reported in 1989 (6) and follow-up information was reported in 1990 (7).

PATIENT CHARACTERISTICS

From 1985 to 1990, 33 patients with classical Paget-Schroetter syndrome were treated according to our clinical algorithm at the UCLA Medical Center (five additional patients were in various stages of treatment). Twenty men and 13 women, who otherwise were in excellent general health, had spontaneous or ef-

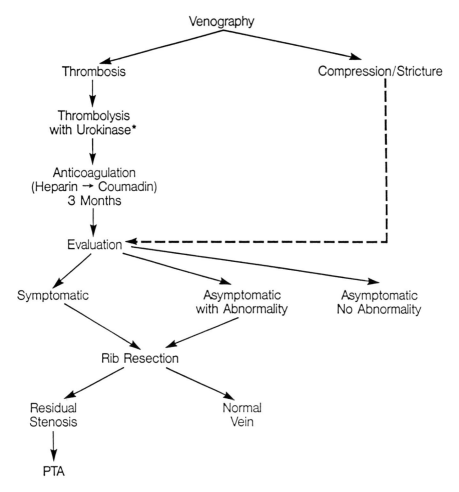

Figure 31–1. Clinical algorithm for management of suspected thrombosis of the axillosubclavian vein. *PTA*, percutaneous transluminal balloon angioplasty.

fort-related upper extremity axillary-subclavian venous thrombosis unrelated to intercurrent illness or iatrogenic manipulation. Only two patients, a fire captain and an elite college athlete, had an episode of trauma even remotely connected with the thrombotic event (8).

Ages of the men ranged from 15 to 41 years, with a mean of 23 years and a median of 20 years. Women were older as a group ($p<.0001$), with ages ranging from 23 to 51 years, with a mean of 39 and a median of 43 years. Thirty patients were right-hand dominant, with the initial episode of thrombosis occurring in the right arm in 24 patients (14 males and 10 females) and in the left arm in nine patients (six males and three females). Three patients had a prior history of axillosubclavian vein occlusion in the contralateral extremity (two males and one female).

Fifteen patients were tradesmen engaged in occupations involving upper ex-

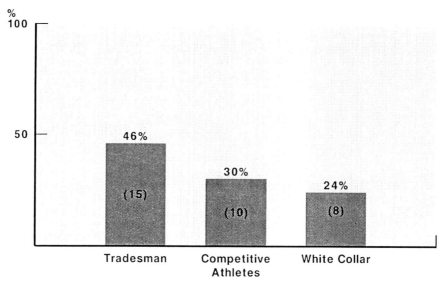

Figure 31–2. Vocation or avocation of study patients.

tremity labor. Eight were so-called white collar workers or the equivalent and 10 were engaged in competitive athletics (Fig. 31–2). Twenty-five patients (76 per cent) had been engaged in competitive sports or manual labor, with the thrombotic event following strenuous effort [20 males (100 per cent of the men), and four females (31 per cent of the women)]. Nine patients were engaged in relatively sedentary activity, with no recognizable precipitating event (all females) (Fig. 31–3).

One male patient had the fist episode of spontaneous thrombosis in the right arm while working as a framer on a construction project. Bilateral venograms revealed a contralateral venous deformity at the thoracic outlet that we have come

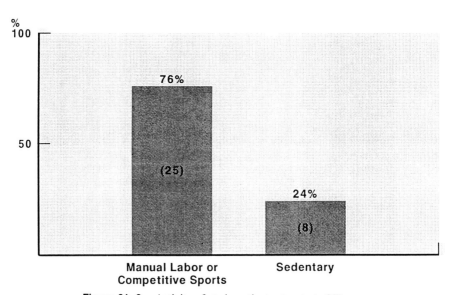

Figure 31–3. Activity of study patients at outset of illness.

to recognize as a precursor to the thrombotic event. One year later spontaneous thrombosis occurred in the contralateral axillosubclavian vein when the patient was working as a cashier in a record store. A second man had contralateral axillosubclavian vein thrombosis 18 months after the first episode under identical circumstances during a camping trip at the same campsite. A female patient had two episodes separated by 17 years.

When seen for consultation, all of these patients were disabled for the performance of their usual occupations. In seven the disability was considered to be work-related by a state worker's compensation board.

LABORATORY EVALUATION

All patients should have venography of the affected upper extremity to confirm the diagnosis. Thirty patients in our series (91 per cent) had complete thrombotic obstruction and three had evidence of external compression or stricture without evidence of residual thrombus (two males and one female). This characteristic of high-grade stenosis with probable intermittent occlusion was suspected in 14 of Hughes' collected cases (in which exploration of the vein failed to reveal any thrombus) (1). This phenomenon was analyzed later in more detail by McCleery et al. (9).

After we encountered three patients with separate thrombotic events involving both upper extremities, bilateral upper extremity venography was included in the patient evaluation. In the 19 patients so studied, abnormalities were found in the contralateral vein in 13 (65 per cent). This included 11 of 13 males studied (85 per cent) and two of the six females studied (33 per cent).The contralateral vein was found to be thrombosed in three, normal in six, and compressed at the thoracic outlet in 10 (Fig. 31–4). The occurrence of bilateral abnormalities corroborates the findings in other reports of Paget-Schroetter syndrome (10).

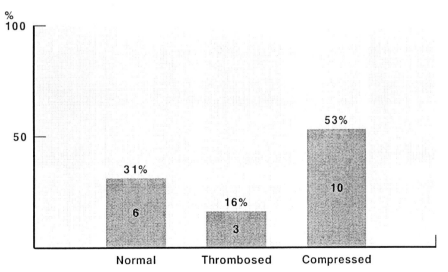

*19 Patients Studied

Figure 31–4.   Results of venography in contralateral vein in 19 study patients.

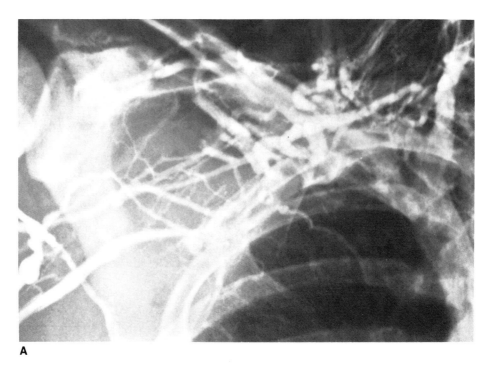

A

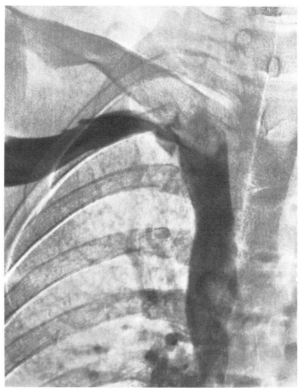

Figure 31–5. *A*, Extensive spontaneous thrombotic occlusion of right axillosubclavian vein seen on basilic venogram in a young male athlete. *B*, Venogram after successful local thrombolytic therapy with urokinase, revealing the typical compressive anomaly at the thoracic outlet.

B

To evaluate symptoms of brachial plexus compression at the thoracic outlet, somatosensory-evoked potentials were studied in 20 patients according to a previously described protocol (11). N9 brachial plexus potentials were measured for median and ulnar nerves in both the neutral and stress positions. These tests were found to be abnormal on the affected side in nine patients [six males (55 per cent of those studied) and three females (33 per cent of those studied)] and were normal in five males and six females.

TREATMENT

The algorithm for management that we have followed includes verification of the diagnosis by venography followed by local thrombolytic therapy and anticoagulation for 3 months (Fig. 31–1). After that time patients with stable occlusion of the axillosubclavian vein are evaluated for residual symptoms. For those patients with significant residual disability, thoracic outlet decompression via transaxillary first rib resection is recommended. Patients with patent but compressed axillosubclavian veins are likewise treated with first rib resection (Fig. 31–5). Following that procedure, percutaneous transluminal balloon angioplasty (PTA) was utilized to correct residual venous stenosis or stricture when this was demonstrated on follow-up venogram.

Local Thrombolytic Therapy

In recent years the superiority of local thrombolytic therapy over systemic infusion of fibrinolytic agents has been demonstrated, particularly for the treatment of axillosubclavian vein thrombosis (12,13). Venography should be performed via the basilic vein of the affected extremity. A separate retrograde innominate or superior vena caval injection from a transfemoral approach can be utilized in selected cases to obtain better visualization of the central veins.

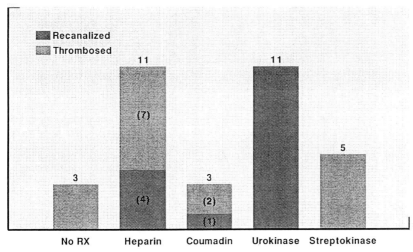

Figure 31–6. Results in patients given no treatment or definitive anticoagulation or thrombolytic therapy.

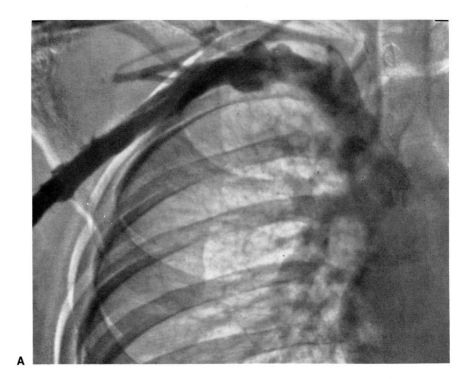

A

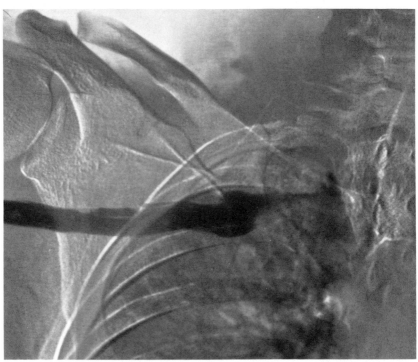

B

Figure 31–7. *A,* Venogram 3 months after successful thrombolytic and anticoagulation therapy in a 28-year-old man with spontaneous axillosubclavian vein thrombosis after a basketball game (arm in neutral position). *B,* A second contrast injection, with arm in the outstretched position, showing a compressive abnormality of the vein at the thoracic outlet. (We believe this to be the predisposing lesion to episodes of spontaneous effort-related thrombosis). *C,* Venogram after transaxillary first rib resection and removal of subclavius tendon. *D,* Second contrast injection, with arm in the outstretched position. Note correction of positionally related compressive abnormality seen in *B* (follow-up venography in 6 months showed a normal vein in both neutral and stressed positions).

440

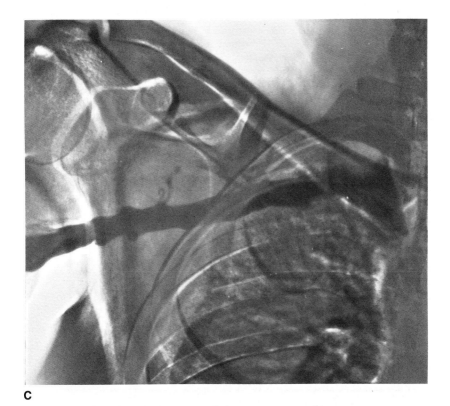

C

D

Figure 31-7. (*continued*)

When thrombus is visualized in the brachial, axillary, or subclavian veins, a small catheter is positioned in the clot via the percutaneous basilic vein approach. An attempt is made to traverse the clot with either a guidewire or a catheter to establish a channel prior to infusion. An earlier therapeutic regimen utilized urokinase in a dose range of 20,000 to 40,000 units/hr (14). Later in our experience optimal therapy was considered to include traversing the thrombus with a guidewire and then infusing a loading dose of 250,00 units urokinase into the clot over 1 hr (4000 units/min). Infusion at this rate can be continued for an additional hour and then changed for 1000 units/min for up to 24 hr (15). Systemic heparinization sufficient to maintain the partial thromboplastin time at 1.5 times control value was used if there was any evidence of thrombus formation in the segment of vein traversed by the catheter or if a prolonged thrombolytic infusion was anticipated. After discontinuation of the fibrinolytic agent, full heparinization was maintained until anticoagulation with warfarin to a prothrombin time of 1.5 to 2 times control values was established. Warfarin anticoagulation was continued for 3 months. Eleven of our patients treated initially with local high-dose urokinase had successful clot dissolution and recanalization (Fig. 31–6).

Eleven patients were treated solely with heparin followed by warfarin anticoagulation. Four of these patients had evidence of recanalization on follow-up venograms. Of three patients treated with warfarin alone, one showed evidence of recanalization. Three patients who were referred for protracted disabling symptoms had no specific thrombolytic or anticoagulant therapy as primary treatment (Fig. 31–6). Following initial treatment, 22 patients were maintained an average of 17 weeks on warfarin anticoagulation. This regimen was planned to allow resolution of the thrombophlebitic process prior to a decision regarding definitive treatment of the underlying abnormality.

We found it particularly noteworthy that three patients had successful surgical thrombectomy (at a referring hospital) as part of their initial treatment, and all experienced rethrombosis of the vein in the early postoperative period, as verified by follow-up venography. Upon completion of thrombolytic therapy and visualization of the underlying compressive lesion, four patients had percutaneous transluminal balloon venoplasty as part of their initial therapy. These procedures, performed at the referring hospitals without prior surgical decompression, resulted in the thrombotic reocclusion of the previously patent but stenotic axillosubclavian vein in all cases. The futility of this approach as a definitive procedure has been documented by others (16).

At the conclusion of anticoagulation therapy, patients who had failed attempts at recanalization of the vein but had a stable nonprogressing venous thrombus were advised to resume normal activity, with the intention of demonstrating the presence or absence of residual symptoms. Patients with continued disability restricting them from their usual occupation or avocation were offered the option for surgical decompression of the thoracic outlet. The rationale for this therapy, in patients with irremediable thrombosis, was based in part on venographic evidence demonstrating compression of the collateral veins at the thoracic outlet when the arm was placed in the elevated position. Additionally, it was evident that the frequent concomitant positionally augmented arterial and brachial plexus compression contributed significantly to the underling symptoms of venous hypertension.

Asymptomatic patients with a compressive abnormality of the vein in either

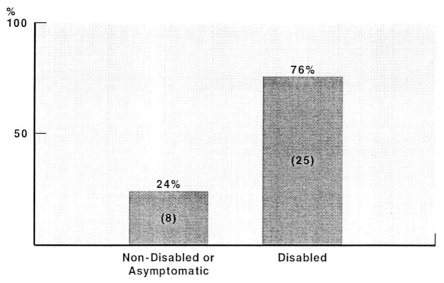

Figure 31–8. Condition of study patients after 3 months of anticoagulation therapy.

the neutral or arm-elevated position were advised to undergo decompressive surgical therapy (at the end of the anticoagulation protocol) to avoid the possibility of future thrombotic events (Fig. 31–7).

At the 3-month follow-up interval eight patients (24 per cent) were either asymptomatic or declined operative intervention for nondisabling symptoms. Twenty-five patients (76 per cent) had residual symptoms that disabled them for their usual occupation or activities (Fig. 31–8). Of the symptomatic patients, 10 clearly had residual symptoms of venous hypertension, with heaviness, edema, and discomfort accompanying exercise. About a third of the patients had symptoms that were more consistent with neurogenic thoracic outlet compression syndrome. These symptoms were predominantly dysesthesias in the course of the brachial plexus, abnormal somatosensory-evoked potential tests, and progressive weakness and evidence of motor or sensory nerve dysfunction.

Surgical Therapy

Nineteen patients underwent transaxillary first rib resection and one had resection of an exostosis of the clavicular head. Six patients had residual vein stenosis after first rib resection and five had successful PTA (Figs. 31–9 and 31–10). One patient failed angioplasty when the stenosis could not be crossed with a guidewire. Despite this failure of angioplasty the patient returned to competitive football after first rib resection and remained asymptomatic without arm edema. Four patients had transaxillary rib resection for correction of the contralateral compressed axillosubclavian vein.

RESULTS

At the last follow-up evaluation (mean of 33 months and median of 24 months), 23 patients had returned to their preillness work or activity (Fig. 31–11). Four

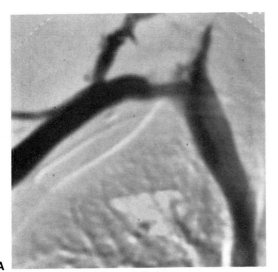

A

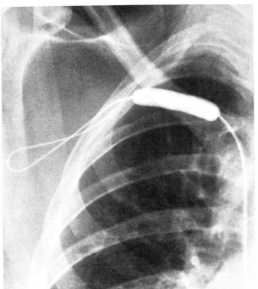

B

Figure 31–9. *A*, Venogram after successful thrombolytic therapy and transaxillary
first rib resection. We recognize this abnormality as representing residual fibrosis and
narrowing of the vein with internal synechia.
B, Balloon angioplasty of stenotic segment.
C, Postangioplasty venogram showing restoration of normal configuration. (Venography and magnetic resonance imaging scans
at 3- to 6-month intervals show continued
patency without restricture. Longer term radiology follow-up is not available in our series.)

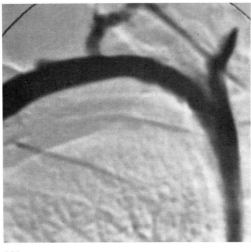

C

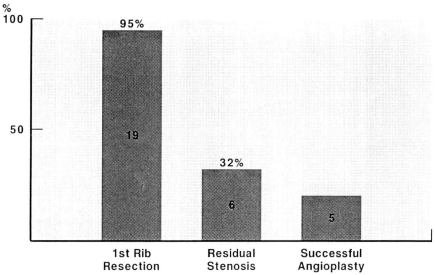

Figure 31–10.   Results in patients undergoing surgical therapy.

laborers were advised to undergo retraining, primarily because of untreated abnormalities of the contralateral thoracic outlet. One patient returned to school,
two of the older women patients did not return to work, and two patients were
awaiting a favorable worker's compensation determination to proceed with surgery. One patient, a laborer referred after failure to achieve recanalization of the
vein, continued to have symptoms after transaxillary first rib resection.

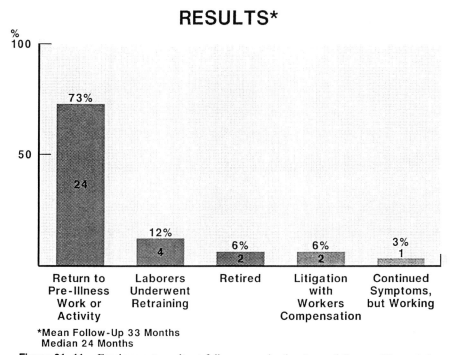

Figure 31–11.   Employment results at follow-up evaluation (mean follow-up 33 months).

SUMMARY

In the natural history of this disorder resumption of normal activity after a period of recuperation (following an episode of thrombosis) frequently leads to symptoms of upper extremity venous hypertension exacerbated by using the arms in the overhead position. This position can be demonstrated venographically to further occlude collateral vessels in the thoracic outlet. A number of patients develop more extensive symptoms of neurogenic thoracic outlet syndrome.

Anticoagulation may protect the collateral vessels and interrupt the period of active clot propagation, resulting in a better functional result than would be expected from the natural history of the thrombotic event. In our experience, local urokinase was the most effective means for reestablishing venous patency. With clot dissolution the underlying compression of the vein at the thoracic outlet can be demonstrated. Balloon angioplasty should not be undertaken in the acute setting nor prior to relieving the tendinous compression. The acute phlebitic process should resolve under the protection of warfarin for about 3 months. At that time it can be determined more effectively which patients require additional therapy. An alternative approach, when it is deemed appropriate to proceed more expeditiously with surgery, would be to continue the patient on warfarin anticoagulation, reversing the anticoagulation with fresh-frozen plasma at the time of first rib resection. We believe that this will reduce the risk of venous rethrombosis when anticoagulation has been carried for an inadequate period of time. The prothrombin time will normalize for a period of about 4 hr without the need to change the anticoagulation regimen. If there is residual venous stenosis on the postoperative venogram, balloon angioplasty can be carried out at the same hospitalization. Warfarin anticoagulation is then continued for a full 3 months postoperatively.

Transaxillary first rib resection will decompress the axillosubclavian vein and the thoracic outlet collaterals, permitting the vein to regain its normal configuration, particularly in younger patients with more acute onset of compression. In those patients with more chronic compression the vein becomes stenotic. Improvement of the luminal configuration has been accomplished with transvenous balloon angioplasty without the necessity for venous reconstructive procedures in this series.

Patients with Paget-Schroetter syndrome have a symptom complex that often reflects more extensive neurovascular compression at the thoracic outlet than that which might result from venous hypertension alone. Although thrombolytic therapy can restore patency of the axillosubclavian vein, first rib resection is necessary to relieve the external compression. This procedure was very effective in patients who had restoration of subclavian vein patency, and to a lesser degree in those with residual occlusion.

REFERENCES

1. Hughes ESR: Venous obstruction in the upper extremity (Paget-Schroetter's syndrome). Int Abst Surg 1949;88:89–127.
2. Daskalakis E, Bouhoutsos J: Subclavian and axillary vein compression of musculoskeletal origin. Br J Surg 1980;67:573–576.
3. DeWeese JA, Adams JT, Gaiser DL: Subclavian venous thrombectomy. Circulation 1970; 42(suppl II):II-159–II-164.

4. Molina JE: Thrombolytic therapy of axillary-subclavian venous thrombosis. Arch Surg 1988; *123*:662.
5. Taylor LM, McAllister WR, Dennis DL, Porter JM: Thrombolytic therapy followed by first rib resection for spontaneous ("effort") subclavian vein thrombosis. Am J Surg 1985;*149*:644–647.
6. Kunkel JM, Machleder HI: Treatment of Paget-Schroetter syndrome: A staged, multidisciplinary approach. Arch Surg 1989;*124*:1153–1158.
7. Machleder HI: Effort thrombosis of the axillosubclavian vein: A disabling vascular disorder. Contemp Ther (in press).
8. Donayre CE, White GH, Mehringer SN, Wilson SE: Pathogenesis determines late morbidity of axillosubclavian vein thrombosis. Am J Surg 1986;*152*:179–184.
9. McCleery RS, Kesterson JE, Kirtley JA, et al: Subclavius and anterior scalene muscle compression as a cause of intermittent obstruction of the subclavian vein. Ann Surg 1951;*133*:588–602.
10. Stevenson IM, Parry EW: Radiological study of the etiological factors in venous obstruction of the upper limb. J Cardiovas Surg 1975;*16*:580–585.
11. Machleder HI, Moll F, Nuwer M, Jordan S: Somatosensory evoked potentials in the assessment of thoracic outlet compression syndrome. J Vasc Surg 1987;*6*:177–184.
12. Zimmerman R, Morl H, Harenberg J, et al: Urokinase therapy of subclavian-axillary vein thrombosis. Klin Wochenschr 1981;*59*:851–856.
13. Becker GJ, Holden RW, Rabe FE, et al: Local thrombolytic therapy for subclavian and axillary vein thrombosis. Radiology 1983;*149*:419–423.
14. Machleder HI: Vaso-occlusive disorders of the upper extremity. Curr Probl Surg 1988;*25*(1):1–67.
15. McNamara TO, Fischer JR: Thrombolysis of peripheral arterial and graft occlusions: Improved results using high-dose urokinase. AJR 1985;*144*:769–775.
16. Glanz S, Gordon DH, Lipkowitz GS, et al: Axillary and subclavian vein stenosis: Percutaneous angioplasty. Radiology 1988;*168*(2):371–373.

X

SURGICAL MANAGEMENT OF VENOUS INJURIES

32

REPAIR OR LIGATION IN EXTREMITY VENOUS INJURIES

Martin I. Ellenby and James J. Schuler

Much confusion and controversy has surrounded the treatment of venous injuries of the extremities. The importance of repairing injured major extremity veins is not empirically obvious. Collateral venous channels provide multiple routes of venous outflow from the extremities such that the initial effect of injury or obstruction to some of the veins may not be very dramatic.

Some authors have discouraged venous repair for fear of subsequent thrombosis, thrombophlebitis, or pulmonary embolus (1,2). Others have expressed the view that venous repair was ineffective, or unnecessary because of the availability of venous collaterals (3–5). Based on his experience in World War I, Makins went as far as to advocate the ligation of an uninjured vein if the companion artery was injured and required ligation (6).

Prior to 1970, there was a paucity of objective data upon which to assess the treatment of venous injuries. This may reflect the lack of interest on the part of some surgeons who viewed the repair of injured veins as futile or unnecessary. In addition, while the consequences of arterial insufficiency tend to be rapid and obvious, the immediate consequences of posttraumatic venous insufficiency are often subtle, and the long-term sequelae may not be evident for 10 to 20 years. Therefore, concern regarding venous injury and its attendant significance has been overshadowed by that regarding arterial injuries.

Ligation of injured veins was the principle method of treatment until the Korean War (7). Venous repairs of injured extremity veins were not performed in sizeable numbers until the Vietnam War (2,8,9). Therefore, information describing the long-term outcome of repaired veins is only now becoming available.

ANATOMIC AND PHYSIOLOGIC CONSIDERATIONS

A single major tributary artery carries most of the arterial inflow to a limb. In contrast, venous outflow is carried by a combination of the superficial and deep venous systems, and is augmented by lymphatic outflow. Furthermore, complete duplication of the major deep venous system of the legs occurs in approximately 2 per cent of individuals. As many as 84 per cent of people have some degree of variation from the classic "textbook" venous configuration in the lower extremities (10). The frequency of these anatomic variations, and the potential for developing compensatory collaterals, have contributed to the uncertainty that surrounds the treatment of venous injuries.

Venous injuries of the lower extremities are more prone to cause long-term sequelae than injuries to the major veins of the arms. The role of the deep venous system and the superficial system are not the same in the arms and legs. Lower extremity veins are subjected to significantly greater hydrostatic forces than those in the arms (11). These basic differences may account in part for the relative rarity of sequelae of upper extremity venous injuries when compared to lower extremity injuries.

During normal function, the deep venous system forms the principle outflow tract from the lower extremities. This is the result of the calf pumping mechanism of the deep veins in conjunction with the normal communications from the superficial system to the deep system. Valves in the perforating veins of the legs direct flow from the superficial veins to the deep veins. In the arms, the orientation of the valves in the perforating veins is in the opposite direction, such that the superficial veins of the arms carry a slightly larger portion of the venous outflow (11).

In addition to the perforating veins, two major connections between the deep and superficial venous systems of the legs are the saphenopopliteal junction and the saphenofemoral junction. The saphenopopliteal junction is located in the popliteal fossa in 60 per cent of individuals (11). The popliteal artery is in close proximity to the popliteal vein in the fossa. There is a paucity of soft tissue outside the popliteal fossa at the level of the knees, limiting the space through which venous collaterals can course. These factors may all contribute to the extreme vulnerability of this area to serious vascular compromise, as reflected by the high rate of limb loss associated with popliteal fossa injuries (12–19).

The position of the saphenofemoral junction relative to the location of a femoral venous injury must be considered. Robinson and Moyer (20) observed that 75 per cent of common femoral vein interruptions for the treatment of deep venous thrombosis resulted in sequelae of venous insufficiency. In contrast, sequelae were observed in only 10 per cent of patients when the superficial femoral vein was interrupted, suggesting that preservation of venous outflow through the superficial saphenous system was important in avoiding functional venous insufficiency (20). Reports of venous complications following "femoral vein" injuries are dependent on the relationship of the saphenofemoral communication to the location of the injury (9,21–24).

The low rate of flow in veins and the propensity for postreconstruction thrombosis discouraged some surgeons from attempting venous repairs. However, there are multiple accounts in the literature of recanalization following thrombosis of a venous repair or venous bypass graft. Recanalization has been documented both in animal models (25–27) and in humans (25,28–30). These observations are not surprising in light of the growing knowledge of the endogenous fibrinolytic activity of venous endothelium (31). Thus, the provision of a potential path for future recanalization should be considered when deciding to ligate or repair an injured vein.

EXPERIMENTAL EFFECT OF VENOUS LIGATION

The immediate effect of acutely interrupting the veins of an extremity has been evaluated in animal models. In a series of experiments reported in 1967, Stallworth et al. (32) acutely occluded all the venous return from the legs of dogs by ligating the femoral vein and applying a tourniquet. A rapid rise in the distal venous pressure was followed by nearly immediate cessation of arterial flow in the femoral artery after venous occlusion. Thrombosis of the occluded femoral vein and the corresponding femoral artery occurred in 60 per cent of the dogs that survived 24 hr of occlusion. Sustained complete venous occlusion was also associated with marked arterial spasm that was unaffected by sympathectomy (32).

Barcia et al. (33) further elucidated the temporal changes in femoral arterial flow after acute femoral vein ligation in 10 dogs. Femoral artery flow rapidly decreased to 33 per cent of baseline following femoral vein occlusion, and then gradually rose to 52 per cent of baseline after 2 hr of vein occlusion. Release of the femoral vein occlusion was followed by a return of arterial flow to 85 per cent of baseline after 10 min (Table 32–1) (33).

Similar experiments performed by Wright et al. (34) also demonstrated an immediate 50 per cent decrease in femoral arterial flow following femoral vein occlusion. Occlusion of any or all branches of the femoral vein alone did not alter arterial flow, nor did occlusion of these branches cause a further decline in arterial flow if the femoral vein was already occluded. Wright et al. also observed a rapid increase in distal venous pressure following venous occlusion, which did not normalize after 4 hr of occlusion, indicating that collateral venous return was inadequate (34).

In a sequel to these experiments performed at the Walter Reed Institute of Research, the femoral veins of dogs and baboons were ligated and the results were studied for longer durations. Femoral arterial flow was significantly and persistently reduced for the first 48 hr following venous occlusion, and then returned to control levels at 72 hr. Venous pressure also tended to normalize by 72 hr, suggesting the development of improved collateral venous outflow at that time (34).

TABLE 32–1.   Effect of Femoral Vein Occlusion on Femoral Artery Flow in Canine Model[a]

INCIDENT	ARTERIAL BLOOD FLOW (ml/min)[b]	PERCENTAGE OF BASELINE
Baseline	53.4	100
Venous occlusion		
Immediate	17.6	33
After 2 hours	28.0	52
Release after 2 hours venous occlusion		
Immediate	41.8	78
After 10 minutes	45.6	85

[a] From Barcia PJ, Nelson TG, Whelan TJ: Importance of venous occlusion in arterial repair failure: An experimental study. Ann Surg 1972;*175*:223–227.
[b] Mean value from 10 dogs.

These experiments demonstrate: 1) the deleterious impact of acute venous interruption on the flow through the companion artery, and 2) the amount of time required for the development of adequate venous collateral outflow. These data provide an experimental rationale for repairing venous injuries in order to maximize the flow and patency of associated arterial repairs, and to optimize perfusion to a compromised limb.

HISTORICAL PERSPECTIVE

The treatment approach to venous injuries of the extremities has undergone an interesting evolution. The pendulum of opinion has swung widely and to opposing extremes. The broad shifts of opinion have been driven in one direction by the development of successful vascular suture techniques during the late 19th and early 20th centuries, in another direction by some spurious conclusions arrived at by surgical leaders after World War I, and in yet another direction by the perceived futility and danger of attempts at venous repair. With the major improvements in vascular surgical techniques that occurred after World War II, along with the systematic means of critically evaluating results from the Vietnam Vascular Registry and recent civilian series, the pendulum may finally be drawing to a more rational central point. A consensus is now surfacing, and the approach to the management of extremity venous injuries is being refined based upon new data.

The first account of a repair of an injured vein is credited to Travers in 1816, when he closed a small hole in a femoral vein. In 1830, G. J. Guthrie applied a lateral ligature to a lacerated internal jugular vein. The first vascular anastomosis is attributed to Eck in 1877, when he experimentally sutured the portal vein to the inferior vena cava. Kummel performed the first end-to-end venous anastomosis in a human in 1889. The techniques of vascular anastomosis and suture were further refined by Murphy, Carrel, and Guthrie at the turn of the century. Several interesting accounts of the early historical development of venous repair are available (35,36).

Controversy surrounding venous ligation was present as early as 150 years ago. In 1833, Gensoul advocated ligation of the intact femoral artery if an injured companion femoral vein required ligation in order to avoid "dangerous" venous engorgement. Dupuytren and Chassaignac viewed interruption of the femoral vein as more deleterious than ligation of the femoral artery. In 1864, Langenbeck recommended the ligation of an intact femoral artery to stem hemorrhage from an injured femoral vein. A school of thought arose that theorized the importance of concomitant arterial ligation in association with ligation of an injured vein to "balance" or "equalize" circulation to an extremity. In contrast, Gross and Nicaise both believed that major veins could be safely ligated without ligation of the companion artery (35,36).

In addition to the concept of "equalization of circulation," Ney (37) outlined a belief in 1912 that ligation of the femoral vein after ligation of an injured femoral artery served to increase the pressure in the arterial system distal to the arterial injury. It was believed that the effective perfusion of an ischemic limb was improved by this increase in pressure in conjunction with the delay in blood transit time following venous obstruction (6,37).

The most famous support for venous ligation, both in response to direct venous injury and as a therapeutic measure following arterial injury, was espoused by Makins in 1917. Based on the British Army experience in World War I, Makins observed that limb salvage was better among soldiers undergoing simultaneous vein and artery ligation than among those undergoing arterial ligation alone. He went on to advocate the ligation of uninjured veins when the associated artery required ligation (6). It is of historical interest that Makins made a basic miscalculation in his data, and there was actually no statistically significant difference in outcome following arterial ligation and combined arterial-venous ligation (12,35).

Following Makins' observations, a variety of anecdotal clinical reports and experimental data were presented during the next 20 years supporting his conclusions. In contrast, Matas stated unequivocally that "the danger of peripheral gangrene is always made doubly worse by the simultaneous injury of the accompanying or satellite vein" (38). Nevertheless, after World War I the preponderance of surgical opinion discounted the need for venous repair and viewed venous ligation as a safe measure (7,12,35).

Makins' views were not clearly refuted until the milestone report in 1946 on vascular injuries from World War II by DeBakey and Simeone. This report stated that "ligation of the concomitant vein furnishes no protection whatsoever against the development of gangrene after acute arterial occlusion and ligation in battle casualties" (12).

While the issue of the therapeutic benefits of venous ligation was laid to rest after World War II, the question of the best treatment of the injured extremity vein remained to be answered.

INCIDENCE OF VENOUS INJURY

The actual incidence of injury to veins of the extremities is difficult to ascertain. Many venous injuries, especially those caused by closed blunt trauma, go unrecognized. However, the frequency of reported venous injuries associated with all forms of trauma during the past 40 years seems to be increasing. The basis for this trend is unclear, but it may reflect in part the growing number of civilian vascular injuries caused by high-velocity weapons, as well as a greater interest on the part of surgeons in diagnosing and treating venous injuries.

Based on his experience in the Korean War, Hughes reported 71 major venous injuries in a series of 180 vascular injuries (39.4 per cent). Sixty-three per cent of the major arterial injuries had an associated venous injury (7,39). In a preliminary report of the Vietnam Vascular Registry, 194 of 718 vascular injuries were venous (27 per cent); 14 per cent of these were isolated venous injuries and 86 per cent were combined arteriovenous injuries (8). A subsequent report of 1000 acute arterial injuries in Vietnam documented concomitant venous injuries in 37.7 per cent of patients. The majority of these injuries were caused by penetrating trauma (9).

Data from civilian series demonstrate similar proportions of venous and arterial injuries (Table 32–2). In Gaspar and Treiman's series in 1960 from Los Angeles County Hospital, 23 per cent of patients with vascular injuries had injuries to major veins (40). More recent accounts of civilian vascular trauma indicate

TABLE 32–2.   Incidence of Venous Trauma in Civilian Series

LOCATION OF TRAUMA	SERIES	YEAR	TOTAL VASCULAR INJURIES	ISOLATED VENOUS INJURIES	ARTERIO-VENOUS INJURIES	TOTAL VENOUS INJURIES	% VENOUS INJURIES
Total body	Gaspar and Treiman (40)	1960	228			52	23
	Kelly and Eiseman (41)	1975	175	31	28	59	34
	Cheek et al. (42)	1975	250			95	38
	Hobson et al. (22)	1983	262			81	31
	Feliciano et al. (43)	1984	408			187	46
Extremity	Cheek et al. (42)	1975	114			25	22
	Hardin et al. (3)	1982	356			86	24
	Agarwal et al. (44)	1982	70			40	57

	Feliciano et al. (43)	1984	163			40	25
	Ross et al. (45)[a]	1985	85	1	20	21	25
	Pasch et al. (46)	1986	204	3	62	65	32
Popliteal	Snyder et al. (15)	1979	81	0	39	39	48
	Lim et al. (17)	1980	40			9	23
	Jaggers et al. (18)	1982	85	5	24	29	34
	Orcutt et al. (19)	1983	56	3	20	23	41
Upper extremity	Graham et al. (47)	1982	85	14	20	34	40
	Ross et al. (45)[a]	1985	36	0	9	9	25
	Orcutt et al. (48)	1986	163			13	8

[a] Blunt injuries only.

TABLE 32–3.   Data on 142 Patients with 158 Venous Injuries[a,b]

MECHANISM		% INJURIES	
Gunshot		57	
Stabwounds		27	
Shotgun		13	
Blunt		3	

LOCATION	VEIN	NUMBER	% TOTAL
Neck			
	Ext. Jugular	13	
	Int. Jugular	18	
	TOTAL	31	20
Upper Exremity			
	Subclavian	4	
	Axillary	5	
	Brachial	11	
	TOTAL	20	13
Abdomen			
	Inf. Vena Cava	23	
	Iliac	10	
	Portal	6	
	Other	6	
	TOTAL	45	28
Lower Extremity			
	Common Femoral	8	
	Superficial Femoral	25	
	Profunda Femoral	6	
	Popliteal	9	
	Tibial	14	
	TOTAL	62	39

[a] From Pasch AR, Bishara RA, Schuler JJ, et al: Results of venous reconstruction after civilian vascular trauma. Arch Surg 1986;*121*:607–611.
[b] Patients seen at University of Illinois Hospital and Cook County Hospital, January 1, 1979 through December 31, 1984.

that major venous injuries occur in 8 to 57 per cent of patients, with rates dependent on mechanism and location of injury (3,15,17–19,22,40–48).

Ross et al. (45) evaluated the incidence of venous trauma among patients suffering vascular injuries due to blunt mechanisms. Nine of 25 patients with upper extremity vascular trauma (36 per cent) and 12 of 38 patients with lower extremity vascular trauma (32 per cent) sustained damage to a major vein (45).

Our experience at the University of Illinois Hospital and Cook County Hospital in Chicago is similar to reports from other centers. Of 139 patients with 204 vascular injuries due to penetrating trauma, 65 major venous injuries were encountered (47 per cent of patients, 32 per cent of injuries) (46). The mechanisms of injury and the vessels injured in 142 patients with 158 venous injuries from our institution are outlined in Table 32–3 (24). The mechanisms and locations of injuries described in Table 32–3 are similar to those in other reports in the literature.

OVERVIEW: LIGATION VERSUS REPAIR

Following World War II, the belief that venous ligation had beneficial effects on the ischemic limb was discredited. However, concern remained that attempts to repair damaged major veins might result in thrombophlebitis or pulmonary embolization emanating from the site of the venous repair. Prior to the Vietnam War, the vast majority of venous injuries were treated with ligation, in part because of fears of the aforementioned complications and in part because of technical limitations of trauma resuscitation and vascular surgical technique (7,8,12). Therefore, little basis existed for comparison of the relative merits of ligation versus repair of injured veins.

The report of Hughes from the Korean War is the first sizable experience with repair of injured extremity veins; 20 major extremity veins were repaired by lateral venorrhaphy (n = 19) or end-to-end anastamosis (n = 1). These repairs were undertaken after it was observed that ligation of major extremity veins resulted in various degrees of venostasis, and on rare occasions this venostasis led to venous gangrene and limb loss. Despite proven thrombosis of some of the repairs, all patients had favorable outcomes without the dreaded complication of pulmonary embolization or significant venostasis at follow-up (7,39).

The initial reports of successful lateral venorrhaphy from the Korean War were corroborated in a civilian series in 1960 from Los Angeles County Hospital. A total of 52 venous injuries were reviewed. Twenty-seven patients were treated with ligation; 21 had "successful" results, three limbs were amputated, and three patients died. Ten veins were treated with lateral venorrhaphy; nine patients had "good" results, and one patient died of associated injuries. Fifteen venous defects went untreated; two patients had "good" results, four died of venous injuries, two died of associated injuries, and seven had subsequent arteriovenous fistulas. Thrombophlebitis was noted in three patients treated with ligation, but in none of those undergoing repair. The authors concluded that lateral suture repair was more effective than ligation in achieving limb salvage and avoiding complications, and that lateral suture repair should be undertaken whenever the patient's condition permits (40).

Interposition grafting of large venous defects was not performed in Korea or in the experience at Los Angeles County Hospital. Inspired by a few scattered anecdotal accounts of success with grafts in the venous system, Dale and Scott (25) undertook a thorough review of available data, and a series of experiments in a canine model examining the efficacy of various grafts in the venous system. Their data favored the use of autogenous venous graft material in all settings with the exception of the superior vena cava, in which they concluded that prosthetic material was satisfactory. They also recognized the potential for recanalization in autogenous grafts and the importance of venous flow rate and pressure, rather than graft rigidity, in the maintenance of patency (25). Further review and experiments by other investigators confirmed the superiority of autogenous material in the venous system (49,50). A recent report by Feliciano et al. also confirmed improved patency with autogenous grafts. However, that report also concluded that polytetrafluoroethylene (PTFE) was acceptable as a temporary venous conduit in proximal extremity veins (51).

The Vietnam Vascular Registry provided more extensive information regarding the management of venous injuries. The interim report included 377 venous injuries, of which 124 (33 per cent) were repaired (Table 32–4). There were no clinically recognized cases of pulmonary embolus or thrombophlebitis following these 124 repairs (9).

The Vietnam era experience dispelled concern of potentially lethal thromboembolic complications after extremity vein repair. The sole benefits of ligation appear to be the rapid establishment of hemostasis and minimization of operative time. The short- and long-term benefits of extremity vein repairs must be weighed against the risk incurred by longer operative time along with, in some instances, the risk of donor vein graft harvest. A growing civilian experience with the management of injured veins and the Vietnam experience provide a basis for the evaluation of the long-term sequelae of venous repair compared with ligation. Repair and ligation may now be assessed for injuries at specific anatomic locations in the venous circulation.

POPLITEAL VEIN INJURIES

The unusually high rate of limb loss associated with popliteal vascular injuries has long been recognized. During World War II, popliteal arterial injuries resulted in loss of limb in 73 per cent of cases (12). During the Korean and Vietnam wars this rate fell to 28 to 32 per cent, but was still greater than other extremity vascular injuries (7,9). Concomitant injury to the popliteal artery and the popliteal vein appears to increase the risks of compartmental hypertension and amputation (13,19,52).

Twenty-six patients were identified with popliteal vein injuries during the early Vietnam experience: eight had isolated venous injuries and 18 had combined arteriovenous injuries. All eight of the isolated venous injuries were repaired, and 13 of the 18 combined injuries underwent venous repair. During short-term follow-up, none of the limbs with venous repairs had edema, while four of five with venous ligation had massive edema. Limb loss occurred in none of the isolated venous injuries, five of the 13 combined arteriovenous injuries with venous repair, and one of the five that had venous ligation (13).

A more extensive report of 110 isolated popliteal vein injuries by Rich et al. (14) warrants special attention. No patients with concomitant arterial injuries were included. Fifty-seven of 110 veins (52 per cent) were ligated. Thirty-two veins (29 per cent) were treated by lateral suture, 15 (14 per cent) by end-to-end anastomosis, and 6 (6 per cent) by interposition grafting. Venous hypertension was observed in 51 per cent of limbs with ligated popliteal veins, but in only 13 per cent of those with venous repairs. There was no limb loss, and no significant difference in rates of thrombophlebitis (5.3 per cent with ligation versus 3.8 per cent with repair). Long-term follow-up was available for 28 patients; chronic edema was noted in 9 of 14 limbs treated by ligation and only 3 of 15 limbs treated with venous repair (degree of statistical significance was not stated by author). These data demonstrate the benefit of repairing popliteal venous injuries when the patient's condition permits (14).

The overall civilian trauma experience with popliteal vein injuries has been comparable to the military experience (Table 32–5). Limb loss rates associated with popliteal vein repair range from 0 to 23 per cent, whereas the rates associated with ligation range from 0 to 60 per cent. The number of veins ligated is becoming smaller in more recent series, as the benefits of repair are elucidated. In general, venous stasis is slightly more common in patients undergoing ligation (4,13–19,52). However, Mullins et al. (53) and Timberlake et al. (4) demonstrated that strict postoperative leg elevation, conservative progressive ambulation, and the liberal

TABLE 32–4. Management of Venous Injuries (Vietnam Vascular Registry, Interim Report)[a]

		ARTERIES	CONCOMITANT VEINS	LIGATION	REPAIR
Neck	Carotid	50	14	10	4
Chest	Innominate	3	1	0	1
	Subclavian	8	4	1	3
Upper extremity	Axillary	59	20	18	2
	Brachial	283	54	42	12
Abdomen & pelvis	Abdominal aorta	3	1	0	1
	Common iliac	9	6	6	0
	External iliac	17	5	3	2
Lower extremity	Common femoral	46	17	8	8
	Super. femoral	305	139	83	56
	Popliteal	217	116	82	34
TOTALS		1000	377	253	124

[a] From Rich NW, Hughes CW, Baugh JH: Management of vascular injuries. Ann Surg 1970;*171*:724–730.

use of fasciotomy resulted in comparable rates of long-term venous stasis sequelae following either venous ligation or repair. However, venous repair does appear to be especially beneficial when there is extensive concomitant soft tissue damage (14–16,19,45).

FEMORAL VEIN INJURIES

Limb loss after femoral venous injury is becoming fairly uncommon (Table 32–6). In a series of 16 common femoral vein or superficial femoral vein injuries at the University of North Carolina, two of nine limbs treated with venous ligation required amputation and none of the seven limbs undergoing venous repair necessitated amputation. Edema was seen in 56 per cent of limbs with venous ligation, and was not reported in any of the limbs that underwent repair (21).

In a series of 25 patients with combined arteriovenous femoral injuries, there were 19 venous repairs (76 per cent) and six venous ligations (24 per cent). Overall, three patients (12 per cent), all of whom had undergone venous ligation, required amputation (23).

Hobson set al. (22) described the outcome of 24 patients with common femoral or superficial venous injuries. All but two were repaired. Seventeen of the 22 repairs were deemed patent at early follow-up. Edema was persistent in six of eight patients initially treated by ligation or with thrombosis of a repaired vein. None of the 17 patients with patent venous repairs had edema at the time of discharge (22).

The series by Timberlake et al. (4) described 79 femoral vein injuries: 62 were ligated and 17 were repaired. There was no associated limb loss. Twelve of 62 limbs (19 per cent) with ligated veins had early edema, all cases of which had resolved within 12 weeks following injury. Four of 17 limbs (24 per cent) with

TABLE 32–5. Popliteal Vein Injury

SERIES (YEAR)	NUMBER OF VEINS INJURED	COMBINED ARTERIO-VENOUS INJURY (%)	TOTAL LIMB LOSS (%)	LIGATION			REPAIR		
				Number	Limb Loss (%)	Edema (%)	Number	Limb Loss (%)	Edema (%)
Sullivan et al.(13) (1971)	26	69	23	5	20	80	21	23	0
Rich et al. (14) (1976)	110	0	0	57	0	51	53	0	13
Snyder et al. (15) (1979)	39	100	13	5	60		34	6	
O'Reilly et al. (16) (1980)	34	76	15	3	33	100	31	13	
Jaggers et al. (18) (1982)	29	83	10	3			26		
Orcutt et al. (19) (1983)	23	87	9	8			15		
Timberlake et al. (4) (1986)	40	78	0	25	0	24[a]	15	0	7[a]
Meyer et al. (52) (1987)	8	100	0	0			8	0	0

[a] Edema resolved by 12 weeks.

TABLE 32–6. Common Femoral and Superficial Femoral Vein Injury

SERIES (YEAR)	NUMBER OF VEINS INJURED	COMBINED ARTERIO-VENOUS INJURY (%)	TOTAL LIMB LOSS (%)	LIGATION			REPAIR		
				Number	Limb Loss (%)	Edema (%)	Number	Limb Loss (%)	Edema (%)
Rich et al. (9) (1970)	156	100		91			65		
Fortner et al. (54)[a] (1977)	7	100		4		100	3	0	0
Mullins et al. (53) (1980)	43		0	21	0	19	22	0	0
Agarwal et al. (44) (1982)	21	71		8		50	13		8
Blumoff et al. (21) (1982)	16	75	13	9	22	56	7	0	0
Hobson et al. (22) (1983)	24	63	0	2	0	50	22	0	36
Phifer et al. (23) (1984)	25	100	12	6	50	50	19	0	
Timberlake et al. (4) (1986)	79	71	0	62	0	19[b]	17	0	24[b]
Meyer et al. (52) (1987)	20	95	0	0			20	0	0

[a] Reconstructions after resection for cancer.
[b] Edema resolved by 12 weeks.

463

venous repair also had transient edema. All patients were treated with strict limb elevation during the postoperative period. No extremity had chronic edema (4).

Femoral vein repair seems to have less impact on limb viability compared to the repair of an injured popliteal vein (Table 32–6). However, most reported instances of amputation after femoral vein injury occurred when the vein was ligated. In addition, there is evidence that long-term venous morbidity is less likely after repair of injured femoral veins (4,9,21,22,44,52–55). Whether these trends are a manifestation of the operative management, the overall severity of vascular and associated injuries, or the functioning of collateral veins remains to be clarified.

AXILLARY AND BRACHIAL VEINS

The upper extremities are not subject to the same hydrostatic pressures that are present in the legs. Consequently, the arms are less susceptible to debilitating sequelae of venous insufficiency. It has also been observed that pulmonary emboli rarely originate from the veins of the arms (11). Therefore, injury to the major veins of the upper extremity has stimulated less interest than injury of lower extremity veins (Table 32–7).

In a study from our institution of venous trauma that included injury to five axillary veins and 11 brachial veins, the only morbidity was one case of severely debilitating upper extremity edema that followed ligation of an axillary vein (24). However, there is no conclusive evidence that ligation of either the axillary or brachial veins predisposes to limb loss or significant swelling (4,9,24,44,47,48,52). For example, none of 38 patients in Timberlake et al.'s series had persistent upper extremity edema, and only one had transient edema of an arm following axillary or brachial vein ligation (4).

Since the axillary vein is formed by the confluence of the deep and superficial venous systems of the arm, it is reasonable to assume that ligation of the axillary vein may have greater attendant morbidity than ligation of the brachial vein or veins of the forearm. Therefore, axillary vein repair seems prudent and is routinely performed at our institution. Injured brachial veins are also generally repaired in hemodynamically stable patients. This approach has not resulted in any venous sequelae in our experience (52). Repair of upper extremity veins may be especially beneficial in the setting of severe soft tissue injury.

FOREARM, PROFUNDA FEMORIS, AND TIBIAL VEINS

Routine ligation of forearm veins, profunda femoris veins, and tibial veins has not been associated with any sequelae (24,48). Injuries to these veins that can easily be repaired by simple lateral venorrhaphy may be best managed by repair rather than ligation to maximize venous return, especially when soft tissue damage is extensive. However, there has not been any critical assessment of the treatment of these smaller veins.

TABLE 32–7. Axillary and Brachial Vein Injury

SERIES (YEAR)	NUMBER OF VEINS INJURED	COMBINED ARTERIO-VENOUS INJURY (%)	TOTAL LIMB LOSS (%)	LIGATION			REPAIR		
				Number	Limb Loss (%)	Edema (%)	Number	Limb Loss (%)	Edema (%)
Rich et al. (9) (1970)	74	100		60			14		0
Graham et al. (47) (1982)	34	59	0	12	0	0	12	0	0
Agarwal et al. (44) (1982)	12	75	0	7	0	0	5	0	0
Pasch et al. (24) (1986)	16		0	8	0	13	8	0	0
Timberlake et al. (4) (1986)	38	100	0	38	0	3[a]	0	0	
Orcutt et al. (48) (1986)	13		0	7	0	0	6	0	0
Meyer et al. (52) (1987)	5	80	0	0			5	0	0

[a] Edema resolved by 12 weeks.

FUNCTIONAL OUTCOME AND SURGICAL TECHNIQUE

The importance of obtaining thorough long-term follow-up of patients with major venous extremity injuries cannot be overemphasized. The basic nature of venous physiology dictates that important differences in outcome may not become clinically evident for years. Since venous repair was not commonly practiced prior to the Vietnam War, follow-up to evaluate long-term sequelae and patency are only now becoming available. Furthermore, most reports rely almost entirely on a subjective evaluation of the clinical manifestations of venous stasis to assess outcome. Objective gauges of patency and function (e.g., impedance plethysmography, photophlethysmography, venous Doppler ultrasound studies, and contrast venography) must be utilized to precisely evaluate long-term outcome, which will in turn allow for the refinement of venous repair techniques and indications.

Meyer et al. (52) performed impedance plethysmography, Doppler ultrasonography, contrast venography, and thorough clinical exams on the seventh postoperative day on 36 patients following venous repair. Venography demonstrated thrombosis of the repair in 14 patients (39 per cent). As shown in Table 32–8, local venous repair had a significantly lower rate of thrombosis (21 per cent) compared with interposition graft repairs (59 per cent; $p<.03$) (52). Data from other studies have also indicated that simple lateral venorrhaphy is the preferred repair technique whenever technically possible (3,50).

Aitken et al. reported on the functional outcome of 26 patients, 6 to 66 months following venous injuries (mean 19.5 months) (55). All patients underwent photoplethysmography (PPG) and Doppler ultrasound reflux studies; 17 underwent contrast venography. Edema was present in five of six patients initially treated with ligation, and in nine of 20 who had repairs. Venograms demonstrated vein occlusion in 11 of 17 patients; nine of 11 with occlusion had edema, including all patients treated with ligation, despite the presence of extensive venous collaterals. Five of six patients with patent repairs were free of edema. The PPG recovery times were significantly shortened in the injured leg compared with the normal contralateral leg (20.6 versus 32.1 sec; $p = .002$). The PPG recovery time also tended to be shorter in limbs with occluded repairs compared with patent repairs (13.4 versus 21.6 sec; $p = .07$).

Aitken et al. devised a system to grade outcome based on the clinical exam and objective tests (Table 32–9). A "poor" outcome was noted in 67 per cent of patients treated with ligation, and in only 35 per cent of those treated with venous

TABLE 32–8. Short-Term Venographic Patency by Type of Repair[a]

	PATENT	OCCLUDED	TOTAL	% OCCLUDED
Lateral repair	5	1	6	17
End-to-end repair	4	0	4	0
Vein patch	6	3	9	33
Vein graft	6	9	15	60
Paneled vein graft	1	1	2	50
TOTAL	22	14	36	

[a] From Meyer JP, Walsh J, Schuler JJ, et al: The early fate of venous repair following civilian vascular trauma. Ann Surg 1987;206:458–464.

TABLE 32–9. Functional Outcome Following Vein Trauma[a]

	ASSESSMENT CRITERIA		
	Good	Fair	Poor
Photoplethysmography Recovery Time	>21s	Abnormal, >17s	Abnormal, <17s
Doppler Reflux	Negative	Positive	Positive
Venogram	Patent	Patent	Thrombosed
Oedema	Nil	Minimal	Severe

	OUTCOME (MEAN FOLLOW-UP = 19.5 MONTHS)		
VENOUS TREATMENT	Good	Fair	Poor
Ligation	1	1	4
Lateral repair	3	2	3
Vein patch	2		1
End-to-end anastomosis		1	2
Interposition saphenous vein	2	2	1
Panel graft		1	
TOTAL	8	7	11

[a] From Aitken RJ, Matley PJ, Immelman EJ: Lower limb vein trauma: A long-term clinical and physiological assessment. Br J Surg 1989;76:585–588.

repair. These data indicate that patients tend to have less severe venous dysfunction following repair than following ligation (55).

The overall efficacy of interposition grafting in the venous system seems to be significantly inferior to that of primary repair (3,50,52). However, interposition grafting is still preferred to ligation in most circumstances in which a disruption of a major extremity vein cannot be repaired primarily, since an occluded graft may ultimately recanalize (28–30). Recanalization is obviously an impossibility if the vein is ligated.

Meticulous surgical technique is essential to produce a successful result following venous repair. Sutures must be placed precisely so that endothelium is in direct apposition with endothelium exclusively on the intraluminal surface. The careless introduction of media or adventitia into the luminal surface will lead to early thrombosis. In addition, the caliber of the repaired segment should ideally match the caliber of the native vein. Since there is a tendency for a continuous running suture to "purse string," narrowing the area of venorrhaphy or anastomosis, an interrupted or partially interrupted suturing technique is usually preferred. A vein patch should be used whenever primary repair with lateral venorrhaphy will result in a stenosis. Likewise, an interposition panel graft should be used if the vein is completely disrupted in order to avoid stenosis or size mismatch.

Autogenous vein is the material of choice for patching injured veins and for interposition grafts (25,27,49). In most instances, the greater saphenous vein can be used. However, vein for interposition grafts or patches must never be harvested from the injured limb. All remaining uninjured veins in the injured limb must be preserved since they may be the major remaining routes of venous outflow. The removal of these intact veins may contribute to subsequent venous insufficiency in the injured limb. Therefore, when vein graft material is needed, it should always be obtained from an uninjured extremity.

ADJUVANTS

A variety of adjuvant measures have been proposed to enhance patency of venous repairs as well as to minimize perioperative sequelae following both repair and ligation.

Timberlake et al. (4) and Mullins et al. (53) showed that postoperative and long-term lower extremity swelling can be minimized by the aggressive use of fasciotomy, and strict limb elevation until ambulation can proceed without resultant swelling. Others have reinforced the importance of relieving compartmental hypertension with complete fasciotomy, in both the upper and lower extremities (44). Meyer et al. (52) reinforced these points, and observed minimal short-term swelling following lower extremity venous repair, despite early thrombosis of the repair in 39 per cent of patients. The low rate of edema was credited to strict leg elevation and appropriate use of fasciotomy.

Intermittent pneumatic compression of the calves has also been advocated to increase venous flow through repaired veins and increase patency (56). There are some indications that the use of anticoagulants may improve outcome and enhance patency through venous repairs. In particular, perioperative low-molecular-weight dextran may improve patency, although this remains to be demonstrated definitively. Perioperative heparin was not beneficial when examined (26,49). The surgical creation of a distal arteriovenous fistula will increase flow through repaired venous segments, and may enhance the ultimate outcome by improving patency (57).

SUMMARY

Most data favor the repair of injured common femoral, superficial femoral, and popliteal veins. Repair may maximize the flow through associated arteries, and reduces the rate of early and late sequelae of venous insufficiency. The importance and necessity of repair of upper extremity veins remains to be demonstrated, although axillary vein repair is considered prudent. Attempts at repair, even if they thrombose initially, provide an avenue for later recanalization. Repair of extremity veins does not increase the risk of thrombophlebitis or pulmonary embolus.

Simple modes of repair such as lateral venorrhaphy or venous patch should be performed whenever the patient's general condition allows. The role of more complicated repairs with autogenous interposition grafts warrants further study, but these repairs are favored over ligation when the patient's condition permits. Follow-up at longer intervals is required to more throughly understand the ultimate outcome of repair and ligation in the treatment of extremity venous trauma.

REFERENCES

1. Cook FW, Haller JA: Penetrating injuries of the subclavian vessels with associated venous complications. Ann Surg 1962;*155*:370–372.

2. Rich NM, Hobson RW, Wright CB, Fedde CW: Repair of lower extremity venous trauma: A more aggressive approach required. J Trauma 1974;*14*:639–652.
3. Hardin WD, Adinolfi MF, O'Connell RC, Kerstein MD: Management of traumatic peripheral vein injuries: Primary repair or vein ligation. Am J Surg 1982;*144*:235–238.
4. Timberlake GA, O'Connell RC, Kerstein MD: Venous injury: To repair or ligate, the dilemma. J Vasc Surg 1986;*4*:553–558.
5. Borman KR, Jones GH, Snyder WH: A decade of lower extremity venous trauma: Patency and outcome. Am J Surg 1987;*154*:608–612.
6. Makins GH: On Gunshot Injuries to the Blood Vessels. Bristol, England, John Wright & Sons, Ltd, 1919.
7. Hughes CW: Acute vascular trauma in Korean War casualties: An analysis of 180 cases. Surg Gynecol Obstet 1954;*99*:91–100.
8. Rich NM, Hughes CW: Vietnam Vascular Registry: A preliminary report. Surgery 1969;*65*:218–226.
9. Rich NM, Hughes CW, Baugh JH: Management of venous injuries. Ann Surg 1970;*171*:724–730.
10. Cockett FB: Abnormalities of the deep veins of the leg. Postgrad Med J 1954;*30*:512–516.
11. Browse NL, Burnand KG, Thomas ML: Embryology and radiographic anatomy, and physiology and functional anatomy. *In*. Diseases of the Veins: Pathology, Diagnosis and Treatment. London, Edward Arnold, 1988;23–70.
12. DeBakey ME, Simeone FA: Battle injuries of the arteries in World War II: An analysis of 2,471 cases. Ann Surg 1946;*123*:534–579.
13. Sullivan WG, Thornton FH, Baker LH, LaPlante ES, Cohen A: Early influence of popliteal vein repair in the treatment of popliteal vessel injuries. Am J Surg 1971;*122*:538–531.
14. Rich NM, Hobson RW, Collins GJ, Andersen CA: The effect of acute popliteal venous interruption. Ann Surg 1976;*183*:365–368.
15. Snyder WH, Watkins WL, Whiddon LL, Bone GE: Civilian popliteal artery trauma: An eleven year experience with 83 injuries. Surgery 1979;*85*:101–108.
16. O'Reilly MJG, Hood JM, Livingston RH, Irwin JWS: Penetrating injuries of the popliteal vein: A report on 34 cases. Br J Surg 1980;*67*:337–340.
17. Lim LT, Michuda MS, Flanigan DP, Pankovich A: Popliteal artery trauma: 31 consecutive cases without amputation. Arch Surg 1980;*115*:1307–1313.
18. Jaggers RC, Feliciano DV, Mattox KL, Graham JM, DeBakey ME: Injury to popliteal vessels. Arch Surg 1982;*117*:657–661.
19. Orcutt MB, Levine BA, Root HD, Sirinek KR: The continuing challenge of popliteal vascular injuries. Am J Surg 1983;*146*:758–761.
20. Robinson JR, Moyer CA: Comparison of late sequelae of common and superficial femoral vein ligations. Surgery 1954;*35*:690–697.
21. Blumoff DL, Powel T, Johnson G: Femoral venous trauma in a university referral center. J Trauma 1982;*22*:703–705.
22. Hobson RW, Yeager RA, Lynch TG, Lee BC, Jain K, Jamil Z, Padberg FT: Femoral venous trauma: Techniques for surgical management and early results. Am J Surg 1983;*146*:220–224.
23. Phifer RJ, Gerlock AJ, Vekovius WA, Rich NM, McDonald JC: Amputation risk factors in concomitant superficial femoral artery and vein injuries. Ann Surg 1984;*199*:241–243.
24. Pasch AR, Bishara RA, Schuler JJ, Lim LT, Meyer JP, Merlotti G, Barrett JA, Flanigan DP: Results of venous reconstruction after civilian vascular trauma. Arch Surg 1986;*121*:607–611.
25. Dale WA, Scott HW: Grafts of the venous system. Surgery 1963;*53*:52–74.
26. Hobson RW, Croom RD, Rich NM: Influence of heparin and low molecular weight dextran on the patency of autogenous vein grafts in the venous system. Ann Surg 1973;*178*:773–776.
27. Hiratzka LF, Wright CB: Experimental and clinical results of grafts in the venous system: A current review. J Surg Res 1978;*25*:542–561.
28. Rich NM, Sullivan WG: Clinical recanalization of an autogenous vein graft in the popliteal vein. J Trauma 1972;*12*:919–920.
29. Phifer TJ, Gerlock AJ, Rich NM, McDonald JC: Long-term patency of venous repairs demonstrated by venography. J Trauma 1985;*25*:342–346.
30. Beggs JH: Recanalization of autogenous vein grafts. South Med J 1988;*81*:1446–1447.
31. Fearnley GR: A concept of natural fibrinolysis. Lancet 1961;*1*:992.
32. Stallworth JM, Najib A, Kletke RR, Ramirez A: Phlegmasia cerulea dolens: An experimental study. Ann Surg 1967;*165*:860–868.
33. Barcia PJ, Nelson TG, Whelan TJ: Importance of venous occlusion in arterial repair failure: An experimental study. Ann Surg 1972;*175*:223–227.
34. Wright CB, Hobson RW, Swan KG, Rich NM: Extremity venous ligation: Clinical and hemodynamic correlation. Am Surg 1975;*41*:203–208.
35. Simeone FA, Grillo HC, Rundle F: On the question of ligation of the concomitant vein when a major artery is interrupted. Surgery 1951;*29*:932–951.
36. Rich NM, Hobson RW, Wright CB: Venous injury: Incidence, etiology, pathology, and historical

perspective. *In* Hobson RW, ed: Venous Trauma: Pathology, Diagnosis, and Surgical Management. Mount Kisco, NY, Futura Publishing Co, Inc, 1983;5–16.

37. Ney E; Du role des veines dans la circulation collaterale arterielle. Rev Chir 1912;*46*:903–913.
38. Matas R: Surgery of the vascular system. *In* Keen WW, ed: Surgery: Its Principles and Practices, by Various Authors. Philadelphia, WB Saunders Company, 1921;17–350.
39. Hughes CW: Arterial repair during the Korean War. Ann Surg 1958;*147*:555–561.
40. Gaspar MR, Trieman RL: The management of injuries to major veins. Am J Surg 1960;*100*:171–175.
41. Kelly GL, Eiseman B: Civilian vascular injuries. J Trauma 1975;*15*:507–514.
42. Cheek RC, Pope JC, Smith HF, Britt LG, Pate JW: Diagnosis and management of major vascular injuries: A review of 200 operative cases. Am Surg 1975;*41*:755–760.
43. Feliciano DV, Bitondo CG, Mattox KL, Burch JM, Jordan GL, Beall AC, DeBakey ME: Civilian trauma in the 1980s: A 1-year experience with 456 vascular and cardiac injuries. Ann Surg 1984;*199*:717–724.
44. Agarwal N, Shah PM, Clauss RH, Reynolds BM, Stahl WM: Experience with 115 civilian venous injuries. J Trauma 1982;*22*:827–832.
45. Ross SE, Ranson KJ, Shatney CH: The management of venous injuries in blunt extremity trauma. J Trauma 1985;*25*:150–152.
46. Pasch AR, Bishara RA, Lim LT, Meyer JP, Schuler JJ, Flanigan DP: Optimal limb salvage in penetrating civilian vascular trauma. J Vasc Surg 1986;*3*:189–195.
47. Graham JM, Mattox KL, Feliciano DV, DeBakey ME: Vascular injuries of the axilla. Ann Surg 1982;*195*:232–238.
48. Orcutt MB, Levine BA, Gaskill HV, Sirinek KR: Civilian vascular trauma of the upper extremity. J Trauma 1986;*26*:63–67.
49. Haimovici H, Hoffert PW, Zinicola N, Steinman C: An experimental and clinical evaluation of grafts in the venous system. Surg Gynecol Obstet 1970;*131*:1173–1185.
50. Rich NM, Collins GJ, Andersen CA, McDonald PT: Autogenous venous interposition grafts in repair of major venous injuries. J Trauma 1977;*17*:512–520.
51. Feliciano DV, Mattox KL, Graham JM, Bitondo CG: Five-year experience with PTFE grafts in vascular wounds. J Trauma 1985;*25*:71–82.
52. Meyer J, Walsh J, Schuler J, Barrett J, Durham J, Eldrup-Jorgensen J, Schwarcz T, Flanigan DP: The early fate of venous repair after civilian vascular trauma. Ann Surg 1987;*206*:458–464.
53. Mullins RJ, Lucas CE, Ledgerwood AM: The natural history following venous ligation for civilian injuries. J Trauma 1980;*20*:737–743.
54. Fortner JG, Kim DK, Shiu MH: Limb-preserving vascular surgery for malignant tumors of the lower extremity. Arch Surg 1977;*112*:391–394.
55. Aitken RJ, Matley PJ, Immelman EJ: Lower limb vein trauma: A long-term clinical and physiological assessment. Br J Surg 1989;*76*:585–588.
56. Hobson RW, Lee BC, Lynch TG, Jain K, Yeager R, Jamil Z, Padberg FT: Use of intermittent pneumatic compression of the calf in femoral venous reconstruction. Surg Gynecol Obstet 1984;*159*:285–286.
57. Schramek A, Hashmonai M, Farbstein J, Adler O: Reconstructive surgery in major vein injuries in the extremities. J Trauma 1975;*15*:816–822.

33

LONG-TERM FOLLOW-UP OF VENOUS RECONSTRUCTION FOLLOWING TRAUMA

Norman M. Rich, Edward R. Gomez, James A. Coffey, Sharon L. Hammond, Carl G. Lauer, and J. Leonel Villavicencio

Unfortunately, long-term follow-up of venous reconstruction following trauma remains largely anecdotal (1–4). This important subject nevertheless mandates periodic review and update because of the continuing controversy that has existed in this century. The nature of the controversy has changed in the past decade from concerns regarding the advisability of performing venous repair, as opposed to ligation, to concerns about the short- and long-term results of repair. This is somewhat ironic since repair of injured veins was determined to be advisable and practical by numerous individuals earlier in this century (2–8). In assessing results, a definition of "long-term follow-up" is necessary because there is no uniformity of opinion on this. Any period of time more than 30 days for the acutely injured patient is acceptable to many investigators. Whether 1 year, 3 years, or more than 5 years should be considered truly long-term remains moot. It is important that follow-up should continue during the life of the patient who has sustained vascular trauma simply because there is minimal information available today regarding the ultimate fate of both arterial and venous repairs. Even sequelae associated with ligation of injured arteries and veins need to be studied continuously (9).

For the purpose of this review any follow-up beyond the initial acute management will be included, in an effort to document the results and/or sequelae associated with the management of venous trauma. Also, the emphasis will be on critical lower extremity venous injuries, with specific emphasis on management of popliteal venous injuries (10–16).

Because as current literature searches by computer often include only the past decade, valuable past knowledge is not easily accessible. Thus the education of each generation redefines and reidentifies necessity for continued observation and evaluation of patients who have sustained vascular trauma. In fact, many factors are changing in the civilian management of vascular trauma. Whereas the paper by Gasper and Treiman (17) from the Los Angeles County Hospital was essentially the only specific report on the management of civilian venous injuries in the 1960s, the past decade has produced more than 10 times the number of publications concentrating on venous injuries in civilian trauma (18–34). Also, penetrating injuries, particularly those produced by missiles, have increased dramatically. Stab wounds of 30 years ago have been replaced by bullet wounds from increasingly sophisticated weaponry. The guns have become more military. Lessons learned and relearned on recent battlefields have become more pertinent to the current experience in urban warfare.

Mattox and coworkers have established a civilian vascular trauma registry at the Ben Taub General Hospital/Baylor College of Medicine in Houston, Texas. There they have evaluated 4459 patients treated for 5760 cardiovascular injuries over a 30-year period from 1958 to 1988 (35). This unique epidemiologic profile provides extremely important details regarding a variety of factors ranging from etiologic wounding agents to specific management of the vascular injuries. However, long-term follow-up information is not included in the design of this registry. Identifying 2135 venous injuries, or approximately 37.1 per cent of the total, this could be an important data base for long-term follow-up for evaluation of the management of venous injuries. Of particular note are 280 femoral vein injuries and 76 popliteal vein injuries.

This chapter makes an effort to emphasize the long-term follow-up of venous injuries. Some background for this is found in references previously cited and others (36–42). Technical considerations, with emphasis on meticulous technique in venous repair, have been emphasized (33,43–45), and a variety of techniques and adjuvants, including distal arteriovenous fistulas, have been utilized (46–54), but it is not the intent of this review to reiterate all of these.

HISTORICAL NOTES

Historical aspects of direct venous reconstruction are well documented (2–8). Travers and Guthrie are given credit for contributions in the early 19th century. However, Schede is credited with the first successful lateral suture repair of a venous laceration in man in 1882, when he repaired a lacerated femoral vein. Eck made an important contribution in 1877 with the first successful experimental anastomosis of two vessels when he produced a lateral communication between the portal vein and the inferior vena cava. In 1899 Kümmel supposedly performed the first clinical end-to-end anastomosis of the vein in repairing an injured femoral vein. In 1897 Murphy documented the first successful clinical end-to-end anastomosis of an injured artery and repaired a laceration of a common femoral vein at the same time. He stressed that similar technique should be utilized in the repair of veins as well as arteries in the future.

There were numerous contributors, led by Carrel and Guthrie, who emphasized basic principles of vascular surgery at the turn of this century. Some had a specific interest in suturing venous lacerations. Among the early clinical contributions were those of Soubbotitch, who repaired veins as well as arteries during the Balkan Wars of 1911 and 1912. Surgical leaders from the capital cities of Europe traveled to Belgrade to witness these pioneering efforts. There were isolated reports of successful venous repairs during the American experience in World War I. Goodman wrote about lateral suture repair of venous lacerations in five patients with lower extremity venous injuries. He noted that four had repair of popliteal and superficial femoral veins. Makins documented the British Army experience in 1917 but reported that injured veins were of minor importance and that ligation was acceptable over repair. There were few changes during World War II. The management of injured veins was largely ligation. However, it was demonstrated that there was no benefit from ligating the concomitant uninjured vein when an injured artery required ligation.

It was during the Korean War, from 1950 to 1953, that repair of injured veins was utilized in select patients. Hughes, Spencer, and others identified various degrees of venostasis associated with ligation of injured veins. Several patients had limb loss after ligation of injured major veins. Selective repair of injured lower extremity major veins was initiated to avoid such complications. Although thrombosis followed some of these repairs, there seemed to be fewer complications. This contributed to the increased interest in repairing veins during the Vietnam War. Specific reports contributed additional valuable clinical information. A retrospective study of 125 failures of popliteal arterial repair identified acute venous hypertension as a significant factor leading to amputation in at least 19 patients (12). Approximately 78 per cent of the patients had concomitant venous injuries in this study group, and surgeons were impressed with the risk factors involved. Sullivan and associates at the 12th Evacuation Hospital emphasized the early influence of repair of injured popliteal veins on the overall treatment of popliteal vascular injuries, and their paper remains extremely important today (16). Subsequent follow-up through the Vietnam Vascular Registry provided early evidence of the value of repairing injured lower extremity veins and substantiated a clinical impression that ligation of these injured veins could lead to sequelae of chronic venous insufficiency and hypertension (2–4,9–15).

The establishment in 1966 of the Vietnam Vascular Registry at Walter Reed Army Medical Center provided the opportunity to document cases and provide long-term follow-up of those who had the misfortune to be wounded while serving in the American military in Southeast Asia (2–4). Questions about the true incidence of venous injuries were to be answered when it was recognized that adequate numbers of reports were being generated. In reviewing 1000 acute arterial injuries, an interim report from the Vietnam Vascular Registry in 1970 noted that 38 per cent had concomitant venous injuries. Even this was believed to be less than the actual experience (3). In a subsequent report in 1974 it was emphasized that a more aggressive approach to the repair of large-caliber lower extremity veins should be considered (11). The precept of life over limb was recognized, but it was recognized that a more aggressive approach could reduce the incidence of acute venous hypertension and prevent the long-term sequela of chronic venous hypertension (3,4). A subsequent report reviewing the fate of 110 isolated popliteal venous injuries corroborated this conclusion (14).

REVIEW OF RECENT RESULTS

Approximately 30 years ago there was concern that patients would have an increased incidence of thrombophlebitis and/or pulmonary embolism associated with attempted repair of injured extremity veins (3,4). This contributed to acceptance of the concept of ligation of injured veins. However, these concerns have been completed refuted by the experience of the past 30 years (1–4). The actual/perceived controversy has moved into the arena regarding whether or not injured veins need to be repaired. In this regard, phlebography can be helpful in determining patency following extremity venous injury and repair. Also, noninvasive tests can assist in monitoring whether or not venous hypertension exists. The practical application and the cost-effectiveness of utilizing these approaches are not established at this time.

It has now been demonstrated that repair of injured veins can be successful and can be performed safely (1–4). Concerns regarding success have been refuted. The physiologic function of the involved venous system remains a concern. It is not well studied in follow-up, except in isolated reports (19,33).

Mullins et al. reported their management of 129 patients with injury to major veins of the lower extremities at Detroit General Hospital/Wayne State University over a 4-year period from 1975 through 1978 (31). Approximately one half of the injuries were treated by primary repair, with the majority treated by simple lateral suture technique. In their report on what they termed "the natural history following venous ligation for civilian injuries," Mullins et al. evaluated those patients who received ligation of injured veins. Excluding nine of 55 patients, they evaluated 46 patients who had ligation of the superficial femoral (13 patients), the common femoral (eight), the profunda femoris (six), the vena cava (six), the external iliac (five), the popliteal (five), and the common iliac (three) veins. They stressed postligation management, which included: 1) early and extensive fasciotomy when indicated, 2) initial strict bed rest with extremity elevation until the patient was edema free, 3) trial ambulation for 2 hr, and 4) added elevation if trial ambulation led to recurrent edema. Forty patients were discharged free of edema and the remaining six had mild edema. In the follow-up examinations, of 39 patients 30 remained edema free. Of the nine patients with edema one was mild without treatment and eight required support stockings for moderate edema. Follow-up was possible for between 3 months and 3 years. None of the patients developed any clinical signs of a pulmonary embolus following venous ligation. Four patients developed thrombophlebitis.

Blumoff et al. reported recanalization of a thrombosed interposition saphenous vein graft in the superficial femoral vein in one of their civilian gunshot wound victims treated at the University of North Carolina, Chapel Hill (22). The phlebogram demonstrating thrombosis at 1 week postreconstruction was followed 6 weeks postoperatively by a second phlebogram that demonstrated recanalization of the venous interposition graft. It was believed that normal-appearing valves in the deep venous system were present both proximal and distal to the interposition graft.

Phifer and colleagues performed a retrospective review of 31 femoral venous injuries from Shreveport over a 20-year period, with 24 undergoing reconstruction (32). Five patients with six reconstructions were located for long-term follow-up to determine patency of the venous repairs by phlebography. This follow-up ranged from 6 to 20 years. Patency and functional valves were found in asymptomatic patients with no clinical evidence of venous insufficiency. One patient with a venous repair with prosthetic material demonstrated thrombosis. In 1985, this appeared to be the only known report of long-term results following venous reconstruction (Table 33–1). There were two repairs by lateral suture technique and one repair with autogenous vein patch graft, end-to-end anastomosis, and interposition saphenous vein graft. In the patient with the failed reconstruction,

TABLE 33–1.   Follow-up Venographic Findings in Six Venous Repairs[a]

TYPE OF REPAIR	FOLLOW-UP (YEARS)	FINDINGS AT REPAIR SITE
Teflon graft (superficial femoral vein)	20	Occluded
Lateral suture repair (common femoral vein)	5	Patent
Saphenous vein graft	11	Patent
End-to-end anastomosis	10	Patent
Lateral suture repair	8	Patent
Autogenous vein patch graft	6	Patent

[a] From Phifer TJ, Gerlock AJ, Rich NM, McDonald JC: Long-term patency of venous repairs demonstrated by venography. J Trauma 1985;25:342–346.

at the end of 20 years there was evidence of chronic venous insufficiency in the involved lower extremity.

Menzoian et al. reported a comprehensive approach to extremity vascular trauma in Boston in 1985 (55). Their review evaluated 368 patients with 382 extremity injuries, including a total of 165 vascular injuries in 136 patients. Seventy of these patients had a total of 88 vascular injuries of the lower extremity, with 18 having a combined arterial and venous injury and 13 a venous injury alone. Table 33–2 outlines the method of management of the 31 venous injuries. Lateral repair was used in nearly 50 per cent of the repairs and ligation was elected in approximately 20 per cent. Ligation was utilized in managing injury to one saphenous vein, two tibial veins, one popliteal vein, and two superficial femoral veins. The popliteal vein was ligated in one patient in whom a second popliteal vein was believed capable of providing sufficient venous drainage. Two superficial femoral veins were ligated in patients with other major traumatic injuries when it was believed that prolonging the operative procedure was not indicated. Venous bypass grafts were used in three popliteal vein injuries and one superficial femoral vein injury. Menzoian and colleagues stressed that major lower extremity venous injuries should be repaired unless there were life-threatening extenuating circumstances. Their experience refuted concern for potential thrombophlebitis and pulmonary embolism. They did use postoperative anticoagulation unless significant soft tissue and/or orthopedic injuries raised concern for associated hemorrhage.

Feliciano and colleagues from Houston reported a 5-year experience with polytetrafluoroethylene (PTFE) grafts in vascular wounds (56). From 1978 through 1983, 206 patients had 236 PTFE grafts used to reconstruct vascular injuries. The

TABLE 33–2.   Lower Extremity Venous Repair Results in Boston[a,b]

	LR	EE	VBPG	VP	L	TOTAL
Common femoral	3	1	0	1	0	5
Superficial femoral	8	1	1	0	2	12
Popliteal	3	4	3	0	1	11
Tibial	0	0	0	0	2	2
Saphenous	0	0	0	0	1	1
TOTAL	14	6	4	1	6	31

[a] Modified from Menzoian JO, Doyle JE, Cantelmo NL, et al: A comprehensive approach to extremity vascular trauma. Arch Surg 1985;120:801–805. Copyright 1985, American Medical Association.
[b] LR, lateral repair; EE, end-to-end anastomosis; VBPG, venous bypass graft; VP, vein patch; L, ligation.

majority of the venous grafts were inserted in injured superficial femoral veins (Table 33–3). It was determined that the non–externally supported PTFE grafts inserted in proximal extremity veins provided excellent temporary conduits that helped decrease hemorrhage in blast cavities and fasciotomy sites; however, all grafts studied by venography at 7 to 14 days were either narrowed or occluded. In the early follow-up edema was not a significant problem in the majority of patients. It was thought that the temporary conduit could provide adequate time for dilatation of venous collaterals and provide benefit from decreased distal hemorrhage.

Timberlake et al. from Tulane University reviewed the medical records of 184 patients with major venous injury, including 43 patients who had isolated venous injury and 141 patients who had combined arterial and venous injury (34). Ligation was utilized in 72 per cent of the injuries in the former group and in 83 per cent of the injuries in the latter group. Injuries were encountered in the inferior vena cava and the iliac, femoral, popliteal, distal leg, and arm veins. Repairs, when done, were performed by end-to-end anastomosis or by lateral phleborrhaphy. Patients were followed for 1 month to 9 years. No permanent sequelae of venous ligation were identified. Timberlake et al. did report that transient extremity edema developed in up to 32 per cent of the patients, regardless of whether the vein had been ligated or repaired. Edema resolved completely within 12 weeks of injury. Their conclusion was that selective management of venous injuries was appropriate.

Meyer and colleagues from Cook County Hospital/University of Illinois in Chicago reported on the early fate of venous repair after civilian vascular trauma in 1987, emphasizing clinical, hemodynamic, and venographic assessment (30). They reviewed the management of 36 patients with major extremity venous injury treated by venous reconstruction during a 27-month period starting in January 1985. Lower extremity veins were involved in 78 per cent of the cases. After operation the venous repair patency was evaluated by clinical examination, impedence plethysmography, Doppler ultrasonography, and contrast venography. Venography performed on the seventh postoperative day demonstrated that 14 venous repairs had thrombosed (39 per cent) and that 22 had remained patent (61 per cent). Meyer et al. believed that, in their experience, clinical evaluation and

TABLE 33–3.   Five-Year Experience with Occlusions of Venous PTFE Grafts in Vascular Wounds (Early Follow-up at 7–14 Days)[a]

LOCATION AND GRAFT SIZE (mm)	DIAGNOSIS BY	OUTCOME
Brachial (4)	Venogram	No edema
Common femoral (12)	Venogram	Edema
Superficial femoral (12)[b]	Palpation (exposed)	Removed; edema
Superficial femoral (12)	Palpation (exposed)	No edema
Superficial femoral (8)	Venogram	No edema
Superficial femoral (8)	Venogram	No edema
Superficial femoral (8)	Venogram	No edema
Superficial femoral (6)	Isotope study	No edema
Superficial femoral (6)	Venogram	No edema
Superficial femoral (6)	Venogram	No edema
Superficial femoral (6)	Reoperation	Removed; replaced with 12-mm[b]

[a] Modified from Feliciano et al. (56).
[b] Same patient: 6-mm graft replaced with 12-mm graft.

noninvasive testing did not provide an accurate assessment of the venous patency after venous repair. In discussion, the authors acknowledged that a 3-month follow-up was insufficient for the total evaluation of patients.

Aitken et al., from the University of Cape Town/Groote Schuur Hospital, described a relatively extensive experience with long-term lower extremity venous trauma evaluation (19). Their experience in managing 26 patients operated upon for lower limb venous trauma was reviewed. A median elapsed time of 19.5 months was cited as follow-up. They reviewed records from 1980 through 1987 and then performed a psychologic assessment using the patients' noninjured limbs as a control. The popliteal vein was involved most frequently (11 patients), followed by the superficial femoral vein (nine), the common femoral vein (four), and the external iliac vein (two). Table 33–4 outlines the clinical assessment criteria utilizing photoplethysmography recovery time, the presence or absence of popliteal reflux, the venographic evidence of thrombosis, and edema. It is particularly pertinent to note that 14 patients had pedal edema, and two had a postphlebitic limb. Table 33–5 identifies the incidence of clinical edema following each method of management (edema is present in the "Fair" and "Poor" outcomes). Since there have been other reports of the management of civilian lower extremity venous injuries without any incidence of lower extremity edema, it is particularly pertinent to note that five of six patients had obvious clinical edema following ligation of a lower extremity vein. That five of eight patients also had clinical edema following lateral suture of a lacerated vein emphasizes the failure of attempted repair. It is important to note that slightly more than 50 per cent of the patients had edema in the overall experience. Aitken et al. believed that vein ligation was associated with considerable morbidity and suggested that all end-to-end anastomoses initially failed. Because of the technical difficulty in providing an appropriate autogenous venous conduit, they determined that the repair of choice was a sephanous vein patch for lacerations of veins and a saphenous panel graft for more extensive injuries. They recommended against ligation of injured veins unless priority had to be given to a life-threatening injury. These authors determined that there were two principle conclusions in their study. First, they thought that 58 per cent of the repaired veins thrombosed, and even if patency was maintained there could be serious physiologic impairment of venous function as assessed by photoplethysmography. Second, they believed that their study confirmed the harmful consequences of popliteal vein ligation with its appreciable clinical morbidity and abnormal physiologic function.

Sharma and colleagues from the Lincoln Medical Center, New York Medical College, gave one of the most recent reports on management of major venous

TABLE 33–4. Assessment Criteria of Final Outcome in Lower Limb Vein Trauma[a]

	GOOD	FAIR	POOR
Photoplethysmography Recovery Time	>21 s	Abnormal, >17 s	Abnormal, <17 s
Doppler Reflux	Negative	Positive	Positive
Venogram	Patent	Patent	Thrombosed
Oedema	Nil	Minimal	Severe

[a] From Aitken RJ, Matley PJ, Immelman EJ: Lower limb vein trauma: A long-term clinical and physiological assessment. Br J Surg 1989;76:585–588.

TABLE 33–5.   Assessment of Outcome in Lower Limb Vein Trauma[a]

	GOOD	FAIR	POOR
Ligation	1	1	4
Lateral repair	3	2	3
Vein patch	2		1
End-to-end anastomosis	1	2	
Interposition saphenous vein	2	2	1
Panel graft		1	
Total	8	7	11

[a] Aitken RJ, Matley PJ, Immelman EJ: Lower limb vein trauma: A long-term clinical and physiological assessment. Br J Surg 1989;76:585–588.

injuries (33). There have been previous valuable contributions from this group, including one by Agarwal and associates reporting a large experience with 115 civilian venous injuries in 1982 (18). In the past 5 years they have addressed various considerations ranging from management of vascular injuries in the lower extremities to limb loss in civilian injuries and compartment syndrome associated with combined arterial and venous injuries in the lower extremities. In their May 1990 presentation at the Fourth Annual Meeting of the Eastern Vascular Society, Sharma et al. reported 38 major venous injuries in 37 patients between January 1981 and December 1989. The majority were associated with gunshot wounds (27) or knife wounds (five). Femoral veins were involved most frequently (27), followed by popliteal veins (10). For retrospective analysis they divided their patients into two groups. Table 33–6 identifies the method of venous repair, including one ligation. Group I (17 patients) had meticulous restoration of the venous lumen, ensured by postrepair phlebography in the operating room. Two of the 17 repairs required revision based on the phlebographic findings. In group II (20 patients, 21 venous injuries) there was no evaluation in the operating room of the repair by phlebography. Late patency of venous repair was confirmed by postoperative phlebography in 10 and duplex scanning in seven patients in group I, demonstrating that all 17 repaired veins were patent. Fifteen of the 20 patients in group II had phlebography and five patients (six veins) had duplex scanning. Eight veins were occluded and 13 remained patent, for a 62 per cent patency rate, compared to the 100 per cent patency rate in group I, in which there was meticulous repair

TABLE 33–6.   Management of Venous Injuries at Lincoln Medical Center, New York Medical College, 1981–1989[a]

TYPE OF REPAIR	GROUP I	GROUP II	TOTAL
End to End	9	5	14
Lat. Venorrhapy	2	10	12
Vein Patch	1	2	3
Vein Compilation	2	2	4
Vein Spiral	1	0	1
Vein Bypass	2	0	2
Gore-Tex	0	1	1
Ligation	0	1	1
TOTAL	17	21	38

[a] From Sharma PVP, Shah PM, Vinzona AT, Pallan TM, Clauss RH, Stahl WM: Presented at the Fourth Annual Meeting of the Eastern Vascular Society, Boston, May 11, 1990.

and phlebographic confirmation ($p < .02$). Sharma and coworkers have thus demonstrated that meticulous restoration to normal caliber of injured veins, confirmed by postreconstruction phlebography in the operating room, can achieve high patency rates in extremity venous injury.

DISCUSSION AND CONCLUSIONS

There are several ways to interpret recent reports. Therefore, the controversy regarding repair of venous injuries continues. It is nevertheless important to emphasize that there is more agreement among all reports that might be obvious initially. For example, it is pertinent to emphasize that early concerns over an increased incidence of thrombophlebitis and pulmonary embolism associated with attempted venous repair have been completely refuted. In fact, no one has expressed this concern in the past 15 years. This is one important area in which the military experience as reported through the Vietnam Vascular Registry has been corroborated repeatedly.

The precept of life over limb remains a requisite in managing injured patients. Therefore reports that include ligating lower extremity injured veins also include repair of injured veins. These repeatedly emphasize that selected management should be utilized. Some patients, particularly those with injuries to a single popliteal vein, will probably benefit from an aggressive attempt at venous repair. Such venous repair, and perhaps even more complex reconstruction, can be successful with meticulous technique and evaluation. Finally, all of the experience of the past 25 years continues to emphasize the necessity for long-term follow-up in evaluation of patients who have sustained lower extremity vascular injuries.

Inconsistencies in venous anatomy remain a central point in the controversy and discussion of venous repair. As has been emphasized, injury to one channel of a bifid popliteal vein can be significantly different in outcome when compared or contrasted to injury of a single popliteal vein. Also, the superficial femoral vein can be duplicated or can have even multiple complete channels. This explains differences of outcome in managing injuries to this axial vein.

It is important to recognize that Danza and colleagues reported one of the earliest lower extremity venous reconstructions in 1970 (57). It would be appropriate to have additional long-term follow-up at this time. In fact, each center that has reported a study of the management of lower extremity venous injuries should make an effort to provide long-term follow-up clinical information. Such an effort continues in the Vietnam Vascular Registry, which recognizes the logistic challenges of locating individuals and securing appropriate evaluation. However, rapidly advancing technology makes accurate noninvasive physiologic assessment practical and valuable. The challenge is to provide such follow-up information. It is hoped that this last decade of the 20th century will see a successful response to that challenge.

REFERENCES

1. Rich NM: Management of venous trauma. Surg Clin North Am 1988;*68*:809–821.
2. Rich NM: Venous injuries. *In* Sabiston DC Jr, ed: Textbook of Surgery, 13th ed. Philadelphia, WB Saunders Company, 1986;2009–2018.

3. Rich NM, Spencer FC: Vascular Trauma. Philadelphia, WB Saunders Company, 1978;156–190.

4. Hobson RW II, Rich NM, Wright CB, eds: Venous Trauma: Pathophysiology, Diagnosis and Surgical Management. Mount Kisco, NY, Futura Publishing, 1983.

5. Haimovici H, Hoffert PW, Zinicola N, Steinman C: An experimental and clinical evaluation of grafts in the venous system. Surg Gynecol Obstet 1970;*131*:1173–1186.

6. Rich NM, Hobson RW II: Historical background of repair of venous injuries. *In* Witkin E, et al, eds: Venous Diseases: Medical and Surgical Management. The Hague, Netherlands: Mouton, 1974;253–261.

7. Rich NM, Hobson RW II, Wright CB: Historical aspects of direct venous reconstruction. *In* Bergan JJ, Yao JTS, eds: Venous Problems. Chicago, Year Book Medical Publishers, 1977; 441–449.

8. Swan KG, Hobson RW, Reynolds DG, Rich NM, Wright CB, eds: Venous Surgery in the Lower Extremities. St. Louis, Warren H. Green Publishers, Inc, 1975.

9. Rich NM, Hughes CW, Baugh JH: Management of venous injuries. Ann Surg 1970;*171*:724–730.

10. Rich NM, Sullivan WG: Clinical recanalization of an autogenous vein graft in the popliteal vein. J Trauma 1972;*12*:929–920.

11. Rich NM, Hobson RW II, Wright CB, Fedde CW: Repair of lower extremity venous trauma: A more aggressive approach required. J Trauma 1974;*14*:639–652.

12. Rich NM, Jarstfer BS, Geer TM: Popliteal artery repair failure: Causes and possible prevention. J Cardiovasc Surg 1974;*15*:340–351.

13. Rich NM, Jarstfer BS, Geer TM: Concomitant popliteal arterial and venous trauma. *In* Swan KG, Hobson RW II, Reynolds DG, Rich NM, Wright CB, eds: Symposium on Venous Surgery in the Lower Extremities. St. Louis, Warren H. Green Publishers, Inc, 1975;29–40

14. Rich NM, Hobson RW II, Collins GJ Jr, Anderson CA: The effect of acute popliteal venous interruption. Ann Surg 1976;*183*:365–368.

15. Rich NM, Collins GJ, Andersen CA, McDonald PT: Autogenous venous interposition grafts in repair of major venous injuries. J Trauma 1977;*17*:512–520.

16. Sullivan WG, Thorton FG, Baker LH, LaPlante ES, Cohen A: Early influence of popliteal vein repair in the treatment of popliteal vessel injuries. Am J Surg 1971;*122*:528–531.

17. Gaspar MR, Treiman RL: The management of injuries to major veins. Am J Surg 1960;*100*:171–175.

18. Agarwal N, Shah PM, Clauss RH, Reynolds DM, Stahl WM: Experience with 115 civilian venous injuries. J Trauma 1982;*22*:827–832.

19. Aitken RJ, Matley PJ, Immelman EJ: Lower limb vein trauma: A long-term clinical and physiological assessment. Br J Surg 1989;*76*:585–588.

20. Barkun JS, Terazza O, Daignault P, et al: The fate of venous repair after shock and trauma. J Trauma 1988;*28*:1322–1329.

21. Bishara RA, Shuler JJ, Lim LT, et al: Results of venous reconstruction after civilian vascular trauma. Arch Surg 1986;*121*:607–611.

22. Blumoff RL, Proctor HJ, Johnson G: Recanalization of a saphenous vein interposition venous graft. J Trauma 1981;*21*:407–408.

23. Blumoff RL, Powell T, Johnson G Jr: Femoral venous trauma in a university referral center. J Trauma 1982;*22*:703–705.

24. Borman KR, Jones GH, Snyder WH III: A decade of lower extremity venous trauma: Patency and outcome. Am J Surg 1987;*154*:608–612.

25. Brigham RA, Eddleman WL, Clagett GP, Rich NM: Isolated venous injury produced by penetrating trauma to the lower extremity. J Trauma 1983;*23*:255–257.

26. Hardin WD Jr, Adinolfi MF, O'Connell RC, Kerstein MD: Management of traumatic peripheral vein injuries: Primary repair or vein ligation. Am J Surg 1982;*144*:235–238.

27. Hobson RW, Yeager RA, Lynch TG, et al: Femoral venous trauma: Techniques for surgical management and early results. Am J Surg 1983;*146*:220–224.

28. Jimenez F, Utrilla A, Cuesta C, et al: Popliteal artery and venous aneurysm as a complication of arthroscopic meniscectomy. J Trauma 1988;*28*:1404–1405.

29. Kropilak M, Satiani B: Combined superficial femoral artery and vein injury with deep venous thrombosis: Elements of proper management. Contemp Surg 1988;*32*:24–28.

30. Meyer J, Walsh J, Schuler J, et al: The early fate of venous repair following civilian vascular trauma; a clinical, hemodynamic and venographic assessment. Ann Surg 1987;*206*:458–464.

31. Mullins RJ, Lucas CE, Ledgerwood AM: The natural history following venous ligation for civilian injuries. J Trauma 1980;*20*:737–743.

32. Phifer TJ, Gerlock AJ, Rich NM, McDonald JC: Long-term patency of venous repairs demonstrated by venography. J Trauma 1985;*25*:342–346.

33. Sharma PVP, Shah PM, Vinzona AT, Pallan TM, Clause RH, Stahl WM: Meticulously restored lumens of injured veins remain patent. Presented at the 4th Annual Meeting of the Eastern Vascular Society, Boston, May 10–13, 1990.

34. Timberlake GA, O'Connell RC, Kerstein MD: Venous injury: To repair or ligate, the dilemma. J Vasc Surg 1986;*4*:533–538.
35. Mattox KL, Feliciano DV, Burch J, Beall AC Jr, Jordan GL Jr, DeBakey ME: Five thousand seven hundred sixty cardiovascular injuries in 4459 patients: Epidemiologic evolution 1958 to 1987. Ann Surg 1989;*209*:698–707.
36. Bergan JJ, Yao JST, eds: Symposium on Venous Problems in Honor of Geza de Takats. Chicago, Yearbook Medical Publishers Inc, 1978.
37. Hiratzka LF, Wright CB: Experimental and clinical results of grafts in the venous system: A current review. J Surg Res 1978;*25*:542–561.
38. Hobson RW II, Croom RD, Rich NM: Influence of heparin and low molecular weight dextran on the patency of autogenous vein grafts: Vein grafts in the venous system. Ann Surg 1973; *178*:773–776.
39. Hobson RW II, Croom RD, Swan KG: Hemodynamics of the distal arteriovenous fistula in venous reconstruction. J Surg Res 1973;*4*:483.
40. Hobson RW II, Howard EW, Wright CB, Collins GJ, Rich NM: Hemodynamics of canine femoral venous ligation; significance in combined arterial and venous injuries. Surgery 1973;*74*:824–829.
41. Wright CB, Swan KG: Hemodynamics of venous occlusion in the canine hindlimb. Surgery 1973; *73*:141.
42. Wright CB, Hobson RW II, Swan KG, Rich NM: Extremity venous ligation: Clinical and hemodynamic correlation. Am Surg 1975;*41*:203–208.
43. Rich NM, Hobson RW II, Wright CB, Swan KG: Techniques of venous repair. *In* Swan KG, Hobson RW II, Reynolds DG, Rich NM, Wright CB, eds: Symposium on Venous Surgery in the Lower Extremities. St. Louis, Warren H. Green Publishers, Inc, 1975;243–256.
44. Rich NM, Collins GJ Jr, Andersen CA, McDonald PT, Ricotta JJ: Venous trauma: Successful venous reconstruction remains an interesting challenge. Am J Surg 1977;*134*:226–230.
45. Rich NM: Principles and indications for primary venous repair. Surgery 1982;*91*:492–496.
46. Dale WA: Chronic iliofemoral venous occlusion including seven cases of cross-over vein grafting. Surgery 1966;*59*:117.
47. Earle AS, Horsley JS, Villavicencio JL, Warren R: Replacement of venous defects by venous autografts. Arch Surg 1960;*80*:119.
48. Gerlock AJ: The use of pedal venous pressure (PVP) as a guide in evaluating the patency of venous repairs. J Trauma 1977;*17*:108–110.
49. Hobson RW II, Wright CB: Peripheral side to side arteriovenous fistula: Hemodynamics and application in venous reconstruction. Am J Surg 1973;*126*:411–414.
50. Hobson RW, Lee BC, Lynch TG, et al: Use of intermittent pneumatic compression of the calf in femoral venous reconstruction. Surg Gynecol Obstet 1984;*159*:284–286.
51. Jacobson JH, Haimov J: Venous revascularization of the arm: Report of three cases. Surgery 1977;*81*:599–604.
52. Johnson V, Eiseman B: Evaluation of arteriovenous shunts to maintain patency of venous autograft. Am J Surg 1969;*118*:915.
53. Levin PM, Rich NM, Hutton JE Jr, Barker WF, Zeller JA: The role of arteriovenous shunts in venous reconstruction. Am J Surg 1971;*122*:183.
54. Richardson JB Jr, Jurkovich GJ, Walker GT, Nenstiel R, Bone EG: A temporary arteriovenous shunt (Scribner) in the management of traumatic venous injuries of the lower extremity. J Trauma 1986;*26*:503–509.
55. Menzoian JO, Doyle JE, Cantelmo NL, et al: A comprehensive approach to extremity vascular trauma. Arch Surg 1985;*120*:801–805.
56. Feliciano DV, Mattox KL, Graham JM, Bitondo CG: Five-year experience with PTFE grafts in vascular wounds. J Trauma 1985;*25*:71–82.
57. Danza R, Mauro L, Arias J, et al: Reconstruction of the femoro-popliteal vessels with a double graft (arterial and venous) in severe injury of the limb. J Cardiovasc Surg 1970;*11*:60–64.

34

MANAGEMENT OF INTRAABDOMINAL VENOUS INJURIES

David V. Feliciano

While abdominal veins are anatomically part of either the caval or portal venous system, it is most useful to discuss injuries to individual veins because of their different locations and associated injuries. Therefore, major abdominal venous injuries are considered to be those involving the superior mesenteric vein, inferior vena cava, renal veins, iliac veins, and portal vein.

As with intraabdominal arterial injuries, little has been written about these injuries in reports of vascular trauma sustained in wartime (1,2). This reflects the wounding power of military firearms and delays in transport to surgical facilities that preceded the Vietnam War. Except for isolated case reports, most of the available literature on intraabdominal venous injuries is from civilian trauma centers and has been published in the past 30 years. For example, 32 per cent of all vascular injuries treated at the Ben Taub General Hospital in Houston during 1982 were intraabdominal in location, and 68.5 per cent of these were to veins; also, 47.6 per cent of *all* venous injuries reported were to intraabdominal veins (3). A 30-year review (1958 to 1988) from the same hospital published in 1989 documented that the inferior vena cava was the most commonly injured vascular structure during the time interval (4).

MECHANISM OF INJURY

Abdominal venous injuries from blunt trauma (5 to 10 per cent) are caused by deceleration, direct blows, or contact with associated bony injuries. A common example of a deceleration injury is the avulsion of small peripancreatic branches from the superior mesenteric vein or portal vein at the lower border of the pancreas (5). With direct upper midline blows, either partial or complete transection of the left renal vein over the aorta has occurred (5). The most classical example of venous injury associated with bony injury is the extensive venous hemorrhage noted wtih pelvic fractures, especially when the sacroiliac joint is disrupted (6).

Penetrating injuries cause 90 to 95 per cent of abdominal venous injuries. The injuries created are similar to those seen in the extremities: lateral wall defects with stable or slowly expanding hematomas *or* free intraperitoneal hemorrhage, complete transection with the same result, blast effects with secondary thrombosis, or, on rare occasions, arteriovenous fistulas.

Iatrogenic injuries are another cause of abdominal venous trauma. Diagnostic procedures such as retrograde venous angiography and laparoscopy and operative procedures such as retroperitoneal node dissections have all been reported to cause abdominal venous injuries (7,8).

DIAGNOSIS

Patients with abdominal venous injuries present with *hematomas* contained by the retroperitoneum, mesentery, or porta hepatis or witih active *intraperitoneal hemorrhage*, much as in patients with abdominal arterial injuries. The ease of diagnosis and urgency of operative intervention will depend on which of these is present. For example, patients with contained hematomas may have only modest hypotension in the field that is often readily reversible with the infusion of fluids. Such patients may remain remarkably stable, even with near transection of a major abdominal vein, until the hematoma is opened at the subsequent celiotomy. In contrast, patients with free intraperitoneal hemorrhage will have profound hypotension and abdominal distention when first seen.

With the exception of those associated with pelvic fractures, abdominal venous injuries from blunt trauma generally occur in the upper abdomen. As previously noted, avulsion of small venous branches off the portal vein will lead to venous hemorrhage, which is usually not exsanguinating, and acute peritonitis. Avulsion of the left renal vein from a direct blow usually leads to exsanguinating hemorrhage and is frequently fatal despite early operation. Because venous injury is much more common than arterial injury when pelvic fractures are present, the hypotension that occurs in such patients is generally considered to be from tamponaded venous injuries that may not be amenable to direct surgical control.

Penetrating abdominal stab wounds cause intraabdominal vascular injuries 10.3 per cent of the time (V. Spjut-Patrinely and D. V. Feliciano, unpublished data, Ben Taub General Hospital, Houston, July 1985 to June 1988), whereas gunshot wounds cause such injuries in 24.6 per cent of patients (9). When an abdominal vascular injury is present in either group, an abdominal venous injury is twice as likely to be present as is an abdominal arterial injury. The higher incidence of abdominal venous injuries in patients with penetrating wounds, especially gunshot wounds, mandates a more rapid diagnostic evaluation and earlier operation than in patients with blunt abdominal trauma.

Preoperative diagnostic maneuvers in patients with abdominal venous injuries are usually limited because the history of hypotension in the field, even if it is partially reversible, or of persistent hypotension in the emergency department suggests the need for early operation. A routine scout film in preparation for an intravenous pyelogram (IVP) is useful in patients with penetrating wounds because the tract of the missile can be predicted from skin clips and the position of the retained missile. A preoperative IVP is performed in stable patients with moderate or marked hematuria after blunt trauma and in all stable patients after penetrating injuries. While this study will not diagnose an isolated renal vein lesion, the documentation that two functioning kidneys are present will make the decision to perform a subsequent nephrectomy for either severe parenchymal or renovascular injury an easier one.

MANAGEMENT BEFORE OPERATION

In the field standard resuscitation is used in patients with suspected abdominal vascular injuries. In patients with blunt abdominal trauma and obvious pelvic fractures, the application of a pneumatic antishock garment (PASG) will be very helpful in controlling hemorrhage (10–13). In contrast, patients with abdominal vascular injuries from other causes actually had a lower survival when the PASG was applied in a recent prospective series from Houston (14). If the patient arrives in the emergency department with marked abdominal distention under the PASG, it is most appropriate to leave the garment inflated during the period of transit to the operating room. When the anesthesiologist and surgeons have completed the usual preparations for celiotomy, the garment is removed and surgery is immediately begun.

The extent of resuscitation in the emergency department depends on the patient's condition at the time of arrival. Emergency department thoracotomy with cross-clamping of the descending thoracic aorta has been used in some centers to maintain cerebral and coronary flow in agonal patients with massively distended abdomens (15). The technique is most useful in patients with some signs of life after penetrating trauma and when the operating room is geographically distant from the emergency department.

Because of the concern about the potential need to cross-clamp the inferior vena cava in the abdomen during a subsequent laparotomy, most trauma centers insert large-bore intravenous catheters for resuscitation into the upper extremities or, if necessary, into the central veins at the thoracic inlet. Most modern trauma centers now have short, large-bore (10-gauge or 8.5 French) catheters, heating elements, and specialized administration sets readily available for the rapid infusion of crystalloids and blood during the preoperative period of resuscitation in the emergency department. With such systems, flow rates of 1400 to 1600 ml/min of crystalloids can be obtained when 300 mm Hg pressure is exerted by an external device (16). Type-specific blood is preferably used during resuscitation of the profoundly hypotensive patient with abdominal vascular injuries; however, universal donor O-negative blood may be used in the patient who is moribund.

OPERATION

Draping and Incisions

The entire trunk from the chin to the middle thighs is prepared and draped in the usual manner. This allows for possible extension of a midline celiotomy incision to a median sternotomy should injury to the retrohepatic vena cava be present, and for retrieval of a saphenous vein from either groin should there be a need for a segmental replacement of an injured abdominal vessel. Before making the incision, the trauma surgeon should confirm that the following items are available in the operating room: blood for transfusion, autotransfusion apparatus, aortic compressor, complete tray of vascular instruments, spongesticks with gauze sponges in place, and appropriate vascular sutures.

Prevention of Hypothermia

Hypothermia is inevitable in shocky patients who are resuscitated with cold-packed red blood cells in either the emergency room or the operating room. Maneuvers to prevent this highly lethal problem (17,18) include the following: use of prewarmed crystalloid solutions, passage of all crystalloids and blood through high-flow warmers, placing the patient on a heating blanket in the operating room, covering the patient's head, covering the lower extremities with plastic bags or a ''space'' blanket, irrigation of the nasogastric tube with warm saline, irrigation of a thoracostomy tube with warm saline, irrigation of open body cavities with warm saline, and use of a heating cascade on the anesthesia machine (19).

General Principles

A midline abdominal incision is made and all clots and free blood are manually evacuated or removed with suction. In patients with blunt abdominal trauma a rapid inspection of all four quadrants is necessary to see if there is a contained hematoma or area of active hemorrhage. In the patient with a penetrating wound these entities are searched for along the tract of the knife or missile.

If active hemorrhage is present it will have to be controlled before any other intraoperative repairs are performed. Hemorrhage from solid organs in the upper abdomen can usually be controlled by packing, while a variety of technical maneuvers may be used to obtain proximal and distal control of actively hemorrhaging major abdominal arteries. Options for proximal and distal control on major veins that are hemorrhaging include manual compression, compression with spongesticks, or the application of vascular clamps.

Once hemorrhage from vascular injuries is controlled, it may be worthwhile to apply noncrushing clamps to as many gastrointestinal perforations as possible to avoid further contamination of the abdomen during the period of vascular repair in patients with penetrating wounds. When only a *few* holes in the gastrointestinal tract are present, rapid one-layer closure using 3-0 polypropylene suture may be performed before the vascular repair. In most patients who have had active hemorrhage upon presentation, the vascular repair is performed first, and it is then covered with soft tissue prior to the repair of other injured viscera.

In the patient with a contained retroperitoneal hematoma over a venous injury, the surgeon may occasionally have time to rapidly perform gastrointestinal repairs in the free peritoneal cavity, change gloves, and then irrigate with a saline solution containing antibiotics. The contained hematoma is then opened as a later step and the vascular injury controlled.

Injuries to the Superior Mesenteric Vein

Injuries to the superior mesenteric vein generally present with contained hematomas in the supramesocolic portion of the abdomen or at the base of the mesocolon *or* with active hemorrhage at either location. Because of the proximity of the superior mesenteric artery, the junction with the splenic and portal veins, and the overlying pancreas and adjacent uncinate process, injuries to the superior mesenteric vein in its proximal portion may be extremely difficult to manage. Injuries underneath the pancreas are managed in a fashion similar to that used for injuries to the most proximal portion of the superior mesenteric artery; that is, the pancreas may have to be transected between noncrushing vascular or intestinal clamps to gain access to the area of injury. Most injuries to the superior mesenteric vein, however, are inferior to the lower border of the pancreas. A perforation in this location may occasionally be amenable to application of a partial occlusion clamp or compression between the fingers of the surgeon or an assistant. Should there be a through-and-through perforation, exposure of the posterior perforation can be accomplished only after multiple venous collaterals in the area have been ligated. In patients with near-transection, reanastomosis is worthwhile. In order to overcome the tremendous ischemic edema of the small intestine present in most of these patients, reanastomosis can be accomplished only when an assistant pushes the small bowel and its mesentery back toward the pancreas to allow the surgeon to reapproximate the ends of the vein without tension.

Ligation of the superior mesenteric vein was performed in 27 patients, of whom 22 survived, in three recent series that reviewed injuries to the portal venous system (20–22). In another review of injuries to the superior mesenteric vein survival was 85 per cent in 33 patients treated with ligation and 64 per cent in 77 patients who underwent repair (23). Stone et al.'s report from Grady Memorial Hospital clearly emphasized the need to use vigorous postoperative fluid resuscitation in patients with ligation of the superior mesenteric vein because splanchnic hypervolemia leads to peripheral hypovolemia for several days after ligation (22).

In four series since 1978, the survival rate for 104 patients with injuries to the superior mesenteric vein was 72.1 per cent (20–22,24) (Table 34–1).

Injuries to the Infrarenal Inferior Vena Cava

When a patient has an inframesocolic hematoma or active hemorrhage coming from the base of the mesentery of the transverse colon, there is always a suspicion that the infrarenal aorta has been injured, particularly in patients with penetrating abdominal wounds. When exposure of the aorta reveals that it is intact and active hemorrhage continues to come from the base of the mesentery of the ascending colon or hepatic flexure of the colon, injury to the inferior vena cava below the liver should be suspected. While it is possible to visualize the infrarenal inferior

TABLE 34–1.   Injuries to the Superior Mesenteric Vein

REFERENCE	YEAR	NO. OF PATIENTS	NO. OF SURVIVORS	% SURVIVAL
Graham et al. (21)	1978	45	31	68.8
Kashuk et al. (20)	1982	10	8	80.0
Stone et al. (22)	1982	37	27	73.0
Sirinek et al. (24)	1983	12	9	75.0
Overall		104	75	72.1

vena cava through a midline inframesocolic division of the retroperitoneum, most surgeons choose to visualize it via mobilization of the right half of the colon and C-loop of the duodenum, leaving the right kidney in place (Fig. 34–1). These maneuvers allow for complete visualization of the entire vena caval system from the suprarenal infrahepatic vena cava to the confluence of the iliac veins.

The inferior vena cava is covered with retroperitoneal fatty tissue that must be stripped away in order to precisely localize a perforation from a penetrating wound or avulsion of a branch from blunt trauma. Should only one area of perforation be present, a Satinsky-type vascular clamp should be directly applied to this perforation as the edges are elevated by a pair of vascular forceps or noncrushing clamps. Through-and-through perforations or more extensive lacerations of the inferior vena cava are not amenable to partial occlusion. In these patients it is helpful to compress the proximal and distal vena cava around the partial transection or extensive laceration using gauze sponges placed in straight spongesticks. This maneuver controls major hemorrhage, while back-bleeding from the lumbar veins may be controlled by having the surgeon place his fingers on either side of the vena cava. This maneuver is obviously awkward and, in many patients, such extensive injuries mandate complete occlusion of the vena cava between large DeBakey aortic clamps. This maneuver will interrupt much of the venous return to the right side of the heart and is poorly tolerated in patients who are already profoundly hypotensive. In order to eliminate this problem, it is worthwhile to simultaneously clamp the infrarenal abdominal aorta throughout the period of clamping of the inferior vena cava.

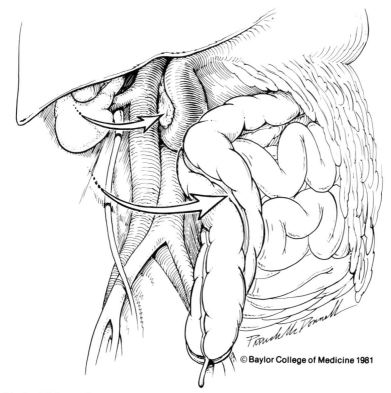

© Baylor College of Medicine 1981

Figure 34–1.   Right medial mobilization maneuver for exposure of infrahepatic inferior vena cava.

The areas where vascular control of the injured inferior vena cava is especially difficult are the caval junction with the renal veins and the confluence of the common iliac veins in the pelvis. With a complex perforating wound at the junction of the renal veins and the inferior vena cava, direct compression at the sites of perforation with either spongesticks or fingers should first be attempted. An assistant can then clamp the infrarenal inferior vena cava and the suprarenal inferior vena cava, followed by looping of both renal veins with umbilical tapes. This will allow for the direct application of angled vascular clamps. Because the dissection is time-consuming in exsanguinating patients, rapid medial mobilization of the right kidney may allow for application of a partial vascular occlusion clamp across the inferior vena cava at its junction with the right renal vein. Medial mobilization of the right kidney is also useful for exposure of posterior perforations in the suprarenal infrahepatic vena cava (25). The first lumbar vein on the right enters the junction of the right renal vein and inferior vena cava, and care must be taken to ligate and not avulse this vessel during the mobilization maneuver.

Another useful technique to control hemorrhage from any location in the inferior vena cava is insertion of a Foley balloon catheter for tamponade (26–28). The technique involves insertion of a 5- or 30-ml balloon catheter into a caval laceration, inflation of the balloon, and then application of traction to the catheter. With the balloon filling the perforation, either a pursestring suture or transverse venorrhaphy is performed, and the balloon catheter is deflated and removed just before completion of the suture line.

Anterior perforations of the inferior vena cava are repaired in a transverse fashion, if at all possible, using running sutures of 5-0 polypropylene; because the caval wall is thin in many patients, a two-layer repair is frequently necessary to attain hemostasis. When vascular control is satisfactory and a posterior caval perforation can be visualized by extending the anterior perforation, repair of the posterior perforation can be accomplished from inside the inferior vena cava. With longitudinal perforations, especially when two adjacent perforations have been joined, the repair will often take on the appearance of an hourglass. It is likely that such a narrowed area of the inferior vena cava will occlude in the postoperative period. Should the patient be unstable and have a coagulopathy, no further attempts should be made to revise the repair at the first operation. In the stable patient, there may be justification for applying a large venous or polytetrafluoroethylene (PTFE) patch to relieve the narrowing.

Ligation of the infrarenal inferior vena cava is the preferred technique in patients who are exsanguinating and who would require an extensive repair to maintain patency. It is of interest that ligation is usually well tolerated in young trauma patients as long as certain precautions are taken in the postoperative period. The first is to maintain circulating volume with appropriate fluids because venous return will be compromised until collaterals in the retroperitoneum develop. The second is to apply elastic compression wraps to both lower extremities and keep them elevated for approximately 5 to 7 days after operation. When the patient starts to ambulate, these wraps should still be worn. The presence of residual edema, even with the wraps in place, at the time the patient is to be discharged should be treated with full-length custom-made support hose.

Ligation of the suprarenal inferior vena cava is performed only when the patient has an extensive injury at this location and appears to have terminal shock at operation. While there have been isolated reports of survivors with ligation at this level, it is best to perform a reoperation on such a patient if his condition stabilizes in the early postoperative period and reconstruct the suprarenal inferior vena cava to prevent postoperative renal failure. Dacron prostheses have been used on an acute basis in the past for injuries at this location, but long-term data on patency are not available (29). At the present time an appropriate choice would be an externally supported PTFE graft, which of course could also be used for replacement of the infrarenal inferior vena cava under the same exceptional circumstances (30).

Survival rates for patients with injuries to the inferior vena cava vary depending on which location of injury is being discussed. If injuries to the suprahepatic and retrohepatic vena cava are eliminated from six recent series, the average survival for 495 patients with injuries to the infrahepatic inferior vena cava was 70.5 per cent (20,25,31–34) (Table 34–2). When injuries to the infrarenal inferior vena cava alone are included, the average survival for 318 patients was 75.5 per cent (20,25,31–34) (Table 34–2).

Injuries to the Renal Vein

If a patient presents with a contained hematoma or active hemorrhage in the lateral perirenal area of the upper abdomen, injury to either the renal artery, renal vein, both, or the kidney should be suspected. In patients who have suffered blunt abdominal trauma and have a normal preoperative IVP, renal arteriogram, or computed tomography (CT) of the kidneys, there is no justification for performing a celiotomy in the absence of other injuries, or for exploring the kidney through its hematoma at the time of celiotomy for other injuries. Presumably, some of these patients have avulsion of branches off the renal vein, but the hemorrhage is contained by the perirenal hematoma and no operative therapy is necessary.

TABLE 34–2. Injuries to the Inferior Vena Cava

REFERENCE	YEAR	VENA CAVAL LOCATION	NO. OF PATIENTS	NO. OF SURVIVORS	% SURVIVAL
Turpin et al. (31)	1977	Suprarenal	9	4	44.4
		Renal	5	3	60.0
		Infrarenal	10	7	70.0
Graham et al. (32)	1978	Renal	30	25	83.3
		Infrarenal	98	74	75.5
Kashuk et al. (20)	1982	Suprarenal	7	4	57.1
		Renal	12	9	75.0
		Infrarenal	22	16	72.7
Kudsk et al. (33)	1984	Suprarenal	18	16	88.8
		Renal	1	0	0.0
		Infrarenal	12	11	91.6
Wiencek and Wilson (34)	1986	Suprarenal	22	10	45.5
		Renal	4	3	75.0
		Infrarenal	14	6	42.9
Burch et al. (25)	1988	Suprarenal	32	17	53.1
		Renal	37	18	48.6
		Infrarenal	129	107	82.9
		Bifurcation	33	19	57.6
Overall			495	349	70.5

As previously noted, blunt avulsion injuries of the left perirenal vein usually result in exsanguination, and early operation with vascular control either by ligation of the left renal vein near the vena cava or by left nephrectomy is necessary to obtain hemostasis.

In the patient with a penetrating wound to the flank and no preoperative staging of a potential renal injury with radiologic studies, the surgeon is obliged to open the perirenal hematoma in order to completely explore the bullet or stab wound tract. If the hematoma is not rapidly expanding and there is no free intraabdominal bleeding, most trauma surgeons will loop the ipsilateral renal artery with an umbilical tape in the midline at the base of the mesocolon. Should the hematoma be in the left perirenal area, the left renal vein can also be looped with an umbilical tape in the midline location; however, vascular control of the proximal right renal vein will have to wait for mobilization of the C-loop of the duodenum as well as unroofing of the vena cava at its junction with the renal veins. Atala et al's recent report from Louisville (35) suggested that preliminary renovascular control is not as critical for salvage of the kidney as has been reported in the past. If there is active bleeding from the renovascular structures in the retroperitoneum, in the renal pelvis, or from the kidney itself, no central renovascular control is necessary. Rather, the retroperitoneum lateral to the injured kidney is opened and the kidney is elevated directly into the midline wound with blunt and sharp dissection. A large vascular clamp can be applied proximal to the hilum either at the midline of the body on the left or just lateral to the inferior vena cava on the right to control any further bleeding. The preferred technique for the usual lateral perforation of the renal vein from a penetrating wound is venorrhaphy with 5-0 polypropylene suture in a transverse fashion. If an extensive injury of the right renal vein is present and ligation is necessary to control hemorrhage, nephrectomy should be performed. Many authors, however, believe that the medial left renal vein over the aorta can be ligated as long as the left adrenal and left gonadal veins are intact (36). In some series of elective vascular procedures in which this maneuver has been used, postoperative renal complications have been noted to occur (37).

The survival rate for patients with injuries to the renal veins from penetrating trauma has ranged from 42 to 88 per cent in the recent literature, with the differences due to magnitude and number of associated visceral and vascular injuries (38). In Brown's series from the Ben Taub General Hospital in Houston, patients with isolated renal vein injuries had a 12 per cent mortality rate. In those patients with injuries to both the renal artery and renal vein, mortality was 17.4 per cent (38).

Injuries to the Iliac Vein

In patients with blunt trauma, the presence of a pelvic hematoma in the absence of diminished pulses in the femoral arteries in the groins suggests injury to branches of the iliac veins secondary to the fracture. It is generally accepted that hemorrhage from sites of fractures may be slowed or stopped by the application of a PASG (10–13,39) or early skeletal fixation (40–42), whereas venous hemorrhage from venous plexuses or smaller veins should be tamponaded by the intact retroperitoneum (6,39). Therefore, stable patients without evidence of intraperitoneal injuries on physical examination, diagnostic peritoneal lavage, arteriography, or CT can be managed nonoperatively when retroperitoneal hematomas overlying iliac venous injuries from pelvic fractures are present. In rare patients, exsanguinating hemorrhage from a major injury to an iliac vein associated with rupture of the retroperitoneal hematoma may demand immediate laparotomy.

In the patient with a pelvic hematoma or hemorrhage after penetrating trauma, compression with a laparotomy pad or finger is maintained as proximal and distal vascular control is attained. Because it is frequently unknown whether the iliac artery, iliac vein, or both are injured under the hematoma, it is common practice to gain proximal and distal vascular control of both vessels if the hematoma is intact. The proximal common iliac arteries and veins are exposed by eviscerating the small bowel to the right and dividing the midline retroperitoneum over the aortic bifurcation. In the usual young trauma patient, there is no adherence of the common iliac artery and vein and umbilical tapes can be passed rapidly around the proximal arteries at this location. As passage of an umbilical tape around the proximal common iliac vein is somewhat more dangerous because of its thin wall, a vascular clamp can be applied at this point should injury to the iliac vein be found. Distal vascular control of the external iliac vessels is obtained where both come out of the pelvis proximal to the inguinal ligament. Because of the difficulty in gaining proximal control of the right common iliac vein underneath the right common iliac artery, it has been suggested that this artery be transected and the aortic bifurcation mobilized to the left to allow for complete visualization of the vein at its junction with the inferior vena cava (43). In a similar fashion, transection and ligation of the internal iliac artery on either side of the pelvis will allow for improved exposure of an injured ipsilateral internal iliac vein (44).

Injuries to the iliac veins are treated with either lateral repair using 5-0 polypropylene suture or ligation. Lateral repair frequently results in extensive narrowing and, much as with the inferior vena cava, thrombosis underneath the repair is likely in the postoperative period. Therefore, with an extensive injury, ligation is used because it is well tolerated in younger patients in the author's experience. Should ligation be chosen the same precautions that have previously been described after ligation of the inferior vena cava are applied. The survival rate of patients with injuries to the iliac veins once again depends on whether an associated injury to the iliac artery is present, but has been approximately 75 per cent in 141 patients reviewed in four recent series (24, 45–47) (Table 34–3). When isolated injury to the iliac vein is present, survival has been as high as 95 per cent.

TABLE 34–3.   Injuries to the Iliac Vein

REFERENCE	YEAR	NO. OF PATIENTS	NO. OF SURVIVORS	% SURVIVAL
Mattox et al. (45)	1978	16 (8)[a]	11 (8)[a]	68.8 (100.0)[a]
Millikan et al. (46)	1981	97 (48)[a]	71 (45)[a]	73.2 (93.8)[a]
Ryan et al. (47)	1982	28	23	82.1
Sirinek et al. (24)	1983	141 (56)[a]	105 (53)[a]	74.5 (94.6)[a]

[a] Isolated injury to iliac vein.

Injuries to the Portal Vein

A hematoma or area of hemorrhage in the region of the portal triad may contain an injury to the portal vein, hepatic artery, both, or vascular injury in combination with an injury to the common bile duct. When a hematoma is present, the proximal hepatoduodenal ligament should be looped with an umbilical tape or a noncrushing vascular clamp should be applied (Pringle maneuver) before the hematoma is entered. If hemorrhage is occurring, finger compression of the vessels will suffice until the vascular clamp is in place. Because the porta is short in many patients, it may be impossible to place a distal vascular clamp right at the edge of the liver. Therefore, manual compression with forceps may allow for distal vascular control until the area of injury can be isolated. Because of the proximity of the common bile duct, vascular repairs should not be performed in the porta until the exact area of injury is precisely defined.

The posterior position of the portal vein in the hepatoduodenal ligament makes exposure somewhat more difficult than it is for injuries to the hepatic artery. An extensive Kocher maneuver, coupled with mobilization of the common bile duct to the left and the cystic duct superiorly, usually allows for excellent visualization of any suprapancreatic injury after proximal (and, if possible, distal) vascular control has been obtained. Should there be a perforation in the retropancreatic portion of the portal vein, the neck of the pancreas may need to be divided for full exposure of the injury. This is performed by having an assistant compress the superior mesenteric vein below and applying a vascular clamp to the hepatoduodenal ligament above while the surgeon divides the pancreas over the portal vein using two straight, noncrushing intestinal or slightly angled vascular clamps.

Injuries to any portion of the portal vein are difficult to manage because of its posterior location, the friability of the wall, and the volume of blood flow. Lateral venorrhaphy with 5-0 polypropylene suture is preferred. Other extensive maneuvers that have been attempted and occasionally used with success include resection with an end-to-end anastomosis, interposition grafting, transposition of the splenic vein down to the superior mesenteric vein, an end-to-side portacaval shunt, or a venovenous shunt from the superior mesenteric vein to the distal portal vein or inferior vena cava. Such vigorous attempts at restoration of flow have resulted from a concern about viability of the midgut if the portal vein is ligated. It should be remembered, however, that ligation is compatible with survival, as

TABLE 34–4.   Injuries to the Portal Vein

REFERENCE	YEAR	NO. OF PATIENTS	NO. OF SURVIVORS	% SURVIVAL
Graham et al. (49)	1978	37	18	48.6
Petersen et al. (50)	1979	28	17	60.7
Stone et al. (22)	1982	41	22	53.7
Kashuk et al. (20)	1982	9	3	33.3
Sirinek et al. (24)	1983	5	0	0.0
Ivatury et al. (51)	1987	14	7	50.0
Overall		134	67	50.0

both Pachter et al. (48) and Stone et al. (22) have emphasized in recent years. The series by Stone et al. in 1982 included nine survivors out of 18 patients who underwent ligation of the portal vein (22). Ligation should be restricted to those patients who have an extensive injury to the portal vein and are hypothermic and acidotic. The surgeon must then be prepared to infuse tremendous amounts of fluids to reverse the transient peripheral hypovolemia secondary to splanchnic hypervolemia, as previously mentioned for ligation of the superior mesenteric vein.

The survival rate of 134 patients with injuries to the portal vein in recent series has been approximately 50 per cent (20,22,24,49–51) (Table 34–4).

Injuries to the Retrohepatic Vena Cava and Hepatic Veins

Juxtahepatic venous injuries are extraordinarily rare, even in the busiest trauma centers. When patients with these injuries present, the intraoperative diagnosis is often delayed and exsanguination occurs before vascular control can be obtained. The indecision of the surgeon in caring for patients like these is compounded by the complex anatomy surrounding the retrohepatic vena cava and hepatic veins.

Injuries to the retrohepatic vena cava or hepatic veins are characterized by massive dark venous bleeding from beneath the liver that increases as the overlying lobe is mobilized out of its fossa. Should the surgeon recognize this injury, there are a number of options that are available to perform venorrhaphy and prevent further exsanguination. Direct lateral approaches to the hepatic veins and retrohepatic vena cava are successful in some children because of the lack of surrounding soft tissue and the ease of mobilization of the overlying lobe of the liver. In adults, direct approaches laterally and through a deep hepatotomy site have been successful in salvage of critically injured patients in recent years (52). Other authors have chosen to use sequential vascular clamping of all major inflow and outflow structures of the liver, or insertion of an internal caval shunt through the inferior vena cava below the liver. Recent reports, however, continue to suggest that the atriocaval shunt originally described in 1968 is the most effective way to divert venous flow away from the area of the perforation.

If the surgeon chooses to use an atriocaval shunt the midline laparotomy incision is extended to a median sternotomy. If a no. 36 French chest tube is to be used as the shunt, an umbilical tape loop is passed around the suprarenal inferior vena cava in the abdomen and another around the intrapericardial inferior vena cava (Fig. 34–2). A 2-0 silk pursestring sutuure is then placed in the right atrial appendage of the heart over a Satinsky vascular clamp. Prior to insertion of the no. 36 chest tube an extra hole must be cut in the chest tube approximately 20 cm from the last hole and a clamp should be applied to the open end of the chest tube. The Satinsky clamp is removed and the atriocaval shunt is rapidly inserted into the right atrium and directed into the infrarenal inferior vena cava in the abdomen. Care must be taken not to have the shunt exit through a perforating wound in the retrohepatic vena cava during passage (53). When all holes in the shunt are outside of the umbilical tapes and the newly cut hole is at the level of the right atrium, the umbilical tapes are pulled tight, thereby forcing blood from the lower half of the body and the kidneys through the shunt. The operative field is far from bloodless at this point because of the large number of hepatic veins

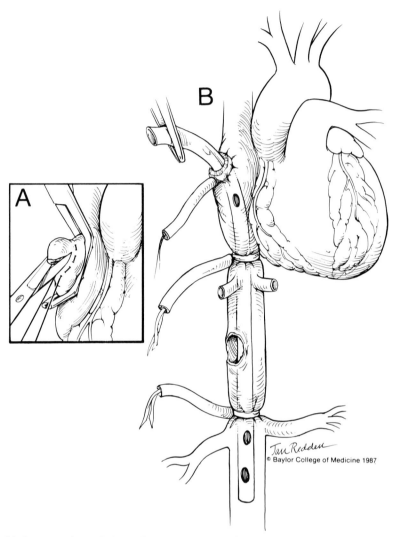

Figure 34–2. *A*, Atriocaval shunt: Satinsky clamp applied to right atrial appendage, and 2-0 silk pursestring suture inserted. *B*, Final position of no. 36 chest tube. All holes in the shunt, including the extra one cut at the level of the right atrium, are outside the umbilical tapes. This forces blood from the lower half of the body and the kidneys through the shunt.

that enter into the retrohepatic vena cava, many of which will still be flowing despite the use of a Pringle maneuver. More recently Rovito has described the use of an endotracheal tube shunt inserted through the atrium, with inflation of the balloon just above the renal veins in the abdomen (54) (Fig. 34–3).

In Burch's report from the Ben Taub General Hospital in 1988, six of 18 patients who had a chest tube atriocaval shunt inserted for penetrating wounds and did not require resuscitative thoracotomy survived during an 11-year period (53). Rovito has had even more impressive results using an endotracheal tube shunt, with four of eight patients surviving after insertion of the shunt for blunt juxtahepatic venous injuries during a 5-year period (54).

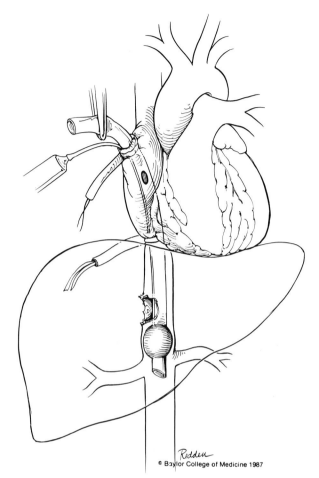

Figure 34–3. No. 8 or 9 endotracheal tube used as an atriocaval shunt.

© Baylor College of Medicine 1987

ACKNOWLEDGMENT: The author acknowledges the technical assistance of Bonnie Landrock.

REFERENCES

1. DeBakey ME, Simeone FA: Battle injuries of the arteries in World War II. An analysis of 2,471 cases. Ann Surg 1946;*123*:534–579.
2. Rich NM, Baugh JH, Hughes CW: Acute arterial injuries in Vietnam: 1,000 cases. J Trauma 1970;*10*:359–369.
3. Feliciano DV, Bitondo CG, Mattox KL, et al: Civilian trauma in the 1980's. A 1-year experience with 456 vascular and cardiac injuries. Ann Surg 1984;*199*:717–724.
4. Mattox KL, Feliciano DV, Burch JM, et al: Five thousand seven hundred sixty cardiovascular injuries in 4459 patients. Epidemiologic evolution 1958 to 1987. Ann Surg 1989;*209*:698–707.
5. Feliciano DV: Abdominal vascular injuries. Surg Clin North Am 1988;*68*:741–755.
6. Mucha P Jr: Pelvic fractures. *In* Mattox KL, Moore EE, Feliciano DV, eds: Trauma. East Norwalk, CT, Appleton & Lange, 1988;505–518.
7. Rich NM, Hobson RW II, Fedde CW: Vascular trauma secondary to diagnostic and therapeutic procedures. Am J Surg 1974;*128*:715–721.
8. McDonald PT, Rich NM, Collins GJ Jr, et al: Vascular trauma secondary to diagnostic and therapeutic procedures: Laparoscopy. Am J Surg 1978;*135*:651–655.
9. Feliciano DV, Burch JM, Spjut-Patrinely V, et al: Abdominal gunshot wounds: An urban trauma center's experience with 300 consecutive patients. Ann Surg 1988;*208*:362–370.

10. Batalden DJ, Wickstrom PH, Ruiz E: Value of the G-suit in patient with severe pelvic fracture. Arch Surg 1974;*109*:326–328.
11. Flint LM Jr, Brown A, Richardson JD, et al: Definitive control of bleeding from severe pelvic fractures. Ann Surg 1979;*189*:709–716.
12. Yap SNL: The management of traumatic pelvic retroperitoneal hemorrhage. Surgical Rounds 1980;*3*:34–42.
13. Dove AF, Poon WS, Weston PAM: Hemorrhage from pelvic fractures: Dangers and treatment. Injury 1982;*13*:375–381.
14. Mattox KL, Bickell W, Pepe PE, et al: Prospective MAST study in 911 patients. J Trauma 1989; *29*:1104–1112.
15. Feliciano DV, Bitondo CG, Cruse PA, et al: Liberal use of emergency center thoracotomy. Am J Surg 1986;*152*:654–659.
16. Fried SJ, Satiani B, Lech P: Normothermic rapid volume replacement for hypovolemic shock: An in vivo and in vitro study utilizing a new technique. J Trauma 1986;*26*:183–188.
17. Luna GK, Maier RV, Pavlin EG, et al: Incidence and effect of hypothermia in seriously injured patients. J Trauma 1987;*27*:1014–1018.
18. Jurkovich GJ, Greiser WB, Luterman A, et al: Hypothermia in trauma victims: An ominous predictor of survival. J Trauma 1987;*27*:1019–1024.
19. Feliciano DV, Pachter HL: Hepatic trauma revisited. Curr Prob Surg 1989;*26*:453–524.
20. Kashuk JL, Moore EE, Millikan JS, et al: Major abdominal vascular trauma—a unified approach. J Trauma 1982;*22*:672–679.
21. Graham JM, Mattox KL, Beall AC Jr: Portal venous system injuries. J Trauma 1978;*18*:419–422.
22. Stone HH, Fabian TC, Turkleson ML: Wounds of the portal venous system. World J Surg 1982; *6*:335–341.
23. Donahue TK, Strauch GO: Ligation as definitive management of injury to the superior mesenteric vein. J Trauma 1988;*28*:541–543.
24. Sirinek KR, Gaskill HV III, Root HD, et al: Truncal vascular injury—factors influencing survival. J Trauma 1983;*23*:372–377.
25. Burch JM, Feliciano DV, Mattox KL, et al: Injuries of the inferior vena cava. Am J Surg 1988; *156*:548–552.
26. Ravikumar S, Stahl WM: Intraluminal balloon catheter occlusion for major vena cava injuries. J Trauma 1985;*25*:458–460.
27. Linker RW, Crawford FA Jr, Rittenbury MS, et al: Traumatic aortocaval fistula: Case Report. J Trauma 1989;*29*:255–257.
28. Feliciano DV, Burch JM, Mattox KL, et al: Balloon catheter tamponade in cardiovascular wounds. Am J Surg (in press).
29. Mattox KL, McCollum WB, Jordan GL Jr, et al: Management of upper abdominal vascular trauma. Am J Surg 1974;*128*:823–827.
30. Dale WA, Harris J, Terry RB: Polytetrafluoroethylene reconstruction of the inferior vena cava. Surgery 1984;*95*:625–630.
31. Turpin I, State D, Schwartz A: Injuries to the inferior vena cava and their management. Am J Surg 1977;*134*:25–32.
32. Graham JM, Mattox KL, Beall AC Jr: Traumatic injuries of the inferior vena cava. Arch Surg 1978;*113*:413–418.
33. Kudsk KA, Bongard F, Lim RC Jr: Determinants of survival after vena caval injury. Analysis of a 14-year experience. Arch Surg 1984;*119*:1009–1012.
34. Wiencek RG, Wilson RF: Abdominal venous injuries. J Trauma 1986;*26*:771–778.
35. Atala A, Miller FB, Richardson JD, et al: Preliminary vascular control for renal trauma: Is it necessary? Presented at the 68th Annual Meeting, American College of Surgeons Committee on Trauma, 1990 Residents' Trauma Papers Competition, Washington DC, March 15, 1990.
36. James EC, Fedde CW, Khuri NT, et al: Division of the left renal vein: A safe surgical adjunct. Surgery 1978;*83*:151–154.
37. Rastad J, Almgren B, Bowald S, et al: Renal complications to left renal vein ligation in abdominal aortic surgery. J Cardiovasc Surg 1984;*25*:432–435.
38. Brown MF, Graham JM, Mattox KL, et al: Renovascular trauma. Am J Surg 1980;*140*:802–805.
39. Moreno C, Moore EE, Rosenberger A, et al: Hemorrhage associated with major pelvic fracture: A multispecialty challenge. J Trauma 1986;*26*:987–994.
40. Mears DC, Fu FH: Modern concept of external skeletal fixation of the pelvis. Clin Orthop 1980; *151*:65–72.
41. Wild JJ, Hanson GW, Tullos HS: Unstable fractures of the pelvis treated by external fixation. J Bone Joint Surg [Am] 1982;*64*:1010–1020.
42. Gylling SF, Ward RE, Holcroft JW, et al: Immediate external fixation of unstable pelvic fractures. Am J Surg 1985;*150*:721–724.

43. Salam AA, Stewart MT: New approach to wounds of the aortic bifurcation and inferior vena cava. Surgery 1985;98:105–108.
44. Vitelli CE, Scalea TM, Phillips TF, et al: A technique for controlling injuries of the iliac vein in the patient with trauma. Surg Gynecol Obstet 1988;166:551–552.
45. Mattox KL, Rea J, Ennix CL, et al: Penetrating injuries to the iliac arteries. Am J Surg 1978; 136:663–667.
46. Millikan JS, Moore EE, Van Way CW III, et al: Vascular trauma in the groin: Contrast between iliac and femoral injuries. Am J Surg 1981;142:695–698.
47. Ryan W, Snyder W III, Bell T, et al: Penetrating injuries of the iliac vessels. Am J Surg 1982; 144:642–645.
48. Pachter HL, Drager S, Godfrey N, et al: Traumatic injuries of the portal vein. Ann Surg 1979; 189:383–385.
49. Graham JM, Mattox KL, Beall AC Jr: Portal venous system injuries. J Trauma 1978;18:418–422.
50. Petersen SR, Sheldon GF, Lim RC Jr: Management of portal vein injuries. J Trauma 1979;19:616–620.
51. Ivatury RR, Nallathambi M, Lankin DH, et al: Portal vein injuries. Noninvasive follow-up of venorrhaphy. Ann Surg 1987;206:733–737.
52. Pachter HL, Spencer FC, Hofstetter SR, et al: The management of juxtahepatic venous injuries without an atriocaval shunt. Preliminary clinical observations. Surgery 1986;99:569–575.
53. Burch JM, Feliciano DV, Mattox KL: The atriocaval shunt. Facts and fiction. Ann Surg 1988; 207:555–568.
54. Rovito PF: Atrial caval shunting in blunt hepatic vascular injury. Ann Surg 1987;205:318–321.

XI

SURGERY OF THE VENA CAVA

35

NONTHROMBOTIC DISEASE OF THE INFERIOR VENA CAVA: Surgical Management of 24 Patients

Edouard Kieffer, Amine Bahnini, and Fabien Koskas

Surgery of the inferior vena cava (IVC) has long been limited to ligation, resection, or lateral suture. Although these techniques have been successful in a number of patients with diseases of the infrarenal segment of the IVC, reconstructive surgery remains mandatory in most patients with diseases of the retrohepatic or suprahepatic segments of the IVC.

A large variety of replacement material has been tried both experimentally (1–4) and in a few clinical cases (5–11). Only recently has some success been obtained with reinforced polytetrafluoroethylene (PTFE) grafts in experimental animals. This has led us to extend our indications for prosthetic replacement or bypass for the IVC. The present chapter is a review of our recent experience with the surgical management of nonthrombotic diseases of the IVC, with special emphasis placed on reconstructive procedures.

PATIENTS AND METHODS

From January 1981 to May 1990 we have surgically treated 24 patients with nonthrombotic diseases of the IVC (Table 35–1). Among the 17 patients with tumors of the IVC, seven had primary tumors (i.e., leiomyosarcomas) and 11 had secondary tumors (10 arising from renal carcinoma and one from a nonsecreting adrenal carcinoma). Six patients had membranous obstructions of the IVC at the diaphragmatic level, with hepatic consequences similar to the Budd-Chiari syndrome. The upper level of caval involvement was used to classify these lesions, with the IVC being divided into three segments: infrarenal, suprarenal (retrohepatic), and suprahepatic (Fig. 35–1). Most tumors involved the retrohepatic segment (Figs. 35–2 through 35–4). All the membranous obstructions were located in the suprahepatic segment (Figs. 35–5 and 35–6). Two of them were associated with occlusion of the entire IVC due to secondary thrombosis (Fig. 35–7).

All patients underwent inferior vena cavography. In patients with complete occlusion of the IVC, retrograde cavography was used in an attempt to define

TABLE 35–1.   Personal Experience with Nonthrombotic Diseases of the Inferior Vena Cava (1981–1990)

SEGMENT	PRIMARY TUMORS (n = 7)	SECONDARY TUMORS (n = 11)	MEMBRANOUS OBSTRUCTIONS (n = 6)
I. Infrarenal	1	1	—
II. Suprarenal	5	6	—
III. Suprahepatic	1	4	6

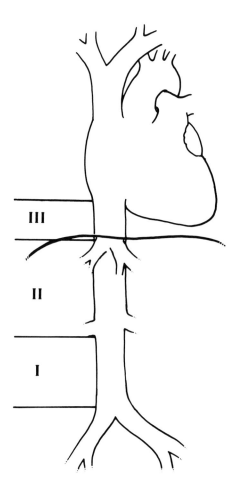

Figure 35–1.   Classification of IVC into three segments: I (infrarenal), II (suprarenal), and III (suprahepatic).

Figure 35–2.   Tumor extension into IVC from right renal carcinoma. *A*, Inferior vena cavography showing thrombus into suprarenal IVC. *B*, Computed tomography scan showing right renal carcinoma and tumor thrombus in IVC.
This patient had right radical nephrectomy and resection of the infra- and suprarenal IVC without reconstruction.

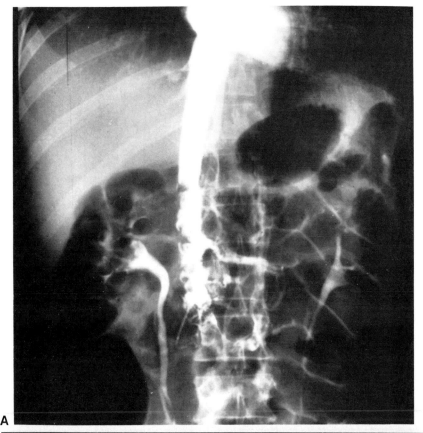

A

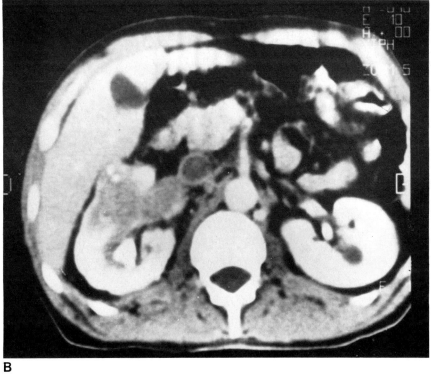

B

Figure 35–2. See legend on opposite page.

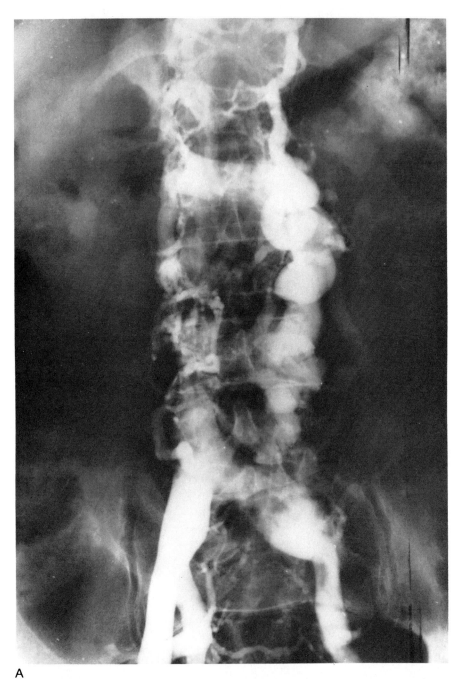

A

Figure 35–3. Leiomyosarcoma involving IVC to segment II. *A*, Ascending inferior vena cavography showing complete obstruction of infrarenal IVC and collateral circulation through left iliolumbar and left renal veins. (*continued*)

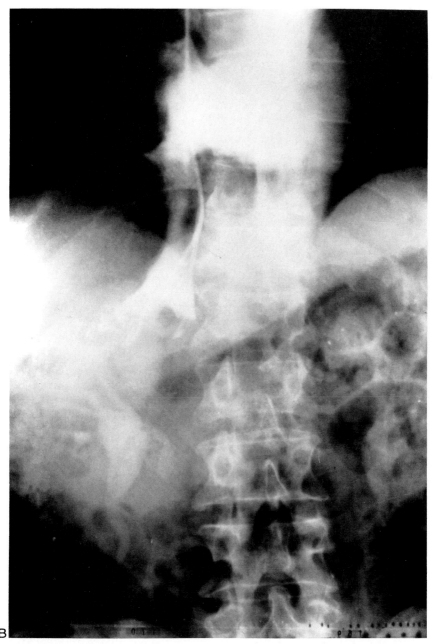

Figure 35–3. *B*, Descending inferior vena cavography showing proximal extension of the tumor. (*continued*)

the upper limit of caval occlusion and possible involvement of the hepatic veins (Fig. 35–3). Selective celiac and mesenteric arteriography as well as computed tomography (CT) scan proved very useful in patients with primary or secondary tumors involving the retrohepatic segment of the IVC (Figs. 35–2 through 35–4). Magnetic resonance imaging was used in five recent cases (Fig. 35–4).

Infrahepatic tumors were approached through a midline or bilateral infra-

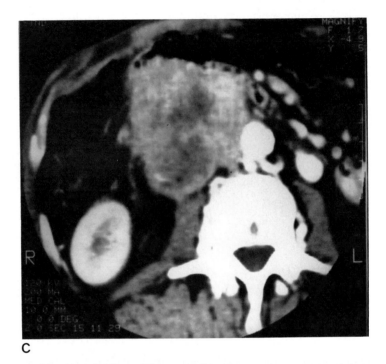

C

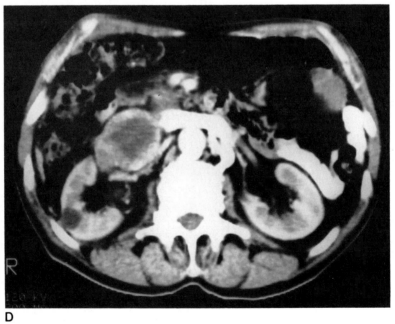

D

Figure 35–3. *C,* Computed tomography scan showing large tumor of the infrarenal IVC. *D,* Computed tomography scan showing upper part of the tumor distending the IVC. The left renal vein is patent. This patient had right radical nephrectomy and resection of the infra- and suprarenal IVC without reconstruction.

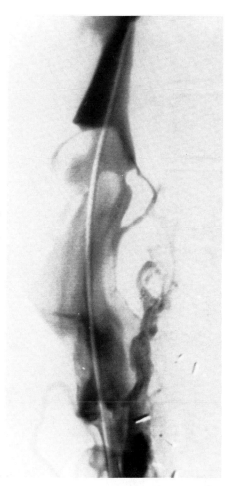

Figure 35–4. Leiomyosarcoma extending to segment III of the IVC. *A*, Inferior vena cavography showing tumor of retrohepatic segment of the IVC. *B*, Computed tomography scan showing large tumor extending to the left hepatic lobe. (*continued*)

A

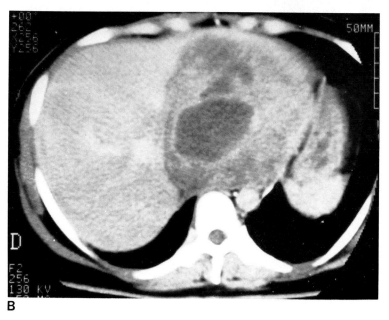

B

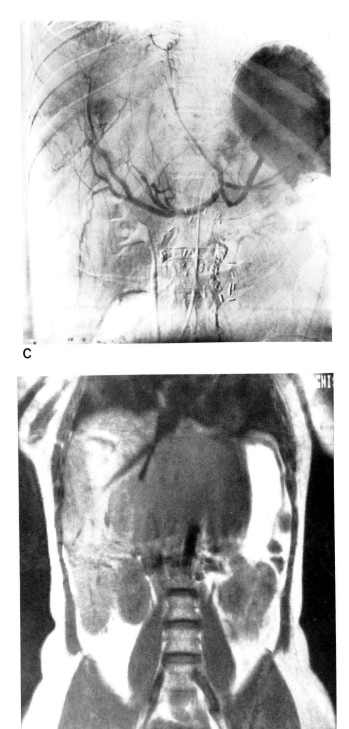

Figure 35–4. *C*, Selective arteriography delineating a large hypovascularized tumor of the left hepatic lobe. *D*, Magnetic resonance imaging scan showing extension of the tumor up to the left and median hepatic veins. This patient had resection of the tumor, including left hepatic lobe, and reconstruction of segments II and III of the IVC using PTFE (Gore-Tex) graft.

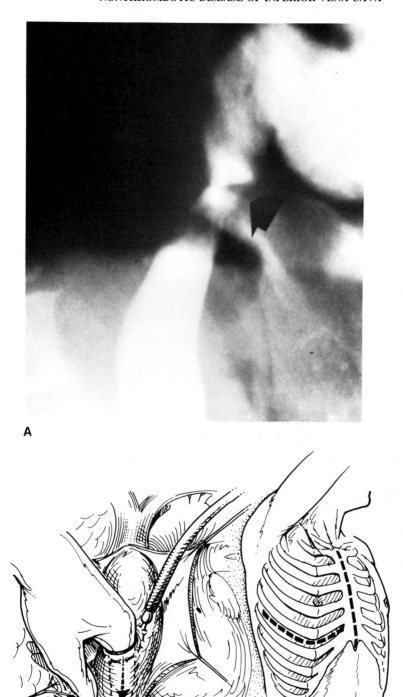

Figure 35–5.   Incomplete membranous obstruction of the suprahepatic IVC. *A*, Inferior vena cavography showing stenosis of the suprahepatic IVC (arrow). *B*, Diagram showing treatment by transatrial membranotomy.

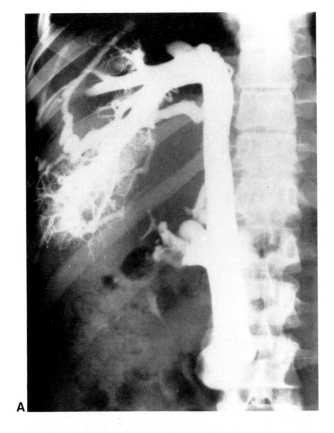

A

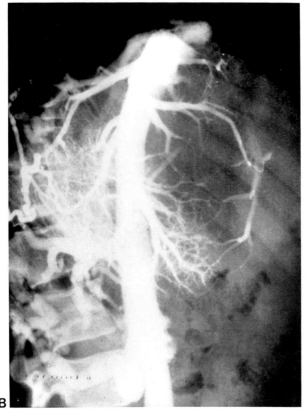

B

Figure 35–6. Complete membranous obstruction of the suprahepatic IVC. Inferior vena cavography in anteroposterior (*A*) and lateral (*B*) views shows occlusion of the suprahepatic IVC with massive reflux into the right hepatic vein. (*continued*)

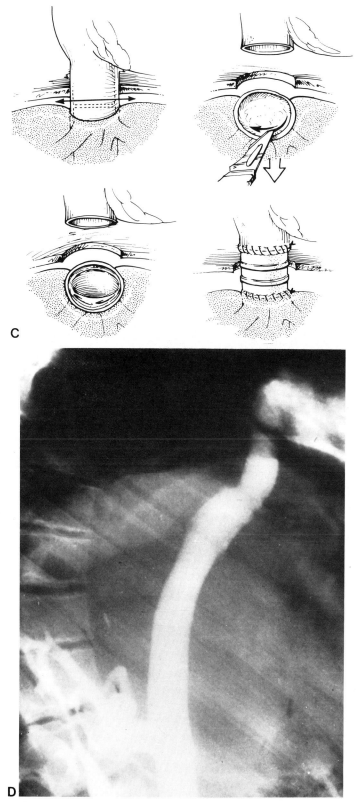

Figure 35–6. *C*, Diagram showing treatment by resection of the membrane, direct control of hepatic veins, and segmental replacement using reinforced PTFE (Gore-Tex). *D*, Postoperative inferior vena cavography showing patency of the reconstruction.

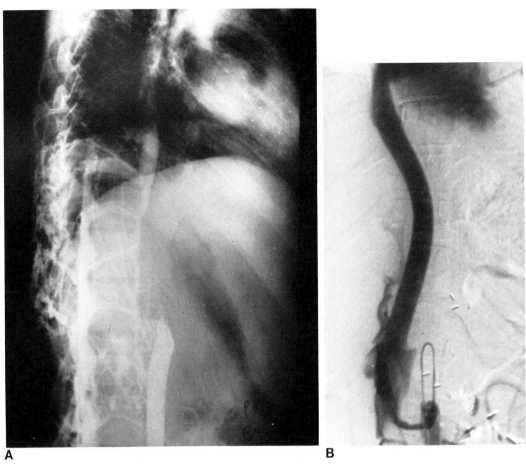

Figure 35–7. Complete membranous obstruction of the IVC with distal thrombotic occlusion. *A*, Lateral view of inferior vena cavography showing extensive occlusion of the IVC with collateral circulation through the spinal veins. *B*, Postoperative inferior vena cavography showing patency of cavoatrial bypass using reinforced PTFE (Gore-Tex) with proximal arteriovenous fistula.

costal laparotomy. Lesions of the retrohepatic or suprahepatic segments of the IVC were approached using a thoracoabdominal incision. Right thoracophreno-laparotomy was used in the earlier cases, whereas midline sternotomy combined with either midline or bilateral infracostal laparotomy was preferred in the more recent ones. Vascular exclusion of the liver was performed without cardiopulmonary bypass, external shunts, or cold hepatic perfusion (8). An autotransfusion device (Cell-saver, Haemonetics) was used during the last 5 years. Surgical management varied according to the nature and site of the caval lesions (Table 35–2). Thrombectomy was performed in five patients with secondary renal (four) or adrenal (one) tumors. Resection of the IVC was performed in seven patients with primary (four) or secondary (three) tumors (Fig. 35–3). In a patient with leiomyosarcoma of the anterior aspect of the IVC at the level of the renal veins, reconstruction of the IVC using autogenous vein patch angioplasty obtained from the infrarenal IVC was performed in order to preserve patency of the right renal vein, thus avoiding unnecessary right nephrectomy (9). Four patients with primary (two) or secondary (two) tumors had PTFE (Gore-Tex) replacement of the IVC,

TABLE 35–2. Vascular Procedures Performed in 24 Patients with Nonthrombotic Diseases of the Inferior Vena Cava

PROCEDURE	PRIMARY TUMORS ($n = 7$)	SECONDARY TUMORS ($n = 11$)	MEMBRANOUS OBSTRUCTIONS ($n = 6$)
Resection	4	3	—
Thrombectomy	—	5	—
Membranotomy	—	—	1
Patch angioplasty	1	0	0
Graft replacement[a]	2	2	3
Bypass[a]	—	1[b]	2

[a] PTFE (Gore-Tex).
[b] Palliative mesoatrial bypass.

using a nonreinforced graft in one case and a reinforced graft in the three most recent cases. Finally, one patient with secondary Budd-Chiari syndrome due to caval extension of renal carcinoma had a PTFE (Gore-Tex) mesoatrial shunt.

All patients with membranous obstructions had reconstructive procedures. One patient with a tight, short stenosis at the diaphragmatic level had a transcardiac membranotomy using a mitral commissurotomy dilator (Fig. 35–5). Three patients with complete occlusions limited to the suprahepatic segment of the IVC had short prosthetic replacements using reinforced PTFE (Gore-Tex) grafts (Fig. 35–6). Two patients with extensive retrograde occlusions complicating membranous obstructions had long cavoatrial bypasses. One had a prehepatic bypass using a nonreinforced PTFE graft and the other had a left retrohepatic bypass using a reinforced PTFE graft (Fig. 35–7).

Associated procedures (Table 35–3) included two right and one left hepatic lobectomy, all in patients with leiomyosarcomas involving the retrohepatic segment of the IVC. Right nephrectomy was performed in 10 patients with either right renal carcinoma or secondary involvement of the right renal pedicle. Right adrenalectomy was performed in the patient with adrenal tumor. In one patient with extensive occlusion of the IVC due to membranous obstruction a significant portocaval gradient persisted following reconstruction of the IVC. Associated portal decompression was therefore performed using an "H"-shaped PTFE graft inserted between the mesenteric vein and the caval bypass. An arteriovenous fistula using a calibrated saphenous vein graft was constructed immediately distal to the lower anastomosis in the last four patients with prosthetic reconstruction of the infrarenal or retrohepatic segments of the IVC (Fig. 35–7).

TABLE 35–3. Associated Procedures Performed in 24 Patients with Nonthrombotic Diseases of the Inferior Vena Cava

ASSOCIATED PROCEDURE	PRIMARY TUMORS ($n = 7$)	SECONDARY TUMORS ($n = 11$)	MEMBRANOUS OBSTRUCTIONS ($n = 6$)
Hepatic lobectomy	3	0	—
Right nephrectomy	2	8	—
Right adrenalectomy	—	1	—
Portal decompression	—	—	1
Distal arteriovenous fistula	1	2	1

TABLE 35–4. Surgical Results in 24 Patients with Nonthrombotic Diseases of the Inferior Vena Cava

	TUMORS (n = 18)	MEMBRANOUS OBSTRUCTIONS (n = 6)
Postoperative mortality	2	0
Mean follow-up (months)	52.8	27.5
Late mortality	7	1
Patent caval reconstructions	5/5	5/6

RESULTS

Two patients died in the early postoperative period (Table 35–4). One patient died from hepatic failure following palliative mesoatrial shunt for Budd-Chiari syndrome due to caval extension of renal carcinoma. The other patient developed a duodenal fistula following removal of a large leiomyosarcoma that was adherent to the duodenum and pancreas. Despite reoperation and initially adequate control of the fistula, he died on postoperative day 15 following massive gastric hemorrhage due to acute stress ulceration. One patient with graft replacement of the retro- and suprahepatic segments of the IVC remained comatose but without focal neurologic deficit for 2 days before she progressively regained normal consciousness. This complication was interpreted as being secondary to air embolization during surgery. All other patients survived the postoperative period without significant complications.

The 16 surviving patients with primary or secondary tumors have been followed for a mean period of 52.8 months. Seven (54 per cent) of them died during the follow-up period, all as a result of recurrence or dissemination of their malignant tumors. Two of these patients underwent reoperations for local recurrences of their leiomyosarcomas. The nine other patients that were operated on for tumor involvement of the IVC are presently alive, although two of them are currently undergoing chemotherapy for pulmonary metastases.

The six patients with membranous obstructions of the IVC have been followed for a mean period of 27.5 months. The patient with a long cavoatrial bypass using nonreinforced PTFE suddenly developed recurrence of symptoms 8 months postoperatively. Cavography disclosed a thrombosed cavoatrial bypass. She died a few weeks later from a secondarily infected ascitis while under evaluation for a splenoazygos anastomosis. The five other patients with membranous obstructions have remained alive and well. This patient represents the only late anatomic failure in our group of 11 patients with reconstructive procedures of the IVC.

DISCUSSION

Although membranous obstructions of the IVC are rare in Western countries (8,12), their natural history is known from large published series of patients originating from various countries of the Far East or Africa (13–15). Liver congestion is the main feature of disease. It may cause a combination of necrosis and fibrosis of the liver. Death usually occurs during the third or fourth decades of life as a result of liver failure or bleeding from esophageal varices. Occasional patients may develop liver carcinoma (14). This dire prognosis can be prevented by vascular operations directed either to reconstruction of the suprahepatic segment of the IVC or to decompression of the portal circulation (5).

Surgery for tumors of the IVC is more debatable in view of the poor results of surgery in this setting. However, although long-term survivals following surgery for leiomyosarcomas of the IVC remain anecdotal (9), experience with renal carcinoma involving the IVC has shown a 5-year survival rate of approximately 50 per cent, the main prognostic factor being associated lymph node invasion (16–18). Provided the patient is a good surgical risk without (or sometimes despite) distant metastases, we believe that surgery should be offered to all surgically fit patients with both primary and secondary tumors of the IVC.

The classical vascular operative procedure in patients with renal or adrenal carcinoma complicated by tumor thrombus of the IVC has been thrombectomy followed by lateral suture of the IVC (16). Whenever feasible, this approach remains preferable to more complicated procedures. Segmental resection of the IVC has usually been performed in patients with primary tumors of the IVC or invasion of the venous wall by secondary tumors. Although resection of the IVC is well tolerated in patients with complete occlusion and adequate collateral circulation, it may cause chronic venous insufficiency in patients with a patent IVC and poor collateral circulation. Furthermore, because of poor or nonexistent collaterals of the right renal vein, resection of the segment of the IVC into which both renal veins terminate may compel the surgeon to perform an unnecessary right nephrectomy (9). Reconstruction is obviously necessary in patients with tumors involving the suprahepatic segment of the IVC. Besides being mandatory in patients with membranous obstructions, reconstruction of the IVC is thus indicated in a large number of patients with tumors, especially in those involving the suprarenal and suprahepatic segments (9,17). Recent experimental studies have shown that both autogenous vein grafts and reinforced PTFE grafts are satisfactory for replacement of the IVC. The use of composite spiral vein grafts obtained from autogenous saphenous veins is usually impractical in clinical situations, when long segments of the IVC have to be replaced or bypassed. We have therefore used PTFE grafts in our patients. The recent introduction of ring reinforcement has proved very useful in maintaining the graft open against intraabdominal pressure.

We believe that the shorter the graft the better. Segmental replacement of the IVC is thus preferred in patients with tumors or limited membranous obstructions (8,10). This necessitates a direct approach to the IVC using a midline sternotomy and various types of associated abdominal incisions. Vascular exclusion of the liver is feasible and safe using simple clamping with close monitoring of hemodynamic parameters (8). The only logical indication for cardiopulmonary bypass is involvement of the right atrium by a tumor thrombus, usually originating from right renal carcinoma (8,17,18). Long cavoatrial bypasses are easier to construct. However, they should be performed only in patients with extensive occlusion of the IVC due to secondary thrombosis complicating membranous obstructions.

Experimental results have shown a significant improvement in patency with complementary distal arteriovenous fistulas (19). Although it is probably unnecessary in patients with direct reconstruction of the suprahepatic segment of the

IVC, we believe that an arteriovenous fistula should be constructed in patients with long cavoatrial bypasses or segmental replacement of the infrahepatic IVC. The most widely used technique has been to construct a femoral arteriovenous fistula. We prefer a calibrated interposed vein graft placed immediately distal to the lower anastomosis. This allows for optimal flow in the graft while avoiding troublesome venous hypertension in the lower limbs. Calibration of the venous graft prevents excessive flow due to dilatation of the vein and allows for simple secondary nonoperative closure using balloon occlusion whenever indicated.

To date our clinical experience with this modern approach to reconstruction of the IVC has been satisfactory. Although further experience with more patients and a longer follow-up is necessary, we feel encouraged to continue our efforts in this exciting area.

REFERENCES

1. Fiore AC, Brown JW, Cromartie RS, et al: Prosthetic replacement of the thoracic vena cava: An experimental study. J Thorac Cardiovasc Surg 1982;*84*:560–568.
2. Gloviczki P, Hollier LH, Dewanjee MK, et al: Experimental replacement of the inferior vena cava: Factors affecting patency. Surgery 1984;*95*:657–666.
3. Herring M, Gardner A, Pegh P, et al: Patency in canine inferior vena cava grafting: Effects of graft material, size, and endothelial seeding. J Vasc Surg 1984;*1*:877–887.
4. Plate G, Hollier LH, Gloviczki P, et al: Overcoming failure of venous vascular prostheses. Surgery 1984;*96*:503–510.
5. Ahn SS, Yellin A, Sheng FC, et al: Selective surgical therapy of the Budd-Chiari syndrome provides superior survivor rates than conservative medical management. J Vasc Surg 1987; *5*:28–37.
6. Gloviczki P, Pairolero PC, Cherry KJ, Hallett Jr JW: Reconstruction of the vena cava and of its primary tributaries: A preliminary report. J Vasc Surg 1990;*11*:373–381.
7. Katz NM, Spence IJ, Wallace RB: Reconstruction of the inferior vena cava with a polytetra-fluoroethylene tube graft after resection for hypernephroma of the right kidney. J Thorac Cardiovasc Surg 1984;*87*:791–797.
8. Kieffer E, ed: Chirurgie de la Veine Cave Inférieure et de ses Branches. Paris, Expansion Scientifique Française, 1985.
9. Kieffer E, Berrod JL, Chomette G: Primary tumors of the inferior vena cava. *In* Bergan JJ, Yao JST, eds: Surgery of the Veins. New York, Grune & Stratton, 1985;423–443.
10. Laurian C, Cormier JM, Guilmet D: Traitement chirurgical direct des occlusions congénitales de la veine cave inférieure rétrohépatique. Chirurgie 1985;*111*:429–437.
11. Victor S, Jayanthi V, Kandasamy I, et al: Retrohepatic cavoatrial bypass for coarctation of inferior vena cava with a polytetrafluoroethylene graft. J Thorac Cardiovasc Surg 1986;*91*:99–105.
12. Marion P, Vial P, Villard J, et al: Syndrome obstructif du confluent hépato-cave (syndrome de Budd-Chiari): Résultats du traitement chirurgical (à propos de 15 observations). Chirurgie 1982; *108*:365–367.
13. Kimura C, Matsuda S, Koie H, Hirooka M: Membranous obstruction of the hepatic portion of the inferior vena cava: Clinical study of nine cases. Surgery 1972;*72*:551–559.
14. Simson IW: Membranous obstruction of the inferior vena cava and hepatocellular carcinoma in South Africa. Gastroenterology 1982;*82*:171–178.
15. Takeuchi J, Takada A, Hasumura Y, et al: Budd-Chiari syndrome associated with obstruction of the inferior vena cava: A report of seven cases. Am J Med 1971;*51*:11–20.
16. Schefft P, Novick AC, Straffon RA, Stewart HB: Surgery for renal cell carcinoma extending into the inferior vena cava. J Urol 1978;*120*:28–31.
17. Smith BM, Mulherin JL, Sawyers JL, et al: Suprarenal vena caval occlusion: Principles of operative management. Ann Surg 1984;*199*:656–668.
18. Vaislic CD, Puel P, Grondin P, et al: Cancer of the kidney invading the vena cava and heart. J Thorac Cardiovasc Surg 1986;*91*:604–609.
19. Wilson SE, Jabour A, Stone RT, Stanley TM: Patency of biologic and prosthetic inferior vena cava graft with distal limb fistula. Arch Surg 1978;*113*:1174–1179.

36

RECONSTRUCTION OF THE SUPERIOR VENA CAVA AND CENTRAL VEINS

William M. Moore, Jr. and Larry H. Hollier

Partial or complete obstruction of the superior vena cava and its major tributaries occasionally results in incapacitating venous hypertension of the upper extremities and/or head and neck. Factors intrinsic and extrinsic to the central veins play a role in the pathogenesis. Medical therapy is indicated in the acute setting of central venous obstruction and usually allows the time necessary for development of collateral drainage routes. However, approximately 20 per cent of these patients will develop persistent or progressive, symptomatic venous hypertension, and approximately 10 per cent will remain incapacitated. It is difficult to establish strict criteria for patient selection for central venous reconstruction but, in general, all patients who remain incapacitated from symptomatic venous hypertension should be considered for operative intervention.

Early clinical progress in venous reconstruction was retarded by the search for an adequate conduit for venous bypass or replacement. Accelerated interest in the field of large vein reconstruction followed the 1976 report by Doty and Baker (1) that described their success with superior vena cava (SVC) bypass utilizing a spiral vein graft constructed from autogenous saphenous vein. That report represented the first clinical account of this technique, which had been previously described by Chiu et al. in the canine model in 1974 (2). Multiple other biologic and prosthetic conduits have been investigated for their effectiveness in large vein reconstruction (Table 36–1). Encouraging results have been observed with externally reinforced polytetrafluoroethylene (PTFE). A considerable number of small clinical series and laboratory studies have reported the use of a variety of conduits and adjunctive measures to enhance patency rates. The following discussion will identify the major advances in SVC reconstruction and recommend a regimen for the management of these difficult cases.

ETIOLOGY AND PATHOGENESIS

Incapacitating venous hypertension of the upper extremities and/or head and neck may develop as a result of a wide variety of pathologic conditions (Table 36–2). Historically, the most common causes of central venous and SVC obstruc-

TABLE 36–1. Potential Conduits for Vena Cava Reconstruction

Biologic materials
  Autogenous vein
    Spiral vein graft
    Translocated nonreversed saphenous vein
    Reversed saphenous vein
  Arterial allograft
  Other
Prosthetic materials
  PTFE
  Dacron (woven/knitted)
  Teflon

tion have been neoplastic and inflammatory masses. These space-occupying lesions progress at various rates of enlargement. The mechanism of interference with venous return is usually extrinsic compression; however, malignant neoplasms and inflammatory masses are notorious for transmural invasion. Direct trauma may also cause acute or subacute thrombosis, as will venous entrapment, such as in effort thrombosis of the subclavian and/or axillary veins.

An increased incidence of central venous occlusion due to intrinsic causes has paralleled the increased use of intermediate- to long-term catheters placed for hemodialysis, central hyperalimentation, chemotherapy, and invasive monitoring (3,4). Mechanical or chemical intimal injury may result in acute venous thrombosis or progressive stenosis with or without delayed thrombosis, ultimately causing venous hypertension. Although the thrombogenic properties of currently available catheters have been greatly reduced, the mere presence of a foreign body in the low-velocity venous system establishes a thrombogenic nidus, especially if concomitant intimal injury exists.

Idiopathic mediastinal fibrosis is manifest as an intense inflammatory process resulting in dense fibrosis of the mediastinal structures, probably in response to an autoimmune reaction. This process may progress to cause partial or complete obstruction of the innominate veins, SVC, or supradiaphragmatic segment of the inferior vena cava (IVC) (5,6).

Obstruction of the great veins of the chest may occur suddenly or may have a more insidious onset. The development of venous hypertension as a result of this obstruction depends on the anatomic location, degree of obstruction, and rate

TABLE 36–2. Common Causes of Central Venous Occlusion/Obstruction

Extrinsic
  Neoplastic masses ⎫
  Inflammatory masses ⎭   External compression, direct extension
  Trauma
Intrinsic
  Intimal Injury
    mechanical ⎫   Resultant sclerosis,
    chemical ⎭   fibrosis, or thrombosis
  Relatively thrombogenic intraluminal foreign bodies
    catheters placed for hemodialysis, chemotherapy, total parenteral nutrition, monitoring
Other
  Spontaneous thrombosis in hypercoagulable states
  Idiopathic mediastinal fibrosis
  Idiopathic thrombosis

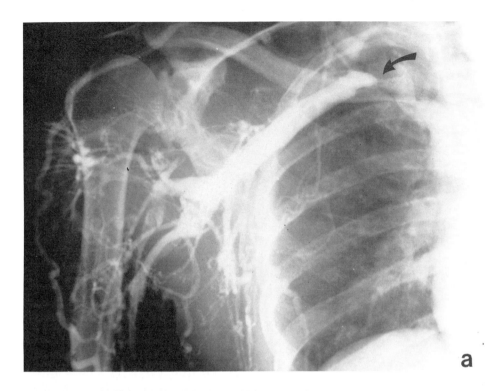

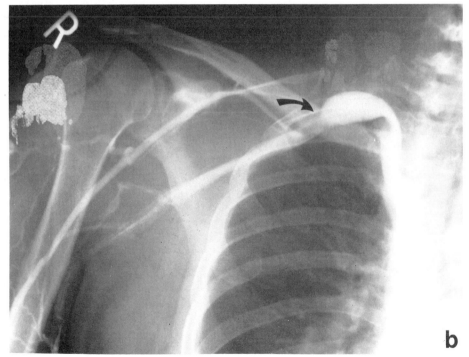

Figure 36–1. *A*, Venogram demonstrating high-grade stenosis of the distal right subclavian vein (arrow) and poorly developed collateral venous network. *B*, Postoperative venogram of patient shown in *A* following right internal jugular–to-subclavian vein transposition. The anastomosis is widely patent (arrow) and there is obvious decompression of the previously engorged tributaries.

of progress of the lesion. These factors directly affect the ability of the regional tributaries to provide adequate collateral drainage.

DIAGNOSIS

Initial presentation and physical examination usually incite a high index of suspicion of the diagnosis of central venous occlusion. Signs and symptoms include upper extremity and/or head and neck swelling, skin discoloration, superficial venous distention, and pain or discomfort that is exacerbated by dependent positions. Although several noninvasive techniques of venous assessment have been described, venography remains the gold standard for diagnosing venous occlusion. Venography permits the identification of the location and extent of the obstructing lesion, as well as assessment of the regional collateral venous network (Fig. 36–1a). Digital venous imaging techniques provide excellent definition of the obstructing lesion and reasonable visualization of the collateral bed. Nuclear scans may also identify the level of obstruction, but do not provide accurate details of the collateral circulation or the length of the obstructing lesion.

INITIAL THERAPY FOR COMPROMISED VENOUS OUTFLOW

The cause of the obstruction and associated pathology must be considered when determining appropriate initial therapy. If SVC syndrome results from a progressive malignant mediastinal neoplasm, external beam readiation should be implemented promptly, with the possible addition of chemotherapy. Acute and subacute thromboses have traditionally been treated by anticoagulation. Initial therapy with intravenous sodium heparin stabilizes the thrombus, impedes propagation, facilitates resolution of acute symptoms, and permits collateralization. Oral warfarin therapy is implemented 7 to 14 days later and continued for approximately 6 months, with close follow-up at regular intervals. Elevation of the involved extremity or head is an important component of medical therapy and will decrease venous pooling, edema, and discomfort. Physical therapy consisting of hand exercises (e.g., compressing a tennis ball) may be implemented several weeks following the acute episode. These exercises increase blood flow to the extremity and activate the musculovenous pump, thereby expediting development of collateral channels. The clinical course during medical therapy will dictate what additional measures must be taken, if any.

Investigations are currently underway to determine the effectiveness of venous thrombolysis using urokinase, streptokinase, and tissue plasminogen activator; however, the data are not sufficient to permit analysis at this time. Clinical trials with percutaneous angioplasty of isolated stenoses of the subclavian and axillary veins have been discouraging (7).

OPERATIVE INTERVENTION

Patient Selection

Proper selection of patients is of critical importance to successful surgical management. The development or the recurrence of incapacitating venous hypertension is the most common indication for central venous reconstruction. The patient must have a general health status that will permit him/her to undergo a major surgical procedure. Patients with malignant disease should have a reasonable expected survival, at least 3 to 6 months, and minimal symptoms related to remote residual tumor. Although clinically evident pulmonary emboli emanating from an SVC thrombus are much less common than those emanating from lower extremity or IVC sources, recurrent pulmonary emboli constitutes an uncommon indication for ligation-in-continuity and venous bypass. With the exception of patients with idiopathic mediastinal fibrosis, or other causes of venous obstruction that have no known medical treatment, all patients being considered for SVC reconstruction should have an adequate trial of conventional medical therapy prior to operative intervention.

Perioperative Management and Surgical Technique

We recently conducted a retrospective review of 10 patients who underwent central venous reconstruction for refractory, incapacitating venous hypertension of the upper extremities or head and neck (8). Six patients had chronic renal failure, were on hemodialysis, had a functional ipsilateral arteriovenous fistula, and had documentation of at least one previous central venous line in the affected vessel. Two patients had idiopathic mediastinal fibrosis and one patient experienced idiopathic spontaneous thrombosis of the SVC, IVC, and portal vein. The only patient with malignant disease had previously undergone an ipsilateral radical mastectomy and postoperative external beam radiation, with resultant subclavian and axillary vein sclerosis and thrombosis, presumably due to radiation phlebitis.

Preoperative imaging studies included venogram or digital venous imaging (Fig. 36–1a) in all cases. The levels of venous obstruction and the method of reconstruction are shown in Table 36–3. Selection of the method of reconstruction was based on the location and extent of obstruction. Occlusions involving the innominate veins and/or the SVC were reconstructed with externally reinforced PTFE bypasses from the internal jugular and/or subclavian veins to the SVC or right atrium. Lesions involving the subclavian vein at the junction with the internal jugular vein were managed with internal jugular–to-subclavian vein transposition. The patient with occlusion of the entire subclavian and axillary vein was managed

TABLE 36–3 **Superior Vena Cava and Central Venous Reconstruction**[a]

PATIENT #	LOCATION OF LESION	METHOD OF RECONSTRUCTION	AVF
1	L. innominate vein at SVC	L. SC → SVC, R-PTFE	Yes
2	SVC and l. innominate vein	L. IJ/SC → R. atrium, R-PTFE	Yes
3	SVC and r. innominate vein	R. IJ/SC → SVC, R-PTFE	Yes
4	SVC and r. innominate vein	R. IJ → R. atrium, R-PTFE	Yes
5	SVC	R. IJ → R. atrium, R-PTFE	No
6	SVC	R. IJ → R. atrium, R-PTFE	Yes
7	R. subclavian vein at IJ	R. IJ → SC transposition	Yes
8	R. subclavian vein at IJ	R. IJ → SC transposition	Yes
9	L. subclavian at IJ	L. IJ → SC transposition	Yes
10	L. subclavian and axillary to IJ	L. axillary → IJ, RSVG	No

[a] *AVF*, arteriovenous fistula; *IJ*, internal jugular vein; *R-PTFE*, reinforced PTFE graft; *RSVG*, reversed saphenous vein graft; *SC*, subclavian vein.

with a reversed saphenous vein graft extending from the axillary to the internal jugular vein.

All patients were begun on aspirin (325 mg/day) and dipyridamole (100 to 150 mg/day) prior to surgical intervention, and this regimen was continued indefinitely postoperatively. All patients were systemically heparinized with 5000 units of sodium heparin prior to reconstruction and maintained on warfarin (5 to 15 mg/day) for 6 weeks following central vein reconstruction. All but two patients either had a preexisting functional ipsilateral, distal arteriovenous fistula or had one established prior to or at the time of venous reconstruction.

Superior vena cava bypass was accomplished by ligation and transection of the occluded innominate vein with the distal anastomosis placed at the internal jugular/subclavian junction in an end-to-end fashion with 10-mm externally reinforced PTFE presoaked in heparinized saline. The anastomosis was performed with running 5-0 polypropylene suture and secured at the heel and toe to avoid decreasing the anastomotic diameter. Similarly, the proximal anastomosis was made to the superior vena cava (two patients) or right atrium (four patients) in an end-to-side fashion (Fig. 36–2). Three patients undergoing reconstruction by this method were managed with continuous infusion of heparinized saline into an ipsilateral facial vein cannula for 48 hr postoperatively (200 to 500 units/hr).

Venous transposition was accomplished in three patients by ligation and transection of the ipsilateral internal jugular vein, with anastomosis of the subclavian vein in an end-to-end or end-to-side fashion to the patent proximal jugular vein. Radiographic confirmation of graft patency was obtained in all patients at 1 week, 1 month, and 6 to 12 months postoperatively by venous imaging (Figs. 36–1b,

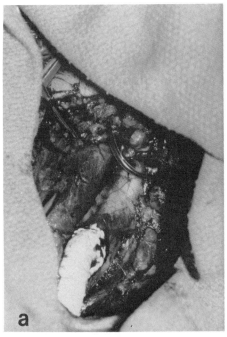 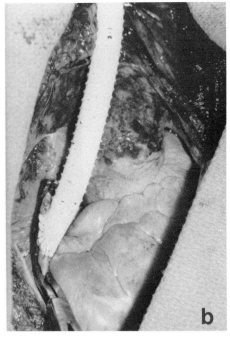

Figure 36–2. *A*, Intraoperative photograph of proximal end-to-side anastomosis of externally reinforced PTFE graft to internal jugular vein. *B*, Intraoperative photograph of distal end-to-side anastomosis of externally reinforced PTFE graft to right atrial appendage.

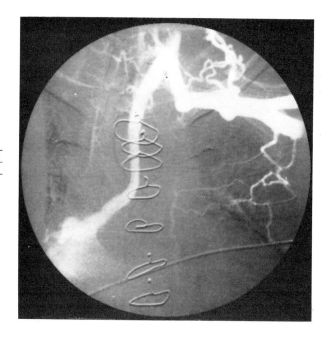

Figure 36–3. Postreconstruction subtraction venogram revealing patent left internal jugular–to–right atrial PTFE bypass graft.

36–3, and 36–4) or contrast-enhanced computed tomography (Fig. 36–5). There were no perioperative deaths or major complications related to the procedure, with the exception of one patient who underwent SVC reconstruction with PTFE. In this instance graft thrombosis occurred early in the postoperative period. This was a 10-year-old child with idiopathic thrombosis of the SVC, IVC, and portal

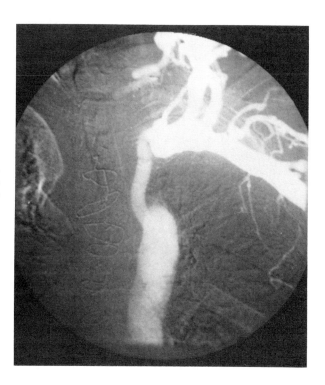

Figure 36–4. Postreconstruction subtraction venogram revealing patent left innominate vein–to-SVC PTFE bypass graft.

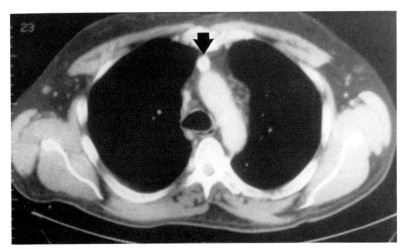

Figure 36–5. Postreconstruction contrast-enhanced computed tomography scan revealing patent internal jugular vein–to–right atrial PTFE bypass graft within the mediastinum (arrow).

vein. Thrombectomy and cannulation of the ipsilateral facial vein for continuous heparin infusion for 48 hr resulted in graft patency, confirmed at 36 months. Two late deaths at 3 and 9 months following reconstruction were due to causes unrelated to venous disease or the operative procedure. All grafts remained patent, with a mean follow-up of 30 months. The arteriovenous fistulas were left intact in all patients undergoing hemodialysis for chronic renal failure.

DISCUSSION

Significant progress has been made in the field of venous reconstruction over the past several decades. This progress has been facilitated primarily by the development of conduits that permit venous replacement with materials that provide adequate diameter and length, resist collapse, and are relatively nonthrombogenic. Table 36–1 lists the materials most commonly reported in vena cava reconstructions. Poor patency rates have been reported with most of these conduits as a result of a myriad of factors, including size mismatch, inadequate flow, relative thrombogenicity in a low-pressure system, anastomotic thrombosis or stenosis, and material collapsibility.

The problem of low-velocity blood flow in a low-pressure system can be eliminated by developing an ipsilateral arteriovenous fistula, which significantly enhances flow through the reconstructed vessel (9–12). This appears to decrease stasis and collapse, and improves early graft patency rates. Six of the 10 patients in our series were on chronic hemodialysis and alrady had a functional fistula.

Reversed or nonreversed, translocated saphenous vein grafts perform well when used to bypass medium-sized veins, but require the more tedious technique of developing a spiral vein graft if used in the central venous system. Success with this technique, developed by Chiu et al. (2) and popularized by Doty and Baker (1), has been reported in several clinical series and laboratory studies (4,12–16).

Utilizing synthetic grafts for central venous reconstruction is an attractive alternative because of convenience and the variety of available sizes, both of which serve to decrease operative time. Early reports of central venous reconstruction with Dacron and Teflon grafts revealed poor patency rates. The development of externally reinforced PTFE has provided a relatively nonthrombogenic material that is resistant to collapse and compression. SVC and IVC replacement with externally reinforced PTFE in the canine model has resulted in patency rates comparable to those with spiral vein grafts when performed in conjunction with distal arteriovenous fistula and antiplatelet therapy (12,17–20). Prior to the development of externally placed rings on PTFE and prior to material alterations that enhanced the thromboresistance of PTFE, Smith et al. (21) reported excellent long-term patency (83 per cent) when PTFE was used to replace the IVC in the canine model; PTFE was superior to lyophilized venous homografts and autogenous fibrocollagenous tubes in their series.

Controlled trials comparing the various types of antiplatelet or anticoagulant therapy have not yet been conducted in the clinical or laboratory setting. Canine studies have demonstrated a 13.5-fold decrease in platelet and fibrin deposition on PTFE when placed in animals receiving intravenous ibuprofen (18) and decreased platelet deposition if the PTFE was presoaked in heparinized saline (17).

Internal jugular transposition for the treatment of symptomatic upper extremity venous hypertension due to chronic subclavian vein obstruction was described by White and Smith in 1966 (22) and again by Jacobson and Haimov in 1977 (23). This represents a safe, efficient method of treating the patient with isolated subclavian vein occlusion that does not involve the internal jugular, innominate, or SVC. This technique is particularly attractive since it may be accomplished without entering the chest or mediastinum and does not require remote vein harvest, spiral vein graft construction, or the use of prosthetic materials. Excellent relief of symptoms and long-term patency may be expected with this technique.

Percutaneous transluminal angioplasty has been attempted on isolated subclavian vein stenoses, but early results are disappointing. Glanz and colleagues reported their experience with 29 such patients (7). The initial success rate was 76 per cent, with a 1-year patency rate of 35 per cent and a 2-year rate of only 6 per cent. Additionally, there was a 7 per cent incidence of postdilatation venous rupture of the distal axillary/proximal subclavian vein. This complication could result in a potentially fatal situation if it occurred following dilation of one of the large veins within the thorax, especially if the patient had a functioning arteriovenous fistula in the ipsilateral extremity.

Adjunctive techniques appear to be very imporant to the success of central venous reconstruction. Three patients in our series underwent placement of an ipsilateral facial vein cannula for continuous infusion of heparinized saline (200 to 500 units/hr). This is easily performed and should theoretically decrease platelet deposition upon the freshly placed PTFE graft. The catheter is empirically discontinued at 48 hr.

Regardless of the method of reconstruction, care must be taken to avoid iatrogenic intimal injury during operative repair for venous occlusion. The most atraumatic occlusive device should be selected based on the limits of exposure and contiguous structures (24).

TABLE 36–4. Measures That Appear to Influence Patency following Central Venous Reconstruction

Patient selection
Externally supported graft material
Autogenous vein
Distal arteriovenous fistula
Anticoagulation (intraoperative/postoperative)
Antiplatelet therapy
Low-molecular-weight dextran
Heparin infusion via facial vein
Nonsteroidal antiinflammatory agents

SUMMARY

We currently believe that any patient with incapacitating symptoms of venous hypertension of the upper extremities and/or head and neck should be considered for surgical intervention if significant disability persists following 8 to 12 weeks of medical therapy. Medical therapy will be ineffective in patients with idiopathic mediastinal fibrosis; therefore surgical intervention should be considered early. When venous transposition for an isolated lesion is not an option, central venous and SVC reconstruction with externally reinforced PTFE can result in patency rates comparable to those of spiral vein grafts, if performed in conjunction with ipsilateral, distal arteriovenous fistula and managed with anticoagulant and antiplatelet therapy and selective facial vein heparin infusion (Table 36–4). This alternative is of particular importance in patients with conditions that prevent the use of the saphenous vein (i.e., lower extremity deep venous thrombosis and inadequate or absent saphenous vein).

REFERENCES

1. Doty DB, Baker WH: Bypass of superior vena cava with spiral vein graft. Ann Thorac Surg 1976;*22*:490–493.
2. Chiu CJ, Terzis J, MacRae ML: Replacement of superior vena cava with spiral composite vein graft. Ann Thorac Surg 1974;*17*:555–560.
3. Greene FL, Moore WM, Strickland GF: Comparison of implantable venous access device (Port-a-cath) versus long-term percutaneous catheterization (Broviac-Hickman) for chemotherapy or hyperalimentation. South Med J 1987;*81*:580–583.
4. Jain KM, Smejkal R: Use of spiral vein graft to bypass occluded subclavian vein. J Cardiovasc Surg 1988;*29*:572–573.
5. Herse B, Dalichau H, Mennicken U: Idiopathic mediastinal fibrosis. A case reort on its surgical treatment. Thorac Cardiovasc Surg 1984;*32*:35–40.
6. Gupta DK, Mathur AS: Cervical and mediastinal fibrosis presenting with vena caval syndrome. Indian Heart J 1979;*31*:302–304.
7. Glanz S, Gordon DH, Lipkowitz GS, et al: Axillary and subclavian vein stenosis: Percutaneous angioplasty. Radiology 1988;*168*:371–373.
8. Moore WM, Hollier LH, Pickett TK: Superior vena cava and central venous reconstruction. Surgery 1991 (in press).
9. Smith CA, Schisgall RM: The effect of a distal arteriovenous fistula upon an autogenous vein graft in the venous system. J Surg Res 1963;*3*:412–414.
10. Johnson V, Eiseman B: Evaluation of arteriovenous shunt to maintain patency of venous autograft. Am J Surg 1969;*118*:915–918.
11. Hobson RW, Croom RD, Swan KG: Hemodynamics of the distal arteriovenous fistula in venous reconstruction. J Surg Res 1973;*14*:483–486.
12. Gloviczki P, Hollier LH, Dewanjee MK, Trastek VF, Hoffman EA, Kaye MP: Experimental replacement of the inferior vena cava: FActors influencing patency. Surgery 1984;*95*:657–666.

13. Doty DB: Bypass of superior vena cava: Six years experience with spiral vein for obstruction of the superior vena cava due to benign and malignant disease. J Thorac Cardiovasc Surg 1982; *83*:326.
14. Smith ER, Brantigan CO: Bypass of superior vena cava obstruction using spiral vein graft. J Cardiovasc Surg 1983;*24*:259–260.
15. Anderson RP, Li W: Segmental replacement of the superior vena cava with spiral vein graft. Ann Thorac Surg 1983;*36*:85–88.
16. Gloviczki P, Pairolero PC, Cherry KJ, Hallett JW: Reconstruction of the vena cava and of its primary tributaries: A preliminary report. J Vasc Surg 1990;*11*:373–381.
17. Plate G, Hollier LH, Gloviczki P, Dewanjee MK, Kaye MP: Overcoming failure of venous vascular prostheses. Surgery 1984;*96*:503–510.
18. Lovaas ME, Gloviczki P, Dewanjee MK, Hollier LH, Kaye MP: Inferior vena cava replacement: The role of anti-platelet therapy. J Surg Res 1983;*35*:234–242.
19. Bernstein EF, Chan EL, Bardin JA: Externally supported grafts for inferior vena cava bypass. *In* Bergan JJ, Yao JST, eds: Surgery of the Veins. Orlando, FL, Grune & Stratton, Inc, 1985; 33–45.
20. Fujiwara Y, Cohn LH, Adams D, Collins JJ: Use of Goretex grafts for replacement of the superior and inferior venae cavae. J Thorac Cardiovasc Surg 1974;*67*:774–779.
21. Smith DE, Hammon J, Anane-Sefah J, Richardson RS, Trimble C: Segmental venous replacement: A comparison of biological and synthetic substitutes. J Thorac Cardiovasc Surg 1975; *69*:589–598.
22. White LC, Smith AC: Single anastomosis vein bypass for subclavian vein obstruction. Arch Surg 1966;*93*:664.
23. Jacobson JH, Haimov M: Venous revascularization of the arm: Report of three cases. Surgery 1977;*81*:599–604.
24. Moore WM, Bunt TJ, Hermann GD, Fogarty TJ: Assessment of transmural force during application of vascular occlusive devices. J Vasc Surg 1988;*8*:422–427.

XII

SURGICAL MANAGEMENT OF VENOUS THROMBOEMBOLISM

37

EMBOLECTOMY FOR ACUTE PULMONARY EMBOLISM

Pat O. Daily

HISTORICAL PERSPECTIVE

In 1983 Sabiston (1) described in detail the 1908 landmark paper in which the physical findings of acute massive pulmonary embolism and the technique for pulmonary embolectomy were delineated by Trendelenburg (2). After numerous laboratory simulations of pulmonary embolectomy, Trendelenburg performed the first procedure at the Leipzig Hospital. That patient died intraoperatively of hemorrhage from a laceration of the posterior aspect of the pulmonary artery when a sling was passed around the aorta and pulmonary artery. A second patient survived for 16 hr, succumbing to right heart failure. A third patient died at 37 hr postoperatively from hemorrhage of the internal mammary artery.

It remained for Kirschner (3) in 1924 to perform the first successful pulmonary embolectomy using the technique described by Trendelenburg. The first successful embolectomy performed in the United States was reported by Steenburg et al. (4) in 1958, and at that time only 12 other successful procedures had been reported in the world literature.

In 1960 Lewis (5) described pulmonary embolectomy with inflow occlusion, and Allison et al. (6) reported pulmonary embolectomy utilizing inflow occlusion combined with hypothermia for central nervous system protection. Sharp performed the first pulmonary embolectomy utilizing cardiopulmonary bypass in February of 1961 (7) and Cooley et al. reported a similar procedure performed in April of 1961 (8).

The conception of the use of extracorporeal circulation by Gibbon (9) was a major, but indirect, consequence of pulmonary embolism. The desirability to provide cardiovascular and pulmonary support until embolectomy could be performed was recognized while observing a patient dying acutely of pulmonary embolism in 1931. In 1965, Beall and Cooley (10) reported the use of partial cardiopulmonary bypass instituted peripherally for support of patients after hemodynamic collapse secondary to pulmonary embolism until pulmonary embolectomy could be performed.

Following the initial reports of Sharp (7) and Cooley et al. (8), there have been numerous articles of pulmonary embolectomy utilizing cardiopulmonary bypass. However, recently Clarke (11) described his results utilizing inflow occlusion.

INCIDENCE OF PULMONARY EMBOLISM AS IT RELATES TO POTENTIAL PULMONARY EMBOLECTOMY

There is general agreement that the only suitable candidates for pulmonary embolectomy are those who have sustained massive pulmonary embolism as defined by "at least 50% or more obstruction of the pulmonary vasculature" (12). In the frequently quoted report of Dalen and Alpert (13), it was estimated that approximately 630,000 cases of pulmonary embolism occurred in the United States annually. Of these, 11 per cent of the patients died within 1 hr, precluding management. Of the 89 per cent surviving more than 1 hr, diagnosis and institution of therapy occurred in only 29 per cent (163,000), and of these patients 92 per cent (150,000) survived. Of the 163,000 patients in whom the diagnosis was made, it was not possible to determine the percentage with massive pulmonary embolism, who were potential candidates for embolectomy.

In a review of pulmonary embolism, Del Campo (14) estimated that 2 to 6 per cent of patients failed to improve with thrombolytic therapy and would be potential candidates for pulmonary embolectomy. This was estimated to represent 1000 to 3000 patients per year in the United States.

The most recent data concerning massive pulmonary embolism as a cause of death were reported by Rubinstein et al. (15). They reviewed the postmortem examinations of patients hospitalized at St. Michael's Hospital in Toronto from 1980 through 1984. Of 1276 patients autopsied, 44 had major pulmonary embolism, an incidence of 3.4 per cent. Furthermore, only 31.8 per cent ($^{14}/_{44}$) of these patients had the diagnosis made premortem. Assuming that the years 1980 through 1984 were inclusive, there was an average of eight patients per year dying of massive pulmonary embolism. In all likelihood, this was an underestimation of the total number of patients with massive pulmonary embolism in that, undoubtedly, some survived. One could estimate that approximately eight to 12 patients per year may be encountered in a typical tertiary referral center. The authors concluded that major pulmonary embolism is still underdiagnosed in hospitalized patients despite the availability of lung scanning and pulmonary angiography.

Perhaps a more specific estimate regarding the number of pulmonary embolectomies performed per hospital per year can be made from the report of Mattox et al. (16). From 1961 through 1981, 40 pulmonary embolectomies were performed at Ben Taub Hospital in Houston, Texas, a 460-bed hospital with more than 17,000 acute admissions and 4000 operations per year. There was an average of two embolectomies annually, which perhaps more realistically represents the small number of patients per year potentially salvageable by embolectomy in comparable hospitals.

In summary, while massive pulmonary embolism is found in 2 to 14 per cent of autopsies, it appears that the diagnosis is estblished premortem in only one third of the patients. Given these data, it is not surprising that only an average of two pulmonary embolectomies per year were reported in the Ben Taub experience. The current general trend is to treat patients with massive pulmonary embolism and hemodynamic compromise initially with thrombolytic agents. Most patients respond to this therapy (17). Consequently, patients requiring embolectomy will be a distinct minority since only those who have contraindications or fail to respond to thrombolytic therapy are potential candidates. Gray et al. (18), however, suggested that up to 32 per cent of patients with massive pulmonary embolism may be too unstable hemodynamically to institute thrombolytic therapy.

INDICATIONS

There is a broad spectrum of recommended indications for pulmonary embolectomy for acute pulmonary embolism. At one extreme Pisko-Dubienski (19) suggested that pulmonary embolectomy should be performed for all but minor emboli, presumably regardless of hemodynamic state. At the other extreme, Oakley (20) stated that "Not only is there no place for acute pulmonary embolectomy but also, there is probably no need for thrombolytic agents." Between these extremes there has been a variety of recommendations. Saylam and associates (21) suggested performing pulmonary embolectomy in patients in shock but without regard to the degree of obstruction, specifically not requiring that massive pulmonary embolism be present. Conversely, Glassford and associates (22) and Lund et al. (23) have recommended pulmonary embolectomy for central emboli even though there may be no circulatory impairment. Sautter et al. (24) and Crane and associates (25) suggested that pulmonary embolectomy was not indicated if the patient could tolerate pulmonary angiography. Several authors (17,25,26) have recommended pulmonary embolectomy only for cardiac arrest or imminent cardiac arrest.

Perhaps a more rational and realistic approach, as illustrated in Table 37–1, would be to consider pulmonary embolectomy in patients with angiographically documented massive pulmonary embolism who are in shock and who 1) have an absolute contraindication to thrombolytic therapy, or 2) have no response or are deteriorating with thrombolytic therapy, or 3) are in a hemodynamic state suggesting impending cardiac arrest and trial of thrombolytic therapy should not be instituted, or 4) have echocardiographically demonstrated right atrial emboli that may be "in transit." With minor variations, these recommendations have been supported by multiple authors (14,18,27–31).

A special consideration for pulmonary embolectomy is the echocardiographic demonstration of right atrial thrombi. Farfel and associates (30) reviewed 49 cases collected from the literature of echocardiographically demonstrated right atrial emboli or thrombi that, presumably, were emboli in transit. Medical management, consisting of cardiac support only, was associated with six of 13 patients dying and thrombolytic therapy plus anticoagulation was associated with a 50 per cent mortality in 16 patients. However, of 20 patients undergoing thrombectomy and pulmonary embolectomy, there was an 85 per cent survival rate. Consequently, Farfel and associates (30) stated that "thromboemboli entrapped in the right heart

TABLE 37–1. Pulmonary Embolectomy Indications in Patients with Angiographically Documented Massive Pulmonary Embolism in Shock

1. Absolute contraindication to thrombolytic therapy
2. No response or deterioration with thrombolytic therapy
3. Impending cardiac arrest
4. Right atrial emboli "in transit" (need *not* be in shock)

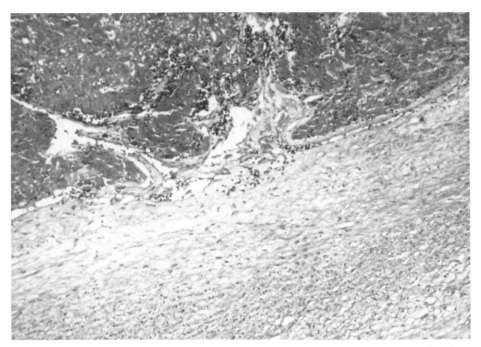

Figure 37–1. This is a cross-section of a pulmonary artery stained with hematoxylin and eosin at approximately 1 week after embolization. Significant ingrowth of fibrous tissue from the arterial wall into the embolus can be seen. Consequently, embolectomy by simple removal is no longer possible and thromboendarterectomy techniques are necessary.

chambers are best handled by a surgical emergency.'' Bloomfield and associates (31) have supported this recommendation.

Suggested contraindications for pulmonary embolectomy relate to the possibility of chronic, rather than acute, pulmonary embolism. It is apparent that after 72 hr pulmonary emboli may become quite adherent to the pulmonary arterial wall, and by 1 week considerable tissue ingrowth into the embolus can be demonstrated, as shown in Figure 37–1. Consequently, the contraindications for acute pulmonary embolectomy suggesting the presence of chronic pulmonary embolism are 1) the presence of symptoms for 7 days or more, 2) more than two recurrent embolic episodes prior to the acute event, and 3) a pulmonary artery systolic pressure of more than 60 mm Hg (32). However, if chronic pulmonary embolism is unexpectedly encountered, pulmonary thromboendarterectomy, as described in Chapter 38, can be performed.

SURGICAL TECHNIQUE

Since the reports of Sharp (7) and Cooley et al. (8) suggesting the use of cardiopulmonary bypass for pulmonary embolectomy, the majority of reported cases have been associated with that method. However, Clarke and Abrams (33) have obtained excellent results utilizing inflow occlusion (5).

The early institution of partial cardiopulmonary bypass for circulatory support is an important consideration. This concept has had a number of early proponents (34,35) and was particularly popularized by Beall et al. (10,36). In a review by Del Campo (14), partial cardiopulmonary bypass prior to sternotomy was utilized in 26 per cent of 537 patients. More recent experience with percutaneously instituted partial cardiopulmonary bypass (37) suggests that this modality be considered in patients with severe hemodynamic compromise prior to angiography if the clinical setting suggests a high likelihood of pulmonary embolism. Furthermore, because of right heart obstruction, the use of cardiopulmonary support is more appropriate than closed-chest cardiac massage for resuscitation after cardiac arrest.

The standard approach with cardiopulmonary bypass involves median sternotomy, typically with transatrial, bicaval cannulation with caval snares. The primary need for bicaval cannulation is to allow inspection of the right atrium and ventricle and inferior vena cava for the possibility of retained emboli. Typically, with or without aortic cross-clamping, an incision is made in the pulmonary artery just beyond the pulmonary valve extending to the pulmonary bifurcation. Using a variety of curved forceps, attempts are made to extract the emboli. Additional maneuvers include opening of the pleural spaces and massaging of the lungs to facilitate the centripetal removal of emboli (38). The use of balloon catheters has been reported but has not been found to be particularly effective (39). Research suggests (40) that retrograde pulmonary vein perfusion to flush out pulmonary arterial emboli can be performed without causing pulmonary edema provided that appropriate pulmonary vein pressures and times of exposure to associated pressures are maintained. However, this method has not been clinically evaluated.

Currently, a more effective technique for removal of pulmonary emboli involves an approach identical to that previously described (41) for chronic pulmonary embolism. An incision is made in the right pulmonary artery extending into the right lower lobe artery and another incision beginning in the right pulmonary artery is extended into the upper lobe artery. On the left side only a single pulmonary arterial incision is made. With these incisions, each bronchopulmonary segmental arterial orifice can be inspected directly and additional emboli removed. Furthermore, if chronic pulmonary embolism is present, thromboendarterectomy would be the only possible mechanism for relief of obstruction and, if indicated, that procedure can be performed as well. If this more peripheral approach is utilized, it should be emphasized that it is necessary to inspect the area immediately above the pulmonary valve via an incision in the main pulmonary artery, as well as the right atrium and ventricle and inferior vena cava, as described previously.

RESULTS FOR ACUTE PULMONARY EMBOLECTOMY

Early Results

For current decision making, it is appropriate to consider the results of pulmonary embolectomy in three different eras. In 1967 Cross and Mowlen (42) reported a survey of centers in North America for experience with pulmonary embolectomy. Responses were obtained from 28 centers in which 1 to 15 patients were reported per center. Overall, 137 patients underwent surgery with 43 per cent survival. Using cardiopulmonary bypass in 115 patients 43 per cent survived, while 40 per cent of 22 patients survived with one of three closed procedures

TABLE 37–2.   Early Results of Pulmonary Embolectomy[a]

	OPERATIONS	SURVIVORS	
		No.	%
Cardiopulmonary bypass	115	50	43
Without cardiopulmonary bypass			
Unilateral embolectomy	11	6	54
Bilateral embolectomy (inflow occlusion)	6	1	16
Classical Trendelenburg	5	2	40
Subtotal	22	9	40
Total	137	59	43

[a] From Cross FS, Mowlen A: A survey of the current status of pulmonary embolectomy for massive pulmonary embolism. Circulation 1967;35(suppl I):I-86–I-91.

(unilateral embolectomy, bilateral embolectomy with inflow occlusion, and the Trendelenburg procedure). These results are summarized in Table 37–2. In a review published in 1985, Del Campo (14) combined the reported results of pulmonary embolectomy performed with and without cardiopulmonary bypass prior to 1984 (see Table 37–3), which included the results reported by Cross and Mowlen (42). Survival with pulmonary embolectomy was 60.1 per cent ($^{323}/_{537}$). However, there was only a 49 per cent ($^{56}/_{114}$) survival in patients having embolectomy without cardiopulmonary bypass (statistically significant at $p < .05$). Several authors (17,24–26,42) have utilized these earlier results with survivals ranging from 30 to 60 per cent as justification for recommending the use of pulmonary embolectomy in only the most dire of circumstances, specifically in patients with impending or present cardiac arrest. For example, Moser (43), in a 1990 "state of the art review" of venous thromboembolism, essentially dismissed the use of pulmonary embolectomy by quoting papers published in 1967 (42) and 1975 (17) wherein the operative mortality for pulmonary embolectomy was 57 and 60 to 70 per cent, respectively. No reports subsequent to 1975 were considered.

Results since 1984 are summarized in Table 37–4. Gray and associates (44) reported 41 of 46 patients who had not had prior cardiac arrest survivng pulmonary embolectomy, an 89 per cent survival rate. However, after preoperative cardiac arrest only 36 per cent ($^{9}/_{25}$) survived. The aggregate survival was 70 per cent. Lund and associates (23), in a comparison of pulmonary embolectomy to treatment with heparin and streptokinase, had 80 per cent ($^{20}/_{25}$) survival for embolectomy. Clarke and Abrams (33) utilized inflow occlusion without hypothermia and obtained 80 per cent ($^{28}/_{36}$) survival for embolectomy without prior cardiac arrest but, similar to Gray and Miller (44), had only 26 per cent ($^{5}/_{19}$) survival in patients

TABLE 37–3.   Early Survival (Prior to 1984) following Pulmonary Embolectomy[a]

	NO. OF PATIENTS	NO. OF SURVIVORS	%
With CPB[b]	537	323	60.1[c]
Without CPB	114	56	49.1[c]

[a] From Del Campo C: Pulmonary embolectomy. Can J Surg 1985;28:111–113.
[b] CPB, cardiopulmonary bypass.
[c] Significantly different ($p < .05$).

TABLE 37–4. Early Survival (Since 1984) following Pulmonary Embolectomy

SERIES	NO. OF PATIENTS	NO. OF SURVIVORS	%
Gray and Miller (44)			
Preop arrest	25	9	37 } 70
No arrest	46	41	89
Lund et al. (23)	25	20	80
Clarke and Abrams (33)			
Preop	19	5	26
No arrest	36	28	80
Last 13 patients	13	12	92

with a preoperative arrest. In their last 13 patients there was only one death, for a survival of 92 per cent. It is apparent that since 1984 survivals in the 80 to 90 per cent range have been obtained in patients without prior cardiac arrest.

There has been only one reported study (32) comparing the early results of treatment with heparin, streptokinase, and embolectomy (see Table 37–5). However, in this study assignment to groups was based on symptomatology and degree of pulmonary vascular obstruction rather than randomization. Consequently, patients assigned to the heparin group had substantially less pulmonary vascular obstruction than those assigned to the streptokinase or embolectomy group. The preoperative level of pulmonary vascular occlusion, as defined by the authors with respect to "embolic score," was 5 ± 4 for the heparin group, 9 ± 3 for the streptokinase group, and 13 ± 3 for the embolectomy group. The difference between the heparin group and the streptokinase and embolectomy groups was statistically significant.

In comparing the streptokinase and embolectomy groups early postoperatively, it was seen that the posttreatment obstruction in the streptokinase group was higher, with a score of 6 ± 4 compared to 3 ± 2 for the embolectomy group ($p < .01$). The hospital mortalities were 21 and 20 per cent for the streptokinase and embolectomy groups, respectively. Additionally, Lund et al. observed that, in five of seven cases, after an initial reversible fall in blood pressure irreversible shock developed, presumably because of secondary embolization. Consequently, the authors recommended pulmonary embolectomy in all cases with emboli in the main branches of the pulmonary artery. They suggested that the primary contraindication to embolectomy was the presence of chronic pulmonary em-

TABLE 37–5. Early Results After Treatment with Heparin, Streptokinase, or Embolectomy[a]

	HEPARIN (*N* = 34)	STREPTOKINASE (N = 25)	ENDARTERECTOMY (*N* = 25)
Hospital mortality	2 (6%)	6 (21%)	5 (20%)
Rx			
Pre-embolic score	5 ± 4 $p < .05$	9 ± 3	13 ± 3
Rx			
Post embolic score (massive PE)	—	6 ± 4 ($N = 7$) $p < .05$	3 ± 2 ($N = 15$)

[a] From Lund O, Nielsen TT, Schifter S, Ronne K: Treatment of pulmonary embolism with full-dose heparin, streptokinase or embolectomy—results and indications. Thorac Cardiovasc Surg 1986;*34*:240–246.

bolism as identified by symptoms of more than 7 days' duration, multiple recurrent episodes, and a systolic pulmonary artery pressure of more than 60 mm Hg.

An alternative approach to pulmonary embolectomy has been described by Greenfield et al. (45). A suction catheter is inserted transvenously and directed fluoroscopically into various pulmonary arterial branches to remove emboli by aspiration. In the more recent report (46), 22 patients underwent this procedure with an overall mortality of 44 per cent. Interestingly, no subsequent reports utilizing this procedure have been forthcoming, possibly because the mortality was not significantly different from that reported with pulmonary embolectomy before 1984 and is worse than that reported since 1985 (10 to 15 per cent).

Complications

In spite of the fact that as a group these patients are severely compromised at the time of surgery, significant complications have been relatively few and reported even less frequently (47). One of the most significant complications, however, is that of neurologic damage, which is nearly always associated with preoperative cardiac arrest. Obviously, because of the obstructive emboli in the pulmonary arteries, standard cardiopulmonary resuscitation is not effective in restoring adequate blood flow. Consequently, this complication represents one of the principal reasons for the suggestion of early institution of cardiopulmonary support when patients are hemodynamically compromised and not responsive to optimal inotropic support.

Severe endobronchial hemorrhage has been reported on several occasions (47–50) but appears to occur in 1 per cent or less of patients. Right ventricular failure is not infrequent and is usually manageable after embolectomy, but may be quite severe and preclude survival unless a right ventricular assist device is utilized to allow recovery of a severely decompensated right ventricle. Localized and systemic bleeding are usually associated with the use of heparin and thrombolytic therapy.

Late Results

Surprisingly, there is only one report of long-term follow-up after pulmonary embolectomy (see Table 37–6). Lund and associates (23) studied 74 patients that were alive 30 days after the start of treatment for pulmonary embolism: 20 patients underwent pulmonary embolectomy, 22 had treatment with streptokinase, and 32 were tested with heparin. The follow-up period ranged from 6 months to 8.7 years, with an average follow-up of 3.6 years. The 5-year survival in the embolectomy

TABLE 37–6.   Long-Term Follow-up after Treatment with Heparin, Streptokinase, or Embolectomy[a]

	HEPARIN (N = 32)	STREPTOKINASE (N = 22)	ENDARTERECTOMY (N = 25)
5 Year survival	71 ± 14%	80 ± 13%	100%
Medical Rx		75 ± 7%	Surgical Rx 100% p < .05

[a] From Lund O, Nielsen TT, Ronne K, Schifter S: Pulmonary embolism: Long-term follow-up after treatment with full-dose heparin, streptokinase or embolectomy. Acta Med Scand 1987;*221*:61–71.

group was 100 per cent compared to 71 ± 14 per cent for the heparin group and 80 ± 13 per cent for the streptokinase group. Combining the medically treated groups, the survival was 75 ± 7 per cent. The difference in the embolectomy-treated group and the medically treated group was significant ($p < .05$).

At follow-up the significant differences were that all patients in the pulmonary embolectomy group were in the New York Heart Association functional classification I or II, whereas some patients in the heparin and streptokinase groups were in classification III or IV. Also, no patients in the embolectomy group had crural ulcers, contrasted to an 8 and a 64 per cent incidence for the heparin and streptokinase groups, respectively.

Prognostic factors for late survival related to pulmonary embolism were the number of recurrent episodes of pulmonary embolism and the degree of cardiac decompensation prior to treatment. Chronic pulmonary hypertension was present at follow-up in 75 per cent of patients who had three or more embolic episodes before treatment, compared to only 8 per cent of those who had two or fewer embolic episodes ($p < .001$). All patients in irreversible shock preoperatively had elevated pulmonary vascular resistance at follow-up as well as decreased ventilatory function and more than 25 per cent reduced pulmonary perfusion. Because the embolectomized patients, in spite of having more severe pulmonary vascular obstruction preoperatively, had a better long-term prognosis, the authors extended their indications for embolectomy to include all patients with central emboli irrespective of the degree of circulatory impairment.

SUMMARY

More recent results for pulmonary embolectomy, with mortalities in the 10 to 15 per cent range for patients who have not had preoperative cardiac arrest, suggest that reconsideration should be given to the role of pulmonary embolectomy in acute massive pulmonary embolism. Late results, with respect to survival and functional status, also support this contention. The increased use of cardiopulmonary support, which can be instituted percutaneously, may substantially improve the outlook for patients with massive pulmonary embolism who are severely decompensated hemodynamically. This point is further underscored by the fact that, in most series, patients who have had a preoperative cardiac arrest have an operative morality of 60 to 75 per cent. Early use of cardiopulmonary support should substantially decrease the incidence of cardiac arrest. Additionally, it is important to identify patients who may have chronic pulmonary embolism that are undergoing embolectomy for acute pulmonary embolism. The simultaneous performance of pulmonary thromboendarterectomy may further improve both early and late results.

REFERENCES

1. Sabiston DC Jr: Trendelenburg's classic work on the operative treatment of pulmonary embolism. Ann Thorac Surg 1983;*35*:570–574.
2. Trendelenburg F: Ueber die operative behandlung der embolic der lungenmarterie. Arch Klin Chir 1908;*86*:686–700.
3. Kirschner M: Ein durch die Trendelenburgsche operation geheilter fall von embolic der art. pulmonalis. Arch Klin Chir 1924;*133*:312–359.

4. Steenburg RW, Warren R, Wilson RE, Leslie ER: A new look at pulmonary embolectomy. Surg Gynecol Obstet 1958;*107*:214–220.

5. Lewis I: Problems in diagnosis and management of pulmonary embolism. *In* Harley HRS, ed: Modern Trends in Cardiac Surgery. London, Butterworth, 1960;64.

6. Allison PR, Dunnill MS, Marshall R: Pulmonary embolism. Thorax 1960;*15*:273–283.

7. Sharp EH: Pulmonary embolectomy: Successful removal of a massive pulmonary embolus with the support of cardiopulmonary bypass—case report. Ann Surg 1962;*156*:1–4.

8. Cooley DA, Beall AC, Alexander JK: Acute massive pulmonary embolism. JAMA 1961;*177*:283–286.

9. Gibbon JH Jr: The development of the heart-lung apparatus. Am J Surg 1978;*135*:608–619.

10. Beall AC Jr, Cooley DA: Experience with pulmonary embolectomy using temporary cardiopulmonary bypass. J Cardiovasc Surg 1965; Sept 5–18 (suppl):201–206.

11. Clarke DB: Pulmonary embolectomy has a well-defined and valuable place. Br J Hosp Med 1989; *41*:467–468.

12. Dalen JE, Banas JS, Brooks HL, Evans GL, Paraskos JA, Dexter L: Resolution rate of acute pulmonary embolism in man. N Engl J Med 1969;*280*:1194–1199.

13. Dalen JE, Alpert JS: Natural history of pulmonary embolism. Prog Cardiovasc Dis 1975;*17*:259–270.

14. Del Campo C: Pulmonary embolectomy: A review. Can J Surg 1985;*28*:111–113.

15. Rubinstein I, Murray D, Hoffstein V: Fatal pulmonary emboli in hospitalized patients. An autopsy study. Arch Intern Med 1988;*148*:1425–1426.

16. Mattox KL, Feldtman RW, Beall AC, DeBakey ME: Pulmonary embolectomy for acute massive pulmonary embolism. Ann Surg 1982;*195*:726–731.

17. Alpert JS, Smith RE, Ockene IS, Askenazi J, Dexter L, Dalen JE: Treatment of massive pulmonary embolism: The role of pulmonary embolectomy. Am Heart J 1975;*89*:413–418.

18. Gray HH, Morgan JM, Paneth M, Miller GAH: Pulmonary embolectomy for acute massive pulmonary embolism: an analysis of 71 cases. Br Heart J 1988;*60*:196–200.

19. Pisko-Dubienski ZA: A new approach to pulmonary embolism. Br J Surg 1968;*55*:138–145.

20. Oakley CM: There is no place for acute pulmonary embolectomy. Br J Hosp Med 1989;*41*:467–468.

21. Saylam A, Melo JQ, Ahmad A, Chapman RD, Wood JA, Starr A: Pulmonary embolectomy. West J Med 1978;*128*:377–381.

22. Glassford DM, Alford WC, Burrus GR, Stoney WS, Thomas CS: Pulmonary embolectomy. Ann Surg 1981;*32*:28–32.

23. Lund O, Nielsen TT, Ronne K, Schifter S. Pulmonary embolism: Long-term follow-up after treatment with full-dose heparin, streptokinase or embolectomy. Acta Med Scand 1987;*221*:61–71.

24. Sautter RD, Myers WO, Ray JF III, Wenzel FJ: Pulmonary embolectomy: Review and current status. Prog Cardiovasc Dis 1975;*17*:371–382.

25. Crane C, Hartsuck J, Birtch A, Couch NP, et al: The management of major pulmonary embolism. Surg Gynecol Obstet 1969;*128*(1):27–36.

26. Bell WR, Simon TL: Current status of pulmonary thromboembolic disease: Pathophysiology, diagnosis, prevention, and treatment. Am Heart J 1982;*103*:239–262.

27. Buckels NJ, Mulholland C, Galvin I, Gladstone D, Cleland J: Massive pulmonary embolism; the place for embolectomy. Ulster Med J 1988;*57*:161–166.

28. Masters RG, Koshal A, Higginson LAJ, Keon WJ: Ongoing role of pulmonary embolectomy. Can J Cardiol 1988;*4*:347–351.

29. Robison RJ, Fehrenbacher J, Brown JW, Madura JA, King H: Emergent pulmonary embolectomy: The treatmet for massive pulmonary embolus. Ann Thorac Surg 1986;*42*:52–55.

30. Farfel Z, Shechter M, Vered Z, Rath S, Goor D, Gafni J: Review of echocardiographically diagnosed right heart entrapment of pulmonary emboli-in-transit with emphasis on management. Am Heart J 1987;*113*:171–178.

31. Bloomfield P, Boon NA, DeBono DP: Indications for pulmonary embolectomy. Lancet 1988; *2*:329.

32. Lund O, Nielsen TT, Schifter S, Ronne K: Treatment of pulmonary embolism with full-dose heparin, streptokinase or embolectomy—results and indications. Thorac Cardiovasc Surg 1986; *34*:240–246.

33. Clarke DB, Abrams LD: Pulmonary embolectomy: A 25 year experience. J Thorac Cardiovasc Surg 1986;*92*:442–445.

34. Stansel HC Jr, Hume M, Glenn WWL: Pulmonary embolectomy: Results in ten patients. N Engl J Med 1967;*276*:717.

35. Sautter RD: Treatment of massive pulmonary embolism. *In* Ingelfinger J, Ebert RV, Finland M, Relman AS, eds: Controversy in Internal Medicine II. Philadelphia, WB Saunders Company, 1974;293.

36. Beall AC, Collins JJ Jr: What is the role of pulmonary embolectomy? Am Heart J 1975;*89*:411–412.
37. Reichman RT, Joyo CJ, Dembitsky WP, et al: Improved patient survival after cardiac arrest using a cardiopulmonary support system. Ann Thorac Surg 1990;*49*:101–105.
38. Beall AC Jr, Hallman GL, Cooley DA, et al: Surgical considerations in venous thromboembolism. Surg Clin North Am 1966;*46*:1021.
39. Goldman BS, Heimbecker RL: Use of the balloon catheter in successful pulmonary embolectomy. Ann Thorac Surg 1966;*2*:855.
40. Daily PO, Moulder PV: Guidelines for pulmonary vein perfusion dislodgement of emboli. Ann Thorac Surg 1967;*3*:242.
41. Daily PO, Dembitsky WP, Iversen S: Technique of pulmonary thromboendarterectomy for chronic pulmonary embolism. J Card Surg 1989;*4*:10–24.
42. Cross FS, Mowlen A: A survey of the current status of pulmonary embolectomy for massive pulmonary embolism. Circulation 1967;*35*(suppl I):I-86–I-91.
43. Moser KM: Venous thromboembolism. Am Rev Respir Dis 1990;*141*:235–249.
44. Gray HH, Miller GAH: Pulmonary embolectomy is still appropriate for a minority of patients with acute massive pulmonary embolism. Br J Hosp Med 1989;*41*:467–468.
45. Greenfield LJ, Bruce TA, Nichols NB: Transvenous pulmonary embolectomy by catheter device. Ann Surg 1971;*174*:881–886.
46. Stewart JR, Greenfield LJ: Transvenous vena caval filtration and pulmonary embolectomy. Surg Clin North Am 1982;*62*:411–430.
47. Masters RG, Koshal A, Higginson LAJ, Keon WJ: Ongoing role of pulmonary embolectomy. Can J Cardiol 1988;*4*:347–351.
48. Rice PL, Pifarre R, El-etr A, et al: Management of endobronchial hemorrhage during cardiopulmonary bypass. J Thorac Cardiovasc Surg 1981;*81*:800–801.
49. Makey AR, Bliss BP, Ikram H, Sutcliffe MML, Emery ERJ: Fatal intra-alveolar pulmonary bleeding complicating pulmonary embolectomy. Thorax 1971;*26*:466–471.
50. Brown S, Mulder D, Buckberg G: Massive pulmonary hemorrhagic infarction. Arch Surg 1974;*108*:795–797.

38

SURGICAL MANAGEMENT OF CHRONIC PULMONARY EMBOLISM

Pat O. Daily

HISTORICAL PERSPECTIVE

In 1956 Hollister and Cull (1) elaborated upon the syndrome of chronic thrombosis of the major pulmonary arteries. They described a case report (2) of a patient who underwent pneumonectomy because of presumed aneurysm of the right pulmonary artery. In actuality there was aneurysmal dilatation secondary to thrombosis of that artery, presumably secondary to pulmonary embolism. Rather than pneumonectomy, they suggested embolectomy or endarterectomy as a preferable treatment, thus preserving pulmonary tissue. Consequently, this represents the first suggestion that endarterectomy might be feasible for surgical management of chronic pulmonary embolism.

The first attempt at removal of chronic thrombotic pulmonary obstruction was reported by Hurwitt et al. (3) in 1958. They utilized inflow occlusion under normothermic conditions. The approach was through the main pulmonary artery and incomplete removal of occlusive material resulted. The patient sustained an intraoperative cardiac arrest and could not be resuscitated.

Because of inadequate removal of the obstructive material through a central approach, the authors proposed a unilateral approach dealing with one lung at a time. As an aside, the authors also suggested replacement of the main pulmonary artery and its bifurcation with an aortic homograft in selected cases of congenital stenoses of the pulmonary artery and extensive cases of thrombosis of the pulmonary artery.

The first successful procedure of endarteretomy for chronically occluded pulmonary arteries was reported by Snyder et al. (4) in 1963. Through a right thoractomy the right pulmonary artery was encircled proximal to the occluded area and a longitudinal incision was performed from the upper lobe branches to the superior segmental branch. "The mass was removed with endarterectomy spoons." Follow-up study 3 weeks later revealed the pulmonary artery to be patent. In this particular case, the diagnosis had not been entertained preoperatively and the operation was performed because of a suspected neoplasm. The authors emphasized that the pulmonary alveolar membrane was not irreparably damaged by prolonged pulmonary artery occlusion and that functional return of the affected lung may be expected following chronic pulmonary embolism.

The first report of successful, planned pulmonary thromboendarterectomy was that of Houk et al. (5). Bilateral pulmonary endarterectomies were performed through a transverse anterior bilateral thoracotomy. The authors suggested that a heightened suspicion could result in the identification of patients with chronic pulmonary hypertension that could be surgically managed.

In 1977 Sabiston et al. (6) reviewed 12 cases from the literature and added six more patients with chronic pulmonary embolism. Cardiopulmonary bypass was utilized in only five of these 18 cases. In 1980 we described (7) the use of median sternotomy with cardiopulmonary bypass, deep hypothermia, circulatory arrest, and peripheral incisions in the pulmonary arteries for pulmonary thromboendarterectomy in four patients, the first of whom underwent surgery in February of 1975. In 1987 we described (8) modifications of this procedure with respect to the use of a cooling jacket to maintain myocardial hypothermia (9) for myocardial protection, and intrapericardial and intrahilar dissection of the pulmonary arteries to avoid entrance into the pleural spaces. Specifically, the use of saline slush for myocardial cooling was identified as a high risk factor for phrenic nerve paresis and has been rigorously avoided since.

INCIDENCE AND CLINICAL SIGNIFICANCE

It is generally accepted that in excess of 500,000 patients in the United States annually sustain pulmonary embolism (10). There is, however, some controversy as to the percentage of these patients who progress to chronic pulmonary hypertension. Several authors (10–12) believe that a single episode of massive pulmonary embolism does not lead to chronic pulmonary embolism, but this concept

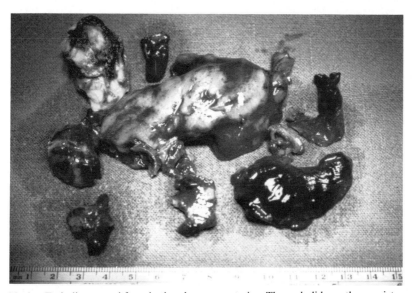

Figure 38–1. Emboli removed from both pulmonary arteries. The emboli have the consistency and appearance of relatively recent thrombosis. Consequently, they would appear to be more susceptible to fibrinolysis.

has not been proven. Consequently, the consensus is that recurrent pulmonary emboli are necessary for the production of chronic pulmonary hypertension.

There is considerable variation with respect to the pathologic aspects of pulmonary emboli. For example, some seem to represent embolization of recently formed clots that are in a "currant jelly" state (Fig. 38–1). Others, however, have been in place quite some time and may be in various degrees of fibrosis. Consequently, the resolution of the latter clots would seem to be substantially more difficult and, therefore, more likely to result in chronic obstruction (Figs. 38–2A and 38–2B).

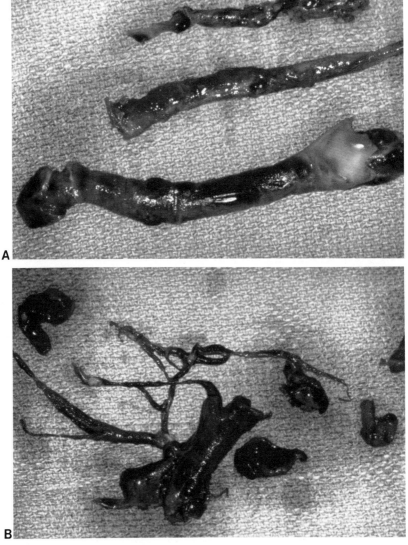

Figure 38–2. *A,* These emboli appear to be much better formed and have a fibrous quality. In the areas of discoloration the emboli are particularly fibrous, suggesting they were older at the time of embolization and that the likelihood of fibrinolysis may be less. *B,* These emboli are also well formed and they represent actual casts of the venous valves. They, too, would appear to be less suceptible to autogenous fibrinolysis.

Additionally, there may be some abnormality in the fibrinolytic system that predisposes to the development of chronic pulmonary arterial obstruction. Probably, some combination of these factors leads to chronic pulmonary vascular obstruction.

Paraskos et al. (13), in a study of pulmonary embolism patients, found that cor pulmonale developed in only 2 per cent. A lesser figure of 0.5 per cent was proposed by Tilkian et al. (14), and Moser (15) suggested an incidence of 0.1 per cent. Using the figure of 500,000 cases per year, this may result in an actual incidence of 500 to 10,000 patients annually developing cor pulmonale. Although this number is quite low, it is much higher than suggested by the number of patients who have undergone surgical procedures for chronic pulmonary embolism. Chitwood et al. (16), in an extensive review of the world literature in 1984, were able to identify only 85 patients who had undergone pulmonary thromboendarterectomy, with an overall operative mortality of 22 per cent. If the above estimates of 500 to 10,000 patients per year developing chronic pulmonary arterial obstruction are reasonably accurate, then one must assume that the diagnosis of chronic pulmonary embolism as the cause of pulmonary hypertension is frequently missed. Furthermore, it is not widely recognized that pulmonary thromboendarterectomy is effective therapy for this problem and, in fact, a number of patients have undergone heart-lung transplantation for pulmonary hypertension secondary to chronic pulmonary embolism.

INDICATIONS

In 1983 (17) we suggested that the indications for pulmonary thromboendarterectomy should include: 1) severe functional disability with patients in New York Heart Association functional classification III or IV; 2) evidence of significant pulmonary arterial obstruction as manifested by resting pulmonary vascular resistance of 300 dynes-sec-cm^{-5} or more; 3) pulmonary angiographic evidence of bilateral obstruction at least as proximal as the lobar level (an exception to this latter indication has been the presence of right or left patient artery occlusion without requiring significant proximal embolic disease on the contralateral side); and 4) institution of an anticoagulant regimen for at least 6 months without a significant decrease in pulmonary vascular resistance. More recently we have omitted this last indication inasmuch as it has been our experience that the majority of patients seen have been on such a regimen and if the pulmonary vascular resistance is chronically elevated, it typically does not regress substantially with long-term anticoagulation.

The most important predictor of success at surgery is the apparent level of pulmonary artery obstructions. In several patients who have had obstructions only at the bronchopulmonary segmental artery, inadequate thromboembolic material was removed, resulting in inadequate relief of pulmonary vascular resistance. This was associated with a prohibitively high mortality.

SURGICAL TECHNIQUE

The pathology of chronic pulmonary embolism necessitates the technique of endarterectomy (18) rather than simple embolectomy. After a period of time, perhaps as short as 3 to 4 days, emboli become adherent to the pulmonary arterial wall by tissue ingrowth. With further time the embolic material is replaced with collagen and elastic tissue and is ultimately adherent to the pulmonary arterial wall. Historically, unilateral thoracotomy was most frequently utilized for pulmonary thromboendarterectomy (16). However, with unilateral thoracotomy only one side of a bilateral problem is addressed. Because of that limitation, we elected to use median sternotomy with both right and left pulmonary thromboendarterectomy as first described in 1980 (7). Other authors (19,20) continue to use lateral thoracotomy, although Jault and Cabrol recently (21) adopted the use of median sternotomy with cardiopulmonary bypass.

An important preoperative consideration is the prevention of subsequent pulmonary emboli. If a Greenfield filter is not in place, it is inserted 3 to 4 days preoperatively. Otherwise, the filter is placed during pulmonary thromboendarterectomy via the right atrium. Correct positioning is aided by radiopaque markers that are placed preoperatively over the spine for fluoroscopical identification of the correct location for the filter.

Consideration must be given to associated diseases such as coronary or valvular disease. When these are present, surgical correction is performed concurrently. The atrial septum is always inspected to identify an atrial septal defect or patent foramen ovale, which must be closed to preclude postoperative right-to-left shunting and consequent hypoxemia as well as paradoxical embolization. In our experience to date, 57.5 per cent ($^{84}/_{146}$) of patients have undergone one or more of these additional procedures concurrently with pulmonary thromboendarterectomy.

For the procedure, the patient is positioned supinely and the chest and both lower extremities are prepped and draped in the event saphenous veins are required for coronary bypass grafting. Median sternotomy is performed and cardiopulmonary bypass is instituted by transatrial, bicaval cannulation and the use of caval snares. Typically, the ascending aorta is cannulated for arterial inflow. As soon as cannulation is performed, systemic cooling to 20°C is initiated. During the cooling process the superior vena cava is dissected free from its adjacent tissues superiorly to the innominate vein and posteriorly to the azygous vein. This allows the superior vena cava to be retracted leftward to facilitate exposure of the right pulmonary artery. The pericardium is divided at its reflection over the right pulmonary artery, with the line of division extending superiorly and inferiorly from the pulmonary artery for a distance of approximately 2 cm in each direction. This line of division results in the incision being made approximately 1 cm posterior to the course of the phrenic nerve, which is essential to protect. Dissection in the right pulmonary artery region is continued beyond the middle lobe branches into the lower lobe artery and also out the upper lobe to its trifurcation (see Fig. 38–3). As systemic cooling progresses, the heart fibrillates secondary to hypothermia; at that time a sump tube is placed in the pulmonary artery and another in the left atrium because of excessive return of bronchial blood flow. If significant left ventricular distention occurs, a cooling jacket is applied to the right and left ventricles, the aorta is cross-clamped, and the aortic root is perfused with 1 liter of hypothermic, cold blood cardioplegic solution. Otherwise, the heart is allowed to fibrillate until just before circulatory arrest is initiated.

When 20°C is reached, the aorta is cross-clamped and myocardial protection, as described previously, is carried out. Because there is some degree of persistent

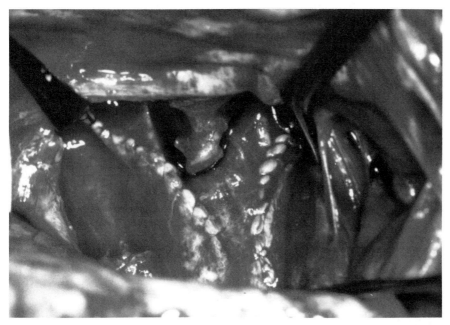

Figure 38–3. Exposure of the right pulmonary artery. The patient's head is to the viewer's right. The superior vena cava has been mobilized superiorly and anteriorly to the innominate vein and superiorly and posteriorly to the azygous vein. The vena cava is then retracted leftward to allow visualization of the right pulmonary artery and the upper lobe branch as well as the continuation of the right pulmonary artery, which supplies the middle and lower lobe bronchopulmonary segmental arteries. The incisions extending from the right pulmonary artery into the lower lobe and from the right pulmonary artery into the upper lobe can be visualized; each has been closed with two rows of continuous 6.0 polypropylene suture.

pulmonary vascular resistance elevation in the early postoperative state, it is essential to maintain optimal preservation of the right ventricle. Primary reliance is placed upon a cooling jacket, capable of maintaining myocardial temperatures at all sites at 10°C or less throughout the period of cross-clamping (8).

For central nervous system protection, when a systemic temperature of 20°C is reached the patient is given intravenous methylprednisolone, phenytoin, and sodium thiamylal to ensure cessation of electrical activity as indicated by the electroencephalogram, which is continuously monitored. The patient is exsanguinated into the heart-lung machine and during this period of time the lungs are hyperinflated repeatedly to facilitate drainage of blood from the pulmonary parenchyma.

An incision is made from the right pulmonary artery into the lower lobe branch that allows direct visualization of each bronchopulmonary segmental artery (Fig. 38–3). Dissection is carried out with a Penfield elevator to establish the correct plane of dissection, which is essential for proper endarterectomy. Once the correct plane is established, dissection is continued distally in a 360 degree circumferential fashion for each bronchopulmonary segmental branch until endarterectomy is complete. The maximum period of circulatory arrest of 20 min is followed by hypothermic (16°C) reperfusion to restore mixed venous oxygen saturation to the prearrest level, which, typically, requires 8 to 10 min. Again, circulatory arrest is obtained for a 20-min period; this process is repeated until endarterectomy is

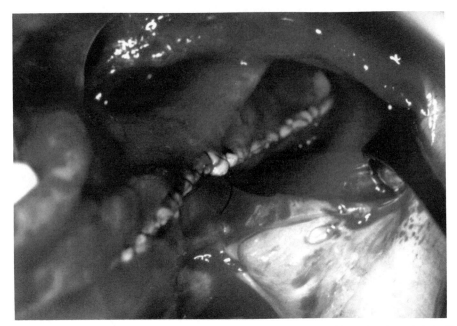

Figure 38–4. Exposure of the left pulmonary artery. The patient's head is to the viewer's left. The incision was started intrapericardially, continued distally into the pulmonary artery beyond the pericardial reflection, and extended distally to the level of the crossing of the left upper lobe bronchus. Through this single incision, all of the bronchopulmonary segmental arteries of the left lung can be visualized. Incision closure was identical to that on the right side.

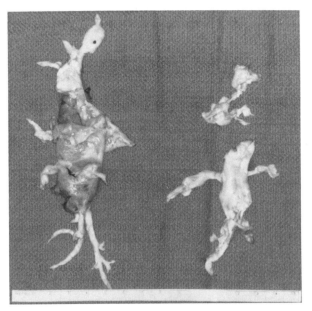

Figure 38–5. Surgical specimen from pulmonary thromboendarterectomy of both pulmonary arteries. This specimen is oriented with the patient's right side to the viewer's left. Essentially all of the bronchopulmonary segmental arteries have been endarterectomized, resulting in a cast of the pulmonary arterial tree.

complete. During a period of rewarming, the incision in the right lower lobe branch is closed with two rows of continuous 6.0 Prolene. A separate incision is made in the right pulmonary artery and extended into the right upper lobe branch to its trifurcation and identical procedures are carried out (Fig. 38–3).

On the left side, the pericardium is freed at its reflection from the left pulmonary artery and the incision is extended superiorly and inferiorly as described for the right side. The left upper lobe bronchus limits the incision on the left side, which is started intrapericardially and extended distally to the left upper lobe bronchus (Fig. 38–4). Again, endarterectomy is performed as described above with closure in the same fashion. Associated procedures, are performed during the process of cooling and rewarming. The above methods recently have been described in detail (22).

A typical endarterectomy specimen is shown in Figure 38–5. It has numerous side branches that correspond with the various bronchopulmonary segmental arteries and subbranches.

EARLY AND LATE RESULTS

In 1984 Chitwood and associates (16) were able to identify 85 patients undergoing pulmonary thromboendarterectomy, with a hospital mortality of 22 per cent. Subsequently, aside from our experience (8,22,23), the only other report of a significant group of patients was that of Jault and Cabrol (21), which added 17 cases to their previously reported 16 (20) for an overall mortality of 20 per cent.

For analysis, our patients have been divided into groups A, B, and C, which are related to methods of myocardial protection and surgical dissection and exposure of the pulmonary arteries. Myocardial protection was obtained in the first group of 16 patients (group A, February 1, 1975, to October 20, 1983) by the use of crystalloid cold cardioplegia and maintenance of myocardial hypothermia with topical saline (24). The method of exposure of the pulmonary arteries involved division of the pericardium to the phrenic nerves. The phrenic nerves were mobilized and retracted from the operative field. The pericardium was further divided to the pulmonary arteries and dissection extended distally, which involved entering the pleural spaces bilaterally.

From March 12, 1984, to September 11, 1984, seven patients (group B) underwent pulmonary thromboendarterectomy with dissection and exposure methods as in group A. Myocardial protection consisted of crystalloid cold blood cardioplegia with maintenance of myocardial hypothermia by saline slush contained in a laparotomy pad wrapped around the right and left ventricles.

Since October 1, 1984, group C patients had the use of cold blood cardioplegia, and myocardial hypothermia was maintained with a cooling jacket encompassing the right and left ventricles. Dissection was started intrapericardially and continued within the hilar tissues (8). Hospital mortality and morbidity for each group, related to phrenic nerve paresis and required ventilatory support, are depicted in Table 38–1. The most significant problem encountered was seen in group B, wherein five of the seven patients had one or both phrenic nerves paralyzed secondary to the use of saline slush. The subsequent rigorous avoidance of saline slush has resulted in a marked diminution of the incidence of phrenic

TABLE 38–1. Hospital Mortality and Morbidity with Chronic Pulmonary Embolism[a]

	N	HOSPITAL MORTALITY[b]	PHRENIC NERVE PARESIS	MEAN NO. DAYS ON RESPIRATOR
Group A (02/01/75–10/20/83)	16	3 (18.7%)	0 (0%)	8.4
Group B (03/12/84–09/11/84)	7	1 (14.3%)	5 (71%)	32.2
Group C (10/01/84–09/18/89)	149	17 (11.4%)	2 (1.34%)	4.5

[a] Data from Daily et al. (8, 23).
[b] All deaths within 30 days or during hospitalization.

nerve paresis. In group C (149 patients), there were two episodes of phrenic nerve paresis, one that was temporary and necessitated mechanical ventilation for 3 days. A second patient underwent repeat pulmonary thromboendarterectomy and had dense adhesions. It was thought that excessive retraction for exposure of the distal pulmonary arteries may have resulted in phrenic nerve paresis.

The surgical procedure has been standardized since October 1, 1984, as characterized in group C, and has been used in 149 consecutive patients extending to September 18, 1989. Preoperative and postoperative patient details are illustrated in Tables 38–2 and 38–3, respectively. Hospital mortality, as defined by death within 30 days or during hospitalization, occurred in 11.4 per cent ($^{17}/_{149}$) of patients. In three patients death occurred intraoperatively from severe intratracheal

TABLE 38–2. Preopertive Patient Descriptors (N = 149)[a]

Gender
  Male: 94 (63.1%)
  Female: 55 (36.9%)
New York Heart Association functional classification
  I: 1 (0.7%)
  II: 13 (8.7%)
  III: 66 (44.3%)
  IV: 69 (46.3%)

	Mean	Range
Age (years)	51 ± 15	20–82
Duration of Symptoms (months)	61.1 ± 66.3	1–432
PaO$_2$, at rest, room air (mm Hg)	68 ± 19	29–104
Mean pulmonary artery pressure (mm Hg)	45.9 ± 13.8	18–105
Pulmonary vascular resistance (dynes-sec-cm^{-5})	806 ± 348	170–2000

	No.	%
Other diseases/conditions	54	36.2
Coronary artery disease	17	11.4
Previous myocardial infarction	6/17	4.0
Renal failure	8	5.4
Peripheral vascular disease	13	8.7
Diabetes (insulin dependent)	3	2.0
Ascites	13	8.7

[a] Data from Daily et al. (23).

TABLE 38–3.   Postoperative Patient Descriptors ($N = 146^a)^b$

	No.	%
Associated procedures		
Coronary artery bypass	13	8.9
Coronary artery bypass/aortic valve replacement	1	0.7
Coronary artery bypass/mitral valve replacement	1	0.7
Tricuspid valve annuloplasty	4	2.7
Aortic valve débridement	1	0.7
Patent foramen ovale or atrial septal defect closure	41	28.1
Caval procedure	23	15.4

	Mean	Range
% Reduction in pulmonary vascular resistance	67 ± 28	0–93
Last pulmonary vascular resistance (dynes-sec-cm^{-5})	236 ± 139	
Total cardiopulmonary bypass time (min)	185 ± 42	113–344
Total circulatory arrest time (min)	58 ± 21	16–129
Total aortic cross-clamp time (min)	115 ± 33	51–207
Days on respirator	4.5 ± 5.4	1–35
Days in hospital, postoperative	19.6 ± 12.3	2–71

[a] Operative deaths excluded.
[b] Data from Daily et al. (23).

hemorrhage in two and acute right heart failure in another. The causes of death are described in Table 38–4.

The most significant morbidity encountered in group C was that of reperfusion pulmonary edema, as manifested by the necessity for mechanical ventilation. Ventilator dependency, as an indicator of pulmonary edema, was defined as the need for mechanical ventilation for 5 or more days. We examined a number of preoperative and operative considerations as potential predictors of hospital mortality and ventilator dependency (22). Multivariate analysis revealed that hospital mortality was predicted by increased cardiopulmonary bypass times, failure to reduce the pulmonary vascular reistance by 50 per cent or more, and increased preoperative levels of pulmonary vascular resistance. Ventilator dependency was predicted by preoperative presence of ascites, prolonged cardiopulmonary bypass time, and requirement of more than four blood product units in the intraoperative

TABLE 38–4.   Causes of Death following Surgery[a]

	NO.	%	POSTOP DAY(S) OF DEATH
Respiratory and multiorgan failure	10	58.8	19.9 (range, 4–47)
Pulmonary hemorrhage	3[b]	17.6	1
Acute myocardial infarction	1	5.9	3
Right heart failure	1[c]	5.9	0
Pulmonary artery thrombosis	1	5.9	6
Late cardiac tamponade	1	5.9	17

[a] Data from Daily et al. (23).
[b] Two intraoperative.
[c] Intraoperative.

TABLE 38–5. New York Heart Association Functional Classification ($N = 35$)[a]

	BEFORE SURGERY (NO.)	AFTER SURGERY (NO.)
IV	22	0
III	13	1
II	0	18
I	0	16

[a] Data from Moser et al. (25).

or postoperative period. Failure to reduce pulmonary vascular resistance by 50 per cent or more nearly reached statistical significance ($p = .08$). Univariate analysis revealed trends that did not reach statistical significance but suggested that an increased data base may allow preoperative prediction of ventilator dependency and hospital mortality. Trends for ventilator dependency were duration of symptoms, New York Heart Association functional classification IV, and presence of associated diseases. Potential preoperative factors for prediction of hospital mortality were age, New York Heart Association functional classification IV, and presence of associated diseases.

Previously we described the long-term follow-up results in 35 survivors of 42 patients undergoing pulmonary thromboendarterectomy (25). There was a mean follow-up period of 28 months. The pre- and postoperative New York Heart Association functional classifications of these patients are illustrated in Table 38–5 and the hemodynamic characteristics before and immediately after pulmonary thromboendarterectomy, and at follow-up, are described in Table 38–6. It is noteworthy that at follow-up there was an additional reduction in pulmonary vascular resistance beyond that seen in the early postoperative period. Although additional follow-up is needed, it is apparent that hemodynamics and functional capability are restored to near-normal levels after pulmonary thromboendarterectomy. If postoperative levels of mean pulmonary artery pressure have predictability for late survival approximating that described by Reidel and associates (26) (Table 38–7), one may conclude that late survival is substantially enhanced by pulmonary thromboendarterectomy as compared to the natural history.

TABLE 38–6. Hemodynamics ($N = 35$)[a]

	PREOP	IMMEDIATE POSTOP	FOLLOW-UP[b]
Mean pulmonary artery pressure (mm Hg)	50.2 ± 8.2	30.4 ± 8.6	24.6 ± 10.4
Cardiac output (L/min)	3.95 ± 1.07	5.75 ± 1.15	5.71 ± 0.77
Pulmonary vascular resistance (dynes-sec-cm^{-5})	985 ± 439	302 ± 146	220 ± 138
Pulmonary capillary wedge (or left atrial) pressure (mm Hg)	7.8 ± 3.4	9.4 ± 1.7	7.3 ± 6.2

[a] From Moser KM, Daily PO, Peterson K, Dembitsky W, Vapnek JM, Shure D, Utley J, Archibald CA: Thromboendarterectomy for chronic, major-vessel thromboembolic pulmonary hypertension. Immediate and long-term results in 42 patients. Ann Intern Med 1987;*107*:560–565.
[b] Mean time to follow-up is 28 months. Range is 7 months to 16 years.

TABLE 38–7. Survival Related to Mean Pulmonary Artery Pressure[a]

MEAN PULMONARY ARTERY PRESSURE (mm Hg)	5-YEAR SURVIVAL (%)
<30	>90
31–40	45
41–50	35
>50	10

[a] Data from Reidel et al. (26).

SUMMARY

There is a small but indeterminate percentage of patients who are significantly disabled with pulmonary hypertension secondary to chronic pulmonary embolism. Currently, pulmonary thromboendarterectomy is associated with a hospital mortality of 11.4 per cent compared to 24 per cent for heart-lung transplantation (27), the only other therapeutic modality for patients with chronic pulmonary embolism. While not complete, early follow-up information following pulmonary thromboendarterectomy indicates a 1-year survival of 87.3 per cent and a 3-year survival of 85.3 per cent. These data compare to 65 and 50 per cent 1- and 3-year survival, respectively, for heart-lung transplantation in the Stanford series (27). These data suggest that patients with severe pulmonary hypertension secondary to chronic pulmonary embolism should be managed with pulmonary thromboendarterectomy when the obstructive material is sufficiently proximal to allow endarterectomy. However, in those patients with more distal disease, lung or heart-lung transplantation should be considered.

REFERENCES

1. Hollister LE, Cull VL: The syndrome of chronic thrombosis of the major pulmonary arteries. Am J Med 1956;*21*:312–320.
2. Boucher H, Protar M, Bertein J: Aneurysme de la branche droite de l'artere pulmonaire par embol latent postphlebitique. J Franc Med Chir Thorax 1951;*5*:421.
3. Hurwitt ES, Schein CJ, Rifkin H, Lebendiger A: A surgical approach to the problem of chronic pulmonary artery obstruction due to thrombosis or stenosis. Am Surg 1958;*147*:157–165.
4. Snyder WA, Kent DC, Baisch BF: Successful endarterectomy of chronically occluded pulmonary artery. J Thorac Cardiovasc Surg 1963;*45*:482–489.
5. Houk VN, Hufnagel CA, McClenathan JE, Moser KM: Chronic thrombosis obstruction of major pulmonary arteries. Am J Med 1963;*35*:269–282.
6. Sabiston DC, Wolfe WG, Oldham HN, et al: Surgical management of chronic pulmonary embolism. Ann Surg 1977;*185*:699–712.
7. Daily PO, Johnston GG, Simmons CJ, Moser KM: Surgical management of chronic pulmonary embolism. J Thorac Cardiovasc Surg 1980;*79*:523–531.
8. Daily PO, Dembitsky WP, Peterson KL, Moser KM: Modifications of techniques and early results of pulmonary thromboendarterectomy for chronic pulmonary embolism. J Thorac Cardiovasc Surg 1987;*93*:221–233.
9. Daily PO, Pfeffer TA, Wisniewski JB, Steinke TA, Kinney TB, Moores WY, Dembitsky WP: Clinical comparisons of methods of myocardial protection. J Thorac Cardiovasc Surg 1987; *93*:324–336.
10. Dalen JE, Alpert JS: Natural history of pulmonary embolism. Prog Cardiovasc Dis 1975;*17*:259–270.

11. Sautter RD, Myers WO, Ray JF III, Wenzel FJ: Pulmonary embolectomy: Review and current status. Prog Cardiovasc Dis 1975;*17*:371–382.

12. Sabiston DC Jr, Wolfe WG: Experimental and clinical observations on the natural history of pulmonary embolism. Ann Surg 1968;*168*:1–15.

13. Paraskos JA, Adelstein SJ, Smith RE, Rickman FD, Grossman WG, Dexter L, Dalen JE: Late prognosis of acute pulmonary embolism. N Engl J Med 1973;*289*:55–58.

14. Tilkian AG, Schroeder JS, Robin ED: Chronic thromboembolic occlusion of main pulmonary artery or primary branches. Am J Med 1967;*60*:563–573.

15. Moser KM: Venous thromboembolism. Am Rev Respir Dis 1990;*141*:235–249.

16. Chitwood WR, Sabiston DC, Wechsler AS: Surgical treatment of chronic unresolved pulmonary embolism. Clin Chest Med 1984;*5*:507–536.

17. Moser KM, Spragg RG, Utley J, Daily PO: Chronic thrombotic obstruction of major pulmonary arteries. Results of thromboendarterectomy in 15 patients. Ann Intern Med 1983;*99*:299–305.

18. Daily PO, Dembitsky WP, Iversen S: Technique of pulmonary thromboendarterectomy for chronic pulmonary embolism. J Card Surg 1989;*4*:10–24.

19. Dor V, Jourdan J, Schmitt R, Sabatier M, Arnulf JJ, Kreitmann P: Delayed pulmonary thrombectomy via a peripheral approach in the treatment of pulmonary embolism and sequelae. Thorac Cardiovasc Surg 1981;*29*:227–232.

20. Cabrol C, Cabrol A, Acar J, et al: Surgical correction of chronic postembolic obstructions of the pulmonary arteries. J Thorac Cardiovasc Surg 1978;*76*:620–628.

21. Jault F, Cabrol C: Surgical treatment for chronic pulmonary thromboembolism. Herz 1989; *14*:192–196.

22. Daily PO, Dembitsky WP, Iversen S, Moser KM, Auger W: Risk factors for pulmonary thromboendarterectomy. J Thorac Cardiovasc Surg 1990;*99*:670–678.

23. Daily PO, Dembitsky WP, Iversen S, Moser KM, Auger W: Current early results of pulmonary thromboendarterectomy for chronic pulmonary embolism. Eur J Cardio-Thorac Surg 1990; *4*:117–123.

24. Shumway NE, Lower RR, Stofer RC: Selective hypothermia of the heart in anoxic cardiac arrest. Surg Gynecol Obstet 1959;*109*:750–754.

25. Moser KM, Daily PO, Peterson K, Dembitsky W, Vapnek JM, Shure D, Utley J, Archibald CA: Thromboendarterectomy for chronic, major-vessel thromboembolic pulmonary hypertension. Immediate and long-term results in 42 patients. Ann Intern Med 1987;*107*:560–565.

26. Reidel M, Stanek V, Widimsky J, Preroesky I: Long term follow-up of patients with pulmonary thromboembolism. Late prognosis and evolution of hemodynamic and respiratory data. Chest 1982;*81*:151–158.

27. McCarthy PM, Starnes VA, Stinson EB, Oyer PE, Shumway NE: Improved survival following heart-lung transplant. J Thorac Cardiovasc Surg 1990;*99*:54–60.

39

VENA CAVA INTERRUPTION: Devices and Results

Lazar J. Greenfield

Considerable progress has been made in the control of pulmonary thromboembolism since the initial approach of operative ligation of the vena cava. Recognition of the advantages of preserving inferior vena caval blood flow and normal distal venous pressure led to the development of suture plication techniques and external smooth or serrated clips, which are now utilized only under unusual circumstances. The early transvenous devices, such as the Hunter balloon and the Mobin-Uddin umbrella, either were susceptible to proximal migration or produced unacceptable morbidity from occlusion of the vena cava and have been withdrawn from the market. What might be considered as the modern era of transvenous devices intended to trap emboli while preserving inferior vena caval blood flow and patency began in 1973 with the introduction of the Greenfield filter (1). This stainless-steel device was designed for operative insertion via either the jugular or femoral vein and has been proved to be safe and effective by long-term follow-up evaluation (2). Since 1984, however, some radiologists have employed percutaneous techniques for insertion of the Greenfield filter and have developed similar designs or alternative types of filters that could be inserted more readily through smaller carrier systems (Fig. 39–1).

Percutaneous insertion of devices designed to provide effective filtration of thromboemboli in the vena cava offers a number of potential advantages for the patient, including reduced discomfort, time, and cost due to the use of the radiology suite rather than the operating room. It is made possible by the Seldinger technique, which allows the percutaneous insertion of progressively larger dilators and a sheath over a Teflon-coated guidewire. The usual route of access is the femoral vein, but the jugular vein also can be used. Once a guidewire has been inserted, enlarging the skin incision permits expansion of the track either by balloon or dilators to permit the insertion of a large sheath. A 26 French size is required for percutaneous insertion of the standard stainless-steel Greenfield filter (SGF), which utilizes a 24 French carrier system (1). This approach is customarily employed from the right groin, and although the jugular vein can also be used, it is less desirable because of the risk of air embolism. Several series have been reported showing a favorable experience in terms of ease of insertion. However, the trauma to the vein would appear to be increased since the follow-up of these patients has shown a high incidence of venous thrombosis at the insertion site, as high as 41 per cent in one series (2). In view of these problems and the me-

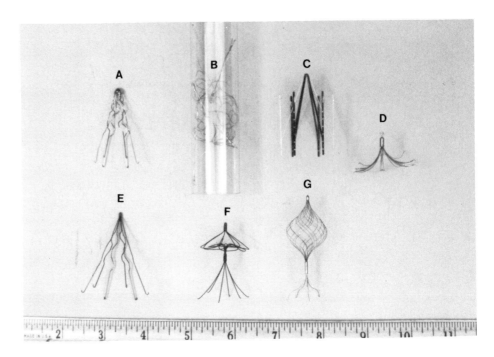

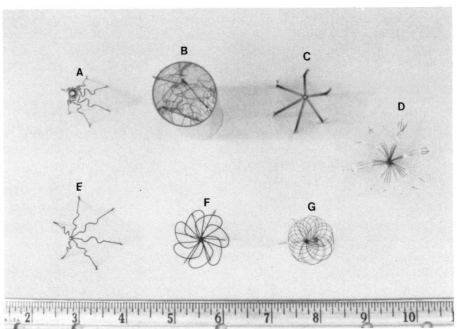

Figure 39–1. *A*, Lateral view of available and experimental vena caval filter devices, including the standard stainless-steel Greenfield filter (*A*); the bird's nest filter (*B*); the Venatech filter (*C*); the Amplatz filter, which is designed to be inserted inverting the cone (*D*); the titanium model of the Greenfield filter (*E*); the nitinol filter (*F*); and the Gunther filter, which is also designed to be inserted in an inverted position (*G*). *B*, Axial view of vena caval filters, shown with labels *A* through *G* as identified in *A*.

TABLE 39–1. Comparison of Inferior Vena Caval Filter Devices

FILTER DEVICE	LARGEST EXPERIENCE	FAILURES TO INSERT	MISPLACEMENT	TILT	PATIENTS FOLLOWED	FOLLOW-UP PERIOD	FILTER-CAVAL OCCLUSION	RECURRENT PE	PROXIMAL MIGRATION	VENOUS STASIS
Standard Greenfield	469	0.6%	2.5%	1.7%	146	12 yr	2%	4%	0	5% new
Bird's nest	568	0	NR[a]	NA[b]	37	6 mo	19%	12 1 death	5 (16%)	NR
Titanium Greenfield	50	1 (2%)	0	1 (2%)	29	5 mo	0	1	0	0
Amplatz	52	NR	2 (4%)	1 (2%)	42	11 mo	21%	1	0	NR
Nitinol	103	0	3 (3%)	Frequent	44	6 mo	18%	2	1 (2%)	13
Venatech	100	2 (2%)	18 (18%)	16 (16%)	90	1 yr	8%	2	4 (4%)	29 (32%)

[a] NR, not reported.
[b] NA, not applicable.

chanical advantage of a smaller carrier system, a titanium version of the Greenfield filter (TGF) has been developed that allows the carrier system to be reduced in diameter to size 12 French (3). With a carrier system of this size, a 14 French sheath is required for percutaneous insertion. Our preliminary experience with this device in 40 patients at three different institutions has been reported and indicates that this technique has not been associated with significant insertion site venous thrombosis (4). The TGF filter can also be inserted at the time of laparotomy either through a pursestring suture in the vena cava or through a smaller venous tributary. Under these circumstances, fluoroscopy is not necessary since the position of the carrier can be determined by palpation and the filter discharged at the appropriate level. Several other devices have been introduced to achieve vena caval filtration using a smaller catheter insertion system; the status of these devices will be reviewed as well (Table 39–1 and Fig. 39–1).

TITANIUM GREENFIELD FILTER

The TGF (MediTech, Incorporated) is made from a titanium alloy previously described (5). Its cone shape is similar to that of the SGF but it is 8 mm wider at the base and 0.5 cm taller (Fig. 39–1). It weighs 0.25 gm as opposed to 0.56 gm for the SGF, and can be compressed to a diameter of 0.144 inch. Mechanical properties of the TGF have been tested extensively and it shows remarkable resistance to flexion fatigue and induced corrosion (5). It exerts a force of fixation on the wall of the vena cava that is measurably greater than the SGF at diameters over 22 mm but less than the SGF at diameters less than 22 mm.

The technique for placement is a guidewire inserted from either the left or right femoral vein over which a dilator system and attached 14 French sheath can be passed. Once the sheath and dilator are in the inferior vena cava at the level of desired filter placement, the dilator is withdrawn and the TGF carrier is then passed under fluoroscopic control to the level of intended insertion. Both the carrier catheter and sheath are retracted as a unit to release the filter. After discharge, the carrier and sheath are withdrawn and gentle pressure is applied to the insertion site. An additional advantage to the use of the sheath is the fact that premature discharge of the filter would result in filter misplacement into the sheath rather than into the patient. Premature discharge is unlikely since a new control handle has been added that allows no manipulation other than retraction of the carrier for discharge of the filter. The filter is also preloaded into the carrier system, obviating concern about crossed limbs.

In our initial clinical experience, titanium filters were inserted successfully in 51 of 52 patients (98 per cent). In one patient previously reported, there was a very tight stricture of the inferior vena cava at the level of the hepatic veins that prevented operative passage of the carrier catheter. This 56-year-old woman had terminal adenocarcinoma and it was thought that her stricture would prevent massive embolism from occurring. At autopsy 10 days later, there was no evidence of pulmonary thromboembolism. In one other patient, an attempt had been made to insert the SGF operatively via the jugular vein, but this was prevented by thrombosis at the junction of the jugular with the subclavian vein. A TGF was inserted operatively from the right femoral vein. All percutaneous insertions were successful in filter placement.

The indications for filter insertion were a contraindication to anticoagulation in 34 patients (65 per cent), recurrent thromboembolism in spite of anticoagulation in nine (17 per cent), a complication of anticoagulation in seven (13 per cent), and adjunctive prophylaxis in two patients (4 per cent). Filters were placed below the level of the renal vein in 46 patients (90 per cent) and above the renal vein in five patients (10 per cent).

There were 19 deaths (36 per cent) during follow-up, only one of which could be attributed to recurrent thromboembolism. In this particular patient, previously reported, there was uncontrollable thrombosis involving her subclavian veins and progressive pulmonary hypertension. Although the patient died at home and no autopsy was permitted, it is likely that she died of recurrent thromboembolism. At the time of development of her subclavian vein thromboses, there was no access that would have permitted insertion of a filter in her superior vena cava, since both iliac veins were thrombosed and she had a filter in position in her inferior vena cava. Recurrent thromboembolism occurred in one other patient, for a rate of 4 per cent.

There were 30 patients who returned for follow-up laboratory examinations at an average interval of 5.2 months. Four patients refused to return for follow-up study. Follow-up duplex examination showed thrombosis in the vein used for insertion in two patients (7 per cent), both of whom were asymptomatic. Although there was no proximal migration, distal migration was seen in nine patients (30 per cent) for distances of 9 to 64 mm (average of 23 mm), usually with an increase in limb diameter. Eight filters had a slight tilt at the time of insertion, varying from 4 to 30 degrees. The frequency of tilting was increased at the time of follow-up to 12 filters showing an angulation of 5 to 23 degrees. Penetration of the filter beyond the wall of the vena cava was suspected in nine patients (30 per cent), and the follow-up CT scan was confirmatory in the four patients in whom it was obtained. There was significant mobility of the TGF noted with respiration, particularly in the suprarenal position, where it is likely that diaphragmatic motion added direct pressure. In one patient, caval perforation by the apex of the filter occurred at the time of insertion from the left femoral vein when it was not appreciated that the apex of the filter was impinging on the wall of the vena cava. At the time of discharge it was noted that the filter did not open, so a second titanium filter was placed below it from the right common femoral vein at the level of L-3. There were no sequelae following this misplacement, and at follow-up examination 4 months later the filters were stable and the vena cava was patent. There were no adverse sequelae from any of the penetrations, from the tilting, or from distal migration; however, the frequency of migration makes this device unacceptable for widespread use.

The present carrier used for the SGF is large enough to present mechanical problems occasionally during both introduction into the vein and passage through the eustachian valve at the atriocaval junction or into the vena cava from the pelvis. Reducing the diameter of the carrier system from 24 French to 12 French has facilitated both entry and positioning and completely eliminated bleeding during percutaneous filter insertion. The mobility of the TGF, however, suggests that it has less initial purchase on the wall of the vena cava than the SGF in spite of the measured greater lateral forces. There is still no evidence that the TGF will migrate proximally or that it will fail to remain secure after entrapping a thromboembolus. In order to correct the problems of migration and caval wall pene-

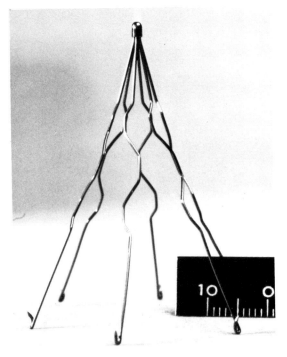

Figure 39–2. Lateral view of the titanium Greenfield filter with modified hook design. The recurved and 80 degree angled hook appears to limit caval wall penetration and distal migration in preliminary clinical trials.

tration, the design of the hook has been changed to a recurved form with an 80 degree hook (Fig. 39–2). In experimental studies and current clinical trials, this modified TGF appears to be stable and has shown no significant caval wall penetration.

BIRD'S NEST FILTER

The bird's nest filter was reported initially in 1984 and a larger series of 568 patients was reported in 1988 (6). The device is constructed of four stainless-steel wires, each of which is 25 cm long and 0.18 mm in diameter. The wires are preshaped with nonmatching bends and each end of each wire is attached to a strut that ends in a hook for fixation to the wall of the vena cava (Fig. 39–1). One strut is "Z"-shaped so that a pusher wire can be screwed onto it. The original model was preloaded into an 8 French Teflon catheter, but in 1986 the struts were modified with the use of a stiff wire measuring 0.46 mm to improve fixation in an attempt to prevent the proximal migration that had occurred with the original design. The broader struts required an increase in diameter of the preloaded catheter to size 12 French. The insertion procedure consists of pushing the first set of hooks into the wall of the vena cava, after which the wire is extruded in an effort to pack the loops of wires closely in the vena cava. Finally, the second pair of hooks is pushed into the vena cava wall. The pusher wire is rotated to free it and allow removal of the catheter. The intention is to pack the wires into approximately a 7-cm length of the vena cava in order to provide multiple barriers to the passage of emboli (Fig. 39–1B).

Follow-up information on the bird's nest filter is limited, since only 37 of the

481 patients in whom the filter had been in place for 6 months or more had objective evaluation of their vena cavas by means of cavography or ultrasound (7). Seven of the patients (19 per cent) had caval occlusion. Three symptomatic patients had pulmonary angiograms for recurrent thromboembolism, which was confirmed in one of them. In addition to problems with thrombosis, the bird's nest filter has demonstrated migration proximally following what appeared to be secure placement. This has been seen both experimentally and clinically, with reports of five patients and one death. In the latter patient, the bird's nest filter was found with a massive embolus in the pulmonary artery 10 days after placement. It was this experience that led to modification of the struts to prevent inversion in the vena cava. In a subsequent report from the University of Arkansas, the experience with three cases of filter migration out of 32 placements was described (8). The two cases identified within 24 hr were successfully retrieved percutaneously and the partially migrated filter was retracted to the intrahepatic segment of the inferior vena cava. The third case of migration was not detected for 6 months, at which time the filter was embedded in the right atrium and ventricle and could not be recovered. This experience was prior to the change in hook design. Additional clinical studies of the modified filter are in progress.

AMPLATZ FILTER

The Amplatz filter was introduced in 1984, and clinical experience has been reported in 52 patients (9). This filter is also cone shaped and made from a stainless-steel alloy, but is designed to be inserted in an inverted position in the vena cava, with pronged loops designed to limit caval wall penetration to 2 mm in order to avoid injury to pericaval structures (Fig. 39–1). A loop has also been added at the apex to allow for repositioning or retrieval. One patient in this series had repositioning from a suboptimal position immediately after insertion, and of the eight patients who were considered candidates for retrieval because of their short-term high risk for anticoagulation, retrieval was actually performed in five patients at 1 to 16 days after insertion. After retrieval, two patients demonstrated intramural abnormalities suggesting local hemorrhage.

The follow-up experience was for a mean of 11 months and showed one insertion site venous thrombosis (3 per cent). Distal migration occurred in one patient and tilting of the filter was observed in another patient. Thrombi in the apex of the filter cone were demonstrated in nine of 34 patients (25 per cent) at venocavography, but the authors believed that these were not likely to produce embolism in spite of the fact that they were on the unprotected side of the filter. Larger thrombi trapped by the filter were seen in four of 34 patients (12 per cent), and in two of them there was propagation through the filter. The third patient had thrombus propagating through the filter with a benign course, but a fourth patient with thrombus on both sides of the filter was found to have pulmonary embolism at autopsy. Overall, nine of 42 patients (21 per cent) had thrombosed vena cavas at follow-up exmaination. Two patients required Greenfield filter placement above the original Amplatz filter. The authors believe that the denser arrangement of wire results in greater clot trapping efficiency, but at the expense of a higher rate of filter and caval occlusion. Of particular concern is the tendency for trapped thrombi to propagate through this particular device. Retrievability is also of only marginal benefit since a filter that has remained patent during the period of risk should not pose any long-term risk to the patient.

NITINOL FILTER

Nitinol is a nickel-titanium alloy that can exist as a pliable straight wire when cooled but rapidly transforms nto a previously imprinted rigid shape when warmed. Although a filter made of this material was described in 1977, clinical experience with the device has only recently been reported (10). The filter design includes a 28-mm dome with eight overlapping loops, and below that the wire is shaped into six diverging legs with terminal hooks to engage the vena caval wall in the configuration of a cone (Fig. 39–1). The preliminary report on the clinical experience with this device indicated that it was inserted in 103 patients in 17 participating centers. Detailed information, however, was only available on 44 patients. The procedure utilizes iced normal saline infused through a 9 French delivery catheter. The filter wire is advanced rapidly with the feeder pump and then discharged from the storage tube. It is said to expand instantly into the appropriate shape and lock into place. In the multicenter study, for the brief period of follow-up there were three cases of recurrent pulmonary embolism and seven cases of confirmed vena caval occlusion with two additional suspected occlusions on the basis of clinical findings. Five of 18 patients studied by ultrasound showed thrombosis at the site of insertion. Of the 44 patients followed, 10 were studied at 3 months but only four completed the 6-month follow-up. Within this group, six occlusions of the vena cava were documented and two additional were suspected, for an occlusion rate of 18 per cent. An additional five patients developed edema with signs of thrombus within the filter. In one of the two patients with recurrent embolism, a proximal propagating thrombus above the filter was identified by venacavography. Migration of one of the filters was mentioned in an addendum to the report.

A more recent update on the clinical experience shows that 224 patients have received nitinol filters, 102 are being followed, and 65 have completed 6 months' follow-up. There were four patients who sustained recurrent embolism, with one fatality, and 20 documented caval occlusions, to which the author added three deaths associated with massive caval thrombosis (11). The high rate of vena caval thrombosis in this series with very short follow-up suggests that the filter material and/or design may be thrombogenic.

VENATECH FILTER

In 1986, another cone-shaped filter with added stabilizing struts on each limb was introduced from France as the "LGM" filter (12). It is currently being marketed in the United States as the Venatech filter, designed for percutaneous introduction. The filter is made of Phynox, which is said to be similar to Elgiloy, used in temporary cardiac pacing wires. It is a stamped, six-pronged device on which there are hooked stabilizers with sharp ends intended to center and fix the device (Fig. 39–1). It is inserted through a 12 French single-use catheter system, preferentially via the right internal jugular vein. A guidewire is used and the filter is ejected after it has been passed through the full length of the catheter. The only reported experience is from France and consists of 100 attempted insertions resulting in 98 filters discharged, 82 of which were positioned correctly. Eight filters had a 15 degree or greater tilt, five opened incompletely, and an additional three were both incompletely opened and tilted. All of the filters were implanted via the jugular route. Nine of the filters were observed to migrate distally and four in a cephalad direction, for a 13 per cent migration rate.

The follow-up experience is limited to 1 year, at which time there were seven occlusions, for a 92 per cent patency rate. Recurrent pulmonary embolism was seen in two patients, both of whom had incompletely opened filters. At the end of 1 year, 13 filters were observed to have migrated, nine to the iliac vein and four to the renal veins. Twenty-nine patients had lower limb edema in spite of the use of elastic support hose, and seven of them had vena caval thrombosis. Another report had a 13 per cent rate of tilting or partial opening and a caudal migration rate of 13 per cent. Caval occlusion was seen in 8 per cent at follow-up and there was a 2.5 per cent incidence of recurrent embolism (13). There are isolated reports of breakage of the stabilizer struts, and it is surprising that the incidence of tilting has been so high in a device that was designed to prevent a tilt.

GUNTHER FILTER

The Gunther filter was described in 1987 as a percutaneous removable filter consisting of a helix of wires with an inverted cone above (14) (Fig. 39–1). It has been tested in Europe but is not available in the United States. There is no long-term follow-up information available on the device, but preliminary results show a 7 per cent caval thrombosis rate and a disturbing caudal migration rate of 70 per cent (15). In addition, caval penetration by the struts was seen in 20 per cent of patients and perforation by the retrieving hook in 78 per cent. Proxmial migration of the device into the right ventricle has also been reported (16), which raises concern regarding its ability to trap thromboemboli safely.

CONCLUSIONS

There is considerable ingenuity in the number of devices now available for clinical trial as vena caval filters. The primary objective—to provide a safe and effective device for permanent implantation—should lead to continued evolution of materials and design. The issue of retrievability, however, is overrated since any implanted device should not represent a long-term risk to the patient and the assumption that thromboembolism can be predicted as a short-term risk is incompatible with the unpredictability of the disorder. The standard for comparison should remain the Greenfield filter, with a recurrent embolism rate of 4 per cent and a long-term patency rate at 12-year follow-up of 98 per cent. The present concern regarding the percutaneous insertion of the SGF overlooks the fact that it can be inserted quite safely at operation under local anesthesia with minimal morbidity. It seems clear that advances in percutaneous techniques will make this the obvious choice for the future, but the safety and efficacy of the conical design of the Greenfield filter suggests that a new design may not be needed.

REFERENCES

1. Tadavarthy SM, Castaneda-Zuniga WR, Salmonowitz E, et al: Kimray-Greenfield vena cava filter: Percutaneous introduction. Radiology 1984;*151*:525–526.
2. Kantor A, Glanz S, Gordon DH, Scalfani SJA: Percutaneous isertion of the Kimray-Greenfield filter: Incidence of femoral vein thrombosis. Am R Roentgenol 1987;*149*:1065–1066.
3. Burke PE, Michna BA, Harvey CF, Crute SL, Sobel M, Greenfield LJ: Experimental comparison of percutaneous vena caval devices: Titanium Greenfield filter vs. bird's nest filter. J Vasc Surg 1987;*6*:66–70.
4. Greenfield LJ, Cho KJ, Pais SO, Van Aman M: Preliminary clinical experience with the titanium Greenfield vena caval filter. Arch Surg 1989;*124*:657–659.
5. Greenfield LJ, Savin MA: Comparison of titanium and stainless steel Greenfield vena caval filters. Surgery 1989;*106*:820–828.
6. Roehm JOF Jr, Gianturco C, Barth MH, Wright KC: Percutaneous transcatheter filter for the inferior vena cava: A new device for treatment of patients with pulmonary embolism. Radiology 1984;*150*:255–257.
7. Roehm JOF Jr, Johnsrude IS, Barth MH, Gianturco C: The birds nest inferior vena cava filter: Progress report. Radiology 1988;*168*:745–749.
8. McCowan TC, Ferris EJ, Keifsteck JE, Lin GC, Baker ML: Retrieval of dislodged birds nest inferior vena caval filters. J Intervent Radiol 1988;*3*:179–183.
9. Epstein DE, Darcy MD, Hunter DW, Coleman CC, Tadavarthy SM, Murray PD, Castaneda-Zuniga WR, Amplatz K: Experience with the Amplatz retrievable vena cava filter. Radiology 1989;*172*:105–110.
10. Simm M, Athanasoulis CA, Kim D, Steinberg FL, Porter DH, Byse BH, Kleshinski S, Geller S, Orran DE, Waltman AC: Simon nitinol inferior vena cava filter: Initial clinical experience. Radiology 1989;*172*:99–103.
11. Dorfman GS: Percutaneous inferior vena caval filters. Radiology 1990;*174*:987–992.
12. Ricco JB, Crochet D, Sebilotte P, Serradimigni A, Lefebvre JM, Barisson E, Geslin P, Virot P, Vaislic C, Gallet M, Biron Y, Lefant D, Dosmarq JM, DeLaFaye D: Percutaneous transvenous caval interruption with the "LGM" filter: Early results of a multicenter trial. Ann Vasc Surg 1988;*3*:242–247.
13. Maquin P, Fajadet P, Railhac N, Bloom E, Brunet M, Railhac JJ: LGM and Gunther: Two complementary vena cava filters. Radiology 1989;*173*(p):476.
14. Gunther RW, Schild H, Hollman JP, Vorwerk D: First clinical results with a new caval filter. Cardiovasc Intervent Radiol 1987;*10*:104–108.
15. Fobbe F, Dietzel M, Korth R, et al: Gunther vena caval filter: Results of long term follow-up. AJR 1988;*151*:1031–1034.
16. Johnson SG, Pickford M, Wilkins RA: Migration of a Gunther filter to the right ventricle. J Intervent Radiol 1988;*3*:33–36.

INDEX

Note: Page numbers in *italics* refer to illustrations; page numbers followed by t refer to tables.